DATE DUE

JE 17 95			
MR 10 95			
AP 3 96			
MY 3 96			
JE 27 07			
MR 12 98			
JY 29 98			
NO 11 98			
NO 11 98			
DE 8 98			
AG 3 00			
JA 28 02			
NO 11 04			

CURRENT RESEARCH IN ARTS MEDICINE

*A Compendium of the
MedArt International
1992 World Congress
on Arts and Medicine*

Fadi J. Bejjani, M.D., D.E.M., M.A., Ph.D.
Associate Professor of Physical Medicine and Rehabilitation
Director, Occupational/Musculoskeletal Diseases
University of Medicine and Dentistry—New Jersey Medical School

a cappella books

Library of Congress Cataloging-in-Publication Data

Bejjani, Fadi J.
    Current research in arts medicine / Fadi J. Bejjani.
    p.   cm.
  ISBN 1-55652-187-1 (pbk.) $29.95
  1. Arts medicine.   2. Art therapy.   3. Dance therapy.   4. Music therapy.   I. Title.
R702.5.B45   1993
615.8'515—dc20   93-20251
                                                                       CIP

© 1993 MedArt International, Inc.
a cappella books
an imprint of Chicago Review Press, Incorporated
Editorial offices:
P.O. Box 380
Pennington, NJ 08534
Business/sales offices:
814 N. Franklin St.
Chicago, IL 60610

Printed in the United States of America

The author dedicates this book

to

Elaine Lee Bejjani

and

Justin-Joseph Bejjani

. . . and acknowledges

the invaluable work

of

Lyann Starkweather

and assistance

of

James Sibrel

Acknowledgments

The author especially wishes to acknowledge the Whitaker Foundation for their funding of his pioneering research in kinematics and kinetics of musicians. Their visionary support helped establish his Human Performance Analysis Laboratory at New York University, where this innovative research took place initially. Many of the national and international scholars who have authored and co-authored chapters in this book had the opportunity to visit the Laboratory and participate in the research over the years. Finally, the Laboratory was the birthplace of MedArt International, the non-profit professional and academic multidisciplinary organization that brought together the impressive body of knowledge that made the 1992 World Congress and this book possible.

By the same token, the author extends his gratitude and appreciation to Dr. Lawrence Ferrara, a great friend, pianist and scholar, who introduced him to the Department of Music and Music Professions at New York University; Dr. John Gilbert, Chairman of this Department, who made the Human Performance Analysis Laboratory project possible; and Dr. Mathew H. M. Lee, Chairman of the Rusk Institute, who later helped introduce the Laboratory to the NYU School of Medicine.

Foreword

There are many unique features to this impressive work, not the least of which is the distinguished body of national and international talents representing many reputable academic institutions, assembled by the editor. A wealth of state-of-the-art research — in medicine, basic sciences, allied health sciences, the arts and arts therapies — is blended together to offer a most comprehensive compendium on the emerging field of Arts Medicine. This unprecedented scholarly endeavor deserves the full respect and recognition of the medical, scientific and artistic communities. This work is indeed genuinely multidisciplinary, offering different yet complementary perspectives on similar or related topics. It allows an approach very similar to that which is practiced within Physical Medicine and Rehabilitation, where ideas are exchanged freely between physicians and non-physicians for the benefit of patient care.

In addition to thoroughly addressing the occupational diseases that can afflict performing and visual artists in a way that will certainly help their diagnosis, prognosis and treatment, this work is the first to introduce the benefits of the creative art therapies to the medical community in a scholarly and well-documented style. This makes it a unique and timely resource to be consulted not only by the physicians and other health professionals treating artists, but also by those treating the disabled and chronically ill. It undoubtedly will inspire researchers for years to come from both the basic sciences such as biomechanics, ergonomics and the neurosciences, and the social sciences such as medicine and allied health sciences.

Joel A. DeLisa, M.D., M.S.
Professor and Chairman
Department of Physical Medicine and Rehabilitation
University of Medicine and Dentistry-New Jersey Medical School

Chief Medical Officer and Medical Director
The Kessler Institute for Rehabilitation, Inc.

Foreword

This book shows the progressive development of medicine in our society in sharing wtih all prople throughout the world the very high value and essential nature of art and medicine in our lives. Dedicated efforts are ensuring that the field of medicine embraces all dimensions of our being — that art and medicine together should play a significant role in new approaches and solutions to ensure progress in a new direction toward achieving good health and well-being for all people. This book shows the necessary and noble work being carried on to cement art and medicine as an important approach.

The history of the world is a book filled with pages about men and women wtih great intellect and insight and imagination who have given birth to ideas that they have pursued and made into reality for the betterment of society. One day in the future, we will look back on these days and will know will certainty that the efforts described in this book have also earned a page in the book of world history.

To you who read this: I want you to know that you can contribute to a miracle of progress by joining in this work. In this rapidly unifying world, it is so important for all of us to mobilize minds in the worlds of science and the arts to begin a rational approach to the advancement of medicine and its uses for the benefit of each of us as a whole person.

So, in a variation on Shelley, I know that I can hear now the words that flow from this book when it is said:

> *Drive my thoughts over the universe*
> *Like withered leaves to quicken a new birth!*
> *And, by the incantation of this verse,*
> *Scatter, as from an unextinguished hearth*
> *Ashes and sparks, my words among mankind!*
> *And through my lips to unawakened earth*
> *The trumpet of a prophecy!*

Hon. Leonard J. Suchanek
Counsel
American World Services, Inc.

Former Chief Judge and Chairman
United States Board of Contract Appeals

Former Chairman
Council on Accessible Technology

Contributors

Jean C. Abell
Consultant VISD
Victoria, Texas

J. Ackerman, M.A.
Art Therapist
Louisville, Kentucky

S. Ahmedzai, M.B., Dh.B., M.R.C.P.
Medical Director
The Leicestershire Hospice
Leicester, England

Karen Allen, Ph.D.
Associate Professor
Research and Training Center on Brain Injury
State University of New York at Buffalo
Buffalo, New York

Kai-Nan An, Ph.D.
Professor of Bioengineering
Mayo Medical School
Rochester, Minnesota

Margo K. Apostolos, Ph.D.
Director of Dance
School of Theatre
University of Southern California
Los Angeles, California

Jon S. Baily, Ph.D.
Department of Psychology
Florida State University
Tallahassee, Florida

Guillermo Bajares, M.D.
Hospital Centro Médico de Caracas
Caracas, Venezuela

Barbara S.J. Balch, R.N.
Independent Midwife
Central Vermont Hospital
Northfield, Vermont

Dietrich Balser
Institut für Arbeitswissenschaft der Technischen
Hochschule Darmstadt
Darmstadt, Germany

Nell Aird Bateman, A.T.R.
Art Therapy Supervisor
Toronto Art Therapy Institute
Toronto, Canada

Dennis Bathory-Kitsz
Composer/Performer, Author, Technologist
Northfield, Vermont

Fadi J. Bejjani, M.D., D.E.M., M.A., Ph.D.
Associate Professor of
Physical Medicine & Rehabilitation
Director, Occupational/Musculoskeletal Diseases
University of Medical and Dentistry-
New Jersey Medical School
Newark, New Jersey

Miriam Roskin Berger, A.D.T.R.
Acting Director, Dance Therapy
New York University
School of Education, Health, Nursing
and Arts Professions
New York, New York

Bradley R. Biedermann, R.M.T.-B.C.
Graduate Student
Music Therapy Department
Temple University
Philadelphia, Pennsylvania

Florence B. Blager, Ph.D.
Research Associate
The Recording and Research Center
Denver Center for the Performing Arts
Denver, Colorado

Willem C.G. Blanken, M.D.
Department of Rehabilitation
University Hospital Rotterdam
Rotterdam, Netherlands

H.M. Borchgrevink, M.D., B.A.
HQ Defence Command Norway
Joint Medical Service
Oslo, Norway

Ann C. Bowman
Psychotherapist
New York, New York

Edith Hillman Boxill
Founder-Director
Music Therapists for Peace, Inc.
New York, New York

Laurie Brand
Music Therapist
Department of Therapeutic Recreation
Rusk Institute of Rehabilitation Medicine
New York University Medical Center
New York, New York

Kenneth D. Brandt, M.D.
Professor of Medicine and
Head, Rheumatology Division
Director, Performing Arts Medicine Program and
Multipurpose Arthritis Center
Indiana University School of Medicine
Indianapolis, Indiana

Lilita Branka-Bakajeva
Research Fellow
Physical Cultural Institute of Latvia
Riga, Latvia

M.P. Brocaar
Department of Otorhinolaryngology
University Hospital Rotterdam
Rotterdam, Netherlands

Sally Brucker, M.S.W., M.A., A.T.R.
Co-Director/Social Worker/Art Therapist
The Women's Growth & Therapy Center
Washington, D.C.

Madeline Bruser, M.M.
Pianist
New York, New York

Kathleen C. Bryant
Speech-Language Pathologist
Denver, Colorado

Mary B. Burch, Ph.D.
Behavior Management Consultants, Inc.
Tallahassee, Florida

Cathy Callis, D.M.A.
Consultant on Call
Riverside Methodist Hospitals
Columbus, Ohio

Peifang Chen, M.D.
Director, Art Phoniatrics Laboratory
Shanghai Conservatory of Music
Shanghai, People's Republic of China

Michelle Chin
Medical Student
New York University Medical School
New York, New York

Marie-Sophie Colas
Artist
Nancy, France

Kerong Dai, M.D.
Professor and Chairman
Department of Orthopedics
Shanghai Second Medical University
Shanghai, People's Republic of China

Katherine E.B. Davis, M.S.W.
Psychotherapist
Whitney Associates
New Haven, Connecticut

William J. Dawson, M.D.
Assistant Professor of
Clinical Orthopaedic Surgery
Northwestern University Medical School
Wilmette, Illinois

Paolo Di Marco, M.D.
First Department of Orthopaedic Surgery
University of Rome 'La Sapienza'
Rome, Italy

Donnatella Di Mastromatteo
Department of Physical Medicine
and Rehabilitation
University of Rome 'La Sapienza'
Rome, Italy

Linda Marie Di Noto, M.A., D.T.R.
Dance Therapist
Boulder, Colorado

Kate T. Donohue, Ph.D.
Psychologist
West Portal Counseling Associates
San Francisco, California

Richard G. Eaton, M.D.
Clinical Professor of Surgery
Columbia University
College of Physicians and Surgeons
New York, New York

Berenice Espejo, M.D.
Dancesport: Dance and Sports
Rehabilitation Clinic
Caracas, Venezuela

Federico Fernandez-Palazzi, M.D.
Director of Orthopedics
Hospital St. John of God
Caracas, Venezuela

Anne-Marie Ferrand-Vidal
Founder
International Association for
Melody-Programmed Therapy of Speech
Pointherry, France

Andrea Ferretti, M.D.
First Department of Orthopaedic Surgery
University of Rome 'La Sapienza'
Rome, Italy

Bella Abramowitz Fisher, P.T.
Physical Therapist
Albert Einstein College of Medicine
Bronx, New York

Ingeborg Formann-Radl
Professor
Psychiatric University Clinic Vienna
Vienna, Austria

Michael A. Franklin, A.T.R.
Director, Art Therapy Program
Bowling Green State University
Bowling Green, Ohio

Diane Lynch Fraser, Ed.D.
St. John's University
School for Language and
Communication Development
North Bellmore, New York

Linda Gantt, Ph.D.
Clinical Instructor
West Virginia University
Morgantown, West Virginia

Millicent Gappell, I.F.D.A.
Delineations
Los Angeles, California

Kay Gardner, M.M.
Composer
Stonington, Maine

Joanna Gburek
Szpital Uzdrowiskowy
Ustron, Poland

Hollister Gignoux
Art Therapist
Department of Therapeutic Recreation
Rusk Institute of Rehabilitation Medicine
New York University Medical Center
New York, New York

Margaret Gold, B.A.(Hons)A.T.
Art Therapist
The Leicestershire Hospice
Leicester, England

Jonathan S. Goldman, M.A.
Founder and Director
Sound Healers Association, Inc.
Boulder, Colorado

Melanie Graham, M.A.
Speech Pathologist
Laguna Hills, California

Helen M. Grob, M.M., R.M.T.-B.C., C.Pv.T.
Director of Music Therapy and Clinical Training
New York Medical College/
Terence Cardinal Cook Health Care Center
New York, New York

Lionel Guibert, Ph.D.
Conservatoire de Musique
Paris, France

John H. Gundy, M.D.
Clinical Associate Professor of Pediatrics
Yale University School of Medicine
New Haven, Connecticut

Shalini Gupta, Ph.D., M.H.Sc.
Health and Welfare Canada
Environmental Health Centre
Ottawa, Ontario, Canada

William G. Hamilton, M.D.
Assistant Clinical Professor of Orthopedic Surgery
Columbia University
College of Physicians and Surgeons
New York, New York

Linda Hamilton, Ph.D.
Research Associate and Clinical Psychologist
Miller Health Care Institute
for Performing Artists
New York, New York

Ineke Hansson-Bosma, O.T.
Adjunct Professor
Conservatory of Alkmaar and Maastricht
Maastricht, Netherlands

John R. Harrison, M.Sc., M.S.
Health and Welfare Canada
Environmental Health Centre
Ottawa, Ontario, Canada

R.I.P. Hayman
Composer/Event Producer
Editor, *Ear* Magazine
Pomona, New York

Ronald E. Hays, M.S., A.T.R.
Assistant Professor
Director of Creative Arts in Therapy
Director of Art Therapy Education
Hahnemann Medical University
of the Health Sciences
Philadelphia, Pennsylvania

Junzhi He
Jin He Orthopaedic Hospital
Sichuan, People's Republic of China

Tianxiang He
Standing Council Member
China Arts-Medical Science Society
Sichuan, People's Republic of China

Marianne Hieb, R.S.M., M.F.A., A.T.R., C.E.T.
Coordinator, Wellness Spirituality Programs
Our Lady of Lourdes Wellness Center
Camden, New Jersey

Ben M. Hillberry, Ph.D.
Professor of Mechanical Engineering
Purdue University
West Lafayette, Indiana

S.L. Hiner
Coordinator
Performing Arts Medicine Program
Indiana University School of Medicine
Indianapolis, Indiana

Xiaokui Hou, M.D.
Associate Professor and Vice Chairman
Department of Orthopaedics
Ninth People's Hospital
Shanghai Second Medical University
Shanghai, People's Republic of China

Bryan C. Hunter, Ph.D., R.M.T.-B.C.
Assistant Professor
Coordinator of Music Therapy
Nazareth College
Rochester, New York

Jennet Inglis
Visual Artist
Sante Fe, New Mexico

Rubén Jaén, M.D.
Orthopedic Surgeon
Hospital Centro Médico de Caracas
Caracas, Venezuela

Olu-Birgit Jeppson, M.A.
Department of Musicology
Universitetet I Lund
Lund, Sweden

Caryl Johnson, O.T.R., C.H.T.
Hand Therapist
St. Luke's-Roosevelt Hospital Center
New York, New York

Tedd Judd, Ph.D., A.B.P.P.
Clinical Neuropsychologist
Good Samaritan Neuropsychological Services
Puyallup, Washington

Lynn Kable
Arts Administrator
Hospital Audiences, Inc.
New York, New York

Lois Kaggen
Founder and President
Resources for Artists with Disabilities
New York, New York

Vara Kamin
Author/Consultant
Deephaven, Minnesota

B. Kap, M.D.
Department of Rehabilitation
University Hospital Rotterdam
Rotterdam, Netherlands

Pieter Kark, M.D.
Performing Arts Medicine Association
of Central New York
DeWitt, New York

M.S. Keane
Graduate Research Assistant
School of Mechanical Engineering
Purdue University
West Lafayette, Indiana

C. Regina Kelley
Associate Professor
Portland School of Art
Portland, Maine

Robert B. Kent, Ed.D., A.T.R.
Department of Art
University of Georgia
Athens, Georgia

L.Y. Kirienko
Department of Biomechanics
Byelorussian Institute of Physical Culture
Minsk, Byelorussia

Ewa Klimas-Kuchtowa, Ph.D.
Department of Psychology
Jagiellonian University
Krakow, Poland

Charlotte Kollmorgen, Dipl. Des. L.
Designer/Artist/Art Therapist
Berlin, Germany

Joanna Kossewska
Master of Psychology
Department of Psychology
Higher Pedagogical School
Krakow, Poland

Casimir Kowalski, M.D.
Orthopaedist
Retinne, Belgium

Michael Kriegsfeld, Ph.D.*
Psychologist
New York, New York

M. Kuijers
Mensendieck Therapist
The Hague, Netherlands

Judith R.F. Kupersmith, M.D.
Department of Psychiatry
Michigan State University
East Lansing, Michigan

Machteld Kuypers
Visual Artist
Amsterdam, Netherlands

Gustaaf J. Lankhorst, M.D., Ph.D.
Rehabilitation Department
University Hospital Rotterdam
Rotterdam, Netherlands

Johan Leanderson, M.D.
Department of Orthopaedics
Karolinska Hospital
Stockholm, Sweden

*Deceased

Mathew H.M. Lee, M.D., M.P.H.
Professor and Acting Chairman
Rusk Institute of Rehabilitation Medicine
New York University Medical Center
New York, New York

Paul Lehrer, Ph.D.
Clinical Psychologist and Professor of Psychiatry
Robert Wood Johnson Medical School
University of Medicine and Dentistry
of New Jersey
Piscataway, New Jersey

Samuel Lehrer
Performing Arts Medicine Association
of Central New York
Riverdale, New York

Jon N. Lemke, Ph.D.
University of Iowa
Iowa City, Iowa

Marcia B. Leventhal, Ph.D., A.D.T.R., C.M.A.
Co-Editor
American Journal of Dance Therapy
Sherman Oaks, California

Kinga Lewandowska
Institute of Psychology
University of Gdansk
Gdansk, Poland

You Xia Li
People's Theatrical Company of Jiangsu
Nanjing, People's Republic of China

Sammi S. Liebman, Ph.D., R.M.T.-B.C.
Director of Music Therapy
University of Windsow
School of Music
Windsor, Ontario, Canada

Lynne A. LiGreci-Mangini, M.S., M.A., P.T.
Physical Therapist
Westside Dance Physical Therapy
and New York City Ballet
New York, New York

Paul Linden, Ph.D.
Columbus Center for Movement Studies
Columbus, Ohio

Barbara Lister-Sink, M.A., A.B.
Dean, School of Music
Salem College
Winston-Salem, North Carolina

Jeanette L. Lovetri
Director
The Voice Workshop
New York, New York

Isabel Luñansky, M.T.
Professor of Music Therapy
Buenos Aires, Argentina

Grethe Lund, L.G.S.M.(M.T.)
Music Therapist
Viborg Psychiatric Hospital
Viborg, Denmark

Vija B. Lusebrink, Ph.D., A.T.R.
Professor and Director
Department of Expressive Therapies
University of Louisville
Louisville, Kentucky

Sherry Lyons, M.S., A.T.R.
Director, Art Therapy Education
University of the Arts
Philadelphia, Pennsylvania

Aileen MacLaren, C.N.M., M.S.N.
Assistant Professor, Clinical Nurse Midwifery
University of Miami
School of Nursing
Miami, Florida

Giuseppe Martini, M.D.
First Department of Orthopaedic Surgery
University of Rome 'La Sapienza'
Rome, Italy

Barbara Mathis, Ph.D.
Music Department
Lamar University
Beaumont, Texas

Lorene McClintock
Teacher and Author
New York, New York

Joan McConnell, A.B., M.A., Ph.D.
Language Program Director
Stanford University
Centro di Studi
Florence, Italy

Teena McConnell, A.O.S.
Former Soloist
New York City Ballet
Glen Ridge, New Jersey

Juanita McElwain, R.M.T.-B.C.
Phillips University
Enid, Oklahoma

Donald E. McGill, B.A., M.D.
Clinical Psychiatrist
St. Mary's Hospital
Passaic, New Jersey

Dalia Merari, M.A., O.T.R., A.T.R.
Department of Occupational Therapy
Sackler Faculty of Medicine
Tel-Aviv University
Tel-Aviv, Israel

Ulrich Moritz, M.D., Ph.D.
Department of Physical Therapy
Lund University
Lund, Sweden

Elizabeth T. Morris, B.S., P.T.
Physical Therapist
Salt Lake City, Utah

Paul G.H. Mulder, M.Sc.
Rehabilitation Department
University Hospital Rotterdam
Rotterdam, Netherlands

Nurit Mussen, Ph.D.
Adjunct Professor
John F. Kennedy University
Orinda, California

Karin Naimark
Hahnemann University
Philadelphia, Pennsylvania

V. Nasarov, Prof. Dr.
Byelorussian Institute of Physical Culture
Minsk, Byelorussia

Florence Nash
Program Consultant
Cultural Services Program
Duke University Medical Center
Durham, North Carolina

Devora Neumark, B.F.A.
Art Health and Safety Consultant
Montreal, Quebec, Canada

Briony Nicholls
Psychopharmacology Group
Psychology Department
University College London
London, England

Charlotte Nilsson, M.D.
Department of Orthopaedics
Karolinska Hospital
Stockholm, Sweden

William B. Nolan, M.D.
Plastic Surgeon, Hand Center
St. Luke's-Roosevelt Hospital
New York, New York

Mary Louise O'Brien, R.N., M.A.
Licensed Counselor
Columbia College
St. Joseph's School
Columbia, Missouri

Andrea J. Olsen
Associate Professor of Dance
Middlebury College
Middlebury, Vermont

T.G. Palferman, M.B., M.R.C.P.
Consultant Physician and Rheumatologist
Yeovil District Hospital
Yeovil, Somerset, England

Patrizia Pallaro, M.A., D.T.R.
Psychologist
Dance/Movement Therapist
University of California, Los Angeles
Los Angeles, California

Janice Palmer
Director, Cultural Services Program
Duke University Medical Center
Durham, North Carolina

Marguerite Papadimitriou-Boulenger, D.O.
Professor of Anatomy
State School of Dance
Athens, Greece

Roberta Toby Pashley, A.T.R.
Ridgeview Institute
Smyrna, Georgia

Glen Paul
Geriatric Division Clinical Rehabilitation Worker
Department of Rehabilitation Services
University Hospital
Vancouver, British Columbia, Canada

Kenneth J. Peacock, Ph.D.
Director, Computer Music
and Technology Program
Department of Music and Music Professions
New York University
New York, New York

Yngrid Perez, R.P.T.
Dancesport: Dance and Sports
Rehabilitation Clinic
Caracas, Venezuela

Ginger Perowsky
Dance Therapist
Metropolitan Hospital Center
New York, New York

Lars I. Persson
Swedish Broadcasting Corporation
Department of Health and Safety
Stockholm, Sweden

Jian Pi
Senior Chief Doctor
Voice Department
Drama Institute of Hunan Province
Hunan Province, People's Republic of China

André Picard
Université Laval
Quebec, Canada

Cesare Augusto Pistara, M.D.
Department of Physical Medicine
and Rehabilitation
University of Rome 'La Sapienza'
Rome, Italy

Marcia Plevin
Dancer/Choreographer/Dance Therapist
Art Therapy Italiana
Accademia Nazionale di Danza
Rome, Italy

Julie A. Plezbert, D.C.
Chiropractor
McHenry, Illinois

Luana Poggini, M.D., Ph.D.
First Department of Orthopaedic Surgery
University of Rome 'La Sapienza'
Rome, Italy

Eva Ramel, R.P.T.
Department of Physical Therapy
Lund Universiy
Lund, Sweden

N.N. Ramlakhan
Psychopharmacology Group
Psychology Department
University College London
London, England

César Restrepo, M.D.
Orthopaedic Surgeon
Hospital Centro Médico de Caracas
Caracas, Venezuela

Salvador Rivas, M.D.
Orthopedic Surgeon
Hospital Centro Médico de Caracas
Caracas, Venezuela

Renee Rocklin, M.S.W.
Supervisor
Psychotherapy Training Program
Yale University School of Medicine
New Haven, Connecticut

Gisela Rohmert
Director
Licntenberger Institute of
Functional Voice Training
Darmstadt, Germany

Marcia L. Rosal, Ph.D., A.T.R.
Department of Expressive Therapies
University of Louisville
Louisville, Kentucky

Walter Ruth
Luleå Universiy of Technology
Department of Human Work Sciences
Division of Working Environment Planning
Luleå, Sweden

Jaiyoung Ryu, M.D.
Orthopedic Surgeon
Texas Tech University
El Paso, Texas

Naotaka Sakai, M.D., Ph.D.
Department of Orthopaedic Surgery
Yokosuka Kyosai Hospital
Yokosuka, Japan

Ans Samama
Mensendieck Therapist
Hilversum, Netherlands

Victoria Santa Cruz
Associate Professor of Drama
Department of Drama
Carnegie Mellon University
Pittsburgh, Pennsylvania

Bruce M. Saperston, Ph.D., R.M.T.-B.C.
Director of Music Therapy
Utah State University
Logan, Utah

Robert Thayer Sataloff, M.D., D.M.A.
Professor of Otolaryngology
Thomas Jefferson University;
Chairman, Board of Directors
The Voice Foundation
Philadelphia, Pennsylvania

Ronald C. Scherer, Ph.D.
Senior Scientist
The Recording and Research Center
Denver Center for the Performing Arts
Denver, Colorado

J.M. Schmidt, M.D.
Department of Otorhinolaryngology
University Hospital Rotterdam
Rotterdam, Netherlands

Fred J. Schwartz, M.D.
Department of Anesthesiology
Piedmont Hospital
Atlanta, Georgia

Xueyong Shen, M.D.
Department of Acupuncture-Moxibustion
Shanghai Traditional Chinese Medicine College
Shanghai, People's Republic of China

K. Schikler, M.D.
Kosair Children's Hospital
Louisville, Kentucky

Diane Silverman, M.A., A.T.R., M.F.C.C.
Art Psychotherapist
Los Angeles, California

Benjamin Simkin, M.D.
Attending Physician
Division of Endocrinology
Cedars-Sinai Medical Center
Los Angeles, California

A.S. Skuratovich
Byelorussian Institute of Physical Culture
Department of Biomechanics
Minsk, Byelorussia

Martha Slaymaker
Visual Artist
Aubuquerque, New Mexico

Chris J. Snijders, Ph.D.
Department of Biomedical Physics
and Technology
Faculty of Medicine
Erasmus University
Rotterdam, Netherlands

John Snyder
Composer
New York, New York

Jeffrey Solow
Associate Professor of Music (Cello)
Ester Boyer College of Music
Temple University
Philadelphia, Pennsylvania

H. Stam, M.D., Ph.D.
Department of Rehabilitation
University Hospital Rotterdam
Rotterdam, Netherlands

Hannah Steinberg, Ph.D.
Psychopharmacology Group
Psychology Department
University College London
London, England

David J. Sternbach, M.M., M.S.W., A.C.S.W.
D.C. Institute for Mental Health
Washington, D.C.

Susan Stoltz
Filmmaker/Teacher
Hospital Audiences, Inc.
New York, New York

Beth Ames Swartz
Visual Artist
Scottsdale, Arizona

Elizabeth A. Sykes, Ph.D.
Psychopharmacology Group
Psychology Department
University College London;
School of Psychology
Middlesex Polytechnic
Middlesex, England

Dwight M. Tamanaha, D.C.
Pro Care Chiropractic Clinic, Ltd.
Green Bay, Wisconsin

E. Terpstra-Indeman, M.D.
Department of Rehabilitation
and Physical Medicine
Academic Hospital Maastricht
Maastricht, Netherlands

J. Thomas
Body Revolution Club
Southampton, England

Louis W. Tinnin, M.D.
Department of Behavioral Medicine
and Psychiatry
Chestnut Ridge Hospital
Morgantown, West Virginia

Concetta M. Tomaino, M.A., C.M.T.-B.C.
President
American Association for Music Therapy;
Clinical Music Therapist, Beth Abraham Hospital
Bronx, New York

L. Turner-Schikler, M.A., A.T.R.
Kosair Children's Hospital
Louisville, Kentucky

Henk van der Rijst, M.D.
Rehabilitation Department
University Hospital Rotterdam
Rotterdam, Netherlands

C.N. van Dijk, M.D.
Orthopaedic Surgeon
Academisch Medisch Centrum
Amsterdam, Netherlands

Marjon D.F. van Eijsden-Besseling, M.D.
Department of Rehabilitation
Academic Hospital Maastricht
Maastricht, Netherlands

J.G.M. van Rossum, M.D.
Psychiatrist
Venlo, Netherlands

J. Verschuure
Department of Otorhinolaryngology
University Hospital Rotterdam
Rotterdam, Netherlands

Nina Viscardi, M.A., A.T.R.
Art Therapist
Henry Viscardi School
Albertson, New York

Laura Vitangeli, M.D.
Department of Physical Medicine
and Rehabilitation
University of Rome 'La Sapienza'
Rome, Italy

S.N. Vlasenko
Department of Biomechanics
Byelorussian Institute of Physical Culture
Minsk, Byelorussia

Arkady S. Voloshin, Ph.D.
Professor of Mechanical Engineering
Lehigh University
Bethlehem, Pennsylvania

Michelle P. Warren, M.D.
Director, Reproductive Endocrinology
St. Luke's-Roosevelt Hospital
New York, New York

Janet Weiss
Performing Arts Medicine Association of
Central New York
Oakdale, New Jersey

Leslie B. Weiss, Ph.D.
Clinical Psychologist
Whitney Associates
New Haven, Connecticut

Joan Whitacre, M.A.
Movement Therapist/Somatic Educator
New York, New York

F.G. Wolf
Indiana University School of Medicine
Indianapolis, Indiana

Russell Woodman, P.T.
Director
Masters Program in Orthopedic Physical Therapy
Quinnipiac College
Hamden, Connecticut

Wayne Woodward, Ed.D.
Division of Education
Georgia Southwestern College
Americus, Georgia

Anders Wykman, M.D., Ph.D.
Department of Orthopaedics
Karolinska Hospital;
Orthopaedic Consultant
Royal Swedish Ballet and Swedish Ballet School
Stockholm, Sweden

Lin Yang
Sichuan Provincial Research Institute
Sichuan, People's Republic of China

Hideo Yano, M.D.
Department of Motor Dysfunction
National Rehabilitation Center for the Disabled
Tokorozawa, Japan

Yonjun Zhang
Drama Institute of Hunan Province
Hunan Province, People's Republic of China

Contents

PART I

AESTHETICS/
ARTS AND MEDICINE

CHAPTER 1

Synesthesia: The Context and Artistic Implications

Kenneth J. Peacock

An interesting story related by Alexander Scriabin to his first biographer, Yuri Engle, tells of an evening in 1907. After a rehearsal, Scriabin, Rimsky-Korsakov and Rachmaninov met at the Cafe de la Paix near the grand opera in Paris. They talked about the connection between colors and keys — an idea unknown to Rachmaninov. Rimsky-Korsakov claimed that the predominance of *D* major ("the color of gold") in the cellar scene of Rachmaninov's *The Miserly Knight* proved that the composer was sensitive to color in sound.

Although there is no evidence that Rachmaninov developed his newly discovered color sense, Rimsky-Korsakov is known to have perceived a relationship between specific colors and tonalities as early as 1867. Scriabin believed integration of colored light within a symphonic work would act as "a powerful psychological resonator for the listener," and this belief in correspondence between stimuli was implemented in his 1911 color-symphony, *Prometheus*.

SYNESTHETIC PERCEPTION

A common childhood trick takes advantage of an interaction between the senses: If blindfolded, and deprived of the sense of smell, it is supposedly impossible to tell if one is biting into an apple or an onion — until it's too late! More dramatic is the direct linking of vivid perceptions in one of the senses with a stimulus from another. This has been described in the literature as synesthesia. A synesthete might be blessed — or cursed, according to one's point of view — with the ability to *hear* colors or odors and *see* sounds, and those who habitually perceive stimuli in this manner are often surprised when told that everyone does not share the faculty.

Synesthesia is by no means limited to the association of color and sound, although this seems to be the most common experience. Largely influenced by the writings of Edgar Allan Poe, many examples of associative correspondence can be found in literary works by Baudelaire, Rimbaud, and others.

A delightful example of synesthetic perception occurs in J.K. Huysmans' fascinating novel, *A Rebours*. Chapter four describes how Jean des Esseintes enjoyed "sonorous gustation." An *orgue a bouche* which satisfied sight, taste, and hearing simultaneously was provided by a set of vials of variously colored liquors. By pulling stops labeled "flute," "horn," or "voix celeste," a few drops from each vial could be tasted in various combinations. "Inner symphonies" resulted, since each liquor corresponded to the sound of a musical instrument. Dry curaçao was associated with the clarinet, kümmel with the nasal sound of the oboe, crème-de-menthe and anisette were like sweet and tart qualities of the flute, kirsch recalled the blast of a trumpet, gin and whiskey were cornets and trombones, marc-brandy was analogous to tubas, and the rakis of Chinos and Mastics gave in taste the full force of cymbals and drums. Huysmans explained further, "the music of liqueurs had its own scheme of interrelated tones." Benedictine was the relative minor of that major alcohol known as green chartreuse, for example.

Thanks to a series of erudite experiments, [des Esseintes] had been able to perform upon his tongue silent melodies and mute funeral marches; to hear inside his mouth creme-de-menthe solos and rum-and-vespreto duets.

Beyond entertainment, one of the goals of literary art is the communication of an aesthetic message, and those who succeed in communicating ideas of universal importance are termed great artists. It follows that any work of art may be viewed as a statement of the artist's ideas expressed in the artist's own personal language. Just as Huysmans' narrative, which pairs taste and timbre, reflects an intimate acquaintance with synesthesia, Scriabin's association of colors with tonalities in *Prometheus* mirrors his personal perception.

Many studies of associative perception appeared in medical journals during Scriabin's lifetime, and investigation of related phenomena became a fashionable branch of psychology. One of the most astonishing subjects in an 1881 study, for example, was a twenty-three-year-old medical student.[1] All of his perceptions were accompanied by parallel color imagery. Letters and words were colored according to sound, and slight variations in pronunciation caused a great change in color shading. He sensed that languages each had a characteristic color: French was dark brown; English, light brown; German, green; Italian, bluish; Ancient Greek, yellow. Days and months were also colored, but not according to sound. Color sensations were evoked by numbers as well as geometric patterns. Circles provided a sensation of bright yellow, a long wavy line gave a dark color, and a triangle yielded bright silver — no doubt due to familiarity with the musical instrument. Odors were never perceived without color sensations. The smell of vanilla was light lilac, ammonia was whitish, vinegar was red. These colors changed when the subject was afflicted with a head cold. The sense of taste was also accompanied by color associations. A sweet taste was red, and bitter was dark brown. Vanilla tasted the same color as its odor.

Linking of perceptions was viewed during the nineteenth century as an organic deficiency like red-green colorblindness — a "short circuiting" of nerve endings which survived from an earlier and, presumably, undifferentiated sensorium. The view persisted well into the twentieth century and in a 1933 study, Otto Ortmann concluded that "the probable basis for synesthesia is an interlacing of nerve fibres . . . sensory-reflex describes the phenomenon."[2] This physiological explanation tended to drop out of favor as psychologists pursued linguistic and metaphorical origins for the phenomenon — often using non-synesthetic subjects during the 1970s in an effort to discover general principles of human perception. A neurological explanation for synesthesia was proposed during the 1980s by Richard Cytowic, who published a series of articles on the topic. His 1988 book, *Synesthesia: A Union of the Senses*, provides the most recent thinking from this perspective.[3]

A substantial number of early case descriptions treated the phenomenon as a highly unusual form of perception, but some publications appearing shortly after the turn of the century showed an interest in the various degrees and possible patterns in synesthesia. It is, of course, only within this broader conception that artistic implications can be discussed, since a narrow medical definition of synesthesia precludes the possibility that large numbers of people would be able to share the precise experience of the synesthete.

Charles Myers, a British psychologist who interviewed Scriabin in London and later published his findings, was one of the first to broaden the definition of synesthesia to include color-thinking. This definition recognized those cases in which a subject's response to actual stimuli was the thought of particular colors with no concomitant photism. The term *photism* refers to a sensation of light caused by a change in the retina, not by stimulation by light-waves.

PATTERNS IN SYNESTHESIA

During the 1930s, psychologists began to discern general patterns in synesthetic perception. They also discovered that the phenomenon was not as rare and mysterious as had been assumed.[4] Two fundamental characteristics of synesthetic perception were determined. First, the phenomenon originated in childhood. The second factor emphasized was that every case of synesthesia consists essentially of a parallel arrangement of two gradient series — shapes or colors, for example, which are then paired with letters, words, numbers, intensities, pitches, tonalities, or anything else of interest to the synesthete. How and why particular systems of correspondence are established is an individual and, usually, subconscious process. Thus it is possible to explain many associations on the basis of learning experiences. What "interlacing of nerve fibres" is apparent in the reported case of a man who sees number *1* as yellow, *2* as blue, *3* as red, *4* as purple, *5* as orange . . . and *8* as black? Anyone who has played pool recently may recall that billiard balls are identified by those numbers and colors.

Further substantiation that in a broad way synesthetic perception is related to meaning, and, therefore, to thinking in general, was provided by an extensive study of Dartmouth College students in 1938. Thirteen percent of the students always associated color with music, often gaining increased enjoyment. A much larger percentage employed this association occasionally, and the experimenters concluded that several findings "which are puzzling to the psychologist should be encouraging to the artist."

It also became apparent that many synesthetic associations follow patterns exhibited by language metaphors. Exciting, fast music, for example, might be visualized by a synesthete as a bright red photism cut by jagged lines in sharply etched colors. The less imaginative, non-synesthetic individual would merely agree that verbal metaphors such as "red-hot," "fiery," or "bright" provided a satisfactory description of the music.

TYPES OF COLOR ASSOCIATION WITH MUSIC

The types of synesthesia related to music have been classified into four groups: (1) synesthesia based on compositional styles, (2) synesthesia based on timbre, (3) synesthesia based on pitch, and (4) synesthesia based on tonalities.

The first type of synesthesia is an expanded concept of color-hearing experienced by many individuals. Association of colors with particular compositions, and, in some cases, the entire output of a composer, has often been reported.

The second group of synesthetes (whose color associations are based on timbre) includes laymen in addition to a large number of musicians. This type of synesthesia, connecting certain colors with musical instruments, is the area in which agreement can often be found among various systems of correspondence — probably due to a common interposed association pattern. The color scarlet, for example, is emotionally exciting because of its use by royalty, and its association with pageants. Trumpets, also connected with royalty, are often associated with fanfares in pageants. Hence, both trumpets and scarlet evoke similar emotions and are perceived as analogous.

The third type of synesthesia, color association based on pitch, is quite common. Many individuals consider low sounds analogous to darker colors and higher sounds are perceived as being brighter. As several writers have noted, most opera composers tend to set dark scenes in low registers and light scenes in higher registers. This inclination is also common today in accompanying music for film and television. Psychologists have not convincingly shown why there seems to be general agreement concerning the appropriateness of this association, i.e. whether there is some physiological process resulting in perceived similarity of dark colors and low registers, or whether composers and audiences are simply accustomed to certain conventions.

The final type of synesthesia, in which particular colors and tonalities are analogous, is fairly widespread among musicians. Andre Gretry, the eighteenth-century dramatic composer, assigned colors to keys, and even Beethoven referred in one of his sketch books to B minor as the "black key," although there is no evidence that he regularly associated tonalities and colors. We should recall, however, that prior to the widespread use of equal temperament, "transposed" intervals would be slightly different in size. Musicians have continued to associate particular key-characteristics, even though all transposed intervals are now the same size because of equal temperament.

Like other forms of synesthesia, pairing of colors and tonalities depends on individual experience. Scriabin, for example, considered the tonality of F-sharp to be a bright saturated blue, according to most sources. Rimsky-Korsakov perceived that key as an indefinite gray-green color. Serge Koussevitsky, who conducted the world premiere of Scriabin's *Prometheus*, claimed in an interview, "F-sharp is decidedly strawberry red!"

Sabaneev reported in 1929 that for many of his subjects, colors corresponding to simple harmonies are almost pure, but flat keys are "connected with metallic, glittering colours, with lustre and reflections. The more complex the key . . . the more complex and fantastic is the colour associated with it."[6] This is certainly true for Scriabin and Rimsky-Korsakov. Each perceived tonalities notated in flats as corresponding to dark colors. This can readily be seen when the synesthetic perceptions of the two composers are compared:

C	Red	White
G	Orange	Indefinite Brown-Green
D	Yellow	Yellow
A	Green	Rosy
E	Light Blue	Blue, with glitter
B	Whitish-Blue	Dark Blue, Steel
F-sharp	Blue, saturated	Indefinite Gray-Green
D-flat	Violet	Dark Brown, Metallic
A-flat	Purple	Gray-Violet
E-flat	Dark, Steel-Blue	Dark Gray-Blue
B-flat	Blue-Gray, Metallic	Dark Gray-Blue
F	Red, dark	Green

Attempts to resolve the issue of *correct* color and key association have not been successful because each synesthete believes his particular system of correspondence is *natural* for everyone. Writing over twenty years ago in *Medical Opinion and Review*, Nicolas Slonimsky asked, "What is the color of C major? Four out of five doctors say it is white. Why doesn't the fifth doctor agree? Because he is a violinist."[5] Many musicians consider C major as white because that tonality is represented by the ivory keys on the piano keyboard. Slonimsky wrote that *F*-sharp is naturally associated with dark colors because that tonality is played on the black keys of the piano. *G*-flat, however, "somehow suggests a silvery hue" because flats look less substantial on paper than sharps, thus implying lighter colors. Slonimsky's remarks are interesting because some of his conclusions are supported in the experimental literature.

SCRIABIN'S SYNESTHESIA

While in London for a performance of Prometheus, Scriabin was interviewed by Cambridge Professor Charles Myers.   In his report of the interview, Myers related a version of the discussion which took place in Paris between Scriabin and Rimsky-Korsakov. According to Myers, this was the first occasion Scriabin's attention had been drawn to his own color-hearing. After reporting the agreement with Rimsky-Korsakov concerning *D* major, Myers claimed, "Scriabin has since compared with his compatriot and with other musicians the colour effects of other keys, especially *B*, *C* major and *F*-sharp major, and believes a general agreement to exist in this respect." According to Myers, Scriabin stated that color "underlines the tonality; it makes the tonality more evident." In light of Scriabin's comment to Myers, it is important to note that in *Prometheus*, the root of the famous six-note "mystic chord" transposition heard in the orchestra always occurs in the color-keyboard part at precisely the same time. This well known pitch collection (*C*, *F*-sharp, *B*-flat, *E*, *A*, *D*) forms the melodic and harmonic basis for this composition, and the chord is characteristic of the complex harmonic vocabulary Scriabin employed in all of his late music.

Scriabin spontaneously recognized only three colors. These were red, yellow, and blue, corresponding to the tonalities of *C*, *D*, and *F*-sharp. Other colors he deduced from the presumption that spectral order is the closest relationship between colors, and that tonalities related by fifths represent nearest keys. Hence, when Scriabin heard tonalities in the ascending circle of fifths, it became habitual to associate each of the keys with colors of the spectrum in ascending order.

The Myers report stressed that for Scriabin a single note apart from tonality had no color, and strongest color sensations were experienced with the major keys of *C*, *D*, *B*, and *F*-sharp. The composer related *C* major to matter and the odor of soil.

F-sharp, an important tonal area in *Prometheus* as well as in much of Scriabin's music of the late period, was considered spiritual and ethereal. Scriabin is known to have objected to the terms *major* and *minor* in tonality, and Myers did not pursue specific effects of modal changes on the composer's color audition, but stated an effect of composite color resulted when several tonalities were combined.

While synesthetic perception, especially *colored hearing,* has often been considered unusual, for many individuals this linking of color and sound is a completely natural way of understanding music. In Scriabin's case, this mode of perception resulted in the color-symphony *Prometheus* — a work which included an instrument he called the Tastiera per luce, which would project colored light according to the composer's system of synesthetic association. It was so natural for Scriabin to associate literal color with tonalities that he did not bother to explain the color significance in the published orchestra.

THE TASTIERA PER LUCE

This instrumental part for colored light, which appears at the top of the orchestral score, is written polyphonically in standard music notation on a single staff in the treble clef. It is primarily two-voiced. One voice moves relatively rapidly with note durations ranging from an eighth-note to nineteen measures. The second voice seems to function as a series of pedal points, since these notes are sustained. For example, bright saturated blue (indicated by an *F*-sharp) is projected for the first 86 measures and for the final 146 measures of the composition. The exact midpoint of *Prometheus* (measures 305-308) is marked by the only occurrence of three voices in the luce.

The faster voice of the luce serves two functions. Simultaneously, this part indicates the specific colors which Scriabin synesthetically perceived in his music, while also indicating the transposition level of the mystic chord employed at any given moment. In the opening twelve measures of Prometheus, for example, the sustained *A* in the upper voice of the luce represents green light. *A* is also the root of the mystic chord heard in the orchestra during these twelve measures. This green light is accompanied by a bright saturated blue--indicated by an F-sharp in the slower luce voice.

What is remarkable is that the luce part, which ostensibly reflected the composer's synesthetic perception and which was intended to provide the "parallel symphony" in colored light, also provides the key to the structural organization of a work written in a unique and complex harmonic language. Thus it becomes clear, once one understands the significance of the luce part, that Scriabin's statement about colored light as a "powerful psychological resonator for the listener" was meant to be taken literally. The problem, of course, is that synesthetic perception of specific tonal areas and colors could not reasonably be expected to be the same for all listeners.

During his last years, Scriabin dreamed of an art form which would actively unite dance, colored light, incense, theosophical poetry, and music in the ultimate development of synesthetic experience. This work, entitled *Mysterium*, was to have taken place in the Himalayas. Although during Scriabin's lifetime, effective implementation of his synesthetic ideas was not yet possible, today's technology is capable of realizing his most visionary concepts. Scriabin's premature death in 1915 prevented the fulfillment of his vision which would have undoubtedly placed him among the most important predecessors of today's multimedia artists.

CONTEXT OF SCRIABIN'S TASTIERA PER LUCE

Technological means to implement what was termed *color-music* — the artistic performance of pure color projection from a musical keyboard — had been explored since the middle of the 18th century. While no practical instrument with widespread acceptance had been developed by the time Scriabin wrote *Prometheus* in 1911, many instruments had been proposed, some actually constructed, and the idea was unquestionably "in the air" during Scriabin's lifetime.

The best-known color instrument of the last century was patented in 1893 by Alexander Wallace Rimington (1854-1918). The inventor, a Professor of Fine Arts at Queen's College in London, called his apparatus the Colour-Organ, and this name has become the generic term for all such devices designed to project colored light. Rimington described his instrument and the color theories upon which it was based in a 1911 book, *Colour-Music: The Art of Mobile Colour.*

The Colour-Organ stood over ten feet high. A very complex apparatus, it employed many filters varnished with aniline dye, fourteen arc lamps, and it required a power supply capable of providing 150 amps. The five-octave keyboard resembled that of an ordinary organ and was connected by a series of trackers a corresponding set of diaphragms in front of special lenses. Stops were furnished to control the three variables of color perception: hue, luminosity, and chroma, or color purity. One stop allowed the performer to spread the spectrum band over the entire keyboard instead of one octave — proof of Rimington's flexible attitude concerning the analogy between particular colors and tones.

Like earlier mechanisms, Rimington's instrument was not capable of producing any sounds. He did recommend, however, that compositions played in color be performed simultaneously on sound-producing instruments because this added to the enjoyment of the color. No new notational system was needed because musical compositions were played on the keyboard in a normal manner and thereby "translated" into colored light.

Rimington's efforts attracted considerable attention. On June 6, 1895, Rimington presented a private lecture-demonstration in London, attended by over a thousand people. His Colour-Organ was accompanied by piano, a normal sound-producing organ, and a full orchestra. It is interesting that this is the same instrumentation called for in Alexander Scriabin's famous 1911 color-symphony, *Prometheus*. Scriabin probably knew of Rimington's work, and he was the first composer to include a part for projected light — his Tastiera per luce — in a score for orchestra.

LATER DEVELOPMENT OF COLOR-INSTRUMENTS

While many earlier innovations such as Rimington's Colour-Organ had been conceived to reveal physical connections between light and sound, most instruments built during the early decades of this century were not intended to express direct association. This frequent difference of opinion concerning *correct* color associations prevented the establishment of a consistent aesthetic for performances of color-music. If the same musical composition was performed on separate instruments the resulting translations would yield entirely different colors.

Many color-projection instruments appeared shortly after 1920 — the year generally considered to mark the birth of kinetic art. In 1920, for example, the English painter Adrian Klein designed a color projector for stage lighting. His instrument, which demonstrated a color theory involving logarithmic division of the visible spectrum, was operated from a two-octave keyboard. Leonard Taylor, another English experimenter, built a device whereby twelve colored lights were activated from a thirteen-note keyboard. Although no relay switches were used, various *organ stops* controlled individual colors which could then be diluted with a variable-intensity daylight lamp (the thirteenth note). Similar color experiments were carried out between 1920 and 1925 by Achille Ricciardo, who built a colored-light instrument for the Teatro del Colore in Rome, and Richard Lovstrom in the United States, who patented an apparatus to perform color-music. The Czech artist Zdenek Pasanek worked with a color-keyboard, as did Alexander Laszlo, who introduced his device (called a Sonchromatoscope) in 1925 at the Music-Art Festival at Kiel. Laszlo's book, *Die Farblichtmusik*, was published the same year. His preludes for piano and colored light employed a special system of notation.

From 1920 to 1925, Ludwig Hirschfeld-Mack studied at the Weimar Bauhaus. During the summer of 1922, he and others were rehearsing one of the shadow plays, often presented at the Bauhaus. When one of the acetylene bulbs they were using needed replacement, Hirschfeld-Mack accidentally discovered that shadows on a transparent paper screen were doubled. By using acetylene bulbs of different color, "cold" and "warm" shadows appeared simultaneously. The principle was refined in subsequent years by using a type of color-organ. This device enabled Hirschfeld-Mack to present reflected-light compositions with his own music. The lighting technique was introduced to the public in 1923 at a film matinee at the Berlin Volksbuhne, and later in Vienna with Fernand Leger's experimental films.

WILFRED'S CLAVILUX

The most famous of the experimental color-instruments was the Clavilux, developed in 1922 by Thomas Wilfred at a cost of over $16,000. Wilfred completely rejected theories which presumed correspondence between light and sound. Light alone was the principal feature of a new art form which he named *Lumla*. It is true that Van Deering Perrine, the noted American painter and friend of Isadora Duncan, had experimented with various color-instruments around 1912 —and he may have been the first to reject the direct allusion to music — but Wilfred was able to develop the full implication of pure light manipulation. He considered the term *color-music* a metaphor; yet his art resembled music

by including factors of time and rhythm in live performance.

The Clavilux was introduced to the public on January 10, 1922 in New York, although the first of several instruments had been partially completed in 1919. This was after more than a decade of experimentation. Wilfred's main instrument, employing six projectors, was controlled from a "keyboard" consisting of banks of sliders. An elaborate arrangement of prisms could be inclined or twisted in any plane in front of each light source. Color intensity was varied by six separate rheostats which the performer operated delicately with his fingers. Selection of geometric patterns was effected via an ingenious system of counterbalanced disks. Wilfred's shifting-light performances have been compared by many to the beautiful display of the Aurora Borealis.

During the years 1924 and 1925, Wilfred toured the United States, Canada and Europe. The late Percival Price has told the author about a Clavilux recital (January 5, 1925) he attended in Toronto: "Before the concert there seemed to be an attitude of snobbery toward the art, but after Wilfred began to perform, everyone was spellbound." Nearly all of the published reviews substantiate this conclusion, and the critics' difficulty in finding the right words to describe the effect of the performance is evident. Deems Taylor, for example, wrote:

The fact that Thomas Wilfred's Clavilux is commonly known as the color-organ is not the only reason why a music reviewer should have attended his recital last night in Aeolian Hall. For this new color-art might very aptly be called music for the eye . . . it is color and light and form and motion, but it is not painting, nor sculpture, nor pantomime. It is difficult to convey in words. Describing the Clavilux to one who has not seen it is like describing an orange to an Eskimo.

CONCLUSION

In the decades following Wilfred's introduction of the Clavilux, many artists experimented with the technique of interpreting music in colored light. George Hall, for example, built a device in the 1930s which he called the Musichrome. It was equipped with eight keys to control two sets of four colors each. In a brochure about his instrument, Hall indicated no set rules to follow when interpreting musical compositions. "The accompanist must follow his own color reactions to the music played. Generally speaking, heavy, loud, thunderous music calls for the use of red, although there are times when an intense blue is desirable."

Extensive technical innovation after World War II made possible the permanent installation of a large number of "color-organs" in theaters and galleries all over the world. These instruments have been operated either by live performance or have been programmed to present light sculptures. One such work, Wilfred's *Lumia Suite* (opus 158), was displayed during the late 1960s in New York's Museum of Modern Art. For two decades (and until recently), the engineer and lighting designer Christian Sidenius gave performances of colored light with music at his private installation in Sandy Hook, Connecticut. His elaborate equipment included stereopticon color-projectors, and he called his concerts, *Lumia, the Theatre of Light* in honor of Wilfred's original Lumia Theatre of New York. And today, similar multimedia experimentation is evident. Jan Gjessing and his artistic collaborators in Norway, for example, have presented many concerts using their stereoscopic projectors. Gjessing works with what he has termed *sound-to-light liquid cells*, which modulate visual patterns in real-time.

Within the past fifteen years, the decreasing cost of technology has fired a revival of interest in the practical development of instruments to perform color-music. One result has been that today's consumers of both art and of entertainment events have come to expect that their aesthetic experiences will be generated by mixed-media — often including colored light and sound. In the United States and Europe, many color-music concerts have been presented by various groups. And audiences in our multimedia age have responded enthusiastically to this veritable explosion of activity.

Nor have commercial applications of color-music been neglected. A few years ago, Macy's provided its "gift to New York City — a one-of-a-kind extravaganza with lasers, lights and holiday music to delight one and all." Shoppers could purchase an inexpensive "color-organ" inside the store (the well-known devices are attached to a home stereo and different audio frequencies trigger various colored lights), then they could step outside to witness the display of lasers with music.

Although experimenters during the past two centuries could hardly have anticipated today's widespread use of laser light in combination with electronic computers, these marvelous inventions are in some ways refinements of earlier technological proposals for a viable color-music instrument. The development of this technology has always been intimately associated with interest in what has been termed *synesthetic perception* — especially one of the most common modes, that of color-hearing. This seems the perfect concept to be pressed into the service of "color-music," since it is the association of particular colors with various parameters of sound. Every generation, it seems, must rediscover and redefine the art of color-music for itself. And rarely does there appear to be awareness that previous activity has occurred. The current catalog of one major video company, for example, informs its clients that with their product, "a new art form was born. Blending color, music and movement, this new medium is a marriage of sight and sound."

REFERENCES

1. Bleuler E, Lehmann K: Zwangsmassige Lichtempfindungen Durch Schall Und Verwandte Erscheinungen Auf Dem Gebiete Der Andern Sinnesempfindungen. Leipzig: 1881.
2. Ortmann O: Theories of synesthesia in the light of a case of color-hearing. Human Biology 5:155-211, 1933.
3. Cytowic RE: Synesthesia: A Union of the Senses. New York: Springer Verlag, 1988.
4. Vernon PE: Synaesthesia in Music. Psyche 10:22-40, 1930.
5. Slonimsky N: Colors and keys. Medical Opinion and Review, 24-31, October 1966.
6. Sabaneeev L: The relation between sound and color. Music and Letters 10:266-277, 1920.

CHAPTER 2

Medical Aspects of Synesthesia

Benjamin Simkin

DEFINITION[1]

a. *Synesthesia* derived from the Greek: *syn* = union, and *aisthesis* = sensation; i.e., union of sensation.

b. Synesthesia is a rare condition, found predominantly in women, in which stimulation of one sense produces an involuntary perception in another sense. While any or all of the five senses (sight, hearing, smell, taste and touch) can be combined, the most common combination is sight with sound, or "colored hearing." This occurs when sounds such as music, voices or noises cause the subject to see moving colors and shapes. For synesthetes, the phrase, "I see what you're saying" is literal.

HISTORY[1]

a. Although known to the medical and psychological communities for over 200 years, neurologists have taken no interest until recently.

b. Some distinguished scientists have studied synesthesia:

In 1704, Sir Isaac Newton tried mathematically to correlate the energy of sound and color, the practical application of which was the *clavecin oculaire*, an instrument that plays sound and lights simultaneously.

Erasmus Darwin (1790), grandfather of Charles Darwin, achieved the same effect with a harpsichord.

c. Studies by various observers drew the following conclusions:

· Synesthesia is not learned.

· There are no direct linkages between the different sensory systems, such as auditory and visual systems.

· Language is not the link between the senses.

CRITERIA of SYNESTHESIA[1]

These separate the phenomenon of synesthesia from imagery or artistic fancy:

a. It is involuntary and cannot be suppressed.

b. The sensations are perceived externally as real.

c. Synesthetic sensations are discrete (few in number and generic in nature).

d. Synesthetic sensations are highly memorable.

e. Synesthesia is accompanied by strong emotion, and a sense of conviction.

ETIOLOGY (CAUSES) of SYNESTHESIA[1,2]

a. *Epileptic Synesthesia*[3]

1. Occurs in less than 10% of temporal lobe-limbic seizures.

2. Characterized by gustatory-visual-tactile perceptions.

3. Any or all of the following symptom complex may occur:

· Visceral (epigastric) disturbances.

· Deja vu (re-experiencing the environment).

· Motor movements such as chewing, swallowing, lip smacking, sucking.

· Unpleasant olfactory hallucinations.

· Visual or auditory hallucinations.

b. *Drug-Induced* (Hallucinogens such as LSD, peyote, mescal)

Occurs only infrequently.

c. *Sensory Deprivation*

Ex. Sound-induced photisms (flashes of light) in a blind visual hemifield.

d. *Gross Brain Stem Lesions*

Ex. Cystic tumor of brain stem.

e. *Electrical Stimulation of Temporal Cortex* (Evoked Response)

f. *Cerebral Concussion*

1. Due to blow to head ("I saw stars").

2. 2% of patients react to sudden noises or bright lights with momentary pain extending into trunk or an extremity (Photo- or audio-algesic synesthesia).

g. *Idiopathic Synesthesia*

1. Patients have normal physical and neurologic exams, as well as normal IQs.

2. Trait appears in early childhood.

3. It is genetic in origin, with autosomal dominant inheritance, and 2.5 to 1 predominance in women.

4. Left-handedness or mixed dominance found in 50% of patients or first-degree relatives.

5. Many subjects have exceptional memories.

MEDICAL CONDITIONS ASSOCIATED WITH VISUAL IMAGES

a. *Migraine*[4]

In 10-15% of patients the prodrome (onset) may take the form of scintillating scotomas (flashes of light) or visual field defects, due to transient local constriction of cerebral or retinal arteries.

b. *Cerebral Concussion*

"I saw stars."

c. *Retinal Tears due to Retraction of Vitreous*[5]

Intermittent dots of light, a second or so in duration.

d. *Visual Hallucinations in Non-Psychotic Normal Patients*[5]

1. Due to automatic firing of retinal cones or nerve endings.

2. Various images seen, such as little men, lights, various objects, and geometric figures.

3. Occur at intervals of days, weeks, or months without any apparent triggering factor.

4. According to Dr. James Salz, who has accumulated a collection of such patients in his ophthalmological practice, there is no known cause or treatment.

e. *Psychotic Visual Hallucinations*

1. Commonly seen in organic brain syndromes due to multiple strokes, senile dementia, and alcoholism.

2. Often precipitated by sedative and hypnotic medicaments.

3. In organic brain syndromes, visual and auditory hallucinations are common due to misinterpretation of sounds and visual inanimate objects such as chairs and tables. Ex. In senile dementia, it is very common to report seeing strange men in the room at night. The "pink elephants" of alcoholic DTs are well known.

f. *Hypnogogic Hallucinations*[6]

1. A feature of narcolepsy (sleep seizures), along with cataplexy (localized or generalized muscle weakness), and sleep paralysis (when the patient is either going into or coming out of a deep sleep).

2. Hypnogogic hallucinations are vivid visual or dream-like states which occur while dozing or being aroused. They are so vivid that patients may act out the dream state on awakening.

CASE REPORT of NEUROLOGICALLY DEFINED COLORED HEARING SYNESTHESIA[7]

Purpose: To illustrate clinical colored hearing synesthesia.

Subject: A 17-year-old right-handed high school choirboy who reported "colored hearing" since childhood.

1. The subject did not have perfect pitch, although one of the controls did.

2. Specific musical notes of the 12-tone scale consistently evoked the same color hues or responses; this did not occur in the controls.

3. Unlike controls, he could make new musical note-color associations in a single trial; that is, when presented with triads, the color responses of the additional notes were depicted as bands on the original color.

4. The same color responses were reproduced on the following day, and again five months later, without further training or repetition.

CONCLUSION

This chapter discusses synesthesia from the physician's viewpoint, an outlook much more limited in scope than that of the artist. Much of the recent medical literature is based upon the work of a distinguished neurologist, Richard E. Cytowic, to whom the author is heavily indebted. The brief case report illustrates the tight clinical boundaries and uncommonality of colored-hearing synthesis, in vivid contrast to the broad, free-flowing concepts of artistic synesthesia presented in the chapter, *Synesthesia: The Context and Artistic Implications*.

REFERENCES

1. Cytowic RE: Editorial. Synesthesia and mapping of subjective sensory dimensions. Neurology 39:849-850, 1989.
2. Cytowic RE: Synesthesia: A Union of the Senses. New York: Springer-Verlag, 1988.
3. Glaser G. The epilepsies. *In* Beeson PB, McDermott W, Wyngarden JB (eds), Textbook of Medicine, 855. Philadelphia: WB Saunders, 1979.
4. Plum F: Headache. *In* Beeson PB, McDermott W, Wyngarden JB (eds), Textbook of Medicine, 731. Philadelphia: WB Saunders, 1979.
5. Salz J: Personal communication.
6. Shapiro WR: Sleep and its disorders. *In* Beeson PB, McDermott W, Wyngarden JB (eds), Textbook of Medicine, 653-654. Philadelphia: WB Saunders, 1979.
7. Rizzo M, Eslinger PJ: Colored hearing synesthesia: An investigation of neural factors. Neurology 39:781-784, 1989.

CHAPTER 3

Jazz as a Metaphor of Medicine

John H. Gundy

As medicine can transform illness into health, jazz can transform oppression into music. Medicine is an art that has organized sensations (sights, sounds, smells and touch) to allow the diagnosis, treatment, and prevention of human illness. Born in ancient civilizations, medicine has been nurtured for thousands of years by scientists and practitioners. Despite the recent development of devices that greatly amplify man's sensations and interventions, the thrust of medicine remains the potential for victory over illness. Jazz is a more contemporary art that has organized sound to allow expression of feelings and communication about relationships. Jazz grew out of black America with strong African roots and significant Western European and church influences. The beginnings of jazz were nurtured amidst the oppression of black slavery and black segregation in the United States. A unique verse form, the *blues*, grew out these years of oppression and depression. This paper reviews the origins, components, and dynamic processes of each art as experienced by the author.

Medicine and jazz share a capacity to combat forces adverse to human well-being. Medicine is an art that can transform illness into health. Medical intervention uses information gathered from the combined senses to diagnose, treat, and prevent human maladies. The medical healer listens and observes well, compares his/her observations with scientific data and offers his/her treatment. Jazz is an art that transforms oppression into music. This music has a unique origin and development out of the oppressed lives of black Americans. Both jazz performer and listener enjoy a release of emotions and a sense of freedom.

Medicine, born of fear and empathy, arose in ancient civilizations in response to human illness. Although the natural healing powers, the *vis medicatrix naturae* of Hippocrates, more active interventions such as the use of magic, herbs, divination, and acupuncture grew among Middle Eastern and Chinese cultures. Attempts to organize clinical observations as a way to enhance continued learning about human illness appear to have begun with Hippocrates and were greatly enhanced by the anatomists of the Renaissance. Descriptions of human illnesses from the seventeenth through the twentieth centuries were the beginnings of contemporary medicine: human anatomy, microbiology, psychology, pathology, physical diagnosis, pharmacology, surgery, rehabitation, psychotherapy, and preventive medicine. Medicine has evolved from magical incantation to organ transplants.

The physician's task, however, has much in common with its ancient ancestors'. S/he practices an art of human interaction in which the goals are to seek the truth and to promote healing. S/he uses an ongoing dialogue with his/her patient based upon a trusting relationship to define the person and his/her illness and to communicate healing measures. The skills of the twenty-first century physician will be the same as the healers' through the ages: listening, observing, diagnosing, and then acting in a manner to restore health with follow-up to measure results. Although cure is not always possible, the physician-patient relationship promotes both the hope of the patient and the continued learning of the physician.

The evolution of jazz in the midst of the slavery of black Americans can be inferred from similarities with music from the slaves' West African beginnings. Perhaps the outstanding characteristic of West African music is the close intertwining of everyday life with dance. Rhythm is supplied by hand-clapping or drums, and some instruments, like the African banjo and xylophone, supply both melody and percussion. Melodies tend to be short and repetitive with theme and variation and call-and-response singing. Musical notes tend to be sung off the third and seventh notes of the scale. These and other characteristics of African music, some of which still exist, may include Arabic influences from North Africa, and their further development in the colonies probably were influenced by the countries of their masters: Portugal, Spain, and England.

The earliest American black music available for study are the field hollers of the farm laborers. The blues, originally a lament in verse form of A-A-B pattern, probably arose out of the social isolation of field workers and was influenced by the tradition of Anglo-Saxon ballads. Afro-Christian music began in the church services provided for slaves and added the strong rhythm, off-pitch notes, and call-and-response from African roots to new and existing Christian hymns. The repertoires of the traveling blues singers and the black church music were brought to New Orleans in the middle 1800s where they were mixed with the existing European band music, especially French. As contrasted to European marching bands, "dirty jass bands" did not march but enjoyed the added skills of European-trained musicians to play for dances, funerals, and for fun. Jazz emerged from the New Orleans cradle as "a mixture of mutually influential folk and popular styles systematized by melody, harmony and rhythm, allowing endless growth and diversity." The earliest recordings of jazz music were made by white musicians who imitated the music of black bands. Today, musicians of all races and cultures contribute to the jazz repertoire and experience.

The blues has continued to be a foundation stone of jazz, with its unique scale and chords using flatted thirds and sevenths. Jazz is created at live performances with improvisation on a theme. The improvised dialogue of the members of a jazz band with each other and with the audience can mirror different qualities of human relationships: competitiveness, tenderness, harmoniousness, or anger. The improvising jazz musician reacts to the human condition and expresses outrage, desire, bitterness, humor, mimicry, or joy. Thus jazz is human interaction which expresses feelings in music. It is this dynamism of jazz that can transform the sadness of the blues to the moments of soaring release.

As a physician, the author uses the inheritance from ages of scientists and practitioners to learn the truth about his patients and their illnesses. He sits down with a patient and reviews his/her past, listens to his/her concerns and performs a physical exam, listening, touching, looking, and sniffing. He maps out

a pathway leading to more harmonious living. As a jazz musician, being a student of the basic components of melody, harmony and rhythm, having learned some of the classical jazz pieces, having witnessed both live and recorded performances by jazz master musicians, and continuing to practice the technique of his instrument, the author approaches each opportunity to play jazz as a release from a regimented professional life and sometimes as a search for musical truth. He first tries out a piece, playing the basic melody and chord pattern until they are inside his head. Then he try different ways to make the same musical statement, sometimes reacting to or continuing a colleague's statement, sometimes proudly copying the statement of a master.

Occasionally, the spark of improvisation lights a fire that lifts us for a moment into a new plane of musical space, a new creation, a release from what has gone before. The similarity of jazz and medicine is in the interaction among human beings, transforming the blues of illness and oppression into a healthy release.

SUGGESTED READING

1. Collier JL: The Makings of Jazz. A Comprehensive History. Boston: Houghton Mifflin, 1978.
2. Inglis B: A History of Medicine. London: Weidenfeld and Nicolson, 1965.
3. Jones LR: Blues People. New York: William Morrow, 1963.
4. Marti-ibanez F: Centaur. Essays on the History of Medical Ideas. New York: MD Publications, 1960.
5. Oliver P, Harrison M, Bolcom W: The New Grove Gospel, Blues and Jazz. New York: William Norton and Co, 1986.
6. Roberts, JS: Black Music of Two Worlds. New York: Praeger Publishers, 1972.
7. Schuller G: Early Jazz: Its Roots and Musical Development. New York: Oxford University Press, 1978.

CHAPTER 4

Health — Rhythm — Balance

Victoria Santa Cruz

The forms or disciplines which exist in certain ancient cultures, such as dance, music, and handicrafts, among others, are intimately linked to the process of evolution of the human being, the basis of the cultural structure. Consequently, these forms — as means of integration — are learned in life, through life, and for the purpose of life.

Through these forms, the consciousness of those who practice them is awakened, cultivating the faculties of observation, the discernment of qualities, notions about responsibility, and the uselessness of excess — that is to say, learning how to live. To live means to vibrate, and to vibrate implies transformation.

This transformation starts from the basis, that is, from the physical body, and should gradually unfold through lighter, more subtle bodies or units.

This physical body, this earth-body — in which, as in every human being, the seed of knowledge is already planted — needs to be plowed and watered with great care, since without this vehicle, evolution is not possible.

Before we discover the capacity to connect, the loyalty of this instrument, the physical body, seems unimaginable. We have to learn how to feel it, how to listen to it, and how not to use it the way we usually do.

It is not in isolation, solely from the intellect, that the physical body expresses itself. In this laboratory are gestating the most complex and subtle substances which will manifest themselves — in the presence of certain external stimuli — as qualities of sensations, of perceptions, of temperature, which, in accordance with the process, will determine specific states of being.

It is by starting from the flavor of the state of being that we are able to penetrate the chemistry of health, discovering that the secret is not necessarily *knowing*, but *being*.

In organic understanding, the number-unit is a living entity which reveals its quality as a consequence of its quantity. This is why such understanding does not resort to counting "1-2-3" to determine the unit.

Each rhythmical combination contains ancient and wise secrets of organization which, when they penetrate our senses, pierce the fibers of the tissues of our physical body, in this way teaching us to discover the flavor of the language of connection, like a tuner who tunes a musical instrument. Thus, through a well-tuned intuition, we are traveling toward centers or plexus, learning to discover a special state of being, a special attitude.

This will be the basis from which we later achieve other levels of attitude, until we connect with the germ of harmony, this seed to which we have already alluded.

Knowing the flavor of the states of being is one of the indispensable steps for achieving a level of consciousness, a level of health. We know that we are not healthy only when we are ill, since we do not know the flavor of health — this particular unit, at once active-passive, which knows how to be ready to act without necessarily receiving any gratification whatsoever.

Those of us who have inherited rhythm through an ancestral culture, familiarizing ourselves with it from childhood, coexisting with this living entity, with its tangible nuances, are unable to accept the definition of rhythm as *time and measure*. Rhythm — considering not only the aspects related to certain artistic disciplines — is the key to the connection; it is the element which is able to establish a relationship between opposite forces, and because they are opposite, complementary and indispensable in the unit.

Health is action, action is a unity. A unit, as we know, is made up of an inseparable binomial, positive and negative.

What is the chemistry, the intelligence of this rhythm, which connects the *positive* and the *negative* and which, while respecting their respective qualities, achieves the marvelous phenomenon of *unity*? This is the secret which we must penetrate within the vehicle we call the physical body.

When the balance is altered, the link is broken, and we encounter noise, chaos, and the labyrinth.

Health, rhythm, equilibrium — these are one and the same.

Only what is healthy has the capacity, the rhythm, that fosters integration. Illness is synonymous with separation, isolation, division. Fortunately, division may also, at a certain moment, prepare a new *re-union*.

Upbringing, education, guidance cannot be disconnected from the life of man since he is the only goal. Man, through his work, discovers who he is. The artisan must attain a level of consciousness and become an artist. The artist must rediscover other levels of consciousness, realizing that he himself is a cell in a great organism.

Then and only then will he be able to transform himself, becoming the work of art which he so passionately sought, and from there another path will open up, a new task, another transformation.

When there is internal comprehension, the external accomplishes its role, inviting us to grow in balance. When this interior is not present, the exterior devours us.

Everything is interaction, transformation, vibration equilibrium, in this cosmos. Vibration implies hierarchy; thus, in the area of sound, a high vibration knows that it is supported by a lower vibration and vice versa. Because harmony within the human family has been ruptured, unity and hierarchy have been distorted.

The human instrument is the only one which cannot be tuned by someone else. We are the instrument, we are the tuner, we are the player, we are the dissonance, we are the melody, and we are also the listener.

To deny that those with greater experience and knowledge are able to help and guide us would be absurd, but the responsibility for tuning is the duty of each one of us. Each of us, in relation to himself and to his surroundings, learns how to undertake his task. Only by assuming this responsibility will we be able to be healed. Hence, my interest is focused on those who have not been declared clinically ill; that is, those presumed to be healthy. I say "presumed to be healthy" because I believe that we are all somewhat ill.

Healing represents, for me, the opening up of the possibility of touching, in the apparently sick or the apparently well person, a level of consciousness, beginning with learning how to believe in oneself, starting from one's own vehicle.

What is illness? Is it not perhaps another of the tools of the *law of harmony*, of the *great rhythm*, inviting us to rediscover our own order? The battlefield is this daily life, so minimized in modern civilization.

Health, to a certain degree, is knowledge. Only knowledge has the power to transform, since transformation implies a high level of consciousness. To learn how to be in tune should be our commitment, and for this commitment there are no recipes. The rational must be sustained by live experiences which are never repeated in the same way. Like fingerprints, every human being is different from every other.

If it is true that knowledge does not belong to us, the manner of communicating it is indeed personal. That is why one who copies from another not only runs the risk of misguiding those whom he purports to teach, but also hinders his own possibilities for finding himself in his own process.

To be in tune, then, should be our commitment until we are able to resound in the universal chord.

CHAPTER 5

Robot Choreography as a Vehicle for Studying Creativity

Margo K. Apostolos

Abstract

Robot choreography has been developed to explore an aesthetic dimension of robotic movement. Industrial robots have been programmed to move in a dance-like fashion through techniques developed by programming computers that control robot motion. The resultant form of choreographed robot movement integrates art and technology as a possible new art form with therapeutic applications. The exploration of an aesthetic dimension of robotic movement has been used to study the effects of this qualitative aspect of machine movement on user acceptance of robots. This research includes the use of robots by the severely disabled in a rehabilitative setting. Robot choreography may provide a vehicle for creative artistic expression for the severely disabled. Thus, physical limitations need not exclude the disabled from the experience of creative expression. Robot choreography integrates the sounds of music, the forms of sculpture, and the movements of dance. Choreography, the art of making dances, uses dance as a series of rhythmic motions in time and space to express ideas through movement sequences. The process of choreographing for a robot combines a logical approach with a sensuous approach in a blend of artistic and scientific creativity. The author presents both choreographic techniques and computer-programming methods. An exploration of the creative potential in rehabilitation is discussed with relation to thought patterns.

INTRODUCTION

The programming of robot choreography appears somewhat similar to choreography for humans: an idea is expressed through physical movement and presented to an audience. The intention of the *dance* is to express an idea from the choreography through the representational form of the dancers, either humans or robots. The audience perceives the representation through neural pathways of reflex, conditioning, memory, and conscious awareness to produce new feelings or experiences not otherwise communicable.[1] In dance, the movement communicates what cannot be said with words.

Choreography is representational of the artist and projective for the audience. The experience of the observer is individual and unique, reflected in the interpretation and identification of the dance. If an observer cannot dance, due to injury or illness, the identification of the movement and expression of the choreography may enhance creative and rhythmic thought patterns. Robot choreography is unique in that the performance of the machine is precise, replicable, and programmable by humans. Robot choreography has been used by the disabled as a form of recreational therapy.[2] Thus, a disabled person could use a robot as a vehicle for creative and artistic expression via the application of choreographic techniques.

CHOREOGRAPHIC TECHNIQUES

The development of robot choreography began as an experiment in computer programming techniques for an industrial robotic arm. The idea appeared to be a rather novel approach to the conventional notion of robot motion; that is, contrasting the mechanical actions of robots with graceful motion. The quality of movement discovered through programming choreography for robots was quite unusual in a striking way. Seemingly, the *dancing robots* altered the conventional mechanics of the industrial machines. What appeared to be smooth and fluid motion apparently violated the standard kinematics of the robot design.

The choreographed movement phrases were synchronized with musical phrases to present a composition similar in structural form to a dance choreographed for human dancers. While the choreographic form of the robot dance resembled the form of human choreography, a degree of difference between the dance creations was evident in the art media rather than the artistic forms. The representation of *dancing robots* has been designed to closely resemble choreographic form; thus, the indication is one of an artistic nuance.

As part of this work, an attempt was made to present movement of the robot choreographed and synchronized with music. The mechanical features of the staccato action of the robotic arm were contrasted with what has been defined as *aesthetic maneuvers*. The aesthetic movements feature a more sustained effort in the actions, smoother transitions from point to point, curved lines replacing many of the straight and short angular motions, and a varied sequence in the timing of movement phrases to break up the constant speed characteristic of the practical patterns of robot movement. The aesthetic maneuvers explore the related movement elements of the action quality, flow, shape, and timing in various movement phrases.

Movement elements often used in dance choreography are used in the design of robot tasks. The elements of shape, space, time, and force are used in dance exploration, and these movement elements can be used in both dance and in application to functional robot tasks. The position and actual movements of the robot in vertical and horizontal planes comprise the basis for shape exploration. Space is a factor which further distinguishes movement by direction, dimension, level, path, and focus. The tempo (rate of speed) of the movement, and the subsequent rhythmic pattern of motion are paramount concerns in the development of aesthetic sequences of robotic movement. The elements of force, i.e. energy, effort, weight, and dynamics, relate to the intensity of movement. The quality of movement then results when time, tempo, and intensity are treated in certain relation to both gravity and space.

PROGRAMMING TECHNIQUES

A program for robot choreography consists of various routines and sub-routines. Individual points in space are named and recorded as movement positions. These points are linked into movement phrases which constitute the sub-routines and routines. Individual points in space are recorded in reference to specific joint angles. These joint positions are stored within the system and recorded with specific names as indicated in the steps of each sub-routine. The qualitative aspect of the movement is achieved by varying speeds between points, which can create various rhythmic patterns.

Currently, *dance steps* for robots have been created within available programming languages; that is, each robot has been operated through system-specific software. Through the software, the points in space (robot positions) are recorded and the subse-quent development of intricate computer programs creates the master routines that control the robot. Much of the programming can be done through a teach-pendant that controls the movement of the robot itself — either by independent joint or through Cartesian space.

Individual points are recorded with reference to joint angles. The degrees of freedom refer to specific joints on the limb, each joint representing one degree of freedom. Most of the robots the author has worked with are manipulated with six degrees of freedom: (1) shoulder rotation, (2) shoulder flexion and extension, (3) elbow flexion, (4) wrist rotation, (5) end effector flexion and extension, and (6) end effector rotation. Various positions corresponding to the joint angles can be stored within a system and recorded with point names. The joint angles are in the memory of the system relative to the calibration position of the robot.

CREATIVE EXPRESSION

Performing artists work with various tools and media. The robot as an artistic tool raises new issues. An artist often feels an intimacy and compassion for a new creation; the notion of expression surrounds the development of art. The feelings and compassion of an artist are often wrapped up in the work of art. Robot choreography presents an unusual approach for the artist, as the choreographer is actually expressing ideas through the computer, with the robot as the vehicle for expression. Thus, the artistic thoughts are twice removed. The choreographer must translate the artistic vision into the computer language in order to manipulate the robot.

The development of robot choreography has established an new vehicle for creative expression. The invention and development of new technology are products of human work; thus, the creative application of the technology may also be considered a product of human expression. Expressive arts therapy is of significant value in treating various disorders.[3] Various art forms have been used in both physical and psychological therapy. "Expressive arts therapy is a means of helping persons with clinically defined dysfunctions, or persons who are 'normal' but who may wish to achieve greater awareness and integration." [3]

CONCLUSION

Robot choreography may be used as a means of expression, communication, and redirection in therapy.

The choreographic techniques and computer programming methods are utilized in an activity which uses a robot as a vehicle of expression combining sculpture, music, and dance. Dance choreography for robots may provide additional artistic alternatives in creative expression.

Dance is both an expression of the choreographer's imagination and the audience's perception of the work. Robot choreography demonstrates an artistic-scientific combination that blends various talents and tools into a unitary piece: sculpture of movements in space, the musicality of rhythmic responses in time, and the expression of the symbolic gestures of dance. A dancing robot is possible as the creative expression of both the artist and the scientist as perceived by an audience through the communicative language expressed in the work of art.

In robot choreography, the purpose is not to develop a creative machine, but rather a machine to be used as an expression of creativity. Subsequently, by virtue of robot predictability, repeatability, and reliability, perhaps the robot may become a vehicle of investigation for studying the creative process of the human mind. The object of such an investigation would be to computerize, not humanize, by using advanced technology to probe the human thought process.

REFERENCES

1. Apostolos MK: Presence, premiere issue. MIT Press, Forum, 1992
2. Apostolos MK: Exploring user acceptance of a robotic arm. Doctoral dissertation. Stanford University, December 1984.
3. Rogers MB: The rhythm therapy computer system: A foundation. Proceedings: Delicate Balance: Technics, Culture and Consequences, 318-319. IEEE Society, IEEE-SSIT. Los Angeles, CA, October 1989.

CHAPTER 6

The Neurophysiological Process of Mimicry as a Model for the Aesthetic Response

Louis W. Tinnin

The aesthetic response can be understood in terms of a primitive neurophysiological process involving brain stem, limbic, and peripheral mechanisms that generate *isopraxic* or *imitative* behavior.[1] The neural connections provide a path for communication between the hemispheres that does not depend on the corpus callosum. During infancy, this extra-callosal route is the sole communication between the hemispheres because the unmyelinated corpus callosum does not transmit information until around age three.[2]

Human communication begins with mimicry. The newborn infant responds to faces with mirrored expressions. One can stick out one's tongue to a newborn and get the same salute in return.[3] Babies imitate a multitude of facial expressions within the first few days of life,[4] and long before language develops, the growing child learns the state of mind of the parent by reflecting the facial expression of that state in mimicry.[5]

Just as isopraxic behavior is the basis of cooperation in flocks of birds and herds of animals,[6] so is mimicry the basis of cooperation between the cerebral hemispheres of the infant for the first three years of life, prior to the onset of callosal transmission. The infant would have two separate minds if there was not an extra-callosal linkage between the hemispheres. That linkage is provided by the neurophysiological mechanisms for mimicry.

The infant's imitation of the smiling face is a brainstem-initiated reaction that gives rise to an associated limbic intention to act. The limbic arousal is expressed through the autonomic nervous system acting internally, as well as through skeletal muscle system action. Although the hemispheres cannot exchange messages across the corpus callosum, each will perceive the visceral and skeletal activation generated by the other and will assume a state of mind associated with that pattern of activation in the past (or genetically associated). This process of brainstem response to a stimulus, limbic outflow, peripheral activation, and cortical response to that activation is involved even when the stimulus is internally generated by one of the hemispheres.

An intention to reach for a toy, for example, is formed as part of a state of mind in one hemisphere; an arousal pattern of readiness for that action is transmitted through the skeletal muscular and visceral systems. The other hemisphere, experiencing the activated pattern of the heart and limbs, and automatically assuming the state of mind associated with that pattern in the past, is ready to enter wholeheartedly into the action. In all likelihood, it is this *internal mimicry* that is the major source of volitional coordination prior to maturation of the corpus callosum at age three.

Once the corpus callosum matures and the governing verbal mental system emerges and assumes dominance, the verbal self disavows internal mimicry and claims that all feelings and actions are self-generated — verbal self, that is. It denies the *a posteriori* nature of conscious emotional experience which, in reality, is initiated outside the verbal mental module.[7]

Despite the denial by the conscious self, this callosal *bypass* continues to process nonverbal communication outside of conscious awareness. The infant's sequence of external imitation, which reproduces another's facial expression and bodily state, and internal imitation, which generates the state of mind fitting that bodily state and facial expression, continues throughout life.

THE AESTHETIC EXPERIENCE

Perception of nonverbal communication is an active process in which the receiver creates the percept by active mimicry, whether the message is carried by emotion or by art. The viewer's response to a picture, for example, begins with an active nonverbal experience which is largely outside of consciousness and involves kinesthetic and visceral mimicry preceding verbal interpretation. The viewer circumscribes the lines and volumes with movements of the scanning eyes while mimetic movements of other body parts follow the contours of the figures.[8]

The listener's response to music is played out with body movement.   Observers of sculpture unknowingly imitate the implied movement.[9]   The kinesthetic imitation is automatic and unintended, and seems to predict the person's pleasure in the art.

It is the sensation produced by mimetic motor activity combined with an emotional pattern of visceral arousal that constitutes the aesthetic experience.[8] Any inhibition of either kinesthetic or autonomic mimicry will diminish it.   The mimicry exercised by the viewer determines the extent of the aesthetic response to an art object.

The mimetic response to the art object is not available for verbal reflection not only because it is nonverbal, automatic, and unintended, but also because it is actively denied by consciousness. This is the reason for the enigmatic nature of the aesthetic response which is so resistive to verbal analysis. At the same time, this is a reflection of the special property of the aesthetic experience, in that it contains the direct, uncensored, nonverbal reaction to the stimulus.

REFERENCES

1. MacLean P: The Triune Brain in Evolution. New York: Plenum Press, 1990.

2. Tinnin L: The anatomy of the ego. Psychiatry 52:404-409, 1989.

3. Meltzoff A, Moore M: Imitation of facial and manual gestures by human neonates.   Science 198:75-78, 1977.

4. Field T, Woodson R, Greenberg R, et al: Discrimination and imitation of facial expression by neonates. Science 218:179-181, 1982.

5. Stern D: The Interpersonal World of the Infant. New York: Basic Books, 1985.

6. Scott J: Nonverbal communication in the process of social attachment. *In* Corson S, Corson E, Alexander J (eds), Ethology and Nonverbal Communication in Mental Health: An Interdisciplinary Biopsychosocial Exploration.   New York: Pergamon Press, 1980.

7. Tinnin L: Biologic processes in nonverbal communication and their role in the making and interpretation of art. Amer J Art Therapy 29:9-13, 1990.

8. Papanicolaou A: Emotion: A Reconsideration of the Somatic Theory. New York: Gordon and Breach, 1989.

9. Kreitler H, Kreitler S: Psychology of the Arts. Durham, NC: Duke University Press, 1972.

CHAPTER 7

Humanizing the Health-Care Environment:
Models for a New Arts-Medicine Partnership

Janice Palmer • Florence Nash

Physicians since Hippocrates have recognized the role of spiritual refreshment in physical healing. No similar precedent exists, however, for the degree to which the science and technology revolution has turned medical centers into high-pressured, impersonal environments where the most fundamental human experiences — birth, death, fear, isolation — are rendered nearly voiceless, drowned out by the machine. We are in danger of losing sight of the ultimate mission of the medical center: to heal, comfort, and protect people in need, when they are most vulnerable. Growing recognition of the power of the arts to shape the emotional as well as physical environment has led to a new kind of movement to incorporate the arts into health-care facilities. In contrast to the specifically therapeutic nature of the arts-medicine and arts-therapy traditions, hospital arts programs work to transform the whole facility, to create a climate in which the human processes can be acknowledged and expressed.

This movement goes hand in hand with increased sensitivity to the issues of arts accessibility and integration. Many health-care arts programs have built upon the essentially grass-roots consciousness embodied in community and regional arts networks. Emerging from this matrix, many arts programs tend to have a distinctly individual stamp. An examination of some of the new programs around the U.S. shows that, as often as not, a program is the result of one person's vision and effort. Familiarity with available resources and the capability to use them effectively are key factors in putting art to work in health-care centers; with them, even one person can achieve an enormous amount.

Some programs are originated in local or regional arts organizations; others begin with hospital staff. However diverse their origins, resources, and immediate objectives, they all hold their larger goals in common. They must deal with the same fundamental issues; and, by and large, they begin by confronting the same basic questions, which determine how they will respond to those issues.

Anyone planning to set up a hospital arts program should define at the outset its most specific objectives and, hence, the shape and direction of its operations. Identifying the primary sources of support and of funding (not necessarily the same thing) will affect the answer to the next important questions: Who will make the decisions about what is "best" for the target population? Who will evaluate the program's success? By what criteria? What are the available arts resources in the community? What is the best working relationship with them? How will the program be coordinated, and where will the program fit into the institutional structure?

There are many program models in existence. By design, the Cultural Services Program (CSP) at Duke University Medical Center includes as many art forms as will work in a hospital setting. (There are, of course, physical limitations, such as the fact that there is no place designed for peformance and the only space large enough for dance has a concrete floor.) By intention, the program implements as many existing community arts resources as possible to respond to the needs of the various populations of the medical center, including patients and visitors, medical and support staff, and medical students.

While some performances are held in spaces such as amphitheaters and cafeterias, the CSP's performing arts focus is primarily on the patient units. "Room Service" musicians, magicians, and poets go from door to door offering a bit of refreshment, greatly appreciated not only by patients and visitors but also by staff.

Original works of art, most by North Carolina artists, have been placed in patient rooms and public areas. Changing exhibitions of two- and three-dimensional art are displayed in several specially designed cases. A gallery of touchable art has been opened in the Eye Center to demonstrate to patients with vision impairments that they too have access to the visual arts.

Video tapes about artists and the arts are transmitted on the patient-television channel, and a unique informational TV bulletin board for patients is created by local artists using a computer-graphics system. Presently, the primary thrusts in the visual arts are the acquisition of sculpture, the commissioning of site-specific projects, and the incorporation of aesthetic concerns into the design of space.

A part-time poet in residence reads aloud to patients and their families and organizes journal- and poetry-writing workshops. The poet also coordinates a weekly literary-interest group meeting open to the entire university population. Poets and authors are invited to read and discuss their work with the group. CSP-produced audio tapes of some of these writers are available to patients.

Cultural Services has also helped to establish an arts-medicine program to facilitate access for artists to the clinics and hospital. One important role of this program is to assure performing artists of rapid attention to medical problems that occur immediately preceding a performance.

This burgeoning movement of arts programs in health-care settings is well- and diversely represented across the country. In July 1991, about twenty-five program directors met to establish a formal organization called the Society of Healthcare Arts Administrators. The objectives of their Society are: (1) to promote the integration of the arts in health-care environments; (2) to assist in the development and management of arts programming for health-care populations; (3) to provide resources and education to health-care and arts professionals; (4) to facilitate the exchange of information pertaining to arts in health care; and (5) to encourage and support research and investigation into the beneficial effects of the arts in health care.

One of the founding-member organizations of the society is Hospital Audiences, Inc. (HAI), in New York City. Incorporated in 1969 HAI provides cultural services to people in health-care facilities, drug-treatment and prevention programs, nursing homes, and correctional facilities. Programming includes escort services and free tickets to events, workshops led by artists, performances in institutions where

persons are confined, and loans and donations of visual art works to rehabilitative institutions.

Project Art was established by Joyce Summerwill at the University of Iowa Hospitals and Clinics in 1978 with funds mandated by the Iowa Art in State Buildings Program. In addition to an impressive permanent collection of art, special exhibitions are installed each month and coordinated with demonstrations and lectures. Volunteers circulate an art cart to patient rooms so that patients may choose the art for their walls. Weekly performances are presented in a variety of spaces, and each summer a two-week folk festival presents daily concerts along with lectures and exhibits.

One of the earliest art-cart projects was begun in the 1970s by Lynn Thompson, M.D., at New York Hospital-Cornell Medical Center. Starting with a collection of 100 graphics donated by Touche-Ross, the collection grew to include photography and painting as well. In 1987, Dr. Thompson began a collaboration with HAI to help stimulate the introduction of the art-cart concept into residential health-care settings. With support from Kodak, Dr. Thompson has helped set up programs all over the country.

During the 1980s at UCLA's Jonsson Comprehensive Cancer Center, Devra Breslow secured art donations from galleries, musems, and art dealers for an art-cart project. In addition, Ms. Breslow initiated the first national exhibition by artists with cancer, and developed the Strolling Musicians project, which involved volunteer musicians playing mini-recitals at the bedsides of patients.

Gifts of Art at the University of Michigan Hospitals also operates a well-stocked art cart for patients. In addition, director Gary Smith and his staff coordinate exhibits in four gallery spaces, weekly performances in the main lobby, and outdoor visual- and performing-arts festivals in the summer.

Bill Noonan has developed a program called Planetree, first at California Pacific Hospital and now at four other sites across the country, which focuses a spectrum of arts activities on a single patient unit: visual art in each room; a print, audio, and video library; bedside storytelling and strolling musicians; and artist-volunteers who help patients participate in music and drawing.

Helen Orem introduced the idea of purchasing original art to bring vitality to the bare walls of the outpatient clinics at the National Institutes of Health's

Magnuson Clinical Center. Six galleries display exhibitions of art approved by a jury, and commissions on sales help to support the art program. Ms. Orem now has her own design firm and consults with architects who work in the health-care industry.

Incorporating the arts into facilities planning is gaining ground both in the U.S. and the U.K. The director of the British Health Care Arts Centre, Malcolm Miles, consults on new building and renovation projects for the British National Health Service, involving artists in the earliest phases of the design process.

Another U.K. program, the Arts for Health Centre in Manchester, grew from an effort begun in 1973 by Peter Senior to take a multidisciplinary arts team into area hospitals and health centers. Arts for Health now works with a number of other regional health commissions.

Fifty health-care arts programs are described in The *Hospital Arts Handbook*, recently published by Duke University Medical Center with support from the Mary Duke Biddle Foundation. Also included in the handbook are sections on how to begin a program, with such specific documents as an artist contract which can be removed for copying and personalizing.

For further information about the handbook and/or about membership in the Society of Healthcare Arts Administrators, contact Janice Palmer, Box 3017, Duke University Medical Center, Durham, NC 27710.

CHAPTER 8

Psychoneuroimmunology in Interior Design

Millicent Gappell

A 1964 paper entitled *Emotions, Immunity and Disease: A Speculative Theoretical Integration* suggested a correlation between stress, immunological dysfunction, and disease.[1] Subsequently, a large body of replicable experimental and clinical data proved the connection between biological responses and sensory stimulation — the emerging science of psychoneuroimmunology (PNI). Its application to the design of home and work place is the art and science of creating environments that enhance well-being, creativity and performance.

The six major environmental factors that influence our physical and emotional well-being are light, color, sound, aroma, texture, and space. Environments that do not integrate these factors properly can increase stress, anxiety, and agitation, thereby affecting health, as well as the ability to concentrate, think, learn, and sleep. A well-designed environment, utilizing the principles of PNI, can have such an enormous physiological and psychological impact on the individual that it can literally set the stage for whatever activity is to take place. For a medical facility, good design can be considered good medicine in itself.[2, 3]

Described herein are some principal PNI elements and general guidelines for interiors that provide positive sensory stimulation as well as being aesthetically pleasing.

LIGHT

Artists have always been aware of the importance of lighting to visual perception. The ability to see and function efficiently depends on the quantity and quality of the illumination around us. Now there is a new awareness of the health benefits of lighting — the field of photobiology.

Daylight affects endocrine control, timing of our biological clocks and circadian (sleep/wake) cycles, neonatal jaundice, Seasonal Affective Disorder (SAD), absorption of calcium, prophylactic control of viral and staph infections, and physical and psychological well-being.[4-10]

Ideally, windows, atria, skylights, and clerestories should provide interior lighting. They enhance visual, thermal, and psychological aspects of a space as well as providing the daily variation in light and the touch of nature so important to well-being.[11] Where daylight is not possible, lights approximating the spectra of daylight should be used.[5]

A high level of lighting enhances people's attention when routine tasks are concerned and no decision-making is involved. Low-level lighting, however, has a deeper effect on memory and sensitiveness, thus being more suitable to concentration and decision making.[10] A comfortable visual environment, therefore, can be provided with a balance of indirect lighting joined with direct task light to produce a non-uniform, more natural illumination.

COLOR

It has been demonstrated that color strongly influences our emotions and entire physiology. Red stimulates the sympathetic nervous system, increases brain-wave activity, and sends more blood to the muscles, accelerating heart rate, blood pressure and respiration. Blue triggers the parasympathetic nervous system, and is credited with a tranquilizing effect.[12-14] Lack of stimulation impairs the functioning of the brain's cortex. In a monotonous environment, attention is turned inward, and there is an increase in heart and breathing rates, causing strain and tension, and inhibiting human activity. A more colorful visual environment provides the needed interest and stimulation.[4, 12]

Color affects perception. Warm colors seem to advance and cool colors to recede. With cool colors, time is underestimated, weights seem lighter, objects seem smaller and rooms appear larger; the opposite is true with warm tones.[4, 12]   Thermal comfort is also affected, making us feel cooler in cool-toned rooms and warmer in warm-toned rooms, although the actual temperature may be the same.[11]

Choosing color depends upon the space and type of activity being performed in it. It should be noted that color appearance is affected by adjacent colors, reflectance of surrounding surfaces, and light sources.[4, 12] An environment, in general, should utilize a variety of colors and shades to provide a stimulating and productive space.

ACOUSTICS

An acoustically comfortable environment is now a necessity. We are living in a world of noise pollution that is positively toxic. The most common adverse effect of noise is loss of hearing, but noise can induce changes in blood capillary structure, impeding the flow of red blood cells and constricting the vascular channels. This can cause high blood pressure, heart disease, and ulcers.[15, 16]

High-level noise causes irritation and frustration, aggravates anger,[15, 16] and reduces pain threshold.[17] Not only does noise impair hearing acuity, it has even been proven to adversely affect visual perception.[15, 16] It literally becomes too noisy to think and function.

An acoustically quieter environment can be provided by irregularly recessed walls and ceilings, and by selecting surfaces and furnishings that do not reflect or amplify sound waves. Although surfaces and furnishings can have varying sound-absorbing qualities, an area with adequate amounts of carpeting, fabric, upholstered walls, wood, acoustic tiles, and sound panels can provide a quieter space.[18, 19]

AROMA

Scent may be called the silent persuader, influencing mind, body, and health. Smell impulses travel a faster, more direct route to the brain than visual or auditory ones, going directly to the limbic system. Smell and emotions are very closely inter-twined. Smell is also the most evocative of the senses. One whiff can recall complete memories.[20-22]

Certain odors, like rotting garbage, are inherently unpleasant and can produce nausea. Any smell that is too strong usually will be disagreeable. Unpleasant smells (e.g. ammonia) increase breathing and heart rates. Conversely, pleasant smells (e.g. spiced apple, light floral scents) are stress-reducing.[20-22]

Floral arrangements and bowls of sachet are pleasant ways of adding fragrance to a space. Fresh air in the environment can be enhanced by real plants, which have an added benefit — they can clean the indoor air. Ordinary houseplants have proven effective in removing toxic pollutants like formaldehyde, benzene, and trichlorethylene from the air inside homes and offices.[23]

TACTILE

The skin is the largest sense organ, yet touch is the most neglected sense. The air quality and thermal comfort of an environment are perceived through skin.[11, 24] The accuracy of movement and physical ease are dependent upon the sense of touch. Learning, alertness, and vitality are enhanced through tactile sensations.[24]

Physical comfort and reduced stress injuries are ensured by ergonomically designed furniture.[25] The tactility of the space may be enriched by interesting surface treatments, a variety of fabrics and finishes, and differing scale in furnishings. The interiors then are interesting and aesthetically pleasing, while providing an environment both comfortable and comforting.

SPACE

The space we create controls us, and the way we arrange our physical space affects people and performance.[26, 27] The proportion, the size, the scale of a room, all affect visual interest and the sense of security. A balance is needed between two mental states — stimulation/activity and rest/rejuvenation — to function at an optimal level. Proper space planning recognizes these needs and allows for the right mix of privacy and human contact to enhance individual and/or group interactions.[24, 26, 27]

We need memorable surroundings against which to think and to be creative. Interior design incorporating the principles of psychoneuro-immunology furnishes sensorially rich environments that provide beauty, interest, and variation in stimuli for all our senses, thereby enhancing our well-being, creativity and performance.

REFERENCES

1. Solomon GF: Psychoneuroimmunology: Inter-actions between central nervous system and immune system. Journal of Neuroscience Research, in press.

2. Gappell M: Psychoneuroimmunology: Humanizing the inhospitable hospital. California Hospitals, 45-46, May/June, 1990.

3. Gappell M: Hospice facilities: Design for spiritual healing. Journal of Health Care Interior Design, Vol II, 77-80.

4. Birren F: Light, Color & Environment. New York: Van Nostrand Reinhold, 1982.

5. Hollwich F: The influence of ocular light perception on metabolism in man and in animal. New York: Springer-Verlag, Berlin: Heidelberg, 1979.

6. Wurtman RJ: The effects of light on man and other mammals. Annual Review of Physiology 37:467-483, 1975.

7. Hughes PC: Natural light and the psychobiological system of man. CIE Pub 562, 1983.

8. Lewy AJ, et al: Light suppresses melatonin secretion in humans. Science 210:1267-69, 1980.

9. Maas JB, et al: Effects of spectral difference in illumination on fatigue. Journal of Applied Psychology 59:524-526, 1974.

10. Smith RC: Light and health, a broad overview. Lighting Design + Application, February 1986.

11. Jokl MV: The psychological effects on man of air movement and the colour of his surroundings. Applied Ergonomics, 119-125, June 1984.

12. Birren F: Color and Human Response. New York: Van Nostrand Reinhold, 1978.

13. Plack JJ, Schick J: The effects of color on human behavior. Journal of the Association for Study in Perception, 4-16, 1974.

14. Goldstein K: Some experimental observations on the influence of color on the function of the organism. Occupational Therapy and Rehabilitation, June 1942.

15. Halpern S, Savary L: Sound Health. San Francisco, CA: Harper & Row, 1985.

16. Katsh S, Merle-Fishman C: The Music Within You. New York: Simon & Shuster, 1985.

17. Minckley B: A study of noise and its relationship to patient discomfort in the recovery room. Nursing Research 17:247-250, 1968.

18. Rush R: Technics: Office acoustics. Progressive Architecture, 9(79):196-205.

19. Behm RD: Material selection important in acoustic control. Designers West, 190-194, October 1984.

20. Doty R: Olfactory communication in humans. Chemical Senses 6(4):351-374.

21. Van Toller S, Dodd G (eds): Perfumery, the Psychology and Biology of Fragrance. London and New York: Chapman and Hall, 1988.

22. Ogle J: Exploring scent therapy. New York Times, Nov 17, 1985.

23. Wolverton BC, Johnson A, Bounds, K: Interior landscape plants for indoor air pollution abatement. NASA Office of Commercial Programs-Final Report: Sept 15, 1989.

24. Montagu A: Touching: The human significance of the skin. New York: Columbia University Press, 1973.

25. American National Standard for Human Factors Engineering of Visual Display Terminal Workstations. Human Factors Society, 1988.

26. Alexander C, et al: A Pattern Language. London: Oxford University Press, 1977.

27. Maier HW: The space we create controls us. Residential Group Care & Treatment 1(1):51-59, 1982.

CHAPTER 9

Music, Metaphor and Creative Process in a Health-Care Setting

Cathy Callis

As a musician, program designer, and consultant, the author is privileged to contribute to pioneering work in the health-care field. The goal of this chapter is to share aspects of the philosophy, process models, consulting procedure and program designs used. It is hoped that this information, in turn, will serve as catalyst to the reader's own creative process, suggesting additional images, shapes, and possibilities for the health-care setting and artistry in medicine.

Much of the work described herein revolves around connection points and communication — how we engage and disengage, and how we can be more fully present for ourselves and others. The process is a matter of communication artistry and artful living — both having their places in quality health care. In the author's work, the use of music, metaphor and creative process applies directly to these ends.

Two health care organizations, Riverside Methodist Hospitals in Columbus, Ohio, and Mt. Carmel Hospitals' Center for Human Empowerment, also in Columbus, supply models for this report.

MODEL #1

Mt. Carmel Medical Center, Mt. Carmel East
The Center for Human Empowerment:
The Arts Partnership Program

The Mt. Carmel Medical Center, with its sister hospital, Mt. Carmel East, is a combined facility of just under one thousand beds. Mt. Carmel is part of a larger network of not-for-profit hospitals under the auspices of the Sisters of the Holy Cross.

In 1986, the Center for Human Empowerment was created. Its purpose was to create programs integrating psychological, sociological, spiritual, and aesthetic elements in ways to empower people and facilitate the healing process. In 1987, the author was invited to become the consulting artistic director, program designer and artist-in-residence for the working model and pilot component involving the arts — the *Arts Partnership Program*. This position entailed designing and implementing prototype and ongoing programs for the Arts Partnership; serving as a mentor for artists subsequently joining the program; introducing concepts of the program and building awareness among staff, nurses, physicians, and the artistic and general community.

Mt. Carmel invited local arts organizations, including the Columbus Symphony Orchestra, Players Theater, Ballet Metropolitan and the Columbus Museum of Art, among others, to play a role in the Arts Partnership Program. The long-range intent was to involve the artistic community in a program that would enable the medical community to learn from, explore, utilize, adapt and integrate certain skills, talents, awarenesses and insights which artists could bring to health care.

The target areas of the pilot were oncology, hospice, and Alzheimer's. Programs were to be designed for patients, staff and caregivers. After prototype programs for each of these areas were designed and implemented, visual artists and musicians joined the program as Arts Partners. Each of these artists brought their own perspective and special gifts to the experience.

The Center for Human Empowerment evolved partly out of a desire to counter the dehumanizing influence resulting from the assembly-line application of technology in health care. Emphasis on the technological at the expense of the whole person tends to dehumanize and objectify the patient, often leaving the patient a passive observer, and out of touch with the marvelous healing resources within. As one person described it, "*high tech* needed to be balanced with *soft touch.*"

MODEL #2

Riverside Methodist Hospitals

Riverside Methodist Hospitals is the flagship medical center for U.S. Health Corporation, with over one thousand beds. It provides extensive community outreach programs and services, including the Elizabeth Blackwell Center and an Emmy Award winning television series, *Life Choices*, hosted by Erie Chapman, C.E.O. of Riverside. Committed to building new models of health-care delivery and medical leadership, and, above all, humanizing the patient's experience in a health-care setting, Riverside has been cited as one of the ten most innovative and service-oriented health-care organizations in the United States.

Riverside invited the author to serve as consultant in creative process and artist-in-residence, having expressed interest in "pursuing creative ways to revolutionize the care provided to patients and families and ways to enhance the quality of work life for employees." This interest was very much in keeping with Riverside's Cardinal Value: *To honor the dignity and worth of each person.*

The very real living out of Riverside's Cardinal Value combined with the author's own philosophical view: Living life to its fullest is in itself a creative process of great love, courage, and artistic expression. These two elements, fleshed out by music, metaphor and creative awareness, became the primary colors out of which any number of possibilities, relevant to the broadly based Riverside community, could be derived.

CREATIVE PROCESS IN THE HEALTH-CARE SETTING

Within the hospital setting, creative process, at its best, is a life-affirming celebration of the human spirit. It enables the individual or team to fashion hope from despair, to design new life — often with deeper meaning — from tragedy, to create order out of chaos, to seek meaning and expression, to affirm a sense of integrity, value and purpose. Creative process is fully an integration of mind, body, and spirit.

The work for Riverside Methodist Hospitals reflects both the diversity of programs and the broad commitment Riverside has to serving its entire community. Their scope of vision allowed for the blossoming of programs and projects at all levels of the organization. Among them are:

For the entire Riverside community (patients, families, friends, physicians, staff, volunteers):

- *Sounds and Silence: A Program of Musical Reflection* — held in the chapel and as invited throughout the hospital, i.e. outpatient dialysis, emergency department.

- *Music in the Lobby*

For administration, physicians, staff and volunteers:

- *Shared Resonances* — A program designed to build community and bring together the people who serve and work at Riverside.

- Programs of creative renewal, communication, performance awareness (for housekeeping; outpatient drug and alcohol staff; NICU, nurses and staff on various units on all three shifts).

Courses, in-services, retreats, orientations, seminars:

- Ohio State University College of Medicine: *A Trip to the Right-Brain Lab: Creative Awareness through Music*[1] — A course offered to medical students from Ohio State at Riverside on communication, creativity, and renewal, with personal and professional application.

- Orientation for Family Practice Residents at Riverside — concepts from *Creative Awareness through Music* course.

- Nurse Managers of Riverside — an all-day retreat including concepts from two courses and workshops: *The Creative Use of Anxiety in Performance*[2] (exploring performance skills, and the dynamics of creative process, change and anxiety) and *Creative Awareness through Music*. Given off-site.

- *Caregiver as Customer* — for nurses and staff on various units, all three shifts. This was designed as a part of the Quality of Service Program of Riverside and was presented in the Quality of Worklife areas on each of the participating units.

PARTNERSHIP IN PROGRAM DESIGN

In work as a consultant, building a sense of partnership in program design is an active, ongoing process, often occurring over an extended time frame. It can be a deeply rewarding experience when based on a growing sense of trust and a shared purpose and vision. A program is well on its way when the unit or department takes on ownership of it, or invests in it through a commitment of resources (caring, support, time, presence, or funding).

Identifying what is central to the other (person, group, organization), and what attracts your services to the other party, is instrumental in successfully designing or doing a piece of work. An ideal situation occurs when something of value transpires as a result of the collaboration of all parties concerned.

PERFORMANCE CHECKLIST

The type of interaction required for any type of performance given in a health-care setting requires in-depth background preparation on many levels. The following guidelines may be helpful guidelines for preparation and performance:

● Preliminary Background: Research and familiarize yourself with the population, system, environment. Build a rich ground of awareness and basic understanding.

● Define and know your limits. Recognize the boundaries of your expertise, knowledge, energy and comfort level. Use this information to expand your skills, growth and resiliency, or to affirm the boundaries that you select or identify.

● Explore the possible avenues of growth and development before being in the actual performance situation. Create avenues of direction and sequences of choice to draw upon. This prepares the facilitator or performer to support the process of thematic development within the context of events unfolding.

● Build trust. Assess your resources and collaborative opportunities. Connect with a team when appropriate.

● Develop flexibility and the ability to learn from all prior performances — the successful and the less so. The ability to formulate new plans and strategies in a given situation is a plus.

● Prepare for the unexpected. A good model allows for accommodation of the unexpected. Allow for back-up in both programming (content, order) and equipment (for example, carrying an extension cord with you, or a boom box and tapes. This saved the day when a performance on an electric piano ended in a short-circuit blowout).

● Account for predictable variables within a hospital setting: time, traffic flow, acuity, space. How you incorporate and accommodate these vari-ables will determine the format and, in some cases, the content of your program. (How you account for them may also have a direct impact on your stress level.)

● Content: Less is more. Shorter units of work are more resistant to the variables of time, traffic, acuity and space. The choice of one or two themes or topics provides a more in-depth opportunity for learning, experiencing, and assimilating the meaning or implications of the material.

● Performance skills and awareness include: establishing a sense of presence (yours, theirs); pacing; timing; focusing; attending to connection — self/self, other, purpose or intent, task, material, environment; and body awareness — breathing, letting go of tension, internal speed.

CREATIVE AWARENESS THROUGH MUSIC

Music, as a time art, serves as an excellent metaphor for life and work process. Work with process in the health-care setting is enhanced and facilitated by the use of music and its metaphors. As an integration of artistic, creative and performance process, music and its metaphors may be applied to issues of quality health care, program design, well-being and healing.

In the hospital work and program design, music may be used as a focal point, a catalyst, as metaphor, or not at all. However, by applying John Cage's definition of music to the world, that "everything we do is music and everywhere is the best seat,"[3] events may be experienced and appreciated through the basic parameters of music — namely melody, rhythm, harmony, sound and growth, or form. In *Guidelines for Style Analysis*,[4] music theorist Jan La Rue claims that every musical event can be described through these parameters or their absence (i.e. sound/silence), and coins the acronym "SHMRG." Applying "SHMRG," or the parameters of music to any activity or event (Cage's definition of music), generates an enormous amount of immediate information about process, flow, and style. Through this framework, people quickly experience their own process.

As a result, there is tremendous application and relevance for both program design and creative awareness in performance (communication, stress management, renewal, the process of doing one's job, and the living of one's life) when events are perceived and related to music and its metaphors.

By applying the parameters of music to a relaxation sequence, for example, immediate benefits are apparent. The autonomic body response to anxiety and stress (tension, breathing patterns, speed of process, etc.) may be affected by attending to the framework of music parameters, calling attention to the body process. The parasympathetic nervous system may be directly affected by the application of these parameters. As the individual's awareness level increases, the person can learn to respond with qualitative change in process. For instance, if one is speeding — internally or externally   one could choose to slow down. If one is bombarded by sound, one could cultivate silence. If one is mesmerized by a particular rhythmic flow, one could change the pace when appropriate.

Elements of creative process and specific parameters of music can find their way to center stage of program design related to *quality of process* on the individual, group and organizational levels. For example, the series *Sounds and Silence: A Program of Musical Reflection* and *Music in the Lobby* both are replenishing by providing a change of rhythm, pace, and flow — a "time away."

Sounds and Silence focuses directly on one of the parameters of music, raising the awareness level both through the title and content of the series. Supporting both a time away and a moment of quiet as renewing and restoring, the program is designed for all three shifts. Excepts from a sample program read: "The holiday season is a time for celebration and, in its most intimate sense, a coming together of mind, heart and spirit ... The mini-break experience is designed as mosaic of (both) *sounds* and *silences*. We invite you to savor the blend of the music of Bach, music of the season, and your own inner resonances, as you experience the gift of music."

Music in the Lobby joins two ideas: (1) experiencing a change in the *rhythm* of flow can be replenishing, and facilitate *creative process*; and (2) building a sense of community contributes to a sense of *harmony* which in itself can be renewing and healing at all levels. Riverside's medical director noted that the program helped "... to ease the travail which they as loved ones of the ill were suffering ... Riverside's efforts to produce a welcoming and comfortable environment were clearly appreciated by these visitors."

CREATIVE PROCESS AND WELLNESS

Quality health care includes the tenets of wellness in its foundations. The traditional components of wellness are the social, psychological, environmental, intellectual, emotional, spiritual, and physical.

Omitted from this list is the one element that is both fuel and catalyst to the implementations of a wellness lifestyle — the *creative*.

This formula of well-being could be enhanced by including creativity in its components. Creative process is the element that integrates, synthesizes, relates, and gives meaning and shape to these components within the context of a person's life. The argument for including creativity as one of the basic parameters of wellness can be demonstrated through the impact of creative process in a health-care setting, and by observing certain life-style choices.

The wellness components, when used in complementary fashion, become life-affirming. Conversely, habitual reliance on, overuse or misuse of one component over another tends to create an imbalanced life style. Examples of such imbalance are all too common: the individual who over-intellectualizes and does not recognize this tendency, thus robbing herself of rich experience; the person who becomes addicted to physical exercise or narcissistically preoccupied with self; the caregiver who gives of himself to such a degree that there is precious little emotional or spiritual energy available for self-care and replenishment, too often becoming a ready candidate for burnout or illness.

In *The Courage to Create*, May writes, "Creativity is a necessary sequel to being."[5] Carrying this further, it is necessary even to our very survival. Our ability to be creative is directly related to our ability to live more purposefully. Our innate creativity allows us to ask the appropriate questions, to seek the appropriate choice rather than the habitual response. The more creatively alive we are, the greater our ability to recognize which components of the wellness model need to be called forth, to be strengthened, to be integrated into a life style that enhances a sense of well-being.

CONCLUSION

The word *whole* appears as a theme with increasing frequency in current and innovative models of health care. Riverside Methodist Hospitals speaks of treating the whole person (mind, body, spirit). A whole-brain approach, combining both the right- and left-hemisphere functions, finds its way into the preventive, diagnostic, treatment and healing aspects of medicine and health care. Norman Cousins speaks of the healing qualities of humor, using it as a metaphor for the whole range of emotions. Herbert

Benson,[6] in his work, evokes a response of mindfulness beneficial to the individual and his whole range of activity.

We speak of relating the parts to the whole, and speculate on systems theory. In this era of the specialist, we sometimes wonder whether we are being treated for the symptom and not the cause, and whether the specialist is indeed is indeed able to see the whole picture. In our prayers or meditations, we may recall scriptural accounts of healing the infirm, making the lame whole.

As we move toward contemporary renaissance, ancient perspective once again breathes life into new form. For the Greeks, Apollo was the god of medicine, music, and poetry. For contemporary humanity, the arts and sciences are necessary complements in the quest for preserving and celebrating life. We arrive at a place where technology allows for the marriage of the intuitive and the scientific through specific, measurable phenomena (i.e. data provided by research in psychoneuro-immunology[7] and biofeedback). Furthermore, the intrinsic spirit of the artist — the artist within the patient, the physician, and within the whole spectrum of caregivers — becomes a resource available to support the wide range of experience and perception needed for the total complement of diagnosis, treatment and healing to occur. Finally, in the arena of wellness, the artistic and creative spirit is invited to play an active role in the designing of a wellness life style, and in the living out of experiences contributing to our well-being and renewal.

REFERENCES

1. Callis C: Creative Awareness through Music. Copyright 1986, course copyright 1990.
2. Callis C: Creative Use of Anxiety in Performance. Began as a workshop service developed under the auspices of the Ohio Arts Council in 1986 for the performing arts. It later became a workshop and a course available for all disciplines. A research grant provided by Delta Kappa Gamma International Society for Women in Education in 1988 furthered the work of conceptualizing a system of performance skills based on a performing arts model, and then adapting this model to accommodate other professions, including health care.
3. Cage J. *In* Katch S, Merle-Fishman C. The Music Within You, 13. New York: Simon and Schuster, 1985.
4. LaRue J: Guidelines for Style Analysis. New York: WW Nordon, 1970.
5. May R: The Courage to Create, 8. New York: Bantam.
6. Benson H (with Proctor W): Your Maximum Mind. New York: Avon Books, 1987.
7. Ader R (ed): Psychoneuroimmunology. San Diego: Academic Press, 1991 (first edition, 1981).

ACKNOWLEDGEMENT

Gratitude and appreciation are extended to Tracy Wimberly, Senior Vice President, Riverside Methodist Hospitals, and to the many others whose dedication and vision have made this work possible.

CHAPTER 10

MedArt: A Personal Perspective

Vara Kamin

I write fables for adults. And, for the past few years, I have been using them as a focal point of discussion in seminars, workshops, and lectures. While the fables are now the primary source of my work, they emerged as part of my own process of healing and change.

In the spring, of 1982, I went for a physical examination. Working two jobs at the time, I had been up most of the night before the appointment, writing an article that was due the next day. I was fatigued and irritable, and suffered the effects of too much caffeine and nicotine. The physician, who was not much older than myself, had not even finished the exam before beginning a lecture about the need to change my habits. "Type A," he said, without even looking up from my chart. "You are a Type A personality, and it would do you some good to understand what that means." With my family history of heart disease, cancer, and diabetes, he warned me that I could be dead before age 35 if I didn't change my habits. "We are seeing a high percentage of young career women with heart attacks in their 30s," he warned. He suggested reading a book by Dr. Herb Benson entitled *The Relaxation Response*.

Needless to say, I was anxious to leave his office. A part of me thought the doctor knew nothing of the creative process or the demands of writing; however, there was another part that knew he was right. I was angry for days, yet realized that beneath the anger was fear; the anger simply kept the truth temporarily out of reach.

Since that prophetic visit to the doctor, my life has radically changed. Although it took several months to withdraw from a ten-cup-a-day coffee habit and a number of years to finally stop smoking, quieting down enough to recognize the self-destructive behavior was just the beginning of the process and the changes that have brought me to the point of writing the fables. As a former nurse, I was trained to take care of others, but I never learned how to care for myself. I didn't even know that there was a "myself" to care for.

In the early 1980s, the concept of stress management was emerging. Of the various available resources, my physician suggested biofeedback. As the weeks progressed, the daily headaches from which I suffered lessened. I not only gained more control of my reactive response to life's daily stresses, but my imagination opened up as well.

During this time, a friend suggested that I might enhance what I was doing by joining her for a class in creative visualization. It was this class, and numerous workshops and seminars since then, that introduced me to my vast inner world and helped to create the life I now live. Stimulated by creative visualization, the process of active imagination laid the groundwork for the fables long before I became aware of their existence in my mind.

It was 1985 when I took that very first class, and three years later, after enduring several disappointments in my writing career, my husband said, "Just write from your heart." For years I had focused on outcome, and for once I was actually giving myself permission to fully embrace the creative process. I had notebooks and computer discs filled with mental musings from my ongoing work with creative visualization. It is from these personal files that I drew my inspiration for the fables, but it was in the bathtub that I was truly inspired.

One morning, just before getting into the tub, I looked in the mirror and asked myself not to worry for one week about all the 'what-ifs' and 'maybes' in my life. A simple task for some, but for me it seemed nearly impossible. Yet, as I sank neck deep in the warm water, my mind freed itself from the concerns at hand and gave to me a great gift.

In my mind's ear I heard a siren, and the next thing I knew, an image came to mind of a police car pulling me over. It was the 'spiritual police,' and I was given a citation for worrying. If caught again that same day, I was threatened not with imprisonment, but with a month of no work, filled with only laughter and fun. From that fateful warm in soak in the tub emerged the fable *The Old Man By The Mill*.

As I continued to explore my own feelings and my responses to the changing and chaotic world in which we live, the fables became the vehicle for expression. Along the often arduous road toward self-discovery, I was forced to reconcile my values. And while I dealt with the endless dichotomies which surround us all, the fables became my anchor. Yet, it wasn't until I read a few of the fables aloud for the first time in March 1989 that I began to see that the fables had a life of their own, far beyond my own inner world. It was this reading, and the many programs and workshops since then, that have provided me with the opportunity to be part of a world of people concerned with the awakening of the human spirit and global healing.

As I continue to reach out to various audiences — from incarcerated women to corporate managers to school-age children — I am shown not how different we are, but how connected we are as individuals and as a human race. Whether an individual is locked behind steel bars or locked behind a wall of stilled emotions, there is something magical about a story that transcends our differences and unites us in thought.

There is no one right way to interpret the fables, and the meaning or understanding of the fable may change each time it is read. For one woman in prison, the farmer in the fable *The Farmer And The Plow Horse* reminded her of her pimp and the life she once led as a prostitute. Through the fable, she saw the possibility for change; and, more importantly, she gained an awareness about the concept of self-forgiveness. That very same fable, when read to a group of therapists and counselors, brought a psychiatrist to the point of tears, for he saw how he pushes and drives himself while ignoring the more gentle side of his nature. Once again, this fable, when read to an eight-year-old by his mother, provided an opportunity for a discussion on the values of kindness and compassion toward others.

The fables have provided me with countless opportunities to push past what I once thought were my limitations. There was a time when I questioned what I was doing and, more than once, giving up seemed like the most viable option. But there was a voice within, coached by a power far greater than myself, that encouraged me to continue. It is that voice that speaks to you through the fables.

The collection of fables will be published by the Putnam Berkley Publishing Group in the fall of 1992. For further information regarding programs and workshops, please contact Kamin's Fables, (612) 229-3635.

PART II

ART THERAPY

CHAPTER 11

The Image as Cultural Messenger:
Iconography of the AIDS Crisis

Michael A. Franklin

As we rapidly approach the end of this century as well as the millennium, few things challenge us as a global community as does the AIDS crisis. We are in the throes of an epidemic that has entered our lives in such a ruthless way that it threatens to redefine the timeless human questions associated with ethics, health care, racism, and the rights of the dying. This struggle is further complicated by the unique qualities of our current post-modern world. Due to unending impressive technological developments, we are in the unique position to produce information faster than we can process it. Much of our daily lives is composed of electronic simulations which become our reality. Sorting fact from fiction, simulation from reality, is one of the major challenges facing contemporary society. Images, the inevitable offspring of these now entrenched technologies, have moved us from a culture of printed information to image information. Rather than being influenced by this ageless power of the image,[1] it is in our best interest to study its past and present so that we are not controlled by its future developments.

Perhaps nowhere else in contemporary society is the power of the image more pronounced than it is with the AIDS crisis. The research summarized here began three years ago as the author stood in the checkout line at a neighborhood grocery store. On display was the usual selection of sensational tabloids. One headline in particular was eye-catching: "'Psycho' Star Anthony Perkins Has AIDS." Inside the magazine, a photograph of Mr. Perkins was carefully composed by placing him in the foreground with the Bates Motel in the background. Seeing the topic of AIDS subtly linked with the character of Norman Bates, the ax-murdering psychopath from the *Psycho* film series, was outrageous. Here was a visual manipulation of the worst kind, linking AIDS and people with AIDS (PWAs) to the personification of evil murderers. Why could not the headline have read, "Movie Star Anthony Perkins Has AIDS"? Since AIDS

imagery is created by our culture, it reflects the culture that made it — a simple equation.

This chapter briefly outlines the mechanisms that are operating when looking at visual communication. It then applies that understanding to the subject of AIDS and how it is packaged and presented to the culture at large. After considering the representation of AIDS in mass culture generally, the discussion will turn to three specific settings in which AIDS imagery has been produced: the Quilt Project, art work created in the art-therapy setting, and art work created by professional artists. Although space constraints prevent an in-depth discussion of any of these individual topics, collectively they provide a useful framework for thinking about the iconography of the AIDS crisis.

ICONOGRAPHY AND IMAGERY

Panofsky[2] discussed the term *iconography* in his seminal work, *Meaning in the Visual Arts*. He described iconography as the branch of art history that concerns itself with the meaning contained in works of art. Rather than focusing on issues of form only, he was concerned with subject matter. Although verbal language is our primary form of communication, visual images can convey and communicate just as impressively. Suzanne Langer[3] spent her life writing about the ability of the arts to communicate, particularly the world of emotion. She discussed the differences between discursive and presentational symbols, the latter falling within the camp of the visual arts. Her hypothesis focused on the ability of pictures to contain a variety of images simultaneously, ultimately presenting and articulating a specific theme. These presentational symbol systems are in large part the reason AIDS imagery is so powerful. Composers of these images can pull together a range of ideas, benign or cruel, within the framework of a single space. One picture, therefore, can contain multiple simultaneous complex themes, composed to educate, to shock, or even to destroy. Pictures can also contain oppositional forces simultaneously, due to the nature of the art materials and actual physical structuring of the art work. For example, the darker and lighter sides of life are easily fused into one picture in terms of form and content. Blacks and deep, dark colors can coexist alongside light, warm colors or values. Combining these features and incorporating them into symbolic imagery faithful to the original drama pushing for expression allows for opposites to coexist, to fragment or, possibly, to integrate.

The power of images and their impact on society is well-documented. Joplin[4] and others outline the role of imagery in primitive cultures. Politics and art have had a rich history as well, focusing on the relationship between art, artist, and society.[5] During World War II, for example, artists in occupied Germany who demanded free expression were met with cruel responses. Prior to WW II, Picasso painted *Guernica*, which was motivated not so much by political ideology as by the shock at the human tragedy of being annihilated by an "invisible enemy."[5] This theme is not too far removed from the subject of AIDS, which is often seen as an invisible enemy capable of silently killing millions. In fact, the theme of military metaphors associated with terminal diseases perceived as rotting the body has been discussed by Sontag.[6]

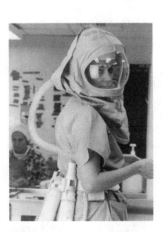

Figure 1: *Suited up for surgery in space-age protective gear.*

Figures 1 and 2 demonstrate how HIV disease can get cast into a theme of war from a variety of perspectives. Surgeons needing to protect themselves from airborne infectious organisms are suiting up in protective gear, looking much like astronauts.[7] The result of such trends casts the person with AIDS into the role of alien. Several weeks after the photo in Figure 1 appeared in print, the one in Figure 2 was published by the Department of Defense. Here, we see the icons of alien and war merging, ultimately furthering the theme of outcast. Numerous subtle connections such as these daily see themselves into our unconscious. Oppressive attitudes often result from these cultural dynamics. Authors such as Debora Silverman[8] have

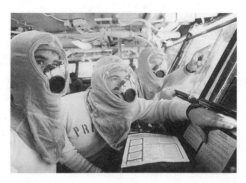

Figure 2

studied various mechanisms at work when visual art is utilized for motives of power. In addition to the brokerage of power, graphic designers, in their attempt to influence and/or educate the public through images, have had immense influence on social attitudes.[9]

AIDS ICONOGRAPHY

The history of the social construction of AIDS and how it has been presented to society at large tells an astonishing story. Gilman[10] points out how the history of sexually transmitted diseases (STDs) such as syphilis, with its 500-year history, and AIDS, with its recent history, closely parallel each other. In addition to these historical trends, recent iconographic examples describe a society being inundated with conflicting messages. All too often, the subject of AIDS is split into various camps of *us* (the healthy, heterosexual, non-drug-consuming public) and *them* (the diseased, homosexual, IV-drug-consuming public). These themes are fragmented even further by separating those infected with HIV into two other negatively labeled groups — *guilty* and *innocent* victims.[11] Innocent victims are distilled into Ryan White-type pictures — children, hemophiliacs, and transfusion recipients. Guilty victims are seen as gay, junkies and, usually, male (although women and AIDS has always been a tragic topic).

The pictures that stem from these unfortunate fragmentations often end up as sad manipulations of the consuming public. The photo in Figure 3, for example, was taken at Ryan White's funeral. Unfortunately, many of those attending the funeral of this exceptional young person were high-profile, well-known public figures. It appears as if it was politically correct for celebrities such as Michael Jackson and Barbara Bush to be present at this media event.[12] One would not expect such an outpouring of public support

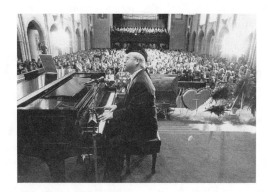

Figure 3: Elton John at Ryan White's funeral.

for those who come from groups operating on the fringes of society. Rather than concern ourselves only with issues of guilt and innocence, or the search to discover the origins of the disease, attention needs to be focused on *all* who are infected, available and accessible treatment strategies, and ways to increase the quality of life for those who test HIV positive (Fig. 4).[13] Artist David Wojnarowicz wrote in the controversial show *Witnesses: Against Our Vanishing* that, "When I was told that I had contracted this virus it did not take me long to realize that I had contracted a diseased society as well" (Fig.5).[14]

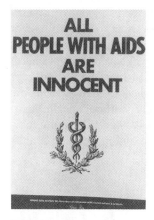
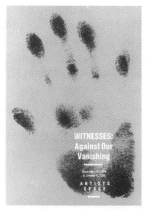

Figure 4   **Figure 5**

After reading statements like this, it occurred to the author that when writing a paper such as this, one walks a fine line between being a sensationalist and an advocate. This topic has often been negatively magnified due to distorted information which is often cruel and calculated. Navigating through this potent subject is never easy, but always necessary. It is hoped that the ideas expressed herein will help to raise awareness and foster a sense of advocacy.

Magazines such as *Time, Newsweek* and *People* have generated abundant imagery (Fig. 6). A handful of pictures has been selected that convey a wide range of themes, each containing multiple messages. Selections have been gathered from printed media, politically active groups such as ACT UP, the popular culture, and the artist community.

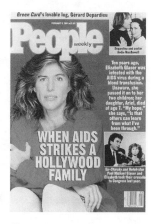

Figure 6

Perhaps the best place to begin this discussion is with the Quilt Project.[15] The range of cultural sublimation infused into this effort is truly admirable. The gamut of human emotions are carefully pieced together containing themes of rage, loss, and grief. The quilt, as all art does, acts as a container for these emotions. This is, in part, the function of the arts. They provide a sense of refuge — a place where we have traditionally gone from the beginning of time when trying to reconcile our human conflicts.[16] Unlike most monuments, however, the quilt has been created by an invested community. It serves as a covering, a blanket of lives connected by death through the metaphor of the quilt. The result is a living visual, tactile organism that evolved through the life-giving force of personal creativity. Giving people power in a powerless situation helps them sense their connectedness to each other. The quilt also helps combat the notion of objectification — the defense mechanism often at work in the cruelest of abuse cases. To see a person as object rather than as human, which is part of the act of casting people into image form, allows for rationalizations of destructive behavior towards them. This is easily seen during times of war. By giving the enemy an objectified name or label, the stigma of killing is made easier. In essence, human beings, not objects or statistics, have empowered themselves to create the quilt as well as other works of art (Fig. 7) This same idea can be witnessed in treatment settings for PWAs.

Art therapists have been studying the treatment as well as diagnostic contributions stimulated by the art work created in medical facilities.[17, 18] These efforts outline the capacity of art work to address the various psychosocial needs of the person. Rosner-

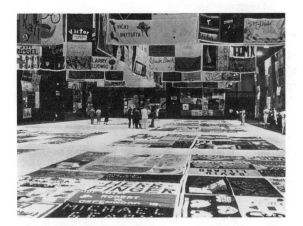

Figure 7: The Quilt Project.   UPI/Bettman Newsphotos

David's[17] research also contains examples of well-defined diagnostic information surfacing as certain opportunistic infections take their toll (Fig. 8).

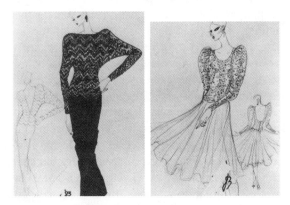

Figure 8: Left: This picture shows how a man who was a successful fashion designer was able to render the human figure competently. As time passed, organic brain impairment resulted, ultimately showing in the art. The picture on the right shows a reversal of the hand, the right hand being placed on the left.

Diagnostic cues such as this are common, since art is very much a combination of cognitive and affective processes. Information of this sort can alert the treatment team to previously undetected advancements of illness, ultimately redefining treatment strategies.

The wealth of material being generated by PWAs in art-therapy settings is staggering. People appear somewhat comforted by their ability to create enduring objects that eloquently reflect their current situation. Spiritual as well as existential concerns can be explored silently and spatially, allowing for a degree of safety and distance from that which hurts, be it social or physical. The refuge offered by art work allows for participation in a process where images are created, their themes accelerated or decreased in time, ultimately allowing for an opportunity to state and restate personal experiences and eventually digest them.

In addition to the art-therapy setting, artists are generating images capable of profound impact. The art world, as would be expected, has turned into a forum with a wide range of artistic responses. Politically motivated and, in some cases, morally corrupt efforts can be observed in the current trends to raise funds through art auctions (Fig. 9).[19] As

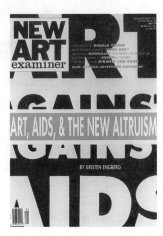

Figure 9

the voice of the times, artists are reflecting to society the sense of urgency felt in communities around the world.[20] The work is often justifiably angry due to the apathy of policy makers. ACT UP and Gran Fury have launched a visual campaign to further their cause of social responsibility.[13, 21] Seeing so many die, members of these organizations appear to feel a sense of desperation as they try to raise awareness, save lives, and challenge current policies. Their images are hard, direct, and calculated (Figs. 10-13).[13] As artist Greer Lankton put it, "Having watched so many friends die from AIDS has been like surgery without anesthesia."[14] This is, in essence, what the AIDS artist community is fighting about — untold losses and inadequate health-care policies.

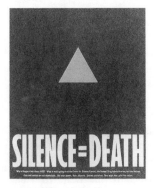

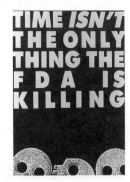

Figure 10   *Figure 11*

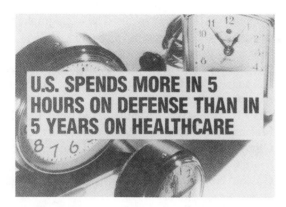

Figure 12

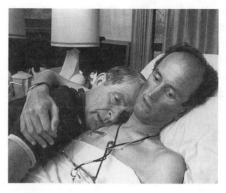

Figure 14: *Robert and Bob Sappenfield, Dorchester, Massachusetts, August 1988.*

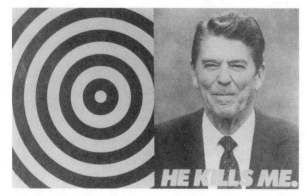

Figure 13

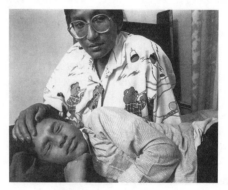

Figure 15: *Elizabeth and Chris Ramos, Cambridge, Massachusetts, August 1988.*

Art shows have been curated with the hope of opening a dialogue that will ultimately influence change.[11] The range of work silences, even numbs. This is due partly to the uncertain direction of current trends in contemporary art. AIDS has surfaced at a time when artists are trying to assimilate elusive modern trends which have been complicated even further by the reality of the disease. This accounts, in part, for the diversity of work. Photography, for example, with its innate ability to make subjects out of all things, has stimulated a wide range of work.[11, 13] As an art form, it slices into life with undeniable accuracy. Not only does it concretize the vision of the artist, it also confronts the audience with a crisp window-like world in which we all live, but which we rarely slow down enough to see. Nick Nixon[22, 23] has carefully photographed PWAs for several years now. His work has been met with appreciation as well as criticism,[13] demonstrating the power of the camera, challenge to the artist, and sensitivity of the subject (Figs. 14-16). Other visual artists continue to produce work based on AIDS; unfortunately, this topic continues to provide tragic subject matter.

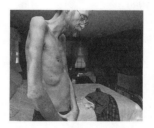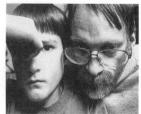

Figure 16: *Donald Perham (left), Milford, New Hampshire, November 1987; Nathaniel and Donald Perham, January 1988.*

CONCLUSION

The image culture that surrounds our daily lives permeates all aspects of contemporary society. The influence of this cultural phenomenon is particularly apparent in the AIDS crisis. Unfortunately, icons of diseases, particularly STDs, often exist independently of the reality of those diseases. Other images, such as those generated by the AIDS community, convey a range of human emotions from rage to emptiness — each camp seems to be reacting to the other. Awareness of these images and their social and cultural impact concerns us all. Although the quantities of images we internalize on a daily basis are vast, perhaps numbing, we must strive to understand their mechanisms of operation. Otherwise, if we ignore these trends, we support a spirit of indifference that avoids the most profound problems of our times — and, ultimately, contributes to them.

REFERENCES

1. Hillman A. A Blue Fire. New York: Harper & Row, 1989.
2. Panofsky E: Meaning in the Visual Arts. Garden City, NY: Doubleday Anchor Books, 1955.
3. Langer S: Philosophy in a New Key. Cambridge, MA: Harvard University Press, 1978.
4. Joplin CF: Art and Aesthetics in Primitive Societies. New York: EP Dutton, 1971.
5. Chipp HB: Theories of Modern Art. Berkeley, CA: University of California Press, 1968.
6. Sontag S: Illness as Metaphor and AIDS and Its Metaphors. New York: Doubleday Anchor Books, 1989.
7. Barnett N: When the Doctor Gets Infected (photograph). Time Magazine 57, Jan 14, 1991.
8. Silverman D: Selling Culture. New York: Pantheon Books, 1986.
9. Helmken CM: Images for Survival. Washington, DC: Shoshin Society, 1989.
10. Gilman S: AIDS and syphilis: The iconography of disease. October Magazine 43:87-108, 1987.
11. Grover J: Introduction to AIDS: The artists' response. *In* Grover JZ, AIDS: The Artist Response, 2-7. Ohio State University: Hoyt L Sherman Gallery, 1989.
12. Shaw B, Yamasaki T: Candle in the wind. People Magazine, 86-97, April 1990.
13. Crimp D, Rolston A: AIDS Demographics. Seattle, WA: Bay Press, 1990.
14. Golden N: Witnesses: Against Our Vanishing. Artists Space Gallery, 1990.
15. Ruskin C: The quilt: Stories from the names project. New York: Pocket Books, 1988.
16. Kramer E: Art as Therapy with Children. New York: Schocken Books, 1977.
17. Rosner-David IR: Psychological aspects of AIDS as seen in art therapy. American Journal of Art Therapy 26(1):3-10, 1987.
18. Fenster GM: Art therapy with HIV positive patients: Mourning, restitution, and meaning. Paper presented at the 20th Annual Conference of the American Art Therapy Association, Chicago, IL, Nov 18, 1990.
19. Engberg K: Marketing the (ad)just(ed) cause. New Art Examiner, May 22-28, 1991.
20. Rosenblum R: Gilbert and George: The AIDS pictures. Art in America 77(11):152-154, 1989.
21. Leigh C: Act up. Art Forum 26:137-138, 1988.
22. Nixon N: Pictures of People. New York: Museum of Modern Art, 1988.
23. Nixon N: People with AIDS. David R. Godine, 1991.

CHAPTER 12

Illustrating the Internal World:
Art Psychotherapy with the Borderline Patient

Diane Silverman

INTRODUCTION

During the past two decades, psychotherapists, especially those who subscribe to the psychodynamic model, have focused considerable attention on the understanding and treatment of patients demonstrating borderline personality organization. Presenting a complex set of dynamics and symptoms neither psychotic nor neurotic, these patients have challenged mental-health clinicians in developing a theoretical basis and effective treatment approach to borderline disorders.

Based on current object-relations psychoanalytic thought, an in-depth understanding of adult borderline syndrome is presented. An overview is offered of the concept of primitive mental states and of the development of two distinct yet parallel personalities in the borderline patient: a neurotic personality and a primitive/psychotic personality that have undergone an interpenetration.

Art psychotherapy provides entry into the internal world of these patients in a way perhaps not possible by other means. Since this process makes available concrete manifestations of the patient's mental processes, particularly material from the unconscious mind, it lends itself to successful treatment. It is generally accepted that the visual image is more powerful than speech because it is less abstract and amorphous. Visualization is the primary mode of conceptualization: infants experience the world through imagery and sensation long before the development of language. Primitive and preverbal psychological constructs become more readily available through the art process. Because of its unique capacity to render or evoke symbols and images related to infantile experience, art psychotherapy is of special value in the understanding and treatment of psychopathology connected with primitive mental states. This modality can be particularly effective in supporting the reparative process of those who have experienced early developmental impairment in their object relations.

The art-psychotherapy process can serve as a *holding environment*[1,2] for those individuals who often experience themselves on the dangerous edge of fragmentation. Through the art modality, the regressed borderline patient can symbolically attempt to control the terrifying experience of dissolution or overwhelming affect. Order can be made of the internal chaos in a concrete, tangible way. The active involvement of the therapist at times can help to further enhance the holding quality of the interaction and the meaningfulness of the therapeutic work within the transference. This parallels the concept of *the container and the contained*.[3] The art-therapy process can allow the diminishment of primitive defense mechanisms and encourage the development of healthy ego functioning.

BORDERLINE SYNDROME

The borderline character presents a deceptive clinical appearance of inconsistent symptoms and a wide variability in adaptive areas. The art work produced by patients in treatment often illustrates, in content as well as in form and structure, the characteristics and dynamics of this personality. The adult patient often describes, or portrays graphically, experiences of emptiness, aloneness, rage, hopelessness, and feelings of unrealness or death. They cannot tolerate being alone;[4] relationships are characterized by dependency, clinging, manipulativeness, and victimization. Their relationships are generally tenuous and shallow, exhibiting little or no capacity for empathic bonding with others. They suffer from a need/fear dilemma: they long for closer relationships yet fear attachment, since separation of any kind is experienced as an abandonment which leaves them vulnerable to experiences of dissolution of the self and psychic fragmentation, i.e. transient psychotic episodes. It is theorized that borderline personalities suffer from a profound dread of annihilation as the result of separation.[5] Frequently, these patients have difficulty in regulating both their affect and their behavior; thus, they exhibit impulsivity in the form of substance abuse, sexual promiscuity or deviation, and multiple, manipulative suicide attempts.

Grotstein's[6-9] concept of primitive mental states and dual personality development is a useful tool for the understanding of borderline pathology. He describes the borderline personality as comprising a primitive personality that often appears psychotic, and a neurotic or normal one as well. These components have undergone an interpenetration as if a symbiosis exists between these *twin* personalities. Art therapy gives access to this dynamic: the art work of many borderline patients often appears to be typical of the psychotic in both content and structure, despite the individual's relatively normal, non-psychotic appearance.

Psychopathology of all disorders can be viewed from the vantage point of the success or failure to achieve bonding between the infant and its mother.[7] It is also viewed as a failure of the adequate negotiation through early separation/individuation phases of development.[10, 11] As a consequence of this failure in mother/infant reciprocity, the infant withdraws, resulting in a precocious closure of a part of the personality from interaction with the normal personality.[7] This is evident when we often see psychotic process in a patient's art work.

The infant who does not succeed in developing a sense of confidence in a maternal container for his psychic content cannot develop a sense of confidence in his own capacity to contain feelings or generate thoughts about these feelings. Consequently, the primary fear of the borderline personality is the experience of danger evoked by a disruption of psychic organization, or mental fragmentation. This can be evoked whenever there is a real or even threatened separation. This loss of a cohesive sense of self becomes apparent in the breakdown of drawing structures, or the need for strong boundary lines as a symbolic attempt to achieve a feeling of containment.   A threatened separation refers ultimately to a rupture in the primary state of *at-one-ment* which evokes a premature psychological birth or sense of *two-ness*.[7-9, 12] In order to cope with this, the child develops two types of pathological reactions: encapsulation, which shuts out the *not-self*

outside world, and confusional reactions, which blur, but do not shut out, the *not-self* outside world.[12] These characteristics are clearly displayed in art work of borderline patients.

The appearance of *black holes* is very common in the art work of these individuals, often portraying the experience of total emptiness — a dissolution of the self into a state of nothingness,[9] the annihilation of the self,[5] the *nameless dread*.[13] Sometimes the black hole appears in the body of a drawn figure. A hole, or *wound*, is experienced by the autistic or psychotic child as a result of a premature rupture of primary oneness with the mother.[12] Separation can produce the feeling that the body or self has open, unprotected holes.

Defective skin boundary formation during the stage of *adhesive identification*[14, 15] inaugurates the later phenomenon of poverty of ego boundaries which characterizes psychotic and regressed borderline personalities. The skin boundary is often perceived as perforated; it no longer functions as a container. It is felt that intruders can enter, or results in the flooding out of internal contents. Several patients have attempted to communicate their sense of permeability by using scissors to cut many little holes into the drawing paper: "... I can't keep anything inside ... I feel void and empty all of the time." The line quality, especially on human figure drawings, is often sketchy, irregular, or not solidly drawn.

Anzieu further elaborates the importance of this phenomenon in a theory of the *skin ego*.[16] Just as the skin is the envelope to the body, he sees the skin ego as a psychic envelope — containing, defining, and protecting the psyche. In this light, their weakened, irregular skin boundaries are responsible for borderline patients' commonly expressed feelings of transparency and corresponding shame and embarrassment. To protect themselves from this impingement and fear of penetration by others, their drawings often portray heavy or excessive outlining, representing symbolic boundaries to defend against the absence of a sense of self-protection. The appearance of eyes, or emphasized eyes, which is common in paranoid ideation, is often present in these drawings. These all-seeing eyes are cruel, penetrating, and inescapable, able to perceive degradation and humiliation. Often, this poverty of ego/skin boundary is revealed by the x-ray phenomenon where the attempt to draw the human form results in a transparency, revealing the contents of the body.

Self-mutilation, which is common among hospitalized borderline patients, can emanate from a desire to reaffirm the presence of a skin boundary. They frequently rake their skin with sharp objects. It is often an attempt to validate their existence and define body boundaries, especially when they are about to fall into a state of deadness, or experience a loosening of cohesion of the self: "...I bleed, therefore I am." This self-mutilation is also seen as a procedure to relieve tension and to cut out the bad parts of the self, as well as an attempt to substitute physical pain for emotional pain, the latter being more frightening and excruciating. At times, patients are able to substitute making a damaging picture for doing damage to their own body. Encouragement of this act of symbolically putting self-destructive impulses onto the paper in therapy sessions allows the patient to discharge those impulses and to convey the enormity of psychic pain. It brings a sense of relief and diminishes the need to enter into a dissociative state of deadness. Psychic pain that is shared is more bearable than pain suffered in silence. Repeated art work containing images of self-mutilation often facilitates the cessation of this acting-out behavior.

IMPLICATIONS FOR TREATMENT

Bion states that raw emotional experience cannot be thought about, but must find a representation.[17] The individual, therefore, needs an apparatus to *think* about emotional processes. Graphic images or plastic forms are representational communication in pictorial form. At the same time, this can become a process by which undifferentiated, disorganized thoughts can be symbolically contained and controlled. Drawings of fragmented and disorganized images can be reduced to segments or compartments as a way to clarify and manage thinking.

Through the art, a patient can symbolically control the dangerous experiences of fragmentation. A strong outline that compensates for weakened boundaries is a common feature of the art work of borderline patients. Such encapsulation in the graphic image functions as a protective maneuver by avoiding impingement from the outside, or total loss of fragmented parts of the self. Both the therapist and the paper or canvas itself help to contain feelings of rage, terror, confusion. The paper serves as a defined space with a boundary. The structure provided in the art process gives a sense of containment and safety. The art materials serve as tools for the expression of these powerful emotions and allow

for the exploration and understanding of them in a safe place where the patient can gain the objective distance that encourages insight. It is often easier to initially talk about the symbolic image on paper than about one's own actual emotions. Anger, for example, is one affect that is easily, and often impulsively, experienced by the borderline patient. Expression of anger on paper serves as more than just an evacuation of primitive rage. The process allows some distance and objectification which, with help from the therapist through appropriate interpretation, allows the patient to derive understanding and meaning. This can be followed by exploration in subsequent drawings of more appropriate means to express these feelings in a constructive, rather than impulsive and destructive, manner. The more complex emotions evoking the angry response, e.g. fear, hurt, disappointment, or guilt, can become available for meaningful use in treatment.

Through the use of a variety of materials and techniques and the graphic expression of emotions and mind states beyond the reach of intellectual verbalization, the therapist has greater access to the patient's internal intrasubjective world in a tangible way. This increases the opportunity for empathic attunement, which is so vitally important in the corrective experience of the treatment process.[18, 19] These patients are very sensitive to rejection, which is often perceived by them as omnipresent in their world. Even the slightest criticism, or even the other individual's preoccupation, can be experienced as a rejection, tantamount to abandonment. Sometimes even the absence of empathy can be experienced as a rejection. Therefore, the pictorial image of an internal state which is shared with another increases the opportunity for empathic attunement and decreases the sense of aloneness.

There are occasions when the therapist will draw on the same paper as the patient, either simultaneously or alternately. The therapist can thus become the *good enough mother* in this *safe holding environment*, which also serves as a *potential space*.[2,20] This direct involvement in the art process can enhance the *holding* quality of the interaction, thereby furthering the development of a sense of self. In discussing his theory of play, Winnicott describes a *potential space* that exists between mother and baby. The ability to form and use symbols brings meaning to the world of a shared reality. Through the art process, the patient develops his own personalized set of symbols, which serve as a nonverbal language.

Within this space, a *play* experience occurs that leads significantly to the formation of the individual's identify, i.e. in the discovery of the self.

This conjoint work parallels the process termed *alpha function*.[17] It is the mother's ability to apply words and meaning to the infant's behavior and internal experiences. The mother/therapist receives and withstands the intolerable, confusing sensations and affects of her child/patient and returns effective, meaningful communication.

A blank sheet of paper, analogous to time and space in life, can be very frightening to an individual already filled with intense fear and aloneness. Initially, it can represent the endless void dreaded by the patient who is on the edge of, or in the midst of, a psychotic episode. A simple mark, a line or squiggle made by the therapist, provides a point of contact. It introduces structure, with which the patient can connect visually. The patient may respond through graphic communication, either by completing the picture alone or by drawing alternately with the therapist. This makes the patient's feelings and internal mental states available for meaningful, shared therapeutic work. Because it is conducive to the differentiation of self and not-self, doing art conjointly can discourage fantasies of merger and help the patient feel less alone and better contained.

Through clinical observation, it has been established that borderline patients have a poorly developed capacity for evocative memory, especially of the holding, soothing experiences. A striking loss of memory for childhood events has been described as typical of the borderline patient.[21] This amnesia may serve as an unconscious defense against all types of negative emotions — guilt, fear, shame, rage, and grief. Art therapy in general, and dyadic art in particular, have led to the revival of significant memories, both positive and negative. This was dramatically illustrated by a 33-year-old female patient who had been raped three times during adolescence and young adulthood. She had totally blocked all memory of the assaults until she produced a series of drawings made in response to the therapist's original mark on paper. The recollection of these traumatic events provided important information for the patient's overall treatment. It also gave her a safe *holding* environment where she found herself able to express the terror and humiliation that had been repressed in the past.

A primary defense of the borderline personality is splitting. An important goal in treatment, and a significant step in patients' emotional growth, is to help them develop the capacity to integrate the positive and negative aspects of significant persons in their lives. The art process can be used to encourage a synthesis through the concrete portrayal of this dynamic and through changes made directly on the drawing itself.

A circle drawn by the art therapist can provide a patient with the special feelings of being held and enveloped. It can become a focused area where scattered, fragmented thoughts and frightening sensation-images can be placed. The therapist establishes a boundary that is round and has no sharp edges, points or corners. The technique of encouraging a patient to draw within a circle is effective when a patient is feeling frightened and on the edge of fragmentation, i.e during an episode of psychotic confusion, fearing being out of control. When the drawing or design within the circle is completed, patients usually appear calmer and report feeling more centered, relaxed, and safe. A series of circle drawings over a period of time can illustrate how a reorganization of disordered thought processes can evolve. A progression in the degree of structure, as well as use of abstract images symbolizing the core issues focused upon in treatment, become apparent.

CONCLUSION

Borderline patients live in a chaotic, confusing world filled with unsatisfying and ineffective interpersonal relationships, plus the consequences of impulsive and acting-out behavior. Many of these patients have difficulty describing their internal experiences effectively, which only intensifies the feelings of hopeless despair and isolation. At times, all they are able to do in art therapy is undifferentiated scribbles, reflecting disorganization, formless chaos and the diffuseness of their psychic state. The art-psychotherapy process can facilitate the articulation and understanding of affective states that the patient has neither the verbal language to describe nor the mental apparatus to process. This can be a wordless state of mindlessness that is essentially dominated by sensations. Eigen refers to mindlessness as a sort of oblivion, a numbing paralysis when intense pain passes a certain boundary.[22]

Through the graphic portrayal of these internal states, the patient is able to externalize his emotional turbulence and develop a form of symbolic communication. In other words, a *visual language* is created that ultimately helps, with the aid of the therapist's interpretations, to develop the verbalization of one's inner experience. The art work enhances the clarity and organization of the treatment issues. In a regressed state, these patients need containment first. They must be given an opportunity to create order out of the formless chaos. *When there is form and structure, meaning follows.* The concrete representation of the internal world makes it easier to *think* about these feelings, rather than be lost in a frightening mindless maelstrom.

REFERENCES

1. Winnicott DW: The Maturational Process and the Facilitating Environment: Studies in the Theory of Emotional Development. New York: International Universities Press, 1965.
2. Winnicott DW: Plavina and Reality. London: Tavistock Publications, 1971.
3. Bion WR: Second Thoughts. London: Heinemann, 1967.
4. Adler G, Buie D: Psychotherapeutic approach to aloneness in the borderline patient. *In* Le Boit and Capponi (eds), Advances in Psychotherapy of the Borderline Patient. New York: Jason Aronson, 1979.
5. Adler G: Borderline Psychopathology and Its Treatment. New York: Jason Aronson, 1985.
6. Grotstein JS: The psychoanalytic concept of the borderline organization. *In* LeBoit & Capponi (eds), Advances in the Psychotherapy of the Borderine Patient. New York: Jason Aronson, 1979.
7. Grotstein JS: A proposed revision of the psychoanalytic concept of primitive mental states, Part 2. The borderline syndrome - Section 1. Disorders of autistic safety and symbiotic relatedness. Contemporary Psychoanalysis 19(4):570-604, 1983.
8. Grotstein JS: A proposed revision of the psychoanalytic concept of primitive mental states, Part 2. The borderline syndrome - Section 2. The phenomenology of the borderline syndrome. Contemporary Psychoanalysis 20(1):77-119, 1984.
9. Grotstein JS: A proposed revision of the psychoanalytic concept of primitive mental states, Part 2. The borderline syndrome - Section 3. Disorders of autistic safety and symbiotic relatedness. Contemporary Psychoanalysis 20(2):266-343, 1984.
10. Masterson J: Psychotherapy of the Borderline Adult: A Developmental Approach. New York: Brunner/Mazel, 1976.
11. Masterson J: The Narcissistic and Borderline Disorders: An Integrated Developmental Approach. New York: Brunner/Mazel, 1981.
12. Tustin F: Autistic States in Children. London: Routledge and Kegan Paul, 1981.
13. Bion WR: Differentiation of the psychotic from the non-psychotic personalities. International Journal of Psychoanalysis 38(3-4):266-275, 1957.
14. Bick E: Experience of the skin in early object relations International Journal of Psychoanalysis 49:484-486, 1968.
15. Meltzer D: Adhesive identification. Contemporary Psychoanalysis 11:289-310, 1975.
16. Anzieu D: The Skin Ego. New Haven, CT: Yale University Press, 1989.
17. Bion WR: Learning from Experience. London: Heinemann, 1962.
18. Kohut H: The Analysis of the Self. New York: International Universities Press, 1971.
19. Kohut H: The Restoration of the Self. New York: International Universities Press, 1977.
20. Winnicott DW: Transitional object and transitional phenomena. International Journal of Psychoanalysis 34:89-97, 1953.
21. Searles H: Some aspects of separation and loss in psychoanalytic therapy with borderline patients. *In* Giovacchini and Boyer (eds), Technical Factors in the Treatment of the Severely Disturbed Patient. New York: Jason Aronson, 1982.
22. Eigen M: The Psychotic Core. New York: Jason Aronson, 1986.

CHAPTER 13

The Curative Role of Color:
An Historical Overview

Jennet Inglis

The history of color as a science and a healing tool begins long before Sir Isaac Newton's 1666 discovery of prismatic light and the properties of color. Centuries before Hippocrates, the Egyptian, the East Indian, and the Chinese cultures, among others, reveal a vast knowledge of color and light. With the advance of civilization, much of this ancient *esoterica* was lost or absorbed into other cultures. For instance, many historians claim that Hippocrates borrowed his *Materia Medica* from India, and that Aristotle is indebted to Hindu physicians. Fortunately, due to the graceful advancement of civilization, we have available today an enormous body of integrated information about healing with color and the role of color in spiritual healing.

A controversial pioneer of color and medicine was the eleventh century Persian Islamic philosopher and physician, Avicenna. Considered by many scholars to be the father of color therapy, Avicenna wrote in his *Canon of Medicine* about the use of color for diagnosis and cure. During his life, Avicenna remained extremely influential throughout all of Europe. Centuries later, the English adopted not his curious medical ideas, but his trademark physician's red cape. Color as a curative tool waned for centuries until the Age of Enlightenment when research began again and, albeit controversially, color was recognized as a curative tool.

Since the Industrial Revolution, there have been many important contributions to the physics and metaphysics of color. In 1810, Johann Wolfgang von Goethe conducted color research that is unrivaled to this day![1] In his *Contribution to Optics. Researches into the Elements of a Theory of Colour,* and his *Moral Effects of Colour,* Goethe established the physical, mental, emotional, and spiritual conceptions of color. Goethe pioneered the first extensive study of the chemistry of color. He established that color is dye and pigments, that in physics color is a spectral composition, and that the psychophysics of color is a science (Fig. 1).

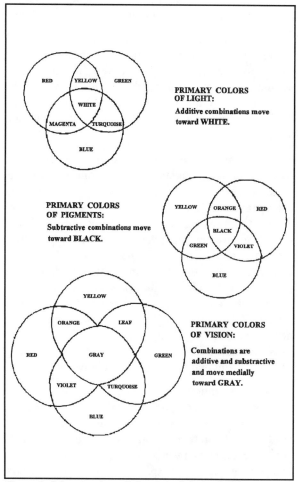

PRIMARY COLORS OF LIGHT:
Additive combinations move toward WHITE.

PRIMARY COLORS OF PIGMENTS:
Subtractive combinations move toward BLACK.

PRIMARY COLORS OF VISION:
Combinations are additive and substractive and move medially toward GRAY.

Figure 1: Primary colors of pigments, light, and vision.

In psychophysics, Goethe explored the study of color in relation to physical stimuli and especially the perception of magnitudes. Goethe also understood the critical curative role color plays in daily life. He realized that color has a positive and a negative effect on the mental and physical attitude of an individual. Goethe, and later other pioneers like Rudolph Steiner,[2] explored the psychospiritual aspects of color and laid the foundation for a western metaphysics of color. Both Goethe and Steiner knew that the subconscious mind can see color, and Steiner, even more than Goethe, explored color as a spiritual curative. Steiner explained that "life radiates color, and out of illness comes a new consciousness that reestablishes its balance in health and healing." As controversial as Rudolph Steiner, yet surely more maligned by the bureaucratic medical establishment in America, are two noteworthy scientists, Dr. Darius Dinshah[3,4] and Dr. Edwin D. Babbitt.[5] These individuals, and many others, have made enormous contributions despite governmental ignorance and harassment.

Contemporary researchers bravely continue to advance our knowledge against interference from the FDA and numerous other governmental bodies. Within the larger crisis of (American) medicine, the battle for truly innovative research monies will no doubt continue, and we can anticipate brilliant advances!

Color could be said to be one of the most dynamic and influential aspects of our history and, quite possibly, our future. Current research promises even greater understanding of the curative role of color. Explorations into ultraviolet and infrared spectrums are revealing yet more curative potential. Great researchers in education, such as the late Faber Birren[6-11] from the University of Chicago, have produced tremendous bodies of work available to the lay person. Color is no longer an abstract or subjective topic only for scientists. Today there is no excuse for not developing a relationship with color — either through fine art in the home, personal projects, study or meditation, and/or a 'conscious' environment!

It is now time for us to realize that the longer we postpone the healing power of *color, light* and *nature*, the closer we come to throwing our psyches, bodies, and culture(s) into imbalance. We live in a natural complete cycle of twenty-four hours of visible light and the complete color spectrum therein. A National Institute of Mental Health study, among many others, indicates that all-around good mental and physical health is critically dependent on full-spectrum light and normal color balance being maintained in our daily life and environment. The natural psychospiritual and physical benefits of color and light cannot be utilized if we are moving more and more rapidly into a technological existence devoid of basic natural elements.

Thus we may assume from the multitude of theoreticians that color as a curative force can be applied on the physical, psychological, and spiritual levels. Because of the perceptual quality of color, it heals both the physical and the higher senses. Many specialists present varied aspects of color or vibrations of consciousness, yet no one seems to have grasped the totality of color like Rudolph Steiner. There have been only a few visual artists who actually and consistently transformed the *body* of color, light, and spirit in their work. The sane holds true in the literary arts and music. Contributions thus far notwithstanding, the modern applications of color healing through the arts and medicine need our enthusiastic attention. We are a planet and a civilization in physical, medical, and spiritual crisis. Color is a gift and a healing force yet to be fully reckoned with. We can begin here and now!

REFERENCES

1. Goethe JW: Theory of Colours (translated by Charles Lock Eastlake). Cambridge, MA.: The MIT Press, 1970.
2. Steiner R: Colour. London: Rudolph Steiner Press, 1935.
3. Dinshah D: Let There Be Light. Malaga, NJ: Spectro-chrome Institute, 1985.
4. Dinshah D: Spectro-chrome Metry Encyclopedia. Volumes 1-3. Malaga, NJ: Spectro-chrome Institute, 1939.
5. Babbitt EG: The Principles of Light and Color. New Hyde Park, NY: University Books, 1967.
6. Birren F: History of Color in Painting. New York: Reinhold Publishing Corp, 1955.
7. Birren F: Color in Your World. New York: Collier Books, 1962.
8. Birren F: The effects of color on the human organism. American Journal of Occupational Therapy, 1959.
9. Birren F: Color Psychology and Color Therapy. Secaucus, NJ: University Books, 1961.
10. Birren F: New Horizons in Color. New York: Reinhold Publishing Corp, 1965.
11. Birren F: Light, Color, and Environment. New York: Reinhold Publishing Corp, 1988.

SUGGESTED READING

1. Abbott AG: The Color of Life. New York: McGraw-Hill, 1947.

2. Adrian ED: The Physical Background of Perception. London: Oxford University Press, 1967.

3. Amber RB: Color Therapy. Santa Fe, NM: Aurora Press, 1983.

4. Anderson M: Colour Healing. New York: Samuel Weiser, 1975.

5. Arnheim R: Art and Visual Perception. Los Angeles: University of California Press, 1974.

6. Bailey A: Esoteric Psychology, Vol l. New York: Lucis Publishing Co, 1936.

7. Basford L, Pick J: The Rays of Light. London: Sampson Low, Narston and Co, 1966.

8. Begbie GH: Seeing and the Eye. Garden City, NY: Anchor Books, 1973.

9. Boos-Hamburger H: The Creative Power Of Colour. London: The Michael Press, 1973.

10. Cheskin L: Colors: What They Can Do For You. New York: Livernight Publishing, 1947.

11. Chevreul MD: The Principles of Harmony and Contrast of Colours. New York: Reinhold Publishing Corp, 1967.

12. Collins JS: The World of Light. New York: Horizon Press, 1960.

13. David W: The Harmonics of Sound, Color Vibration. Marina Del Rey, CA: DeVorss & Co, 1980.

14. Dunlap R: Probing the mysteries of light. Today's Health, March 1963.

15. Edelson R: Treatment of cutaneous T-cell lymphoma by extra-corporeal photochemotherapy. New England Journal of Medicine, Feb 5, 1987.

16. Ellinger EF: The Biological Fundamentals of Radiation Therapy. American Elsevier Publishing Co, 1941.

17. Fletcher J (ed): Goethe's Approach to Colour (translated by Hilde Boos-Hamburger). London: The Michael Press, 1958.

18. Graham CH (ed): Vision and Visual Perception. New York: John Wiley & Sons, 1965.

19. Graves M: The Art of Color and Design. New York: McGraw-Hill, 1941.

20. Gregory RL: Eye and the Brain: The Psychology of Seeing. London: Weidenfeld & Nicholson, 1971.

21. Guptill AL: Color Manual for Artists. New York: Reinhold Publishing Corp, 1946.

22. Hering E: Outlines of a Theory of the Light Sense. Cambridge, MA: Harvard University Press, 1964.

23. Huxley A: The Doors of Perception and Heaven and Hell New York: Harper & Row, 1963.

24. Itten J: The Elements of Color. New York: Reinhold Publishing Corp, 1970.

25. Johnson K: The Living Aura: Radiation Field Photography and the Kirlian Effect. New York: Hawthorn Books, 1975.

26. Judd DB, Wyszecki G: Color in Business, Science, and Industry. New York: John Wiley & Sons, 1963.

27. Kandinsky W: The Art of Spiritual Harmony. Boston: Houghton Nifflin Co, 1914.

28. Kargare A: Color and Personality. York Beach, ME: Samuel Weiser, 1982.

29. Kepes G: The Language of Vision. Chicago: Theopold, 1944.

30. Luckiesh M: Color and Its Applications. New York: Van Nostrand & Co, 1921.

31. Luscher M: The Luscher Test. New York: Pocket Books, 1971.

32. MacIvor V, LaForest S: Vibrations. New York: Samuel Weiser, 1979.

33. Maerz A, Paul MR: A Dictionary of Color. New York: McGraw-Hill, 1930.

34. Mayer G: Colour and Healing. Sussex, England: New Knowledge Books, 1960.

35. Newton I: New Theory About Light and Colors. Munich: W Fritach, 1967.

36. Ostwald W: Colour Science. London: Winsor & Newton, 1931.

37. Ott J: Color and light: Their effects on plants, animals, and people. International Journal of Biosocial Research, special subject issues (1985-1988).

38. Sander CG: Colour in Health and Disease. London: CW Daniel Co, 1926.

39. Sargent W: The Enjoyment and Use of Color. New York: Scribner & Co, 1923.

40. Schindler M: Goethe's Theory of Colour. Sussex, England: New Knowledge Books, 1964.

41. Sight, Light, and Color. New York: Arco Books, 1984.

42 Stevens EJ: Rhythms and Colors. San Francisco: Rainbow Publishing, 1938.

43. Tucci G: The Theory and Practice of the Mandala. Rome, 1949.

44. Wagner C: The Wagner Color Response. Santa Barbara, CA: Wagner Institute for Color Research, 1985.

45. Wright WD: The Measurement of Colour. London: Adam Hilger Ltd, 1944.

CHAPTER 14

Art Therapy in an Orthopedic Hospital

Nell Aird Bateman

In order to assess the usefulness of an art-therapy program in an orthopedic hospital, it is necessary to examine some of the general psychological stresses involved. To doctors, illness and disability are an objective collection of facts, while to patients, they are subjective experiences. The hospital situation, with its unfamiliar demands, requires a shift in attitude to dependency at a time when emotional stability and physical strength are at their most precarious.[1] It is the patient's assessment of his/her illness that should be crucial to the overall consideration of the treatment program. The symbolic significance of an individual's disability must be considered; this is particularly so when the response is out of proportion to what is expected.

Too often, the emotional aspects of hospitalization and surgery are given scant attention in most hospitals.[2] Frequently, patients develop a 'giving-up' syndrome with accompanying feelings of helplessness and hopelessness. In health, patients have protected themselves against these feelings; many find that their usual defenses and reactions do not work when a major life event such as surgery has caused them to be vulnerable. The trauma of surgery can bring old, unresolved fears and conflicts to the surface.

The emergence of unaccustomed fears and loss of capacity to cope goes beyond unpleasant feelings, and includes a disruption of key relationships and a failure of motivation, the latter a critical factor in recovery. As the hospitalized patients' world shrinks, internal determinants of behavior become more important. Thus, regressive behavior is almost inevitable. There are many causes for patients in hospital to be more emotional than under normal circumstances, and both conscious and unconscious factors are involved. Addressing unresolved problems becomes important, for the more issues that are resolved, the more energy there will be for healing.[3]

Kornfeld has studied the psychosocial determinants of recovery, and has found that many environ-mental factors in the hospital can increase emotional distress and thereby adversely influence recovery. Bedside rounds or casual remarks of staff can leave patients subject to vague fears and fantasies. Routine tests — not routine to patients — and the isolation of recovery rooms can generate feelings of insecurity. In addition, many patients who have been very active previously have great difficulty in coping with the enforced inactivity of hospitalization and surgery. A further stress for some patients may be an ill-defined belief that their disability has been visited upon them as punishment for some past misdemeanor. Such doubts and fears can shake a patient's already pre-carious self-confidence.[4] The resulting symptoms of tension and depression can persist and make physical conditions worse. Foster has found that art therapy has particular value in an orthopedic hospital, where, he says, all patients are suffering from some form of emotional distress.[5] Art-therapy sessions can provide these patients with a much needed outlet for the deeply felt emotions that may be triggered by the trauma of surgery.

Essentially, art therapy is based on the belief in the creative ability of all human beings. Symbols, our earliest and most primitive form of communication, provide for the individual a wider means of expres-sion, a means to say in pictures what one is unable to reveal in words.[6] With skill, the art therapist can encourage patients to discover the meaning of their own symbols and uncover, in a non-threatening way, material that may have been previously repressed. Art therapy can also relate to the healthy part of the patient and thereby reveal unrecognized ego strengths.[7]

Robert Coles states that art work is a projection in which deep psychological laws are at work. He finds that pictures "offer solace, comfort, reassurance and a neutral medium for exchange," a means of communi-cation that can cross cultural barriers in a predominantly verbal society. Coles reminds us that, as Jung has stated, "we paint what we see within us, not before us."[8] Creativity arises from the whole of human experience, and drawings and paintings act like dreams, in that they are symbolic representations of the self. Many of Freud's discoveries of the mechanisms of dream analysis can be applied to art.[7, 9]

A hospital art-therapy program can provide a relaxed and therapeutic environment in which patients are encouraged to picture anything they want. In art-therapy sessions, individuals can decide when they feel ready to share their emotions, without feeling a sense of intrusion. All intolerable situations can be dealt with in pictures, and angry and aggressive feelings safely portrayed. Interpretations of the art must be carefully woven into the artist-patient's declared theme. Verbal and nonverbal expressions must be taken into account.[10] First pictures also can be of diagnostic importance and can often contain a map of where the individual is headed.[11]

When time is limited, art therapy can be a particularly beneficial adjunct to the overall treatment program in an orthopedic hospital. In such a short-term program, the art therapist must be mindful of the time constraints and take particular care not to delve too deeply into conflictual material that cannot be resolved in the limited time available.

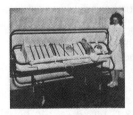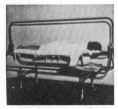

Figure 1: *The Stryker frame is still used in many hospitals after back surgery to stabilize the patient for at least a week. The frame enables the patient to be turned safely and with limited disturbance to the spine.*

It is difficult to generalize about the basic themes that emerged in the patients' art in the art-therapy program at the Orthopaedic Hospital in Toronto, involving, as it did, some 30 patients.[12] While some areas of emotional distress were similar for all patients, understandably, each individual found certain issues more emotionally painful than others. Upon examination of all the art, however, the findings were remarkably consistent. Most often encountered were anger at helplessness, boredom, and fears of an outcome that might be worse than expected. Expressed in the art also were feelings of isolation, of being forgotten and abandoned by loved ones, and, at times, an unfamiliar sense of depression.

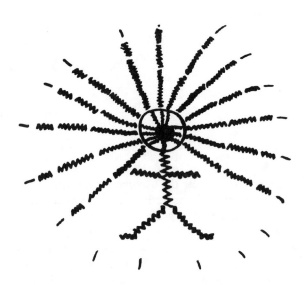

Figure 2: Going Wacky. *Titled by the patient, this is a clear expression of the feelings she was experiencing on the Stryker bed. She stated that it was "feeling like the top of one's head will crack up." She felt "hemmed in," and t was "getting worse." Art-therapy sessions provided an outlet for these intense emotions.*

Shown herein are examples of pictures done in such an art therapy program. They speak clearly of patients' distress at various times during their hospital stay. Most patients were confined to the Stryker frame for a period of several weeks, and most art-therapy sessions were private, usually lasting about an hour. The patients' own verbal associations to their art are included. One patient stated the case for art-therapy sessions: "This is the greatest thing — you never get to talk about feelings."

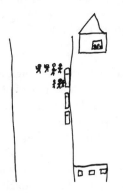

Figure 3: The Dream. *This young police constable was reluctant at first to become involved in the art-therapy sessions because, he said, "art therapy is not my bag." The picture depicts a recurring dream he was having while in the hospital. The dream reenacts an incident that occurred two years prior, in which he and another officer were assaulted by five young men. He had tried to forget the incident, to "put it out of my mind," but had found, after his surgery, that he would "waken in a cold sweat with feelings of fear." The surgery had reawakened these buried feelings. It is hoped that the art-therapy sessions helped to forestall a lengthy traumatic neurosis. He was surprised at his need to express his feelings. Despite his reservations and primitive, he was one of the most prolific participants.*

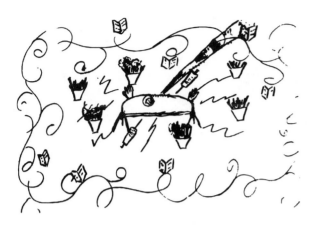

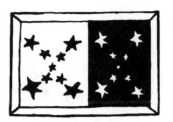

Figure 6: "A window, trying to focus everything — trying to get a center of perspective by making this small window." This patient was striving for some sort of emotional balance at a time when contact with the world had become restricted to the hospital window.

Figure 4: Being Smothered with "needles, helping hands, friends — wishing sometimes they would all leave me alone." The staff reported that this patient never complained. She said of herself and her emotions, "I find it hard to speak my mind." Her picture has spoken eloquently for her about her feelings.

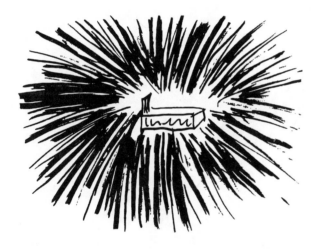

Figure 5: Busting Out of Here. The title was provided by the patient, a girl of 15 who at first was excessively polite and cooperative. After several art-therapy sessions, she felt safe enough to express very different feelings as she worked on this picture. The lines were done in many colors "to show all my feelings," and are going out from her fed. The bed was done in black, she said, "to show I am in prison." She continued that she was angry at many aspects of being in the hospital, where "you have to be so nice." She was particularly upset also by the immobility she was experiencing and somehow had not expected.

REFERENCES

1. Schontz FC: The personal meaning of illness. J Psychosomatic Med, 1972.
2. Schmale AH: Giving-up as a common pathway to changes in health. J Psychosomatic Med, 1975.
3. Barker R: Adjustment to Physical Handicap and Illness. A Survey of the Social Psychology of Physical Disability (revised ed). New York: Social Science Research, 1953.
4. Kornfeld E: Psycho-social determinants of recovery. J Psychosomatic Med, 1972.
5. Foster D: Art therapy in an orthopaedic hospital. Medical and Biological Illustration 20:1970.
6. Naumberg M: Dynamically Orientated Art Therapy. Its Principles and Practices. New York: Grune and Stratton, 1966.
7. Gibson RW: The impact of national policy on the health professions. American Art Therapy Conference, 1976.
8. McNiff S: Artists and psychotherapy: A conversation with Robert Coles. J Art Psychotherapy 3:1976.
9. Freud S: Complete Works. Volume IV. Interpretation of Dreams. Hogarth Press.
10. Fischer M: Consultations and educational material. Toronto Art Therapy Institute, Canada. 1974-1991.
11. Shoemaker R: Significance of the first picture in art therapy. American Art Therapy Conference, 1977.
12. Bateman JE: Personal communication. Toronto, Canada, 1980-1991.

CHAPTER 15

The Healing Power of Art Therapy for Mentally Ill Deaf Adults

Sally Brucker

INTRODUCTION

This chapter demonstrates how art therapy helped a population of hospitalized, mentally ill, deaf adults to express interpsychic conflicts, unconscious feelings, and early issues relating to disturbances in parent/child communication and emotional development. Fifteen patients on a specialized inpatient ward for mentally ill, deaf adults were divided into two art-therapy groups according to diagnostic categories, proficiency in sign language, and overall level of socialization skills. Each group met weekly for 90 minutes for a period of three years, providing a longitudinal sample for analysis of these issues.

A brief review of art therapy, deafness, and historical treatment of this population in the United States provide the context for understanding the significance of art therapy as a treatment modality for these individuals. The common themes which emerged in the art work of one group are discussed. Specific examples of patient art work highlight how art therapy helps to alleviate symptoms of impulsivity, aggression, isolation, and depression often observed in this patient population. Themes relating to oral deprivation and frustration in gratification contribute to our understanding of early psychological development of deaf children raised by hearing parents. The emergence of imagery depicting auditory hallucinations is reviewed to shed new light on how deaf persons experience psychotic symptoms.

MENTAL ILLNESS AND THE DEAF: INCIDENCE AND TREATMENT AVAILABILITY

The incidence of mental illness in the adult deaf population in the United States occurs at the same rate as in the hearing population, roughly ten percent.[1] At least 25,000 of the 250,000 deaf adults in the U.S., therefore, might find themselves in need of mental-health services in their lifetime. Faced with few programs geared to meet their specific needs, many adult deaf persons were and sometimes still are simply misdiagnosed and 'shelved' in state mental institutions where they remain in profound isolation which often exacerbates their symptoms.[2] Several notable exceptions were hospitals which hired deaf mental-health workers and trained others to communicate in sign language and to understand the psychology of deafness. The patients described herein participated in a program of this type established in 1963 at Saint Elizabeth's Hospital in Washington, D.C. This program pioneered in the use of expressive art therapies (art, dance, and psychodrama) as integral to the recovery process for these patients.

PSYCHOLOGY OF DEAFNESS

Inability to communicate desires and feelings to significant others from early infancy, as in the case of these patients, may contribute to secondary symptoms which include behavioral disturbances and social maladjustment.[3] Further contributing factors are said to be inadequate schooling, lack of social input, and emotional and physical isolation. These symptoms have been noted as more apparent in those raised by hearing parents as opposed to those raised by deaf parents, where a common language and culture exist. Secondary symptoms include: (1) impulsivity, (2) lack of introspection, (3) prolonged egocentricity, (4) emotional immaturity, and (5) inability to delay gratification.[3]

ART THERAPY

Art therapy has been found to be of particular value with deaf psychiatric patients, in that visual messages expressed through their graphic and plastic representations often convey heretofore pent-up or inadequately expressed emotions.[4] The artistic expression is often the first step in learning to recognize, conceptualize, and convey important inner experiences. The art materials themselves provide tactile and visual stimulation in accordance with deaf persons' most important mode of perceiving the world and processing information. Art media and art making include structural elements of color, texture, line, form, and composition. In producing art, visual, kinesthetic, and motoric responses merge naturally. Through the pressure of line, selection of color, or choice of composition or theme, deaf patients can frequently express immediate feelings and release tension.

GROUP ART THERAPY

In a group setting, shared art works not only serve to reduce isolation and enhance mutuality and support, but also become a kind of *symbolic speech* and group memory that is tangible.[5] In the course of the session, the art therapist lends her skills and ego strengths to assist patients in merging their pure emotions with the self-control and awareness needed to complete a recognizable or finished image. The image itself may then be reworked or even discarded, allowing the patients to practice their ability to control, make decisions, test reality, or achieve a level of mastery and competency. The completed image becomes a concrete expression and record of the patient's concerns, conflicts, memories, and experiences. More often than not, common themes emerge as shared concerns in discussions of the art work with the group, an important part of the therapeutic process. When this occurs, patients experience relief and feelings of connectedness and enhanced sense of self, thus further reducing their isolation. Ways in which to carry these insights into their relationships outside of the group can then be discussed.

One group consisted of four females and three males ranging in age from 23 to 31 years (Table).

Overall goals for the group included expressing and working through personal conflicts relating to past and present situations, and establishing group trust and exploring group dynamics through self-directed discussions relating to the theme and content of the art work. The mode of communication was American Sign Language. For the most part, the individuals in the group worked on self-directed projects. At times, specific themes were suggested, such as "Draw the group," "Draw your family," etc. The format of the group was established to create a sense of continuity and safety. This included: (1) initial discussion of current issues and events (15 minutes), (2) art-making and clean-up (60 minutes), and (3) group discussion focused on the content and process of individual pieces and the group dynamics (30 minutes).

COMMON THEMES

Many common themes emerged in the patients' art work over the course of three years of art therapy. These included: (1) auditory hallucinations, (2) oral needs, (3) sense of the self as strange, (4) aggressive impulses-anger, and (5) communication.

Auditory Hallucinations

The existence of auditory hallucinations in profoundly deaf patients has been reported in the literature.[6,7] Approximately five such drawings appeared spontaneously in this group. Dan, a profoundly deaf man diagnosed as schizophrenic (acute episode), drew himself as "hearing voices from the devil" (Fig. 1). Similarly, Liza, a 27-year-old woman with a moderate

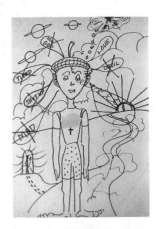

Figure 1:   *Auditory hallucinations — by Dan.*

hearing loss, diagnosed as schizoaffective, drew two self-portraits depicting her wish to "stop the voices" (Fig. 2). The process of externalizing these "inner voices" offered temporary relief and comfort. It remains unclear whether the auditory hallucinations experienced by these patients were actual perceived sounds as reported by them or images of words.[6,7]

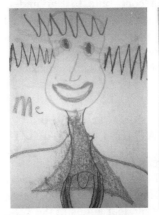
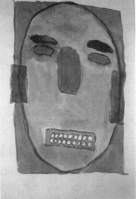

Figure 2: Auditory hallucinations (left), and Liza's wish to "stop the voices."

Table: Description of Art-Therapy Group

	Age	Diagnosis	Etiology/Degree of Hearing Loss	Mode of Communication	Length of Hospitalization (At Time of Group)
Lynn	29	Schizophrenia: Acute episode	Birth/ Profound	*ASL (good)	6 months
Ann	30	Severe depression	Birth/ Profound	ASL (good)	3 months
Joe	23	Chronic undifferentiated schizophrenia	Birth/ Profound	ASL (poor)	2 years
Sandy	27	Borderline psychosis	Birth/ Profound	ASL (good)	2 years
Ralph	31	Paranoid schizophrenia	Birth/ Profound	ASL (good)	6 months
Dan	29	Schizophrenia: Acute episode	Birth/ Profound	ASL (good)	3 months
Liza	27	Schizoaffective disorder	Birth/ Moderate	Voice; some sign language	1 year

*American Sign Language

Oral Needs

The graphic and plastic representations of the mouth in exaggerated and distorted form emerged repeatedly in the group. In discussing the significance of this pattern, the group focused on early frustrating attempts to have needs met and to communicate with hearing caregivers. Lynn, 29, profoundly deaf and diagnosed as schizophrenic, sculpted a baby seal from clay (Fig. 3). The seal was described as "screaming for food, waiting ... crying." The enormous mouth of the seal was seen as "empty and needy," which Lynn was able to identify as representing herself in relation to her mother. Through this image, the group began to understand how their unfulfilled nurturance and dependency needs had left them feeling empty and angry at times.

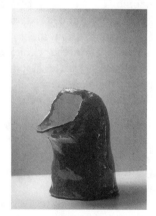

Fig. 3: Oral needs: by Lynn

Sense of the Self as Strange

The art of psychiatric patients often depicts the self as strange or different.[8] Self-portraits done by patients in the group not only contained such distortions, but also conveyed feelings relating to the experience of not being able to hear or communicate with the "hearing world." For example, Sandy, a 27-year-old profoundly deaf woman diagnosed as borderline psychotic, drew several self-portraits depicting herself as a creature from outer space. One such portrait (Fig. 4) was described as "shooting the bad baby martian." This striking image shows a frightened one-eyed creature being shot because it is "different, ugly." Full life body tracings done by other patients show similar depictions of body distortions and self-revulsion.

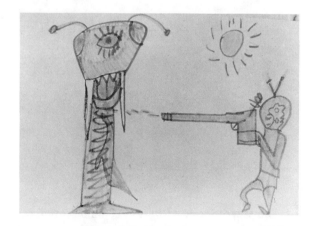

Figure 4: An example of Sandy's sense of herself as strange.

Aggressive Impulses/Anger

Many drawings and paintings produced by group members contained images of covert and overt expressions of rage. Ralph, 31, profoundly deaf and diagnosed as paranoid schizophrenic, had been incarcerated for one year prior to his admission to the hospital. He was described as assaultive and aggressive. Despite these tendencies, he was able to utilize the art media expressively and with control. His self-portrait (Fig. 5) shows a primitive, wild-looking man with long unkempt hair and a green face. Although this portrait in no way physically resembled Ralph, it represented his feelings of being seen as strange, his anger at his continued hospitalization and need to take psychotropic medication, as well as his potentially explosive inner rage. This image provided a means through which he could begin to understand and express his feelings in an acceptable

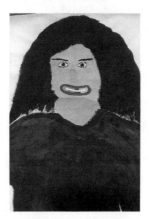

Figure 5: *Ralph's aggressive impulses.*

manner. Other patients frequently drew images of volcanoes or fires and described them in terms of the inner turmoil and rage they had felt for years.

Communication

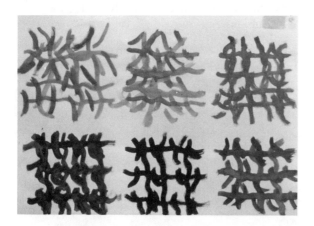

Figure 6: *Ann's "Chinese" communication.*

The search for new forms of communication was an ongoing theme within the group. Often, patients would produce art work which resembled foreign languages or which represented an attempt to create a new one, e.g. an oriental design (Fig. 6). This was described as "Chinese" by Ann, a 30-year-old pro-

foundly deaf and severely depressed woman. When the group commented that they could not speak Chinese, Ann laughed and explained, "That's how I feel trying to talk to my husband and kids!"

Joe, a 23-year-old profoundly deaf man diagnosed as schizophrenic (chronic undifferentiated), attempted to create an entirely new language for himself and the group (Fig. 7). When his symptoms were acute, Joe exhibited bizarre behavior and often lapsed into his own incomprehensible language. This creation of his own language, which

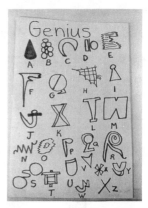

Figure 7: *Joe's "new language."*

not even deaf persons could understand, served to give Joe a sense of power and control lacking in his life.

CONCLUSION

It has been said that the absence of sight cuts one off from the world of things but not the world of people. To see and yet be unable to hear or comprehend sounds and words in the hearing world and to suffer from mental illness creates a profound sense of isolation. For the clinician seeking to establish a relationship with deaf patients and working towards enhancing their sense of self and reducing isolation, the challenges are many.

Group art therapy, in combination with sign-language fluency on the part of the art therapist, served as a catalyst to unlock repressed emotions and reduce behavioral symptomatology. Common themes which emerged in the art work further our understanding of the subjective experience of this patient population. It remains to be seen whether this information can be generalized to the larger patient population of mentally ill, deaf adults. It is hoped that in the future, more systematic and scientific studies relating to the artistic expression of this population might aid in our understanding and design of treatment strategies. From the work described herein, it is clear that a strong need to communicate experiences, thoughts, and feelings was felt by group members. The fact that these patients were able to utilize the art media in their struggle to understand themselves and one another speaks to the power of art as a visual language and therapeutic tool.

REFERENCES

1. Schein J, Delk M: The Deaf Population in the United States. Silver Spring, MD: National Association for the Deaf, 1974.
2. Altshuler KZ, Rainer J: Mental Health and the Deaf: Approaches and Prospects. U.S. Dept. of Health, Education and Welfare, Social and Rehabilitation Service, 1968.
3. Altshuler KZ, Deming WE, Vollenweide J, Rainer JD, Tendler R: Impulsivity and profound early deafness. American Annals of the Deaf 121:331-345, 1976.
4. Silver R: Potentials in art for the deaf. Eastern Arts Quarterly 1(2), 1968.
5. Naumburg M: Dynamically Oriented Art Therapy: Its Principles and Practice. New York: Grune and Stratton, 1966.
6. Cooper AF: Deafness and psychiatric illness. British Journal of Psychiatry 129:216-226, 1976.
7. Critchley EMR, et al: Hallucinatory experiences of prelingually profoundly deaf schizophrenics. British Journal of Psychiatry 138:30-32, 1981.
8. Prinzhorn H: Artistry of the Mentally Ill. New York: Springer-Verlag, 1972.

SUGGESTED READING

1. Altshuler KZ: The social and psychological development of the deaf. American Annals of the Deaf 119:365-376, 1974.
2. Boulton B (ed): Psychology of Deafness for Rehabilitation Counselors. Baltimore: University Park Press, 1976.
3. Brauer B, Sussman AE: Experiences of deaf therapists with deaf client. Mental Health in Deafness, #4, NIMH, DHHS, (ADM) 81-1047, 1980.
4. Dickens D: The mental health program for the deaf at Saint Elizabeth's Hospital. In Bradfords L, Hardy WG (eds), Hearing and Hearing Impaired. New York: Grune and Stratton, 1979.
5. Donahue RJ: The deaf personality. Journal of Rehabilitation of the Deaf 2:37-52, 1968.

6. Furth HG: Thinking Without Language: Psychological Implications of Deafness. New York: Free Press, 1966.
7. Harris RI: Communication and mental health. The Deaf American 34(4), 1982.
8. Levine ES: Psychology of Deafness, 303-308. New York: Columbia University Press, 1960.
9. Lowen A: The Betrayal of the Body. New York: MacMillan, 1967.
10. Lowenfeld V, Brittain LW: Creative and Mental Growth, 4th ed. New York: MacMillan, 1964.
11. Mykelburst HR: The Psychology of Deafness. New York: Grune & Stratton, 1966.
12. Oosterhous S: Dance movement therapy with the deaf: The relationship between dance/movement therapy and American Sign Language. Unpublished masters thesis, Goucher College, Towson, MD, 1985.
13. Robinson LD: Sound Minds in a Soundless World. Dept of Health, Education and Welfare; Public Health Service; Alcohol, Drug Abuse and Mental Health Administration, NIMH, DHEW, (ADM) 77-560, 1978.
14. Rubin JA: Child Art Therapy: Understanding and Helping Children Grow Through Art, 2nd ed. New York: Van Nostrand, 1984.
15. Schiff W, Thayer S: An eye for an ear? Social perception, non-verbal communication, and deafness. Rehabilitation Psychology 21:56-57, 1974.
16. Stein M: Role playing and spontaneity in teaching social skills to deaf adolescents. Unpublished masters thesis, 1976.
17. Swink D: Therapists and therapies with deaf people: The need for specialized training, attitude exploration and novel approaches. Unpublished paper presented at the Southeast Regional Institute on Deafness, Birmingham, AL, Oct 1979.
18. Vernon MC: Techniques of screening for mental illness among deaf clients. Journal of Rehabilitation of the Deaf 2:30, 1969.
19. Vernon MC: Deafness and mental health: Some theoretical views. Gallaudet Today, 9-13, Fall 1978.

CHAPTER 16

Correlation of Psychiatric Diagnosis and Formal Elements in Art Work

Linda Gantt

Over the past century, writers have noted similarities between a patient's mental illness and his or her art.[1-8] It is reasonable to conclude, therefore, that the distinctive features of each illness are encoded in the art in some consistent or law-like way. If psychiatric symptoms have isomorphic equivalents in formal elements (such as use of color or amount of detail) it should be possible to develop a rating instrument based on the symptoms distinctive for each disorder.

METHOD

In this paper, the term *diagnosis* refers to the classifications used by the American Psychiatric Association (third edition of the Diagnostic and Statistical Manual, Revised [DSM-III-R]).[9] Four DSM-III-R Axis I categories were studied — schizophrenia, organic mental disorder, bipolar disorder (mania), and major depression.

Formal Elements Art Therapy Scale

To develop the rating scales, the following steps were taken: (a) assume that specific symptoms are expressed in some regular and predictable way in art work; (b) review previously used scales and rating instruments; and (c) examine global formal characteristics of art which might be analogous to specific symptoms.

Those symptoms which might be expressed in formal elements were selected. Ones which were related or opposites were combined (e.g. "increase in goal-directed activity or psychomotor agitation" in mania and "fatigue or loss of energy" in depression were combined in Scale #3, *Energy*). Each scale reflected a range of possible responses rather than simply *presence* or *absence*.

Pictures

All drawings were done on white drawing paper (12" x 18") with felt-tip markers (red, orange, dark blue, light blue, dark green, light green, hot pink, magenta, purple, brown, yellow, and black), drawn according to the instruction: "Draw a person picking an apple from a tree."[10]

Twenty-five drawings (5 from each diagnostic category and 5 from controls) were selected from the files of a university-affiliated psychiatric hospital. Although the same assessment drawing is requested at admission and discharge, only admission pictures were used. Presumably, the symptoms, assumed to be reflected in the drawings, peak at admission.

From Patients: A computer printout for the calendar year 1989 showed that 547 adults were treated. Records of those with any of the following discharge diagnoses* were reviewed: Schizophrenia (295.1x — disorganized, 295.2x — catatonic, 295.3x — paranoid, 295.6x — residual, 295.9x — undifferentiated); Major Depression (296.2x — major depression, single episode, 296.3x — major depression, recurrent); Bipolar (296.4x — manic, 296.70 — bipolar disorder NOS [not otherwise specified]); and Organic Mental Disorder (290.1x — presenile dementia of Alzheimer's type NOS, 290.4 — arteriosclerotic dementia, uncomplicated; multi-infarct dementia; 290.00 — senile dementia NOS, 290.10 — presenile dementia NOS).

There were 205 patients with the above discharge diagnoses during one or more hospital stays. To obtain a homogeneous sample for the subgroups, records were screened for co-existing disorders likely to affect the drawings. Anyone with the following was dropped: (1) more than one Axis I disorder during any hospital stay (including substance abuse disorders); (2) substantially different Axis I diagnoses

*Note: *The numbers refer to those used in the DSM-III-R. An "x" denotes the inclusion of all the variants of this diagnosis. The other bipolar subcategories were not included because there was no guarantee that the patient might have been manic during the hospital stay. In the other subcategories such as "Bipolar Mood Disorder, Depressed," the bipolar designation might have been made on past history.*

Table I: *Characteristics of Patients Whose Drawings were Used in Study*

Patient	Age	Sex	DSM-III-R Code	Discharge Diagnosis/Admission Diagnosis
				Schizophrenia
A	68	F	295.30 295.30	Schizophrenia, paranoid type, unspecified/ Schizophrenia, paranoid type, unspecified.
B	67	F	295.94 295.92	Schizophrenia, undifferentiated type, chronic, with acute exacerbation/ Schizophrenia, undifferentiated type, chronic.
C	39	M	295.34 295.32	Schizophrenia, paranoid type, chronic with acute exacerbation/ Schizophrenia, paranoid type, chronic.
D	58	M	295.32 295.32	Schizophrenia, paranoid type, chronic/ Schizophrenia, paranoid type, chronic.
E	19	M	295.30 295.95	Schizophrenia, paranoid type, unspecified/ Schizophrenia, undifferentiated type, in remission
				Organic Mental Disorders
F	81	F	290.40 294.10	Multi-infarct dementia, uncomplicated/ Dementia in conditions classified elsewhere.
G	74	M	290.00 294.10	Primary degenerative dementia of the Alzheimer type, senile onset/ Dementia in conditions classified elsewhere
H	73	M	290.00 294.10	Primary degenerative dementia of the Alzheimer type, senile onset/ Dementia in conditions classified elsewhere.
I	59	M	290.10 290.00	Primary degenerative dementia of the Alzheimer type, presenile onset/ Primary degenerative dementia of the Alzheimer type, senile onset.
J	80	F	290.00 294.10	Primary degenerative dementia of the Alzheimer type, senile onset/ Dementia in conditions classified elsewhere.
				Bipolar Mood Disorders
K	34	F	296.40 296.40	Bipolar disorder, manic, unspecified/ Bipolar disorder, manic, unspecified.
L	49	M	296.40 296.70	Bipolar disorder, manic, unspecified/ Bipolar disorder, not otherwise specified.
M	43	F	296.40 296.40	Bipolar disorder, manic, unspecified/ Bipolar disorder, manic, unspecified.
N	55	F	296.40 296.60	Bipolar disorder, manic, unspecified/ Bipolar disorder, mixed, unspecified.
O	69	F	296.40 296.40	Bipolar disorder, manic, unspecified/ Bipolar disorder, manic, unspecified.
				Major Depression
P	19	F	296.20 296.20	Major depression, single episode, unspecified/ Major depression, single episode, unspecified.
Q	48	M	296.20 296.20	Major depression, single episode, unspecified/ Major depression, single episode, unspecified.
R	39	F	296.20 296.23	Major depression, single episode, unspecified/ Major depression, single episode, severe, without psychotic features.
S	33	M	296.30 296.20	Major depression, recurrent, unspecified/ Major depression, single episode, unspecified.
T	52	F	296.32 296.20	Major depression, recurrent, moderate/ Major depression, single episode, unspecified.

during different hospital stays; (3) severe psychotic symptoms along with the mood disorders or the organic mental disorders (e.g. someone with "major depression, severe with psychotic features"); (4) depressive features along with schizophrenia or organic mental disorders; (5) Axis II disorders (personality disorders and/or mental retardation); (6) history of stroke (cardiovascular accident) or seizure disorder; and (7) over 70 years of age (except in the organic mental disorders group) to rule out the possibility of undiagnosed Alzheimer's disease in the other diagnostic groups.

To ensure that the pictures had not influenced the discharge diagnosis, patients who did not have the same or similar diagnosis on both admission and discharge were eliminated. Examples of similar diagnoses are "atypical depression not otherwise specified" and "major depression single episode." Thus, patients whose drawings were rated represented a single Axis I diagnosis without complicating factors. This left a total of 47 patients. Eleven with depression had an admission diagnosis of "atypical depression disorder, not otherwise specified" and were eliminated from the sample. The rest of the 11 patients with depression had a closer match between their admission and discharge diagnoses and made a more homogeneous group.

Records of the 36 remaining patients were checked for Axis III disorders (physical disorders) which might impair drawing ability, and those with serious physical illnesses were excluded. Each subgroup was reviewed for age and sex, and the final sample was selected so as to have a reasonable balance on these variables (Table I).

From Controls: The same drawing was routinely collected from students, visitors, and family members. Most had been done by women. Pictures from the calendar year 1987 had the greatest number done by men, so the control group pictures were taken from that year. The controls ranged from 18 to 70 years of age (Table II).

The judges were three female art therapists with no knowledge of the study's hypotheses. All had a Master's degree in art therapy and had been practicing for one to 15 years.

General Hypothesis

The null hypothesis was that no statistically significant differences would be found among the mean scores for pictures drawn by subjects in five

diagnostic categories as measured on each of the 14 sub-scales of the Formal Elements Art Therapy Scale (FEATS).

Table II: Age and Sex of Controls Whose Pictures Were Used

Control	Age	Sex
U	18	F
V	23	M
W	30	M
X	53	M

RESULTS

Reliability of the ratings was computed using an intra-class correlation and found to be within the range of an earlier pilot study for 8 of the 14 scales (Table III). A one-way analysis of variance (ANOVA) was computed on each scale to see if there were any statistically significant differences between the mean scores of the groups (Table IV). There was a statistically significant difference between the groups at the $p < .05$ level on 10 of the 14 scales. Scheffé post-hoc comparisons $(p < .05)$[11] were made, with each scale being compared with every other scale (Table V).

Table III: Reliability of Judges' Ratings on 23 Pictures

	Scale	Intra-class Correlation	(Range from Pilot Study)
1.	Prominence of Color	.90	(.83 to .98)
2.	Color Fit	.86	(.82 to .97)
3[a].	Energy	.60	(-.54 to .94)
4.	Space	.92	(.90 to .97)
5.	Integration	.94	(.84 to .97)
6.	Logic	.92	(.77 to .96)
7.	Realism	.88	(.93 to .98)
8[a].	Problem-solving	.92	(.79 to .99)
9[a].	Developmental Level	.88	(.80 to .98)
10.	Details	.80	(.93 to .99)
11.	Line Quality	.32	(.73 to .95)
12.	Person	.90	(.94 to .99)
13.	Perseveration	.54	(.57 to .82)
14.	Rotation	.76	(.49 to .88)

[a]Calculated on 21 pictures

DISCUSSION

The drawings of the control group were given the highest mean scores on 10 of the scales and the second highest on the remaining four. Thus, a "normal" drawing would have colors appropriate to the subject matter, would be logical, have a well-integrated composition, show at least the developmental features common to adolescent drawings, have a reasonable amount of detail, color and energy, depict a fairly realistic person, and show a practical way of getting the apple out of the tree.

Table IV: *Analysis of Variance on 25 Pictures in 5 Diagnostic Groups*

Scale	F Ratio	F Probability
1	3.76	.0193
2	1.94	N.S.
3	6.00	.0024
4	2.35	N.S.
5	9.20	.0002
6	7.86	.0006
7	4.78	.0072
8	14.11	.0000+
9	6.62	.0015
10	4.69	.0078
11	1.77	N.S.
12	6.75	.0013
13	2.03	N.S.
14	3.25	.0331

Drawings by the patients with organic mental disorders had the lowest mean scores on 12 of the 14 scales and the next-to-lowest mean scores on the other two. There is relatively little color and the color does not fit the subject. There are few details, little energy, and little use of space. The drawings are poorly integrated and illogical with a low developmental level, little or no problem-solving or realism, and no recognizable person depicted.

There were no statistically significant differences between drawings by patients with depression and those of the control group on any of the scales. The drawings by patients with depression, however, could be distinguished from those of patients with organic mental disorder by significantly increased energy, better integration, greater use of logic, better problem-solving, higher developmental level, and better depiction of person. Drawings by patients with depression were separated from those of patients with mania by significantly greater use of logic and better problem-solving.

Table V: *Scheffé Post-HOC Comparison of 14 Scales*

Scale	Statistically Significant Differences
1	None of the pairwise comparisons were significant at the $p < .05$ level
2	.. a
3	C>O*; D>O*
4	.. a
5	C>M*, C>O*; D>O*
6	C>O*; D>O*, D>M*
7	C>O*
8	C>O*, C>S*, C>M*; D>O*, D>S*, D>M*
9	D>O*; C>O*, C>M*
10	C>O*, C>M*
11	.. a
12	C>O*; D>O*
13	.. a
14	None of the pairwise comparisons were significant at the $p < .05$ level

* $p < .05$

C = Control; M = Mania; S = Schizophrenia;
D = Depression; O = Organic Mental Disorder

[a]The ANOVA was not statistically significant; therefore, the Scheffé test was not computed.

The depressed group had the most interesting and distinct pattern — its pictures were rated closer to the control group on some scales (energy, integration, logic, realism, problem-solving, developmental level, line quality, and rotation) and closer to the other patient groups on others (color prominence, space, and details). The drawings by depressed patients have less color, fewer details, and less use of space, but they are logical and show adequate problem-solving.

The drawings by patients with schizophrenia were distinguished from those of both the controls and the patients with depression by a statistically significantly lower mean score on problem-solving.   They resembled the pictures by the organic patients in their lack of detail, prominence of color, and color fit. They fell midway between the organic group and the control group in realism, integration, logic, use of space, level of energy, problem-solving, depiction of person, and developmental level.

Similarity Between Patients with Mania and Patients with Schizophrenia

The mean scores of the manic and schizophrenic groups were identical on two scales (prominence of color and space) and virtually identical on seven others. Only on the rotation scale was there a difference of any magnitude. Such similarity may be due to the degree of illness, rather than to the type, since it is known that patients with mania and ones with schizophrenia can appear to have some of the same symptoms if the psychosis is sufficiently severe.

The schizophrenic group was homogeneous in that the patients represented only a small number of possible variations in schizophrenia. Four patients had a discharge diagnosis of "schizophrenia, paranoid type" and three had been described as "chronic." The DSM-III-R (p. 197) states that patients with this type of disorder do not exhibit symptoms of loose associations, incoherence, or grossly disorganized behavior. Their drawings, therefore, should not show low scores on the scales for logic and integration. This, in fact, was the case, for the sample had mean scores which fell between the organic and manic patients on one hand, and the depressed patients and controls on the other.

CONCLUSION

The major strengths of this study include (1) quantifying observations made by writers over the past 100 years; (2) holding the content constant so that major structural differences could be compared; (3) controlling for the time at which the drawings were collected; (4) carefully selecting the patients whose drawings were to be used by applying reliable diagnostic criteria; and (5) staying with a descriptive, empirical approach to the drawings which emphasized the isomorphism with symptoms, rather than attempting to tie the art to theories about underlying purported causes of the illnesses. The principle weaknesses are (1) the use of a small sample; (2) two scales (perseveration and rotation) still need additional refinement to be useful; and (3) the scales use imprecise measurements. Twelve of the 14 scales are moderately high to highly reliable and did distinguish some diagnostic groups from each other. One must be cautious, however, in generalizing about formal elements in the art of all members of a specific clinical group because of the relatively small

sample used in the study. The five patients in the subgroup for schizophrenia, for example, did not represent the range of symptoms associated with this illness (none of their pictures showed evidence of the bizarre thinking considered the hallmark of the disorder).

Perhaps by using these scales, art therapists can develop more effective art-based assessments. This study attempted to avoid using the molecular approach, reducing the subject categories to simply "patient/non-patient," failing to separate state- and trait variables, trying to find a single dimension which was presumably higher in patients, and espousing the interpretive approach before extensive work was done on description. It demonstrated that reliable scales for measuring global formal variables in patients' art could be developed and that they can distinguish between certain psychiatric diagnostic groups. Also, such scales could be useful in future research to determine the degree of change in art due to medication effects or other alterations in psychological state.

This is an abbreviated version of "A Validity Study of the Formal Elements Art Therapy Scale (FEATS) for Diagnostic Information in Patients' Drawings," a doctoral dissertation done at the University of Pittsburgh (Pennsylvania). For a copy of the rating scale and the rating manual, write the author at Route 1, Lake O' Woods, Bruceton Mills, WV 26525, USA.

REFERENCES

1. Anastasi A, Foley J: A survey of the literature on artistic behavior in the abnormal: III. Spontaneous productions. Psychological Monographs 52(6):1-71, 1940.
2. Anastasi A, Foley J: A survey of literature on artistic behavior in the abnormal: IV. Experimental investigations. Journal of General Psychology 23:187-237, 1941.
3. Anastasi A, Foley J: A survey of the literature on artistic behavior in the abnormal: I. Historical and theoretical background. Journal of General Psychology 25:111-142, 1941.
4. Anastasi A, Foley J: An analysis of spontaneous artistic productions by the abnormal. Journal of General Psychology 28:297-313,1943.
5. Guttmann E, Maclay W: Clinical observations on schizophrenic drawings. British Journal of Medical Psychology 16:184-205, 1937.
6. MacGregor J: The Discovery of the Art of the Insane. Princeton University: unpublished doctoral dissertation, 1978.

7. Levy B, Ulman E: Judging psychopathology from paintings. Journal of Abnormal Psychology 72: 182-187, 1967.

8. Wadeson H, Carpenter W: A comparison of art expression in schizophrenic, manic-depressive bipolar, and depressive unipolar patients. Journal of Nervous and Mental Disease 162:334-344, 1976.

9. American Psychiatric Association. Diagnostic and Statistical Manual of Mental Disorders (3rd ed, revised). Washington, DC: American Psychiatric Association, 1987.

10. Tabone C, Gantt L: A new art therapy assessment technique. Unpublished paper, 1989.

11. Scheffé H: A method for judging contrasts in the analysis of variance. Biometrika 40:87-104, 1953.

CHAPTER 17

Art Therapy as a Support Group for Adolescent Muscular Dystrophy Students

Nina Viscardi • *Mathew H.M. Lee*

"No one understands what it's like to have muscular dystrophy, except someone else with muscular dystrophy." This statement was made by David Freeman, a graduate of the Henry Viscardi High School on Long Island and currently a student at the University of California, Berkeley. His comment, frequently expressed by adolescents with muscular dystrophy, magnifies the significance of providing a support system for those facing this life-threatening illness.

Muscular dystrophy (MD) refers to a group of forty similar genetically transmitted neuromuscular diseases, characterized by the progressive deterioration of voluntary skeletal muscles. Duchenne muscular dystrophy (DMD) is the most common and most severe type, striking boys almost exclusively and usually appearing between the ages of two and six. Patients are usually exclusive wheelchair users by age twelve and few survive into their early twenties. About one in every 3,500 boys is affected by this deadly disease. The different forms of MD are passed on by one of three inheritance patterns — dominant, recessive, and X-linked. One third of the cases occur by mutation, with no family history of the disease. Females usually transmit the condition to 50% of their male offspring but are not affected themselves. There can be several boys within one family who have DMD, where there are different fathers.

As their disease progresses, adolescents with MD need increased amounts of physical assistance with most, if not all, activities of daily living. The Henry Viscardi School, a division of NCDS, the National Center for Disability Services, is a private, state-supported facility for educating the severely physically and orthopedically impaired child from preschool through high school. A primary objective of this unique school is to provide the best possible education. As part of that mission, the school believes it must help every student understand and adjust to his/her physical disability. For youngsters who have MD, this is often a difficult and challenging task.

The adolescent who is experiencing the development of an adult body needs to adjust to a new self-image, which includes a need for acceptance by peers of both the same and opposite sexes, as well as a desire for independence. It is in this stage of growing up that the onset of a physical terminal illness, upsetting the normal passage into adulthood, tends to promote dependence at a time when independence is so vital. The loss of autonomy can bring loneliness, anxiety, guilt, pain, and feelings of separation and abandonment from family and friends. An increase in the constant dependence on family members for physical care and assistance becomes a necessary part of life. The fear of bodily invasion from medical procedures such as spinal fusion, tracheostomy and respirators comes at the same time as the gradual loss of independence.

Based on observations by the senior author, the school psychologist, teachers, and support staff at the school, the following behaviors were noted as part of the profile of students with MD:

☐ lack of eye contact during a conversation.
☐ speaking in a low, whispering voice, even when they are capable of normal-volume speech.
☐ emotional and social withdrawal from peers and adults.
☐ difficulty breathing when talking.
☐ difficulty maintaining a task when tired.
☐ not asking for assistance when they need it to complete a task and are capable of asking.
☐ giving one-word answers to questions when they are capable of using complete sentences.

The school is concerned about their social withdrawal and their willingness to ask for assistance from others when necessary. Withdrawal may be caused by rage, anger, or depression related to MD or a variety of other factors, such as:

- [ ] a fear of social situations.
- [ ] inability to take a breath.
    feeling constantly fatigued by breathing, talking, or moving even slightly.
- [ ] not wanting to ask for help.
- [ ] feeling humiliated.
- [ ] feeling guilty by the burden they cause others.

The staff is accepting of all of these feelings. The goal is to encourage students to recognize their feelings and to learn how to accept them.

METHOD

Because of the unusual number of students with MD at the school, a group was formed in response to these problems. It was decided that using art therapy might help to encourage more positive behaviors. It was also decided that the group would include girls who had MD but not specifically DMD, and to include students in grades 7 to 12. Basic principles of art therapy were used in this project:

- [ ] Create initially when the student first comes into the group.

- [ ] Develop a keen sense of observation while the group is working: Take note of how they engage in working with the art materials. Do they have difficulty starting or stopping? Are they able to ask for help when materials are out of reach or whenever they need assistance? Do they talk to others?

- [ ] Keep notes of verbal and nonverbal responses and interactions for each session.

- [ ] Develop a strategy of questioning which constantly redirects questions to the art work.

- [ ] Students become engaged with their artistic creating, which affords the therapist the opportunity to observe their social behavior.

During the first meeting of the group, students were presented with a choice of art materials and suggestions for possible projects in order to give them a sense of control. For their first project, they chose clay and completed a family sculpture, one of the diagnostic and treatment methods developed by Keyes.[1] This involved a directed meditation which resulted in a clay model of earliest relationships. It contained clues to present problems and conflicts. The brief explanation was given somewhat as follows:

When you were a child, you received instructions from your family on how to be "you." One way of exploring what these messages were is by sculpting what your family felt like when you were growing up. What we are investigating is how you came to think about yourself in the ways you do and perhaps limit yourself in the ways you do. The idea is not to make a figure, but how the person "felt" to you. When you have sculpted each family member in turn, including yourself, put them in relation to each other to show who seemed closer to you and who was far away emotionally.

The analysis of the family sculpture gave each group member a chance to tell his/her story. One by one, students placed their sculptures in the center of the group. The student who made the sculpture listened, while the rest of the group commented on what they saw. For example: *...you placed your father in the farthest corner of the sculpture...who in the family was touching or not touching...you made yourself the tiniest of all, even smaller than your younger brother...your mother is all sharp angles...you forgot to include yourself...*, etc. Once the group has finished commenting, the student is then able to talk and comment on the significance of what he did. This provides insight to the creator, who might not have seen that which was obvious to others. It also pro-vides insight into how the student behaves within the group.

The second project chosen by the group was sculpture, using light-weight foam core board. The senior author suggested that they work as a group and display their finished sculpture in the school lobby so that everyone would be aware of their meetings and art work. They decided to each work individually and then to assemble and arrange their work together as a finished sculpture. This involved making a decision as a group. Foam core board was light enough to enable the physically weakest students, with extremely limited range of motion, to handle large pieces.

When each student had finished, they took turns placing their sculptures in the center of the group. Again, the student who made the sculpture listened, while the group commented on what they saw. For example: *your sculpture is very flat...your sculpture is symmetrical and looks very organized...your sculpture looks like a plane about to take off...your sculpture has lots of pieces piled up on top of each other as if there is something hiding underneath...your sculpture looks like a tower, it's so tall and thin...your sculpture feels religious, like a temple or a church.* One student's sculpture, titled, actually was a three-foot jet surrounded by a 4.5-inch wall, preventing it from ever taking off. Another reached 14 feet high, made of narrow rectangular strips, supported by a sturdy base. Through dialogue, this student shared that his sculpture was really him. His family was the strong base and he was the part reaching up to the clouds.

RESULTS

Specific behaviors were found to be changing, both during the time when the students were making their projects and during the talking and sharing time:

□ Students made eye contact with each other and with adults.

□ Students initiated verbal interaction. At the beginning, they were very hesitant and needed constant verbal cues and coaxing, often giving only one-word answers. During the family sculpture, some students offered no verbal responses at all. When asked to comment, they would not answer. When coaxed, they gave only one-word answers. Gradually, they were able to give one-word answers about another student's work and, finally, they were able to talk throughout the project, both to others and about themselves.

□ Asking an adult or another student to pass material which was out of reach. During the foam core board sculpture, several students were observed staring at a piece which they wanted but did not ask for help. Gradually, they were able to ask for what they wanted, instead of just staring at it.

□ Students were able to respond to others and give support and encouragement to feelings which they had experienced.

CONCLUSIONS

Art therapy has great promise of bringing students out of their social withdrawal. Painting, drawing, and sculpting serve as a therapeutic expression of themes which reflect inner conflict in the present moment. These particular images provide a deeper understanding of the underlying dynamic, and are a valuable tool for psychological assessments. It also encourages these severely physically challenged students to ask for help when they need it.

This study suggests that the application of the principles of art therapy to students with MD may be important in helping them overcome social and emotional withdrawal. While the evidence clearly points in this direction, further research is necessary to verify these findings in other settings and to address other questions:

□ Is the increase in social interaction exhibited in the art-therapy process generalized to other social settings?

□ Can this process be applied to other progressive disabilities, such as children with cancer or AIDS?

□ Can the principles of art therapy be applied to other disciplines in the school environment?

□ Can the process of art therapy be applied to the increased social interaction between disabled and non-disabled peers?

□ Are there similar themes in the art work of terminally ill adolescents?

REFERENCES

1. Keyes MF: Inward Journey: Art as Psychotherapy. La Salle, IL: Open Court, 1983.

2. Siegel B.: Love, Medicine and Miracles. New York: Harper and Row, 1988.

3. The Arts in Psychotherapy 11:25-28. Ankad International Inc, 1984.

CHAPTER 18

The Art Therapy Concept:
An Alternative View

Joanna Gburek

Art therapy is a form of psychotherapy defined as a healing influence of one psyche on the other. This definition is based on ethical maximalism, and it rules out subjective treatment of a patient.

Art expresses the creative status of contemporary man, and it is understood that artistic activity brings about enhanced values. Thus, the artist is a creator of values.

This discussion focuses on visual art. Let us reflect on the arguments commonly put forth when demonstrating the positive role of art therapy:

● Artistic creation stimulates self-recognition and the self-realization process.

● Creative forces are present in each individual, and it is never too late to activate them. The goal is to achieve a wholly creative personality which is favorable for fighting illness.

● A patient finds relief in his/her own artistic creation, suggested by a therapist.

● Creation is the only way for some individuals to escape their loneliness.

The scene: An open-air sculpture for blind and deaf-mute persons is organized by sculptor W. Janasz. Clay is the material; *Portrait* is the subject. Sculptures larger than life-size are being created. This scene, with disabled people, emotionally involved, creating their huge sculptures, is exceptionally moving. The commentary to the film made to publicize this event includes the following statement: *Such wonderful works are being made because these people have no idea how difficult it is.*

This example can be seen as a starting point for the criticism of an idea of the artist-therapist who makes people aware of their potential creativity — needed, but not yet realized. The disabled sculptors have been treated light-heartedly, like children who should be praised for evidence of creativity.

In spite of the optimism of artists involved in art therapy, one must accept the existence of great difficulties in bringing the values carried by art to people who, in many cases, are completely unprepared for these values. What is meant here is the majority of so-called 'ordinary people,' consumers of popular culture, i.e. the culture prepared in a special way to their order. A danger of kitsch experience being the reaction to a real work of art, or one's own kitsch-like creation analyzed with no regard to the actual intention of the patient, can be the consequence of treating art as a panacea for all problems.

It often happens that the patient finally pours paint on canvas in a *spontaneous* gesture only to give the therapist pleasure or for fear of losing face. The therapist may decide to suggest an easy subject, which is a kind of mishandling and shows a lack of respect for the patient. (S)he may also use his/her experience with contemporary art, which may not be understood. The author's experience in working with elderly patients has shown that accepting impractical art and artistic activity poses the greatest difficulty for them. The artist's anxiety, which is recorded through the act of creation, is a kind of self-therapy, in the common search for the meaning of human existence; it gives him/her the sense of self-salvation. But the usefulness of contemporary artistic achievements in therapy could be questioned, since the perception of this art is difficult as regards both its aesthetic aspect and extra-aesthetic message.

Elderly patients at the Geriatric Hospital in Ivry are advised to take art classes. Some of them, rather than spending their time alone in their rooms and thus losing their sense of reality, find their way to the fine-arts studio, where they create paintings and drawings. Exhibitions are organized in a prestigious Paris gallery. Some patients continue to paint after returning home; others, following discharge, visit the studio regularly, despite transportation difficulties.[1]

One particular fact has drawn the author's attention: The artistic activity in which these elderly people participate does not protect them from feelings of loneliness and dejection. They come back to the fine-arts studio to enjoy the attention and kindness shown to them there. Art may become a pretext under which relationships between people are formed, but it cannot substitute for human interaction and friendship.

The author is attempting to show that love and being understood by others are most important to the patient, regardless of whether he is physically or mentally disabled. It is not the *creative* potential which should be triggered to return the patient to health, but the *humanistic* one, which first should be activated within the therapist him/herself.

All matters that are of the greatest importance to man take place within the sphere of human relationships. The natural ability to communicate with others proves his maturity, in the same way that his involvement in the world of values does. To be human means to have connections to other persons, and to values.

According to E. Dreifuss-Kattan, desirable features of the therapist's personality include the ability to adapt to a current situation, capacity for self-control, profound self-recognition, his identification with the patient, professional competence, and the ability to maintain therapeutic distance.[2] El Fuller Torrey speaks of the healing influence of naturalness, warmth, and empathy.[3]

The author finds the concept of therapeutic distance somewhat disturbing. The characteristics noted by Fuller Torrey would seem to be more conducive to communication. The features of the therapist's attitude that facilitate communication, such as self-command (understood as a form of love), hope for far-reaching contact with others (even in unfavorable conditions), trust, and enabling mutual contact on an equal basis, should be the most natural ones. Otherwise, we deal with spurious conversation, and with spurious therapy.

What is meant by *spurious therapy*? The patient has not been treated openly and sincerely, and the picture of the world which has been suggested to him has no real foundation. The therapist cannot support the model which he designed with his own behavior. Even if a situation of this kind leads to effects considered positive by observers or even by the patient himself, it should not be accepted, since, in doing so,

we would declare for the *lesser evil* principle, which is contradictory to the ethical maximalism assumed herein. A man morally irresponsible in his own life cannot help others, although he may create the illusion of doing so. A man unworthy of trust should not place himself in a situation where he is given someone's confidence. This rule refers in particular to therapists dealing with people whose choices and priorities are specifically determined by their illness. Illness and suffering intensify the need for love; hence, this love can be indispensable in therapy. *To be means to love* becomes an imperative.[4]

In discussing *art therapy*, one must consider the place of an artist and art in the proposed therapy model. The conviction of universality of beneficial contacts with art has already been criticized. So have been declarations of the following kind: *I am an artist; I know that art is something absolute, like religion. It refers to the most profound existential matters. Creative forces of man are most completely and distinctly expressed in it. I have found that art has self-therapeutic values, so why don't we suggest it to patients? Creation has a healing influence."*

The author proposes a different declaration as obligatory: *I am an artist. I am aware of my limited usefulness in our struggle against suffering, and this disturbs my attempts to fully use my creative potential. I do believe that my deep affection for others may give them the strength to fight illness, or at least to light up their faces for a while. It may happen that there will be a place for a conversation about art and for joint artistic activity during my contacts with patients, which is justifiable, for art is a remarkable part of my life.*

In the first case, artistic creation is used as a way of obtaining an intended effect; in the latter, it exists as one of the most natural human abilities, wherein the artist is a person who is predestined and ready to act for the other's benefit. This attitude is possible due to the assumption that life is the work of art, requiring constant creative forming and corrections being made with considerable effort, and with mere hope for ultimate perfection.

One could cite Dufrenne's thesis on art being the cause of ethical attitude, including approval of the model, *life as a work of art*. Ethos of art is *the ethos of the individual who cultivates arts, a way of life in accordance with which he acts and behaves as a man. This sublimation of a human body is the beginning of ethics, an indispensable condition of ethical attitude towards the other man.*[5]

Dufrenne asks as well: *Can I be really free and happy when the others are not free and happy? And how can the poor, starving and oppressed people cultivate the art of life?*[6] This question leads him to the following conclusion: The aim of artistic activity is the sense of community; it is the only instrument that makes true life, *the art of life*, possible.

One can now see how close the anarchistic concept of art is to the personalistic idea of communication, with its ethos of community rather than the ethos of competition.

In summary: The idea of an artist-therapist revealing unrealized creative potential to an ill individual in order to help fight the illness has been criticized. The author has attempted to prove that such an assumption often leads to an instrumental use of art, and this kind of attitude towards art means automatic elimination of all that is brought about with it. This may be the reason for art therapists' reluctance to answer questions concerning the moment when art appears in the process of art-therapy.

The mention of spurious therapy is aimed at drawing the reader's attention to an important and, in the author's opinion, decisive role of love and friendship in all relationships between people — in particular, ill people. *To help means to love* has become a rule.

Finally, it should be stated that being an artist and a therapist is a difficult but still feasible task for those who derive their strength from trust in man and in art.

REFERENCES

1. Colin-Cyvoct B: Artistic expression in elderly subjects during chronic hospitalization. Medicographia 4(1):27-30, 1982.

2. Dreifuss-Kattan E: Praxis der Klinischen Kunstterapie. Bern: Hans Huber, 1986.

3. Fuller Torrey E: Czarownicy i Psychiatrzy (The Mind Game, Witch Doctors and Psychiatrists). Warsaw: PIW, 1981.

4. Mounier E: Wprowadzenie do egzystencjalizmów (An Introduction to Existentialism). Cracow: ZNAK, 1964.

5. Dufrenne M: O Ethosie Sztuki (On Ethics of Art). Warsaw: PWN, 1985.

6. Dufrenne M: Place de l'experience esthetique dans la culture. Esthetique et Philosophie III, 1981.

CHAPTER 19

Art Journaling: A Wellness Model

Marianne Hieb

Journal-art is a meditative modality combining aspects and learnings from the worlds of fine arts; art therapy; relaxation, visualization and stress- reduction techniques; journaling disciplines; spiritual practice and, ultimately, from holistic medicine and wellness. It is a process utilizing simple art materials and facilitated by an art therapist, with a resultant nonverbal experience of accessing a person's inner wisdom at the service of wellness

Over the past ten years, the journal-art has been introduced and facilitated in workshops and retreats sponsored by the Wellness Center of Our Lady of Lourdes Medical Center in Camden, New Jersey. Clients come to the center seeking to move in a positive way toward insight and responsibility for the self.

Sessions using this carefully focused nonverbal modality can help a client to identify, set goals around and, ideally, be moved to make life-enhancing choices and changes in personal, relational, or environmental arenas.

The theoretical framework in which journal-art is presented is wellness. Pilch defines wellness as: *an ever-expanding experience of pleasurable and purposeful living which you and I, especially as motivated by spiritual values and beliefs, create and direct for ourselves in any way we choose.*[1] This choice for life, this deep inner wisdom, exists and can be accessed by a person who comes with a willingness or desire for greater life.

This wisdom can be revealed through a felt body sense as described by Gendlin.[2] It can be discovered and illumined in images that arise in our minds, as was plumbed in the lifework of Jung.

Tauraso[3] illustrates in a simple system these three aspects of our wholeness, our wellness, in three triangular formations (Fig. 1):

In a subsequent diagram, the author gathered the data from Fig. 1 into the mandala, ancient symbol of wholeness, to show how we are unified, centered, dynamic: all aspects of the self present simultaneously (Fig. 2).

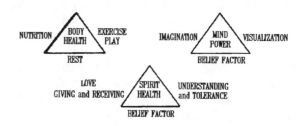

Figure 1: *Aspects of our wholeness, as pictured by Tauraso.*

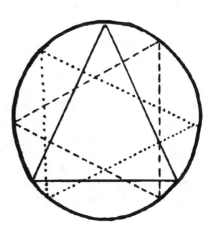

Figure 2:   _____ = Body; . . . . = Mind; _ _ _ _ = Spirit

Someone engaged in the process of journal-art, then, would be a person challenged to be present to all these aspects of the self and the information and imagery arising from the realms of body, mind and spirit.

The client is focused toward a felt sense of his or her body: in a specific way, to begin to slow down, to be conscious and generous with breathing, to identify quality of muscle tension, to be present environmentally and come to rest.

S/he would be invited into the realm of visualization, allowing rich personal and collective imagery to arise.

On the spiritual level, s/he would be challenged to be present to a belief factor: love, of the self and of larger relationships, in order to choose change or seek healing from a place of freedom.

Finally, the invitation would be to be present to these levels of wisdom, to be open to a movement toward change, growth and healing, and to respond with a commitment to some action that would move the client in that direction.

What is the process that facilitates these aspects? A person is seated in an area where pastels, drawing paper and writing implements are available. There would be an introduction, acknowledging body sense, breath and being present. A visualization using the thought of *color* would begin to free the client's imagery into an atmosphere that allows newness to arise, perhaps in a surprising way. Eventually, the client is invited to be present to his or her life as it is now. A meditative question would be posed to help surface in a concrete way aspects of the person's life to which s/he begins to assign a personal color significance.

Although there are many important color theories as well as an archetypal sense of colors, it is the author's experience that people also have an individual color vocabulary that arises from their *own* life experiences. This needs to be validated in order that the limiting, judgmental self that tends to rear up in moments of invitational creativity does not constrict the expression (e.g. "I'd better not use red; it means anger." "I'll stay away from black; they might think I'm depressed," etc.) The invitation to make marks on the paper should be as unconditional and safe as possible.

Sufficient psychic and physical space must be provided in order to allow free expression. A stated time limit continues the theme of safety and structure in the face of what could be sudden unbounded imagery, energy, emotion, and expression.

After the person dialogues with the question nonverbally, using the pastels, s/he is asked to end the first "drawing" and is again brought to a place of visualization, using aspects of color in a mental imagery exercise to deepen the sense of a personally discerned color as energy and healing. The client then is invited to a second drawing, with the focus being more intentionally on a deeper inner awareness

of life-places within which there is a call toward change or growth or healing.

Then, there is a "listening to" that which has been expressed, and a time for quiet written journaling to bring to clarity the nonverbal expression. At this point, that deep inner wisdom seems to emerge in a twilight sense of awakening where we know the edges of our lives that are healing, or are in need of movement or attention. What we have been waiting to tell ourselves is right there, and we are in a structure and attitude to listen.

Eventually, there is an invitation to share verbally in the one-to-one or group context. This frequently brings the revelation into action in the shared acknowledgment that "this is what is going on in my life," "this is relationally where I am healing," "this is where I sense a call to change," etc.

In the written journaling that follows the making of both drawings, the client is invited to look at his or her drawing using some formal elements from the world of visual art — line quality, use of space, intensity of color, size relationships, placement of forms, etc. — in order to expand possible learnings.

One woman, diagnosed with multiple sclerosis (then in remission), holding a responsible position and leading a full life, tearfully shared this after completing the exercise: "When you suggested that I look at my drawing in light of those design elements, I was amazed at how large I had depicted my pain. What I'm struck with now is how much energy I must expend in holding down my experience of that pain, pretending it isn't there. I'm grateful to see how large it really is. I need to consider that and make some choices for myself that allow me more rest and self nurturance."

In drawings by people who are elderly and are experiencing some diminishment in body or mind, what frequently happens is a connection with a spiritual reassurance. Themes of the goodness of life, a sense of something beyond, of how, on reflection, life reveals its meaning, illustrate the opening up and access to that spiritual reality — a belief factor, a universal wholeness.

The artist-poet William Blake tells us, ". . . in your own Bosom you wear your Heaven and Earth and all you behold, tho it appears Without, it is Within, in your Imagination . . ."[4]

The world of art and the world of medicine weave in this healing moment, this healing modality that leads individuals within to their own life force and outward to a lived expression of wellness that finds expression in their own lives, in the context of their families and communities, in the life of our world, in the larger life of the shared environment of our earth.

REFERENCES

1. Pilch JJ: Your Invitation to Full Life. Minneapolis: Winston Press, 1981.
2. Gendlin E: Focusing. New York: Bantam Books, 1982.
3. Tauraso NM: How to Benefit from Stress. Maryland: Hidden Valley Press, 1979.
4. Erdman DV: The Poetry and Prose of William Blake. New York, Doubleday, 1965.

SUGGESTED READING

1. Ardell DB: High Level Wellness. Berkeley, CA: Ten Speed Press, 1986.
2. Collier G: Form Space and Vision. New Jersey: Prentiss Hall, 1972.
3. Emeth EV, Greenhut JH: The Wholeness Handbook. New York: Continuum Publishing Co, 1991.
4 Franck F: The Zen of Seeing. New York: Vintage Books, 1973.
5. May R: The Courage to Create. New York: WW Norton, 1980.
6. Progoff I: At a Journal Workshop. New York: Dialogue House Library, 1975.

CHAPTER 20

Transformations:
Visual Arts and Hospice Care

C. Regina Kelley

When confronting death, a person often responds with a profound search for wholeness, healing life's wounds and making peace with the world. The arts are a vehicle for self-expression and, therefore, a significant tool for transformation during the dying process. The arts assist patients, families, and staff to understand the whole of their own lives, as well as the profound journey towards death which they share. In this way, the arts uniquely fit the mission of hospice care, which is to assist terminally ill patients and their families in maintaining the highest possible quality of life as long as life lasts.

Hospice care generally enters a person's life when a doctor assesses the patient as terminally ill, with less than six months to live. Thereafter, medical care is palliative and medical personnel are joined by hospice professionals and volunteers who offer a range of services for emotional, physical, and spiritual needs. The arts address all of these areas, functioning as an animator, that which endows life or spirit. The arts reawaken the senses often ignored during long illnesses. They address what is possible rather than what is lost. They bring beauty, joy, and every form of expression into a time which we often assume to be unbearably painful.

The arts are an agent of self-expression and, therefore, are transforming in nature. The artist begins with an ephemeral idea — a vision or possibility. Then the artist faces the blank page and, in doing so, his or her fears as well. As the vision meets concrete reality of materials, the artist sheds preconceptions and steps into the unknown. The reality of the evolving art work is a product of growth and discovery. The artist is empowered not only by self-expression, but by tangible nonverbal knowledge. This seed of transformation is present in every art-making process and can help to prepare patients for their final transformation, death. The lessons of letting go and experiencing the present moment are an invaluable component of hospice care.

One patient, Maria, exemplifies the potential of art to transform. Maria, 39, came to the hospice homeless and dying of AIDS. In the arts program, she began drawing butterflies, a universal symbol of transformation. She began to feel fully alive for the first time, and responded to kindness by making gifts of drawings and painted T-shirts for everyone who had befriended or helped her. In her former life as a drug addict, she had stolen from friends and family. Her true spirit of generosity healed many relationships. As her artistic knowledge developed, she began a "master work," an autobiographical journal-sketchbook that included drawings of her daily feelings and experiences, photographs, mementos, letters to her family, and journal entries. Through her art, she found a new way to express both her joy and the pain that once drove her to drugs. It was her hope to eventually publish her book so that "people can understand people with AIDS and be less fearful." Maria was a high school drop-out with a twenty-year drug history; during her last year she became an artist, craftsperson, and author.

Maria exemplifies the two motivations to make art that commonly arise: the desire to summarize one's life experiences and to make gifts for loved ones. Participatory arts offer the opportunity for a patient to resume the role of a participating family member. They are a significant means of nonverbal communication — offering love and, often, forgiveness. Most importantly, they are a way for the patient to reclaim his or her power — to say, *I am.*

The arts function at three levels of comprehension and use in hospice care. Many patients and families believe that lifelong hobbies and craft work are no longer possible with the patients' diminished physical strength. This can result in a loss of identity, as our culture often associates self-worth with work. Many familiar activities can be adapted to new physical circumstances by using lighter weight tools and materials. Simpler crafts can be substituted for complex projects. Often, four hands — a volunteer or family member assisting — can make a special project possible. For instance, a young man in his thirties with AIDS was well-known for his oriental-rug avocation. As he neared death, he began a cross-stitch embroidery project for his mother which he was able to plan and execute with assistance during his last days, although he was feverish and nearly blind. In this first level, patients are invited to continue working with activities they cherish, albeit in a new way.

Mrs. O., an artist and homemaker in her late sixties, wanted to continue in her profession as well as make gifts for her family, since much of her work focused on her family. She was able to complete two crosses for a daughter who was to be ordained to the ministry. The process became one that united friends and family. When hospice care began, Mrs. O. was receiving chemotherapy and was extremely weak. She began drawing and designing the crosses. A neighbor cut the wood in his shop, the author did some of the machine sanding, and Mrs. O. completed the silver work on the first cross as some of her strength returned. She began the second cross, incorporating a design that her other daughter found on her travels in Europe. A jeweler-friend completed the cross by setting a sapphire in the center. Mrs. O. was able to see the finished work and present it to her daughter the week before she died (Fig. 1). The hospice provided encouragement and coordinated the efforts of participants.

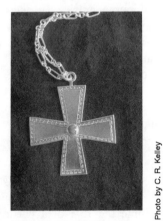

Figure 1: Mrs. O.'s cross.

Photo by C. R. Kelley

The second level is to learn a new art form. It is easy to forget during illness that we all love to learn and grow. Suitable techniques and art experiences can be designed for virtually every level of physical capability. Simply by handling unfamiliar materials the senses are stimulated. Concentration can relieve pain and anxiety as one's focus is directed to the new experience. Patients develop a new sense of confidence as their creativity becomes apparent. A young AIDS patient who collected paintings and prints of clowns was delighted to create his own painting. An

elderly woman enjoyed creating abstract watercolor paintings as thank-you notes.

Finally, art can lead to a profound expression of one's life. This can take many forms, such as a book, a painting, or a video which fulfills patients' desires to collect their experiences — their wisdom in a concrete form. Annie was a 31-year-old ALS patient living in an intensive-care unit. Her only form of communication was to blink her eyes to indicate yes or no, and she was receiving various medications which affected her concentration. She was an anthropologist/archaeologist, and wished to make a significant art work to challenge her keen intelligence, which was locked in a non-functioning body. As a hospice artist, the author invited her to make a traditional native American shield that united her goals of contemplating the important things in her life and continuing to learn about native American customs and artifacts. The author served as her hands, described the process, and framed as many choices as possible in questions that could be answered with a yes or no. Annie also painstakingly spelled out important information letter by letter. The resulting shield (Fig. 2) contains significant animals in her life, the mountains she loved to hike, and an important dream image of an owl. She dreamed that at night her heart burst open and she became an owl that could fly around the hospital. Like many of us, she was very frightened of death and did not wish to speak about it or make decisions while she could still communicate about resuscitation or other details surrounding death.

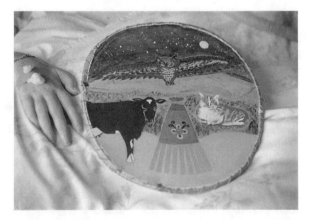

Figure 2: "Annie's Shield."   Photo by C. R. Kelley

One day, however, her breathing machine malfunctioned and she had a near-death experience in which she felt herself to be floating in a night sky. The shield was changed to depict the night sky and was then hung at the foot of her bed, reminding her that death could be peaceful. She died two weeks later.

The arts offer families a way to create special memories and conversations during the dying process and a way to remember and grieve during bereavement. So often our imperfect communication patterns become painfully inadequate during times of crisis. Families in the midst of anticipatory grief find it a relief to be offered an activity to do together. It creates an emotionally neutral situation and family members are gratified to find that making art can be fun, can initiate new conversations and allow participants to assist each other in loving ways. One family gathered in their grandfather's sick room with three generations present. Each member made a paper collage of a favorite memory of grandfather. The collages were united into a paper 'quilt.' This day became a special memory for each one, and the quilt will be a treasured heirloom. Art works like this one can also be part of the bereavement process, uniting a family, sparking remembrances of activities and qualities of the loved one who has died.

A hospice ministers to medical personnel and to its own staff and volunteers as well. Everyone who works with the dying needs to come to terms with his or her own beliefs and understanding of death. The arts are a means to explore this issue and to restore harmony during times of intense grief. Caregivers need multiple ways to remember their experiences with patients. The intensity of caring and resulting feelings of loss when death occurs can become a burden unless we realize all that we receive from the people we assist. The arts allow caregivers to take a moment to honor the special people who pass through their lives, to document the moments of heart-to-heart communication in which patient becomes teacher. In the sculpture, *Annie and The Owl,* the author was able to explore the transformation of death and honor this remarkable young woman, telling both of their stories in the sculpture (Fig. 3).

Art can also be a significant means to build community among people. At the Connecticut Hospice, an in-residence facility, the entire staff helped to create a bronze sculpture. Staff members, from the janitor to the president, were asked to create

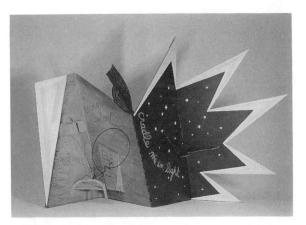

Figure 3: "Annie and the Owl."   Photo and sculpture by C. R. Kelley

small wax sculptures that symbolized how they renewed themselves after a difficult day in the hospice. Responses were both varied and beautifully similar. A nurse discovered that she, a volunteer, a patient, and a doctor all turned to music for solace, yet each pictured it differently. With a jeweler, the author then integrated the wax images into a column that will support a bell. The entire sculpture will be placed in an outdoor garden designed by the staff. The soothing sounds of the bell and the rich imagery will serve to remind the staff of the many ways they can care for themselves and each other. With the arts helping to create a supportive environment, staff members are able to provide ongoing compassionate care for patients without feeling depleted.

The courage of the human spirit is never more evident than when people choose to take creative risks, to transcend physical limitations, to examine their lives through the arts in order to meet death with equanimity. The art work, or gift, becomes a visible symbol of their love and will, a triumph in every case. The whole process of making art is healing, as patients, families and staff experience well-being and heightened awareness during the great mystery of death.

ACKNOWLEDGEMENT

The author is grateful to jeweler Melinda Bridgeman for her assistance in creating the bronze sculpture for the garden at Connecticut Hospice.

CHAPTER 21

Imaging and Drawing as Treatment Vehicles in Art Therapy

Robert B. Kent • Wayne Woodward

This chapter briefly outlines the present status of psychology-immunology and mind/body healing as it relates to investigating new experiences and responsibilities for expressive therapists.

Descarte's famous motto, *Cogito, ergo sum,* is one of the most influential statements in the history of Western philosophy. Cartesian philosophy's dictum of the separation of the mind and body has been a source of continuing argument. Recent studies have seriously challenged Cartesian philosophy. There appears to be conclusive evidence that there is a systems unity to the functioning of mind/body and environment. Recent studies have investigated the intriguing world of psychobiologicial-immunological functioning.[1-3] The use of a variety of creative mental processes — self-hypnosis, imaging, drawings — in conjunction with a positive life style and enlightened medical procedures can radically improve health.

Can the mind — by concentration, meditation, hypnosis, imagery, and drawing — alter the physical status of the body? First, let us look at the never-ending question of the validity and proof of the entity we call the mind. It has been noted that the brain has $2^{100,000,000}$ active connections among its nerve cells.[1] This is the number 2 multiplied by itself a hundred million times. This means that there are more possible mental states in each person's brain than there are atoms in the known universe. This number is staggering. Can one speculate that the energy field generated from this configuration is capable of physically and philosophically assuming a condition we call *mind*? If the answer is in the affirmative, then the above position makes sense.

As we shall see, belief can have an energetic force and, when used creatively, can be an effective part of the therapeutic process.

There are many excellent books on mind-body healing, including two by Rossi which are excellent for both beginning and experienced therapists.[1-11] A major beginning point in Rossi's writings about mind-body healing is the word *transduction,* which refers to the conversion or transformation of energy from one form to another.

A windmill transduces wind energy into the mechanical energy of the turning blades. If the mechanical energy of the turning blades is attached to a generator, it is transduced into electrical energy, which can in turn be transduced into light energy by an electric bulb. In the typical clinical application of biofeedback techniques, the biological energy of the body's muscle tension can be transduced into visible information of a measuring device that enables the subject to alter his muscle tone. These examples, together with the basic concepts of information, communication and cybernetic theories, have led to a view of all biological life as a system of information transduction.[1]

Transduction generally utilizes aspects of hypnosis. It can be safely said that many aspects of therapeutic healing involving imagery, creative imagination, movement, drawing, etc., use hypnosis, directly or indirectly.

It is well-known that hypnosis can be self-induced. Aside from Hollywood's romanticized depiction, we see hypnosis employed in many commonplace activities, e.g. the high jumper visualizing his approach to the bar; waking up at a specific time; programming oneself to curtail smoking, eating sweets, etc. Bowers says that the:

... tendency to split etiological factors of disease into either psychic or somatic components, though heuristic for many purposes, nevertheless perpetuates, at least implicitly, a mind-body dualism that has defied rational solution for centuries. Perhaps what we need is a new formulation of this ancient problem, one that does not presuppose a formidable gap between the separate realities of mind and body.[12]

A major key to understanding this process is to see it as a unified concept of mind/body in which information is a dynamic communicative process.[12] The body is then seen as an interlocking network of informational systems — genetic, immunological, hormonal, etc. Further, each system has its own codes, and the idea of the use of transmission of information between systems necessitates some kind of a transducer which permits the code of one system, e.g. genetic, to be translated into the code of another system, which could be immunological. Bowers asks the intriguing question: How is information received and processed at a somatic level, and vice versa? He proposes that deep hypnosis is an important variable in this transduction process which can result in the start of healing.

Rossi has explained hypnosis as a bridge between the conscious and subconscious, a part of the worlds within worlds which we interpret as an evolutionary process of energized information, growing exponentially, which assumes a life force of its own. This could explain how communication information can be directed in both a macro- and micro manner. Information enhancement (energized by hypnosis, for example) can indeed be directed to communicate with the psychophysiological mechanisms of the immune system. The authors hypothesize that information directed by the expressive therapist to communicate with the mechanism of the immune system can be more powerful when the therapist suggests that the patient visually give shape, color, texture, and velocity to their commands.[13, 14] This can be a more powerful process when the patient is encouraged to visually illustrate this experience.

Recent discoveries of the functions of the limbic-hypothalamic system are of increasing importance to art therapists and expressive therapists. This system of the brain is the major mind-body connector modulating the biological activity of the autonomic, endocrine, and immune systems in response to mental suggestions, beliefs, imagery, and drawings.

The limbic-hypothalamic system is quite complex. It is hoped that a brief description of its main parts and functions will give the reader a basic understanding of its role in mind-body immunology.

Hypothalamus: The portion of the forebrain that forms the floor and part of its side. It has a role in the mechanisms that activate, control, and integrate peripheral autonomic mechanisms, endocrine activity, and many bodily functions (hunger, body temperature).

Pituitary: A small, oval gland attached to the base of the brain, connected to the hypothalamus by a stalk. Sometimes called the *master gland*, the pituitary affects the entire endocrine system through secretion of several hormones.

Autonomic Nervous System (ANS): A portion of the nervous system concerned with the regulation of the cardiac muscle, smooth muscle tissue, and the glandular system. The ANS regulates such things as the rate of heartbeat and digestion.

Endocrine System: This pertains to any of the endocrine glands or ductless glands which secrete internally — thyroid or adrenal, Islands of Langherhans in the pancreas, ovaries (female), testes (male). The secretions pass directly into the bloodstream from the cells of the gland.

Immune System: The anatomy and functions are generally understood but incredibly complex, and many of its interactions are considered mysterious. It is defined primarily in terms of its functions in resisting invading organisms or toxins. The main defenses are the skin, thymus, lymph nodes, and humoral activity from bone marrow.

Selye's monumental research has clearly shown that mental stress, for example, activates the limbic-hypothalamic system of the brain, which converts the neural messages of mind into the neurohormonal messenger molecules of the body.[15] These messenger molecules can then excite the endocrine system to produce steroid hormones that travel into the nucleus of a variety of body cells which can modulate the character of genes. In this dynamic process, the messenger genes can direct the cells to produce a variety of molecules that have the capacity to regulate metabolism, growth, various cellular activity levels, degrees of sexuality, and, most important, the immune response in maintaining wellness and attacking involving organisms and toxins.

New discoveries in the science the of limbic-hypothalamic system are of great excitement and importance to art- and expressive therapists. They open new vistas for therapeutic applications. They accentuate the art in therapy by challenging the therapist to deeply explore the emotions inherent in art expression of both the therapist and the patient. It is truly a creative endeavor, in that the various forms graphic expressions develop are by their very nature therapeutic. The authors believe that the making of art can be healing on both a spiritual and a molecular level.

REFERENCES

1. Rossi E: The Psychobiology of Mind-Body Healing. New York: WW Norton, 1986.
2. Grof S: The Adventure of Self-Discovery. Albany: State University of New York, 1988.
3. Siegel B: Love, Medicine and Miracles. New York: Harper & Row, 1986.
4. Rossi E, Cheek D: Mind-Body Therapy. New York: WW Norton, 1988.
5. Locke S, Colligan D: The Healer Within: The New Medicine of Mind and Body. New York: Mentor, 1987.
6. Benson H: The Relaxation Response. New York: Avon, 1975.
7. Borysenko J: Minding The Body, Minding the Mind. Reading, PA: Addison-Wesley, 1987.
8. Siegel B: Peace, Love & Healing. New York: Harper & Row, 1989.
9. Gendlin E: Focusing. New York: Bantam, 1981.
10. Gazzaniga M, Le Doux J: The Integrated Mind. New York: Plenum, 1978.
11. Soskis D: Teaching Self-Hypnosis. New York: WW Norton, 1986.
12. Bowers K: Hypnosis: An informational approach. Annals of the New York Academy of Sciences 296:222-237, 1977.
13. Kent R: Genesa: An adjunct to art therapy in the treatment of drug and alcohol abuse clients. *In* Einstein S (ed), Drug and Alcohol Use: Issues and Factors. New York: Plenum, 1989.
14. Kent R, Woodward W: Varieties of internal imaging through visualization techniques. Unpublished paper, University of Georgia, 1990.
15. Selye H: Stress Without Stress. New York: Signet, 1974.

SUGGESTED READING

1. Citrenbaum CM, et al: Modern Clinical Hypnosis for Habit Control. New York: WW Norton, 1985.
2. Cousins N: Head First: The Biology of Hope. New York: EP Dutton, 1989.
3. Dwyer JM: The Body of At War: The Miracle of the Immune System. New York: Mentor, 1990.
4. Furth GM: The Secret World of Drawings: Healing Through Art. Boston: Sigo Press, 1988.
5. Johnson DR: Introduction to special issue on creative arts therapies in the treatment of substance abuse. The Arts in Psychotherapy 17(4): 295-29, 1990.
6. Lusebrink VB: Inner guide. Art Therapy 5(3):99-105, 1988.
7. McMurray M: Illuminations: The Healing Image. Berkeley: Wingbow Press, 1988.
8. Ornstein R, Swencionis C (eds): The Healing Brain: A Scientific Reader. New York: Guilford Press, 1990.
9. Samuels M: Healing with the Mind's Eye: A Guide for Using Imagery and Visions for Personal Growth and Healing. New York: Summit Books, 1990.
10. Shorr JE: Psychotherapy Through Imagery. New York: Thieme-Stratton, 1986.

CHAPTER 22

Can the Visual Arts Contribute to Healing?

Machteld Kuypers

This paper represents the point of view of the professional visual artist. About twenty years ago, the author discovered that she was part of a hidden tradition: the arts as a healing medium. For example, in the Middle Ages, Matthias Grunewald was commissioned to create an altar piece for a hospital, where patients would be exposed to the art work, panel by panel (the Isenheimer altar piece in Colmar, France.[1] It is so impressive that one cannot but believe the reports of 'miraculous' healings as a result. Hildegard von Binfgen, a famous visionary nun from the twelfth century, also reports the beneficial influence of color on the *lumen corporis* and most specifically the *greening* quality, which keeps the individual from *sin*, which she equates with drying out or shriveling up.[2] In the Byzantine tradition, the influence of the portable created image or 'icon' was so great that the spirit of the saint depicted was believed to be actually present and could therefore work 'miracles.'[3] In general, artists are credited with special vision. They somehow develop a sixth sense, and become a link between the commoner and the 'Great Spirit.'

In a mechanized society, people have become increasingly dependent, not only for their everyday needs like food and housing, but also on a spiritual healer as well, or rather his/her outcome: a spiritual healing by visual perception. In this respect, art becomes a 'sacred business.' Without religion, people become spiritually starved and increasingly estranged from their essential self. When attention is paid to the material body only, an unbalanced condition will result. The artist, through his/her work, can restore this equilibrium. Sensitivity to color, with shapes, rhythm, and composition following closely behind, plays an important part in the visual arts; this phenomenon has been explored by men like Goethe and Steiner.[4]

In the final analysis, however, it is the artist's mind who is communicating to the perceptive public through his/her medium. The observer is relating to the *spirit* of the painting, which is universal and also within him/herself, although usually in the unconscious realm. Often, people are not aware of a beneficial influence of a work of art — or the reverse, for that matter. Perhaps our sensitivity to color has to do with the fact that we *are* color. According to *The Kingdom and the Power* by Louise Hurlbutt de Wetter, human souls are perceived as color combinations and the intensity changes with their being *tuned in* or *healthy*.[5] Hildegard von Bingen confirms this when she describes the human body as being generated by *colored flames*.[2] Whether or not one believes in these writings, the idea is fascinating and the fact remains that people do respond to color and color combinations, the *tool* by which the visual artist communicates with the public.

In her book *Color and Personality,* Audrey Kargere describes the effects of chromotherapy, which heals by applying the right color to the afflicted area.[6] It is noteworthy that, since colored glass has a different effect from painted glass, stained glass windows, therefore, must have a definite influence on the observer. Regardless of subject matter, people respond to colors for their own sake. This is in favor of abstract art, which relies heavily on colors and their sheer infinite combinations by gradation. Only the primary colors red, yellow and blue are relevant; white is the blending of all hues; black is their absence. All other tones and shades are mixtures.

Light transmitted through a colored surface has healing effects because it coincides with the observer's 'own' natural colors which, by the way, have a universal appeal. Even though people have their own specific and very individual preferences, the meaning of the colors themselves is standard.

Regarding the author's own art work, interestingly enough, her painting evolved, totally intuitively, towards the exclusive use of transparent material with a high shine — be it plexiglass or foil — with the sole use of various shades of the primary colors. Thus, her art seems to be entirely in tune with the aims of a healing function, an effect that is indeed experienced by some of the owners of her paintings.

What the art of bygone civilizations tries to tell us is that the soul does not perish with the body and that, in fact, the body should be subservient to its inhabiting spirit. Thus, it is of vital importance that art stimulates and revitalizes that part in us that is dormant, albeit a healing factor. Short of an organic disorder, can a good picture, worthy of its name, exert a calming, soothing influence and pave the way to total recovery of body and soul?

In conclusion, the author makes the following suggestions to promote healing through the visual arts:

☐   Talented artists, so inclined, should be trained towards this lofty goal.

☐   Support for their efforts should be rallied by public recognition through scholarships, awards, etc.

☐   They should be given the opportunity to serve the public through exhibitions in hospitals and similar places.

☐   The opportunity to study and experiment with the medical staff, should also be provided, in order to document the effect of their art.

REFERENCES

1. Gall R.: Schlüssel zum Isenheimer Altar. Im selbst-verlag des Verfassers, 1960.
2. Mulder E: Hildegard, een vrouwelijk genie in de late middeleeuwen. Ambo/Baarn, 1982.
3. Brion M: La grande aventure de la peinture religieuse. Librairie Académique Perrin, 1968.
4. Steiner, R: De Kleuren. Zeist, Vrij Geestesleven, 1991.
5. Hurlbutt de Wetter L: The Kingdom and the Power. Rindge, NH: CM Randal, 1974.
6. Kargere A: Color and Personality. York Beach, ME: S Weiser, Inc, 1979.

CHAPTER 23

The Teacher in School Children's Drawings: Psychotherapeutic Technique

Kinga Lewandowska

Children's drawings can be studied as to implied concepts and knowledge of the external world, early emotional experiences, actual attitudes, and preferences.[1] The author is interested in measuring students' attitude toward school and considers many psychological factors connected with the school career of a given child.[2] Using the same psychometric scale, it was found that attitudes toward school are less favorable than 20 years ago. The teacher who is too rigorous and critical, giving mostly bad grades, causes negative feelings and a tense classroom atmosphere.

Based on the assumption that there is a correlation between emotional attitude and artistic expression, groups of 15-year-old pupils were asked to draw the teacher whom they like best and the one they like least. The exercises were conducted by the university psychologist who trains students in educational psychology. After drawing, there was a group session in which pairs of drawings were interpreted by the class and the pupil him/herself. The subject of discussion was the way in which the student expressed feelings connected with a particular behavior, situation, etc. On the basis of materials gathered, one can conclude that among the factors influencing emotional attitude toward a teacher, the following are important:

- the teacher's personality, especially his/her ability to create warm relationships with pupils and involvement in didactic process;

- the student's individual experiences in contacts with teachers;

- the degree of the student's emotional sensitivity;

- the level of class expectations and wishes connected with the particular subject and the way of teaching it.

It may happen that the teacher gets opposite appreciation and image in drawings by younger and older children. Insufficient level of acquired knowledge or practical skills in a class affects children's feelings at school. For example, a group of older students, doing poorly academically, rejected the new, rigorous teacher who was loved by younger pupils, doing well in math. Drawings were also an indication of the level of emotional and social maturity, reflecting temper, preferences, wishes, and ideas.

The variety of affective tendencies can be seen in details as well as in the overall composition of the drawings. Positive feelings — love and approval — result in the beauty of the figure, accuracy of the picture, and selection of ornamentation. They are also revealed verbally during psychotherapeutic discussion, when children describe the person as nice, gay, calm, interested in pupils, willing to explain, etc. Negative attitudes — dislike and contempt — are indicated in caricatures of a person behaving in an aggressive way, and ugliness of the details of the face and clothing. The pairs of art works shown herein originated in a class of 12-year-old children:

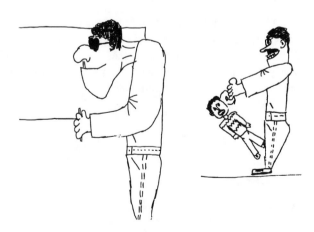

Figure 1: In this pair of drawings, the favorite teacher (left) is perceived as a funny, humped, non-threatening person. The second drawing shows "the teacher whom I dislike the most."

Collected drawings were in the form of realistic portraits, cartoons, and classroom scenes, though sometimes assuming a symbolic character with animals (e.g. cats, pigeon), figures from children's movies, class objects, instruments of torture, musical notes, algebraic signs, and common grades.

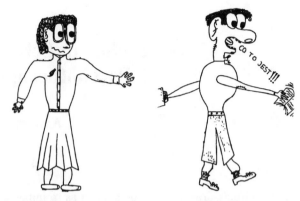

Figure 3: The boy stated that his favorite teacher (left) is pleasantly surprised by his knowledge. In the second situation, the teacher is shouting at the pupil while checking his exercise book.

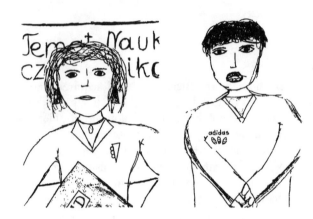

Figure 2: This student depicted his favorite teacher (left) as ornamented with many trinkets. The physical-education teacher is seen as aggressive because she gave the boy, who loves sports, a bad grade.

Some children evaded the theme of a teacher in their drawings by presenting the world of their own highly valued interests or rejected social situations, e.g. a longed-for motor club, peaceful nature, destructive war. Among defense mechanisms, one can see negation ("I have no favorite teacher"), displacement (choice of a person who does not teach the class), and regression (selection of a teacher from preschool).

The technique helps children to reveal their actual emotions and preferences, even when temporarily distorted because of school success or failure. The psychotherapeutic discussion can be aimed at changing the subjective picture of relationships with teachers to realistic ones.

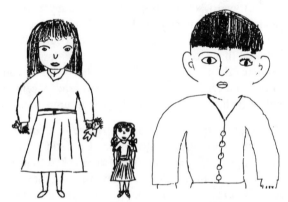

Figure 4: The girl chose a teacher from preschool as her favorite (left), whom she liked because she played with the children. The disliked teacher gives low grades and is severe, in the opinion of the student, who is doing poorly.

REFERENCES

1. Di Leo JH: Children's Drawings as Diagnostic Aids. New York: Brunner/Mazel, 1973.
2. Lewandowska K: Postawy uczniów wobec szkoły. Kwartalnik Pedag Ogiczny 2:77-87, 1972.
3. Lewandowska K: Nauczyciel na rysunkach uczniów z klas V-VIII — technika psychorysunku, manuscript, 1990.

CHAPTER 24

Use of Puppetry to Promote Psychological Resilience in Children

Mary Louise O'Brien

In recent years, the topic of psychological invulnerability, resilience, hardiness or stress-resistance in children has been a focus of attention.[1-10] Some investigators have focused on children who have endured chronic and severe stress such as poverty,[10, 11] Holocaust experiences,[12, 13] divorce,[14, 15] and living with psychotic parents[16-18] and emerged psycho-logically healthy. Other investigators[19, 20] suggest that 'hassles,' or frustrating everyday events, are better indicators of resilience. School is a natural setting to improve tolerance and mastery of 'hassles.'

Junior-high students described by teachers as well-adjusted and students with deficiencies work in small groups to produce puppetry skits to help students in kindergarten through grade 2 cope with 'hassles.' In preparing presentations, students discuss resiliency attributes and coping strategies, and interview younger students to identify specific frustrations young students encounter at school.

The skits consist of three parts: (1) a re-enactment of the stressful situations identified by the young students; (2) audience participation in which the puppets become stationary and younger students are asked, "What would you do if this happened to you?" and (3) puppets demonstrate unsuccessful and successful resolutions in a humorous and enlightening manner.

Katherine Kersey has outlined eleven attributes of resilient children which are used as a basis for the formulation of this prevention program, which encourages the development of resilient qualities in elementary and middle school.[21]

1. *They know how to play vigorously.* Puppets are naturally engaging and facilitate vigorous play. Each junior-high student selects and names his/her puppet for the duration of the project, which further fosters identification.

2. *They are excited about life. They seek out new experiences.* Young audiences respond enthusiastically to the puppets and this enthusiasm has a contagious effect on the preadolescents, who usually respond by suggesting other things they could do to build on elements that were positively received.

3. *They are independent and self-reliant.*[7] Strengthening an internal locus of control is demonstrated in the skits. For example, self-reliant coping strategies such as "You could tell yourself that when he calls you a name it doesn't mean it is true" are acted out. Furthermore, performing before an audience builds confidence. The puppet provides a screen to reduce self-consciousness and the responsiveness of the young audience further encourages pre-teens to become more creative and innovative.

4. *They have a belief in themselves and their ability to make things happen.* Students are usually impressed with their ability to elicit information from younger students in a classroom setting, to help them and to make them laugh.

5. *They know where and how to ask for help.*[7, 21] In the skits, when self-reliant behaviors do not ameliorate the conflict, puppets demonstrate how to identify and approach appropriate adults in order to enlist help.

6. *They have social skills and they are able to attract other people to them.* In addition to modelling communication which attracts others, the role of puppeteer attracts positive attention from young students, teachers, and the principal. The admiration which young children naturally extend to older children has a very powerful effect on socially isolated and estranged students.

7. *They have a sense of humor.* Behind the shield of puppetry, shy and inept preadolescents are usually able to stage humorous encounters and learn

to make funny comments, to entertain and to make others laugh. Each student writes his/her own script with help from the peer group. Audience laughter is a strong social reinforcer, and after shy children experience this response they often revise their scripts to include more humorous material.

8. *They have been required to look out for and help others.*[6] Only-children have an opportunity to help younger children. A preadolescent who was referred to the counselor for help bonded emotionally to a young child with similar problems. She expressed affection and concern which was not observed in the school setting, but is an important part of an individual's repertoire of social skills.

9. *They have a close bond of trust with at least one adult.*[8, 23] Preadolescents help teachers of younger students by addressing areas teachers identify as problems. This reverses their role of receiving assistance *from* teachers to providing assistance *to* teachers. Students also meet with the music teacher to find meaningful songs the children could sing with the puppets.

10. *They have developed skills, talents, hobbies, and interests.* Students are encouraged to write scripts, act, design, and paint scenery, and choose or write songs and poetry. Students who may not be interested in athletics or other well-supported programs find a forum for their interests in the arts.

11. *They have a sense of belonging, a reason for being, and a purpose for living.* Preparation for performances encourages cooperation and a sense of shared purpose to achieve a common goal. Structured tasks in small groups offer shy children a more comfortable environment for developing friendships. In addition, contributing to the well-being of younger students fosters a feeling of belonging to the larger community, namely the school.

Using puppetry is a non-threatening, success-oriented, fun approach to developing attributes of resiliency and strengthening stress-resistance in elementary- and middle- school students.

REFERENCES

1. Anthony E: The Invulnerable Child. New York: Guilford Press, 1987.
2. Garmenzy N, Rutter M (eds): Stress, Coping, and Development in Children. New York: McGraw-Hill, 1983.
3. Luthar S, Zigler: Vulnerability and competence: A review of research on resilience in childhood. Amer J Orthopsychiatry 61(1):6-22, 1991.
4. Johnson J: Life Events as Stressors in Childhood and Adolescence. Newbury Park: Sage Publications, 1986.
5. Miller A: The Drama of the Gifted Child. New York: Basic Books, 1979.
6. Masten A, Garmenzy N, Tellegen A, Pellegrine, Larkin D, Larsen A: Competency and stress in school children: the moderating effects of individual and family qualities. J Child Psychology and Psychiatry 29(6):745-768, 1988.
7. Murphy L, Moriarty A: Vulnerability, Coping and Growth: From Infancy to Adolescence. New Haven: Yale University Press, 1976.
8. Rutter M: Protective factors in children's responses to stress and disadvantage. *In* Kent M, Rolf J (eds), Primary Prevention of Psychopathology: Social Competency in Children. Hanover, NH: University Press in New England, 1979.
9. Rutter M: Psychosocial resilience and protective mechanisms. Amer J Orthopsychiatry 57:316-331, 1987.
10. Werner E, Smith R: Vulnerable but Invincible: A Study of Resilient Children. New York: McGraw Hill, 1982.
11. Sameroff A, Chandler M: Intelligence quotient scores of four-year-old children: social-environmental risk factors.   Pediatrics 79(3):343-350, 1987.
12. Moskovitz S: Love Despite Hate: Child survivors of the Holocaust and Their Adult Lives. New York: Schoeken Books, 1983.
13. Moskovitz S: Longitudinal follow-up of child survivors of the holocaust. J Amer Acad Child Psychiatry 24(5):401-407, 1985.
14. Wallerstein J, Kelly J: Surviving the Breakup: How Children and Parents Cope with Divorce. New York: Basic Books, 1980.
15. Wallerstein J: Children of divorce; stress and developmental tasks. *In* Garmenzy N, Rutter M, (eds), Stress, Coping, and Development in Children.   New York: McGraw Hill, 1983.
16. Anthony E, Koupernick C (eds): The Child and His Family: Children at Psychiatric Risk. New York: John Wiley and Sons, 1974.
17. Fisher L, Kokes R, Cole R, Perkins P, Wynne L: Competent children at risk: A study of well-functioning offspring of disturbed parents. *In* Anthony E, Cohler B (eds), The Invulnerable Child.   New York: Guilford Press, 1987.

18. Rutter M, Quinton D: Longitudinal studies of institutional children and children of mentally ill parents. *In* Mednick S, Baert A (eds), Prospective Longitudinal Research: An Empirical Basis for the Primary Prevention of Psychosocial Disorders. Oxford: Oxford University Press, 1981.

19. Lazarus R: The stress and coping paradigm. *In* Eisdorfer C, Cohen D, Kleinman A (eds): Conceptual Models for Psychopathology. New York: Spectrum, 1980.

20. Lazarus R: Puzzles in the study of daily hassles. J Behavioral Med 7:375-389, 1984.

21. Kersey K: Helping Your Child Handle Stress. Washington, DC: Acropolis Books, 1985.

22. Pines M: Superkids. Psychology Today 12(8): 53-63, 1979.

23. Hunter R, Kilstrom N: Breaking the cycle in abusive families. Amer J Psychiatry 136(10):1320-1322, 1979.

CHAPTER 25

Three Art Therapy Techniques to Facilitate Disclosure

Roberta Toby Pashley

Disclosure of sexual abuse has proven to be a difficult process. Disclosure is defined here as the making known of information to oneself and/or to others. The techniques described herein were developed for in-hospital art-therapy groups.

NO-THOUGHT-MESS DRAWING TECHNIQUE

This technique has been adapted from the *Creativity Mobilization Technique* (C-M-T).[1] The C-M-T is a process-oriented, nonverbal approach to reducing the potency of brain-disturbing material that interferes with optimal functioning. Some assumptions underlying this theory are that (1) the brain contains self-adjusting functions that (2) can find disturbing material within the system and (3) can reduce their potency, (4) resulting in multidimensional therapeutic readjustments.[2]

The C-M-T engages the self-regulatory brain mechanisms and allows them to reduce the potency of functional brain disturbances. When brain-disturbing material is reduced, the unblocking and development of inherent verbal and nonverbal creative potentials can occur.

Luthe has tentatively organized phenomena experienced during C-M-T sessions into five stages of mental reactivity.[1] During Stage 1, the participant is engaged in actively oriented thought processes involving directive thinking. In Stage 2, more passive concentration is experienced, allowing disturbing mental material to surface to the point of awareness. It is important to allow these self-regulatory mental processes to follow their own course in the reduction of the brain-disturbing. In Stage 3, passive concentration is maintained and positive dynamics are released which are more closely linked to creativity. At Stage 4, the return of brain-disturbing material can occur at a less intense level. Here, an increase in passive acceptance and passive concentration is experienced. Stage 5 is deeply relaxing and recuperative. An immersion in the present is experienced along with a freedom from attachment to mind processes.

No-Thought-Mess Technique: *12" x 18" manila paper is used with a 12-color set of Sketcho craypas. The patient is directed to think of a disturbing mental image, and then to make a mess using chosen colors. The patient is free to use as many pieces of paper as needed, and is encouraged to verbalize any mental images that may occur.*

Some patients may need time to progress through Stage 1 with its emphasis on goal-directed striving. The group process can assist patients with the movement into a more passive mode of concentration by providing models of Stage 2 behaviors. At Stage 2, when a more passive mental attitude is attained, disturbing material can reach awareness. Some material may be stronger in content, and may need thematic repetition that can require additional sessions. The disturbing material may be accompanied by a need to cry or unload aggression. These needs are respected and are allowed to occur as long as they do not result in harm to oneself or others. A corollary technique is offered that has proven useful in containing negative affect on paper.

Contained-Scribble-Mess Technique: *A border is drawn around the edges of the paper and the patient is directed to scribble disturbing feelings onto the paper. Verbalization of the material is encouraged. The drawn container/border symbolically contains the negative affect represented by the scribble mess.*

Both of these art-therapy techniques have proven effective in enabling hospitalized psychiatric patients of all ages to uncover brain-disturbing material.

CONTAINED-SECRET TECHNIQUE

Who has not felt the need to keep a secret? The hypothesis underlying this technique is that a secret can be psychically damaging to one who holds it. The secret can have an importance far beyond its actual value when it carries unconscious psychic elements that are projected onto it. As such, the projected contents represent a potential for increased consciousness. The secret is dysfunctional when it remains in the form of an unintegrated content.

VonFranz concurs with Jung's view of the projection as an "unperceived and unintentional transfer of subjective psychic elements onto an outer object."[3] Dysfunctional projection can be disturbing and interfere with adaptation so that the "integration of the projected content into the subject is desirable."

VonFranz has structured a five-stage process in the withdrawal of projections that results in a corresponding increase in consciousness. In Stage 1, archaic identity occurs. This identity of subject and object is seen in the Greek world of antiquity where the world was alive with demons or spirits. In Stage 2, a differentiation and separation take place. The gods live on Olympus but are separate from Olympus. Moral evaluation of the gods takes place at Stage 3. Here, the gods are representative of good or evil principles. In Stage 4, further elucidation takes place and the spirits are defined as illusory. At Stage 5, the gods become psychic qualities and states in the individual. This is known in modern psychology as integration. The previously unconscious psychic content is recognized as belonging to the personality.

This technique has proven effective as a means of relieving accumulated secret-generated stress, while simultaneously effecting a projection of the secret. The secret is not confronted, though stress resulting from keeping it is reduced.

Contained-Secret Technique: *The patient is directed to choose a symbol, or somehow represent the secret, in a disguised form. A container is drawn around the secret. The patient is further encouraged to fold and seal his drawing to "keep it safe." The secret is not discussed, and the patient is directed to keep this secret sealed until he is ready to open it and discuss it. The patient is encouraged to identify feelings surrounding the secret and, if possible, discuss the impact that keeping of this secret has had on his life.*

It is of paramount importance to affirm the patient's control over disclosure of the secret, and to explain clearly that the focus is on the identification and exploration of feelings surrounding the keeping of the secret.

The patient is in the archaic-identity stage, where the secret is fused with the personality. The process of withdrawing projections is initiated to allow the secret's contents to be reclaimed by the patient. Moving into Stage 2, where a separation between the subject and the contained secret is established, the patient verbally identifies and explores feelings surrounding the keeping of this secret. Importantly, the distancing is accomplished in the service of stress-reduction. A movement into Stage 3 can now take place and the patient can place a moral evaluation on keeping the secret. When Stage 3 is positively worked through, a disclosure of the secret can result. With disclosure, the patient has moved into Stage 4, where the need for the secret no longer exists. The further task of therapy is to integrate the content of the secret with the rest of the personality.

Materials chosen for this technique are determined based on the needs of the patient. A very elaborate container can be devised for the secret, which can also be symbolized elaborately. In contrast, typing paper and pencil can be used successfully for this art-therapy technique, which has proven valuable with hospitalized psychiatric patients of any age.

ILLUSTRATE-THE-STORY TECHNIQUE

This technique is grounded in the works of Nucho[4] and Erickson.[5] Both hypothesize that the person is directed by goals that lie within the structure of the person.

Nucho views the mind as a cybernetic control system to process information. This *psychocybernetic* (P-C) model is also one of intervention that combines the verbal-analytic symbol system with the visual-imagistic symbol system in a four-phase therapeutic process. During the *unfreezing* phase, the introduction to art therapy is undertaken and the "psychological and concrete means of getting started" are provided. During the *doing* phase, the specific art-therapy experience is structured. Here, a theme can be specified, or the patient can be directed to pursue his own direction. The *dialoguing* phase begins with discussion about the produced visual image when the visual-imagistic symbols are translated into the verbal-analytic mode of symbolization by the patient. In the *ending* phase, information translated from the visual- to the verbal system is integrated with information previously available to the patient and closure for the session is made.

Erickson believed that the unconscious contains the power and ability to heal itself through inherent patterns of healing that lie within the psyche and are activated by the use of symbolic language. Erickson's work underlies Davis' creation and use of therapeutic stories to metaphorically transfer knowledge that will influence unconscious patterns for healing.[6]

Illustrate-the-Story Technique: *A story is chosen from the Davis collection that relates to the issues of group members. The story is read to the group. Patients are directed to draw a picture, as detailed possible, about the story.*

This technique is used within the structure of the P-C model. In the *doing* phase, the story is read to the group and each participant produces a visual image. During the *dialoguing* phase, the images are verbally processed for their information. Materials suitable for this technique are determined by the needs of group members. Inexpensive art materials are appropriate. This technique is useful for all ages of hospitalized psychiatric patients. It is "in this 'child state' that we are most open to learning, most curious, and most able to change."[5]

REFERENCES

1. Luthe W: Creativity Mobilization Technique. New York: Grune & Stranon, 1976.

2. Luthe W: Dynamics of Autogenic Neutralization. New York and London: Grune & Stranon, 1970.

3. VonFranz M: Projection and Re-collection in Jungian Psychology. La Salle and London: Open Court, 1985.

4. Davis N: Once Upon a Time... Oxon Hill, MD: Psychological Associates of Oxon Hill, 1990.

5. Erickson M, Rossi E: The February Man. New York: Brunner/Mazel, 1989.

6. Nucho A: The Psychocybernetic Model of Art Therapy. Springfield, IL: Charles C Thornas, 1987.

CHAPTER 26

Art and Healing:
Confronting Cancer Through Art

Martha Slaymaker

Since 1960, I have been a professional visual artist. Originally, I worked as a painter and printmaker; I now concentrate primarily on relief sculptures formed of clay and mixed media adhered to a plywood base.

My interests lie in the stratification of the earth's archaeology. Obscured layers of information below the earth's surface relate to existing information remaining on its surface ... I see a relationship between the archaeology of ancient civilizations and an archaeology of my own memories, both conscious and unconscious.[1]

In 1983, I learned that breast cancer, for which I'd had a radical mastectomy in 1972, had metastasized throughout my axial skeleton and lymph nodes. My oncologist felt that my days were numbered.

As a creative person, initially terrified, I sought innovative solutions to my own survival. Along with traditional medicine, plus dietary changes and regular exercise, I began to explore right-brained options. In an attempt to strengthen my immune system, I studied self-hypnosis and visual imagery through a local university psychologist. The process of making art, reconnecting with my musical background, and numerous other imaginative devices, became important outlets and helped dissipate the panic in recognizing my own mortality.

Since my metastasis, my relief sculpture has gradually evolved to another plane. I focus upon what feel to me to be healing images, colors, and materials. Through the art, I am laying claim to the future, as well as the past. I have come to believe that in extending my connection further, I am thus healing myself and becoming more whole. As a result, my relief sculptures are more embellished. I now literally carve into the wood base to another dimension and, on the surface, more complexity has developed with more metaphysical connections to what I have been perceiving. Art has become a means for me to understand myself.

The mandala, that most ancient of symbols, is, in its many forms, an important expression in my work. Conceiving and forming the image in clay is tranquilizing and hypnotic.

The Sanskrit word mandala *means circle in the ordinary sense of the word. In the sphere of religious practices and in psychology, it denotes circular images, which are drawn, painted, modeled, or danced ... Structures of this kind are to be found, for instance, in Tibetan Buddhism, and as dance figures these circular patterns occur also in Dervish monasteries. As psychological phenomena they appear spontaneously in dreams. In Tibetan Buddhism the figure has the significance of a ritual instrument (yantra) whose purpose is to assist meditation and concentration ... The fact that images of this kind have under certain circumstances a considerable therapeutic effect on their authors is empirically proven and also readily understandable ... Even the mere attempt in this direction usually has a healing effect, but only when it is done spontaneously. Nothing can be expected from an artificial repetition or a deliberate imitation of such images.*[2]

Colors which feel healing to me encompass the lighter spectrum, as opposed to my former earth-colored palette. These tones and values have come to me during meditation and visualization. Occasionally, I add stones which seem to have healing properties within the reliefs. These include chips of crystal, amethyst, and turquoise, the last being sacred to Native Americans, with whom I feel a deep empathy.

It is my wish that my work contribute to the healing process of others as well as myself. A recent 4' by 8' commission for the Mayo Clinic in Phoenix, Arizona, was particularly gratifying. It provided the opportunity to reach many patients who are also in need of healing. In the design, I used three mandalas in varied forms, from broken to whole, to signify stages of healing.

Music, which has always been important to my well-being, is now a form of self-therapy. Singing and composing hymn-like chants, only for myself, has become an emotional catharsis.

A cancer support group in New Mexico has helped me realize that I am not alone with my disease, and that a disproportionate number of visual artists develop cancer. It may be that the toxicity of our materials is a major factor, and much research and education are needed. I would recommend that doctors inquire of artists in treatment about their specific art materials and their studio ventilation.

In 1988 and 1989, I curated and chaired invitational art exhibitions for our cancer support group. The shows were entitled *Viva la Vida, Viva el Arte: Confronting Cancer Through Art*. All artists in the exhibits had encountered cancer. This year, the show continued and the group dedicated it to me, which was heartwarming. Each year, the art exhibit has been hung in a heavily trafficked public gallery. Beside each work is a statement by the artist referring to his or her personal experience with cancer. Viewers reading these comments often are visibly moved. The combination of art and word creates a bond between the artists and the public.

Artists dealing with illness concur that art-making is healing, and the creative process is more important than the finished work of art. Making art helps artists regain control of their lives. Art pulls them through their life-threatening, agonizing experience and, afterward, their world is a different place. Each day is a special gift. The ancient Sufis have a saying, "When the body weeps for that which it has lost, the spirit laughs for what it has gained." In exchange for physical loss, artists indeed gain spiritual gifts.

Art is a system invented by nature to enable human beings to come into full possession of their higher senses. It is a form of wealth in which all can share and which is dependent not on ownership but on desire and perception ... It is a way of assigning values to things we think and do. Finally, it is a way of imparting meaning to life and life to meaning.[3]

REFERENCES

1. Nelson MC: Approaching the layer as a formal element and a significant metaphor in artmaking. Leonardo 19(3):223-229, 1986.
2. Jung CG: Mandala Symbolism, 3-5. Bollinger Foundation, Princeton University.
3. Cousins N: Confronting Cancer Through Art. 1987. Los Angeles, CA: Jonsson Comprehensive Cancer Center, University of California, 1987.

CHAPTER 27

A Transitional Journey: A Case Study of Art Therapy in a Hospice

M. Gold • *S. Ahmedzai*

Patients who are living with terminal cancer have not only physical and emotional pain to contend with, but bodily deterioration and often unsightly tumors to accentuate the trauma. When hospice patients are offered the opportunity to engage in art therapy, therefore, many issues must be considered regarding motivation, application, and ultimate involvement.

Creativity responds to our emotional world; thus, inner feelings will be evoked through the process of making art. The boundaries of the picture frame become a safe place to *enact* and resolve unspoken emotional trauma. Encouraging spontaneous expression enables the patient to find his/her own creative language. This can be extremely complex in the sense that it must meet with an unconscious defense strategy in not being too revealing, yet respond to a primitive urge to find a tangible way of expressing and managing unspeakable emotions. Interpretation is unnecessary and possibly destructive of both the process and the therapeutic relationship. The image has evolved in preference to verbal confrontation and creating provides its own catharsis. "Any drawing has a cathartic effect and that catharsis allows the symbol to move inner psychic energy and begin the healing process."[1] Sharing the images and experiencing the feelings with the patient enables the therapist to facilitate the process and accompany the patient through the transition.

This case study illustrates the value of visual art in exploring the physical and emotional world of a female patient with terminal cancer. It shows how she worked through many conflicting issues simultaneously, including organic aspects, through the process of making pictures.

Mary was 49, suffering with invasive squamous cell carcinoma of the pharynx with direct extensions of tumor into the neck. The consequent constriction of the throat area inhibited clear speech, so conversation necessitated written responses. The illness created many distressing symptoms including an offensive smell and incessant sputum. Formerly a physical-education teacher, Mary held strong opinions and was determined that she would get better. Physically, she was anorexic and appeared frail, with a nasogastric tube providing sustenance.

Mary responded immediately to the idea of painting and described, then found, her perfect rose. She started by drawing it in pencil, and made more pictures of the same rose in colored pencil, then paint. The involvement became more intense. The senior author began tentatively to ascribe to the rose in the picture human characteristics such as "gracious" and "elegant." Mary identified with these responses readily, yet any suggestion that the pictures expressed feelings was firmly denied and something she did not want to "dwell upon."

More intense involvement about the stem and calyx of the rose became apparent. In viewing the flower as a symbol of the self, this area could be seen to be related to the throat and neck, the site of Mary's cancer. Her preoccupation suggested an instinctive urge to know more about it, and the emphasis on the *throat* area of the rose where the petals enfolded each other suggested the physical sensation was being instinctively explored in a more visibly accepting and manageable way. Furth describes this phenomenon: "Energy invested in shading may reflect fixation or anxiety about the shaded object or shape represented symbolically."[1]

Experience had shown that Mary was prepared to consciously accept only positive elements in the rose symbol. It was clear that verbal intervention would be invasive and damaging to the therapeutic trust. Yet the considerable energy invested was evidence of a commitment to a process which engendered intense emotional interaction. It seemed, therefore, that the image had evolved as a place of safety where unconscious expressions of psychological and somatic experience could be enacted. The image became an embodiment of the inner struggle, contained and resolved in an evolutionary sequence. This experience is consistent with a description of the embodied image in which "Emotions which were repressed, which felt too difficult, too painful to face, became accessible, contained as they are 'out there' in the image within the frame of the picture."[2]

Mary was due to go home for a visit. Before leaving, she arranged the pictures around the wall and established a secure place for her return. When we next met, she had completed a number of fuchsia flower pictures. They were beautifully drawn but it was hard not to observe that they bore a strong symbolic relationship to her more stooped demeanor. They followed the same evolutionary sequence as the rose drawings and were added to the others on the wall. By now these images were making a powerful impact on the room and the people who visited. Were they there to distract or call attention to the real person, within the sick body? The truth may be seen in Schaverien's words: "In art therapy the client makes an image and in so doing performs an act which very act affirms a sense of self — the 'I' exists."[2]

At this stage, Mary explored the use of different materials and created a series of spontaneous pictures which were more open to interpretation. The first was of four black trees with a blue pathway winding upwards. Others included an explicit picture of a mouse being kicked towards a black hole, a black basket full of black flowers, a weeping willow and, finally, a church with a graveyard. On black paper she painted the churchyard again, in white. This she hung directly in front of her door, making it impossible to ignore. Now, she said, flowers were not suitable. She began to concentrate on abstract shapes and was totally absorbed. She still denied that her works were related to her feelings, although they were, she said, intensive and relaxed. Over the next several days, she created four similar powerful images. Sadly, they proved to be her final pieces. Later, when seeing them in relation to the first rose picture, the same schematic form implied a rose head without a stalk. It was only days before the first abstract image was made that Mary said that her throat was now closing off entirely — a horrific image to contemplate and ultimately experience.

Mary chose to draw the rose with confidence. The repetition of the same imagery was a way of maintaining confidence, both artistically and psychologically, of the experiences engendered by the process. This established control and provoked more intensive evolvement. It is apparent that instinctively, the formation of the rose met the unconscious criteria of being a safe image to explore somatic and inherent emotional experience, while still maintaining defenses. The transitional process is evident — from the initial sense of denial to the conflict and confrontation of the wall pictures — since the movement through the repeated sets of images reflected gradual psychological changes. This repetitive process afforded Mary total command of her subject; using this coping strategy enabled her to reach a gradual acceptance at her own pace. In the first stage, where denial was still in evidence, movement to the drooping flowers showed the initial acceptance of change. With the mixed media and inconsistent images, there was a sense of disintegration and grief, until the graveyard picture issued a final challenge. "If denial is no longer possible, we can attempt to master death by challenging it."[3] In the abstract image there is a total relinquishing of the original skills, yet still a stubborn urge to maintain control. Thus, the ultimate confrontation courageously and vividly portrayed was managed on Mary's own terms.

The senior author worked with Mary over a period of eight weeks. During that time, the energy and courage she expressed through her work was indicative of the determined person she had always been. It would seem that the linking of the first rose image and the final abstract image indicated a *coming together* process: the individuation or wholeness that Jung believed all men strive to achieve.[4]

REFERENCES

1. Furth GH: The Secret World of Drawings, 12, 59. Boston: Sigo Press, 1988.
2. Dalley T, Schaverien J, et al: Images of Art Therapy, 79, 84.. London/New York: Tavistock, 1987.
3. Kubler Ross E: On Death and Dying, 13. London/New York: Tavistock/Routledge, 1989.
4. Jung C (ed): Man and his Symbols. Picador, 1964.

SUGGESTED   READING

Bach S: Life Paints its Own Span: On the Significance of Spontaneous Pictures of Severely Ill Children. Switzerland: Daimon, 1990.

CHAPTER 28

The Expressive Therapies Continuum:
Relationship to the Arts in Medicine

Marcia L. Rosal

The use of image, art, and other expressive media as an integral aspect of behavioral medicine is now widely accepted.[1] Many physicians are aware that the client's affective and psychological states are factors in the healing process. The use of imagery and the arts as a means of addressing psychological concerns in healing is at the heart of the concept of holistic healing. Theoretical models of how to apply expressive media to work with clients experiencing chronic diseases is not as universal, however. A model of how to theorize about the use of artistic expression with clients is explored herein.

BACKGROUND

The Expressive Therapies Continuum (ETC)[2] was developed as a model for understanding clients' interactions with expressive media: visual art materials, music, dance or movement, and drama. The ETC was based on other developmental models including Piaget's model of cognitive growth[3] and Lowenfeld's stages of graphic development.[4]

The ETC consists of four levels of expression: kinesthetic/sensory, perceptual/affective, cognitive/symbolic, and creative. The four levels can be used as guidelines for assessing the client's level of emotional functioning. In addition, each level has specific benefits for a client in terms of the development of expression and in terms of therapeutic value.

THE CREATIVE LEVEL
AS A HEALTH MODEL

The creative level of the ETC is defined as a synthesis between inner experiences and outer realities.[2] The outer realities are most often boundaries or limitations within which individuals must exist. Within the constraints of the ETC model, if one can synthesize and reconcile inner and outer

experiences, one is living creatively and is emotionally healthy. Living creatively and in good health also implies that the individual has accepted his or her affective responses and has an ability to cope with stressors.[5]

If an individual develops a chronic disease, that disease has an impact on the person's inner experiences and outer realities. The various responses an individual may have in reaction to the disease are numerous. A speedy coping adjustment to a disease and a quick synthesis of inner and outer experiences will affect the course of treatment and therapy in a positive manner. The client may be said to be creatively coping with the disease and creatively dealing with the new reality. Although the individual may not be 'cured' or 'the picture of health,' he/she continues to live creatively and in a healthy manner.

Discord results, however, if the inner experience is in conflict with the outer reality of an illness. This discord, perhaps helplessness and hopelessness, may negatively affect the course of treatment, preventing the client from fully benefiting from therapy. Thus, it seems that helping individuals become fully functioning and creative may aid in healing.

Functioning on the creative level of the ETC requires the integration of all other levels into the creative process.[6] This implies that an individual is experiencing a great deal of input and stimulation, although this may be difficult for some individuals. A form of creativity can be experienced on each level of the ETC.[6] Thus, for clients unable to integrate vast amounts of stimuli, using art materials on the other levels of the ETC can lead to creativity without the overpowering punch of the creative level.

CREATIVITY ON EACH ETC LEVEL

On the *kinesthetic/sensory level*, an individual is interacting with media in an exploratory fashion. The kinesthetic aspect of this level involves motor activity and motor actions; the sensory aspect involves the use of touch and other senses to explore media. Both aspects may lead to mental and concrete images. The development of imagery, either through movement and action or through touch and senses, is seen as the creative indicator on this level.

The kinesthetic/sensory level would be useful for clients who may benefit from the discharge of energy. Scribbling or splash painting, for example, may help release tension and anxiety, and sensory touching of clay or painting with large, slow strokes may relax and calm a client.

On the *perceptual/affective level*, the individual interacts with media to find form for ideas and to find a means of expressing emotions. The use of visual elements such as line, shape, and color can facilitate the development of form for images, both mental and concrete. The visual elements give form to feeling states and concretize the images of emotions. An expression of form or image which emits emotion and feeling is the essence of creativity of this level.

Interaction with art materials on this level may be useful for clients who are unsure of how they feel about a disease or the treatment. The use of forms in nature or work with the visual elements may help a client define and understand feeling states.

Interactions with media on the *cognitive/symbolic level* are solution-oriented and/or meaning-seeking. The cognitive aspect of this level involves problem-solving and logical thinking processes. Clients who utilize intellect and rational thinking will begin work with art materials on this level. The symbolic aspect involves the use of global information and intuition to arrive at resolution. Clients attempting to integrate 'self' issues including feelings, body sensations, and spiritual questions will work with media to enhance symbols which may help bring meaning to personal questions.[6]

Clients seeking meaning to illness will work best on this level. Choosing to work with either the cognitive aspect or the symbolic aspect will be dependent upon the client's defense mechanisms and modes of processing information. Collages are excellent tools for cognitive clients who seek meaning and understanding through order, logic, and information gathering. Creativity on the cognitive level occurs when a client is able to resolve an issue through problem identification and solution generation.

Exploration of myths or stories through paintings and drawings may be useful for the client who seeks meaning through global and universal experience. A creative experience on the symbolic level is one in which the client discovers meaning from understanding and integrating experiences, both personal and universal.

SUMMARY

In summary, the ETC is a model for helping the behavioral-medicine community understand and theorize about how art and other expressive techniques can help a client with a chronic illness. The definition of creativity with the ETC model can also be a definition of health. The ETC consists of four levels of interaction with media. Each level can help a client deal with issues related to developing an illness. In addition, on each ETC level, a client can experience creativity which may lead to increased coping and improved response to treatment.

REFERENCES

1. Achterberg J: Imagery in Healing: Shamanism and Modern Medicine. Boston: New Science Library, 1985.
2. Kagin SL, Lusebrink VB: The expressive therapies continuum. Art Psychotherapy 5: 171-180, 1978.
3. Piaget J, Inhelder B: Mental Imagery in the Child. New York: Basic Books, 1969.
4. Lowenfeld V: Creative and Mental Growth, 6th ed. New York: Macmillan, 1970.
5. Ley RG, Freeman RJ: Imagery, cerebral laterality, and the healing process. *In* Sheikh AA (ed), Imagination and Healing, 51-68. Farmingdale, NY: Baywood, 1984.
6. Lusebrink VB: Imagery and Visual Expression in Therapy. New York: Plenum Press, 1990.

CHAPTER 29

A Brief Art-Therapy Intervention with Juvenile Rheumatoid Arthritis Patients

V.B. Lusebrink • M.L. Rosal • L. Turner-Schikler • K. Schikler • J. Ackerman

The present study investigates the effects of art-therapy interventions on the experienced pain and helplessness of Juvenile Rheumatoid Arthritis (JRA) patients.

The chronic pain associated with JRA influences a child's physical activities, psychological adjustment, and overall health. School children with JRA have been found to have lower self-esteem and poorer self-concept than controls.[1] Low self-concept impairs the ability to deal with psychological stress, which influences the onset and severity of illness.[1,2]

The perception, assessment and alleviation of pain in JRA patients depend on the child's cognitive-developmental level, as does the child's perception of illness. The perception of pain by children depends on the meaning children attribute to the sensations in their joints.[3] The differentiation of sensations as pain or as a basis for other emotional experiences helps the child to understand and gain control of his/her internal experiences. Small children may lack the ability to communicate and express their pain verbally, and it is manifested in their externalized or internalized behavior.[4,5]

Rheumatoid arthritis patients may also manifest characteristics of alexithymia, or the lack of ability to express feelings.[6]

Art therapy and imagery intervention have been used to enhance individuals' own healing abilities, to assist medical treatment,[6-9] and to deal with the psychological components of chronic pain.[10] Progressive relaxation and guided imagery have been shown to reduce the level of subjective pain and to increase adaptive functioning.[11-13] Studies with adult rheumatoid arthritis patients indicate that relaxation, identification and expression of feelings, and the use of active coping strategies are associated with decreased levels of pain and functional impairment.

This study used relaxation, visual expressions of feeling, and guided imagery as art-therapy interventions with children who have JRA. Two visual assessments of the child's experience of pain have been used in studies with JRA patients — Visual Analogue Scale (VAS)[14,15] and body outlines with a color coded scale of pain intensity.[4,16] Red and black colors have been selected most often by children to represent pain.[17,18] A graded bar scale (Figs. 1a, 1b),

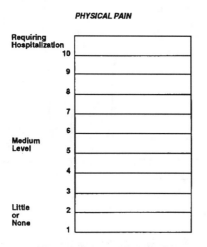

Figure 1a: Visual Pain Scale.

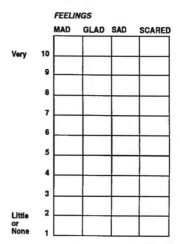

Figure 1b: Visual Basic Feeling Scale.

adapted from the VAS scale[14] was used in this study; in addition, body outlines were used in interventions to differentiate the pain locations and different feelings (Figs. 2a, 2b). The body image, self-image, and mood were also considered in "Draw a Person by Window." The drawing of the human figure was rated for the experience and differentiation of body image, and the window for weather portrayed, reflecting mood, environmental pressures, and internal versus external orientation.

A Disease Awareness Questionnaire (DAS) was adapted for children from the Arthritis Helplessness Index,[19] reflecting relations to locus of control, self-esteem, and helplessness.

The hypotheses was that as a result of the intervention, the subjects would show an increased awareness and differentiation of feelings and sensations of pain, as well as a decrease in the experienced level of pain and helplessness.

METHODOLOGY

Subjects

Twelve patients (7 boys, 5 girls) with JRA were selected as subjects and seen during their regular monthly visits to the Rheumatoid Disease Clinic. Ages ranged from 8-17 years (mean age 12.6 years). Each subject served as his/her own control.

Procedure:

The subjects were seen four times during a four-month period. Upon their first visit, the status of their illness was evaluated the author (KS). During visits 1, 2 and 4, the subjects were asked to complete the set of outcome measures. After completing this set during their second visit, they were asked to portray their intensity and location of pain in a body-outline drawing (Fig. 2a). They also received relaxation- and guided-imagery interventions, including drawing of the imagery.

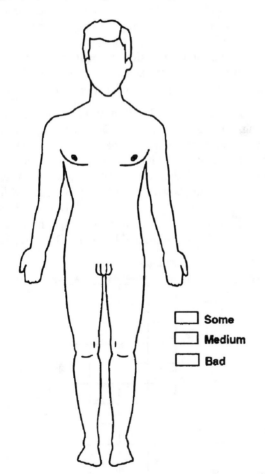

☐ Some
☐ Medium
☐ Bad

Figure 2a: Body Pain Map.

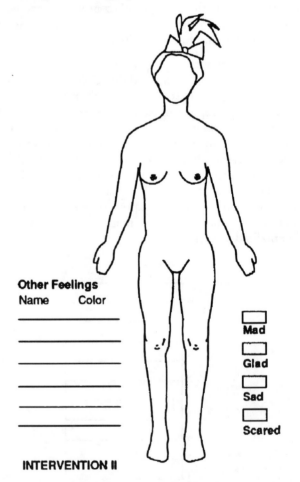

Other Feelings
Name   Color

_____
_____
_____
_____
_____
_____

☐ Mad
☐ Glad
☐ Sad
☐ Scared

INTERVENTION II

Figure 2b: The Feeling Map.

During Session 3, they were asked to complete a Body Feeling Map (Fig. 2b). They also received more relaxation and reinforcement of guided imagery, including drawing it. Colored markers were used to fill in the feeling chart, and to draw "a person by the window" on a 9" x 12" manila paper. At the end of the fourth visit, they completed the outcome measures. During this visit, their clinical status was reassessed by KS.

Measures:

The following measures were used to assess changes in the illness and subjects' responses to it: physician's ratings of restriction of motion, swelling, tenderness, heat, and overall status of the severity of JRA, Disease Awareness Scale, Pain Scale, Feeling Scale, and "Draw a person by window."

RESULTS

The comparison between the change rates for the baseline (B-A) and treatment periods (D-B) were calculated using a univariate repeated-measures test for the numerical data and sign tests for the categorical data.

There were no significant differences between any of the baseline and treatment-period measures for the group; however, inspection of individual case data for some individuals showed changes in the physician's ratings of the severity of symptoms, and on several of the measures used.

Inter-rater reliability for the ratings of figure completeness and weather in the window drawings was highly significant between two raters, as indicated by the Kappa statistics ($p < 0.0001$)

DISCUSSION

Results for the entire group do not show any significant differences between the baseline and treatment period in any of the measures, nor in the physician's ratings in the intensity of the severity of the illness. This is hardly surprising, considering the chronicity of the illness and the few monthly interventions. Prolonged and more frequent interventions would be expected to be more effective. [13]

This study provides information, though, in regard to the measures used. All 12 subjects represented different feelings in the body outline, whereas 6 subjects checked only *glad* on the Feeling Scale on all three collections of the data. The feelings checked by the rest of the subjects were either predominantly *sad* and/or *scared*. The Feeling Scale seemed to project more denial of feelings than reflected in the body outline with the respective feelings. In the case where the feelings were charted more truthfully, the change in feelings reflect the individual's response to the change in the clinical symptoms. The Pain Scale, similarly, does not seem to reflect the subject's experience correctly.

Representations of pain and feelings within the body-outline drawings seemed to provide much more accurate reflection of the inner states and sensations experienced. These outlines were used only for interventive purposes. The measures used to rate the "person by a window" drawing reflected the main changes in the drawings. Three subjects represented inclement weather in their window drawings. Further studies correlating these with the other measures used are recommended.

The greatest drawback of the study was the unavailability of the subjects for interventions more frequent than once a month. Rhodes' study involved 20 weekly sessions, three hours each, [13] as compared to the three one-half- to one-hour interventions in the present study. To counteract this drawback, the subjects were given art materials and paper for expressions of feelings and pain at home, but none complied with this request.

The other drawback was the lack of control subjects due to the limited subject pool available at the clinic.

Regarding guided imagery, 10 subjects were able to imagine a meadow with water nearby in a relaxed state. Six subjects used meadow- or outdoor-tree imagery in the subsequent sessions as an image of a relaxing place. The two subjects who had not been able to visualize the meadow produced images of their rooms with TVs as relaxing places. The guided imagery of a meadow seems to be a valid imagery support for a relaxed state for children and adolescents.

CONCLUSION

Although the results of this study did not indicate any significant changes in the different measures as a result of a brief art-therapy intervention, the study yielded the following important information for future research:

1.   Pain- and feeling measures seem to be more accurately represented in filling in outline drawings than on graded scales.

2.   The effect of imagery and art-therapy interventions for chronic illnesses such as JRA needs to be studied for a prolonged time period. The interventions should be more frequent than once a month.

3.   The changes in the size of the figure drawing, its relationships to the window, and the weather portrayed in the "person by a window" drawing warrant further studies in correlation to the severity-of-illness ratings.

4.   Guided imagery of a meadow by a river appears to be supportive of a relaxed state in children and adolescents. This warrants further systematic study.

REFERENCES

1.   Anderson KO, Bradley LA, Young LD, McDaniel LK: Rheumatoid arthritis: Review of psychological factors related to etiology, effects, and treatment. Psychological Bulletin 98(2):358-387, 1985.

2.   Heisel SH: Life changes as etiologic factors in juvenile rheumatoid arthritis. Journal of Psychosomatic Research 16:411-420, 1972.

3.   Thompson KL, Varni JW: A developmental cognitive-biobehavioral approach to pediatric pain assessment. Pain 25:283-296, 1986.

4.   Varni J, Thompson KL, Hanson V: The Varni/ Thompson Pediatric Pain Questionnaire, I: Chronic musculoskeletal pain in juvenile rheumatoid arthritis. Pain 28:27-38, 1987.

5.   Varni JW, Thompson-Wilcox K, Hanson V, Brik R: Chronic musculoskeletal pain and functional status in juvenile rheumatoid arthritis: An empirical model. Pain 32:1-7, 1988.

6.   Achterberg J, Lawlis GG: Bridges of body mind. Champaign, IL: Institute for Personality and Ability Testing, 1980.

7.   Baron PH: Fighting cancer with images. *In* Wadeson H (ed), Advances in Art Therapy, 148-168. New York: John Wiley & Sons, 1989.

8.   Fleming MM, Cox CT: Engaging the somatic patient through art. *In* Wadeson H (ed), Advances in Art Therapy, 169-180. New York: John Wiley & Sons, 1989.

9.   Lusebrink VB: Imagery and Visual Expression in Therapy. New York: Plenum Press, 1990.

10.   Landgarten H: Clinical Art Therapy. New York: Brunner/Mazel, 1981.

11.   Lovell DJ, Walco GA: Pain associated with juvenile rheumatoid arthritis. Pediatric Clinics of North America 36(4):1015-1027, 1989.

12.   O'Leary A, Shoor S, Lorig K, Holman HR: . A cognitive-behavior treatment for rheumatoid arthritis. Health Psychology 7(6):527-544, 1988.

13.   Rhodes JT, Foard T, Dickstein, L: Professional peer group counseling in the management of rheumatoid arthritis: A clinical trial. *In* Ahmed PI (ed), Coping with Arthritis, 73-106. Springfield, IL: Charles C. Thomas Publishing, 1988.

14.   Abu-Saad H: Assessing children's responses to pain. Pain 1:163-171, 1984.

15.   Beales J, Keen JH, Holt PJL: The child's perception of the disease and the experience of pain in juvenile chronic arthritis. Journal of Rheumatology 10(1):61-65 , 1983.

16.   Thompson KL, Varni JW, Hanson V: Comprehensive assessment of pain in juvenile rheumatoid arthritis: An empirical model. Journal of Pediatric Psychology 12(2):241-254, 1987.

17.   Savedra M, Gibbons P, Tessler M, Ward J, Wegner C: How do children describe pain? A tentative assessment. Pain 14:95-104, 1982.

18.   Unruh A, McGrath P, Cunningham SJ, Humphreys P: Children's drawing of their pain. Pain 17:385-392, 1983.

19.   Nicassio PM, Wallston KA, Callahan LF, Herbert M, Pincus T: The measurement of helplessness in rheumatoid arthritis. The development of the arthritis helplessness index. Journal of Rheumatology 12(3):462-467, 1985.

ACKNOWLEDGEMENT

This study was supported in part by a grant from the Rheumatoid Arthritis Self-Help Group (RASH), Louisville, Kentucky, and Arts in Medicine, Department of Psychiatry and Behavioral Medicine, School of Medicine, University of Louisville, Louisville, Kentucky.

CHAPTER 30

Collage Therapy with Heart Attack Patients

Charlotte Kollmorgen

Stress situations, especially ongoing vocational and family problems, often impair health if an equilibrium is not established. Creativity can relieve the everyday pressures, and the collage technique is both spontaneous and playful, and a simple and effective means of relaxation for patients.

Heart attack patients need to learn to relax. Quite often these patients have a type A personality, as described by English and American authors. They often suffer from the fear of separation and, as a result, compensate by becoming overweight and by smoking too much. There are many more problems, of course. Their problems become so substantial that they do not wish to define them by name. These patients can become masters of denial; they do not have any problems. For, in their perfection, a problem *cannot* exist where it *may* not exist.

The arrangement in the collage with the aesthetic means of printed paper from illustrated magazines and advertisements meets, in a creative way, the perfectionism and the strong defense mechanism of these patients.

In 1981, the author was asked by the physicians at the rehabilitation clinic in Wannsee, West-Berlin, (an institution supported by the BfA, an agency comparable to the National Health Service in England) to work creatively with their heart patients. She found the only suitable technique for this purpose to be the collage.

Collage therapy takes place three times a week and lasts for a two-hour period. Participation is voluntary. All patients receive a written invitation to attend these classes. They are also informed about them by their doctors.

During the course of one year, approximately 10 percent of the total number of heart attack patients took part in the collage-therapy sessions. Since 1981, over 2,000 patients have created collages with spontaneity and creativity. In doing so, they felt, thought, created, observed, and acted profoundly with unexpected perception.

The creation of a collage is simple, stimulating, concrete, and very effective. Just as the consumer may be prompted by an ad into buying a particular product, the patients are stimulated, by the printed black-and-white or colored paper in the magazines, into creating images which convey their wishes, their fears and anxieties, consciously or unconsciously. Thus, this can be actually seen as the reversal of the advertisement effect.

A patient sits alone at a table or with a group of other patients; gradually he begins to see the pictures, forms, colors, and lines displayed in the magazines. Depending on his personality, he will either proceed purposefully or he will let himself be surprised by what appeals to him. Guided only by his personality, or by those forms, shapes, or colors which appeal to him, the patient proceeds. He will be surprised by his creative perspectives. Now, he begins to search, find, cut, tear, take and put aside the various pictures, etc. Who is ever allowed to grasp whatever he wants without encountering boundaries, rules, or commitments, or without causing him pain when separation occurs (tearing out, throwing away)? The voluntary, playful experimental association with the movable elements in collage relaxes and provides joy, positive experience, encouragement, and ultimately self-confidence.

Collage therapy is the quickest and most protective means for people who are under extreme stress to achieve relaxation through creativity and to open up possibilities which were, until then, closed to them. The patient is completely *free* — and in this lies the true meaning of the therapy. There exists *no* obligation, *no* necessity, *no* pressure to perform. *No* instructions are given. Neither artistic skill nor experience in the use of the materials are pre-requisites because the potentiality and possibilities are unending.

All those patients who are in the rehabilitation phase ask what they should do. A patient explained it as follows: "So you want me to do this?" "No, I want you to *want* to do it." Pause — surprise, irritation, relaxed laughter, comprehension. And now the patient 'must' discover only what he wants to seek and find which will benefit him personally. What he does *today* is his life. What will his life be? What he makes of it; with his hands, his mind.

CASE STUDIES

A patient said the following during a collage session: "The forest that surrounds me is dead, but the small tree is alive. The water will come to me." With these words, he showed the key to his positive fantasy, *himself*. His first attempt at collage was a dead black and white forest and dark clouds, both of which he assembled into a form similar to a television picture. All of a sudden a little green tree appeared: "That is I," said Mr. Low. Gradually, intense and impressive ideas were shaping up. Then, suddenly a problem seemed to arise: "I want to build a wall." (He was talking about the middle segment which lay between the top and bottom of the cardboard.) "Should I or shouldn't I? What do you think?" "Build your wall and try by yourself to do what *you* want to do! I don't know what *you* should do. Build your wall and you will see what it looks like and where *you* stand. In front of it, behind it? On top or wherever. *You* will see, observe, perceive, feel, think and know what is the right position for *you*. What *you* eventually do is *your* decision."

Continued communication between the patient and the therapist concerning the collage commences only upon the wish of the patient. It is the task of the therapist to develop the trust which enables the patient to open him/herself. Through verbal communication the creative process is renewed — seeing, searching, finding, nearing, and orienting oneself.

The experience of creative reflection, whether by heart-attack victims or by other people who are in stress situations which cause health disorders, provides one with strength to experiment in daily life, opens new paths for one's senses, leads one out of often self-inflicted isolation, and gives courage and desire to try something new.

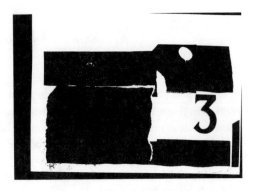

Figure 1: D.G.'s first collage, after her second bypass surgery.

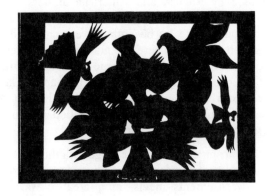

Figure 2: 'Birds are picking my heart.'

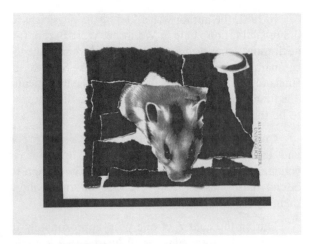

Figure 3: 'I will fight my way through!'

After her second bypass operation, D.G., a 70-year-old female patient, created her first collage during her rehabilitation phase (Fig. 1). Then she was required to decide for or against yet another operation. This prompted the creation of her second collage, 'Birds are picking my heart,' where black birds are picking a red heart (Fig. 2). One week before the new operation, the patient said: "I will fight my way through!" after she had stood at a distance and looked at her third collage from all angles (Fig. 3). The operation was successful. Due to this type of rehabilitation, she had reached the stage where the operation stopped being the most important worry in her mind. Through the creative aspects of collage therapy, she taught herself to open her mind to other creative ways of her life.

REFERENCE

Kollmorgen, Charlotte. Collagen Therapie/ Bildnerische Arbeit mit Herzinfarkt-patienten in der Rehabilitationsklinik. Stuttgart: Hans Huber Verlag, 1989.

CHAPTER 31

Art as a Facilitator
to Communication in Dementia

Melanie Graham • *Kathleen C. Bryant*

Change is one word to describe the New Age in America: change in the aging population, in the methods of health care, and in the attitudes toward the deterioration that is part of increasing longevity. Change manifests itself in terminology — the elderly are now *geriatric*, senility is *dementia*, and the *adult day care center* has emerged.

The community has replaced the family. In some instances, day-care centers operate Monday through Friday from 8 a.m. to 5 p.m. for people who live with relatives, in board-and-care homes, or in their own places with community-based support. Participants in such facilities have received a medical diagnosis and must be under the care of a physician. Physical therapy, speech/language therapy, occupational therapy, and psychological support services are available. Recreational therapy frequently is included in the care plan. Although the stated purpose of the center is to assist the geriatric population, younger individuals who have survived life-threatening disease and/or trauma often present with symptoms that make them eligible for inclusion in the group. It became apparent to the authors that within these 'care' communities, verbal interaction would facilitate the psychosocial needs of this population, stimulated by the technique of encouraging drawing or sketches. As far as could be ascertained, the strategy of drawing in a group setting to meet interaction needs had never been used. A few reports were uncovered that explored drawing with individual stroke patients. Troupe explored drawing with individual nonverbal patients.[1] Yedor and Kedo found notably creative communication through drawing in a severe aphasic patient.[2] Lyons studied the use of sketches as a communication avenue in aphasic adults.[3]

The authors have had considerable experience with the communication value of drawing by young children. Children consistently draw pictures that stimulate communication about themselves, their emotions, and their fantasies. They respond particularly well in group situations. It followed that if groups were successful with children, it should be possible to stimulate communication with adults who appeared mildly depressed, passive, and verbally limited. Precedents were found which clearly indicate that for therapeutic purposes, adults, through drawing, could be as expressive as children.[4,5]

Although the objective was not therapy, the authors elected to present the day-care population with a drawing task for the purpose of facilitating communication among themselves and others. Approximately 30 participants were seated at two long tables and supplied with paper and colored pencils. The instruction given was: "Draw yourself when you were five." The resulting verbal interaction from both tables was surprising. "I can't draw," said one person, whose neighbor replied, "Tell me what you looked like and I will do it for you." Personal interchange flowed among the group. Persons who had been habitually silent carried on animated verbal interchange around personal reminiscences. These responses prompted the authors to develop a study based on *Art as a Medium to Stimulate Conversation*.

METHOD

A protocol based on the use of drawing and clay modelling was developed to elicit creative and verbal expression of universal human themes. Eight sets of instructions were developed based on the human yearning to reminisce. The themes were (1) *When We Were Five*, (2) *Favorite Pet*, (3) *Favorite Animals*, (4) *Favorite Flowers*, (5) *First Ride in an Automobile*, (6) *Houses Remembered*, (7) *Special House*, and (8) *Dolls and Children*. The participants' verbal and nonverbal communications were carefully monitored and recorded.

SUBJECTS

All participants of the day-care center, ranging in age from 32 to 87, were included in the study. Seventy-five percent were female; 25% were male. Medical diagnoses included stroke, trauma, Parkinson's disease, multiple sclerosis, dementia, and Alzheimer's disease. As a group, they appeared mildly depressed, passive, and limited in verbal social interaction.

RESULTS AND DISCUSSION

Verbal behavior ranged from partially intelligible but appropriate utterances to detailed life stories. Telegraphic speech patterns produced by the severely impaired were frequently expanded by others in the group, who in the past had not demonstrated any 'helping' or 'reaching-out' behavior. The drawings ranged from primitive to sophisticated. At times they were incomplete, but usually the form could be recognized. Clinical experience has suggested that internal visualization is expressed in drawing. Thus, reminiscences became concrete and were expanded upon. Thoughts became fixed rather than fleeting and were shared. For example, the response to the remark "That's a nice house" brought the reply, "This is not really a picture. It's just thoughts." During modelling sessions, increases in free- association, conversation, and verbal interchange were observed. Interpersonal relations blossomed with drawings and making of dolls. Discussions of roots, marriages, children, death — all the human ex-periences — were shared compassionately and received emphatically.

The participants were no longer depressed and passive, each reminiscing of his or her personal story. They had actively transferred the auditory-verbal channel to a visual-tactile mode. This mode facilitated communication with staff and volunteers as well as within the group. Changes were apparent in several ways: Patients no longer resisted therapy, their responses were more meaningful, behavior improved, and the staff reported easier access to patients and greater success in filling needs. A window of communication had been opened.

REFERENCES

1. Troupe E: Training severely aphasic patients to communicate by drawing. Annual Convention of the American Speech-Language-Hearing Association, 1986.
2. Yedor K, Kearns, K: Establishing communicative drawing in severe aphasia through response elaborative training. Clinical Aphasiology Conference, 1987.
3. Lyon J, Sims E: Drawing: Its use as a communicative aid with aphasic and normal adults. Clinical Aphasiology Conference, 1988.
4. Furth G: The Secret World of Drawings. Boston: Sigo Press, 1988.
5. Siegel B: Peace, Love & Healing. New York: Harper & Row, 1989.

SUGGESTED READING

Dychtwald K: Age Wave. New York: St. Martin's Press, 1989.

CHAPTER 32

'A Moving Point of Balance':
Introduction to Transformative Art

Beth Ames Swartz

INTRODUCTION

Can art be transformative or healing and if so, for how many people? This is a preliminary analysis of the author's exhibition, *A Moving Point of Balance* (owned by Stanton S. Perry of California), and the participants/viewers reactions to it. Another tour is being planned to collect additional data.

DESCRIPTION of the EXHIBIT

The results of a six year study (1986 - 1991) of viewer reactions to *A Moving Point of Balance* are presented. The exhibit is a contemplative art installation that is both environmental and participatory in nature. It chronicles the author's experiences with the rituals of Native American and East Indian cultures and includes seven 7' x 7' paintings (with light reflective materials), each presenting an East Indian chakra (places in the body that govern emotional, intellectual and spiritual equilibrium). The viewer follows a "journey" from painting to painting. At each station, participants stand within a colored light bath in a darkened room, listening to soothing music. Included in the exhibition is a Navajo medicine wheel by the Native American healer David Paladin and a "balancing room" that combines light and optics technology (Figure 1).

MATERIALS and METHODS

Computer cards were available to be filled out as viewer/participants were leaving the exhibition at each venue. Pencils and pens were provided. Completing the questionnaire was optional. The cards were coded and entered into the computer in 1991.

The Moving Point of Balance Viewer Reaction Card included several questions concerning the demographics of the participants: Age group, sex and marital status. A question designed to gauge overall reaction listed these choices: Uplifted, Centered,

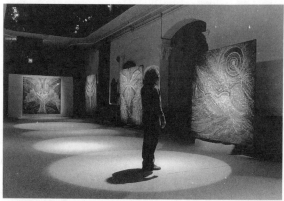

Figure 1: *"A Moving Point of Balance". Installation Photograph at the New House Center for Contemporary Art, Staten Island, 1989.*

Relaxed, Unaffected, Dissatisfied and Other. The card asked the viewer to judge his/her reactions to the Paintings, Music, Color Baths and Balancing Room by checking one of the following: More relaxed and peaceful; Less relaxed and peaceful or Unaffected. There was also space provided at the bottom of the card for additional comments (Charts A and B).

DATA ANALYSIS

Data analysis was performed by sociologist Mary Westcott from Arizona State University and Michael Dornan, sociologist and private consultant, using the statistical package SPSS (P.C. Version).

Approximately 1,468 respondents from seven cities (Staten Island, New York; San Diego, California; Aspen/Snowmass, Colorado; Tucson, Arizona; Palm Springs, California; Tempe, Arizona; and Salt Lake City, Utah) computer the Viewer Reaction Cards.

RESULTS

Demographics of the viewers

1) *Male/Female ratio:* 68% were female; 28% were male; and 4% undetermined.

Chart A: Viewer Reaction Card to "A Moving Point of Balance". Front.

Chart B: Viewer reaction Card to "A Moving Point of Balance". Back.

2) *Age Range*: 56% were between 25-45 years; 29% were over 45; and 15% were under 25.

3) *Marital Status:* 59% were single; 33% were married; and 8% undetermined.

Levels of reaction

1) *Level One*: Of the 96% who responded to the questions, 92% of those had a positive reaction and felt relaxed, uplifted, centered, stimulated or spiritually moved.

2) *Level Two*: Response rate to specific questions about the four parts of the exhibition (paintings, music, color baths and balancing room) ranged from 91-94%. Of those:

- 72% were more relaxed by the paintings
- 80% were more relaxed by the music
- 76% were more relaxed by the color baths
- 76% were more relaxed by the balancing room.

3) *Level Three:* Willingness to be on the mailing list and to find out more about the exhibition: 66%.

4) *Level Four*: This is the most important of the four levels concerning the people who had extraordinary reactions, either healing or transformational: 30% made additional comments; of these 7% had extraordinary reactions, excerpts of which follow:

■ Physical Reactions: "Centered me"; "Internally focused me"; "Gave me a deep sense of wellbeing";

"My body was pain-free"; "Cured my migraine"; "Increased energy"; "Giddy"; "Lighter"; "My sinuses were cleared and I was able to breathe better"; "My hands throbbed with energy"; "Physically warm to perspiring"; "Heightened my usual senses"; "I was in pain when I walked in, now I am no longer in pain"; "Like a treatment of polarizing therapy of balancing out the body"; "Felt movements of energy in my chakras (energy centers)"; "Rejuvenated"; "Cleansed"...

■ Emotional, Spiritual and Transformational Reactions: "My life is changed forever"; "Transcendent"; "Hope-filled"; "Inspired"; "Energized"; "Totally immersed"; "Tuned-in"; "Joyful" "Activated"; "Serene"; "Strengthened"; "Awed"; "Intrigued"; "Overjoyed"; "Peaceful"; "Moved"; "Curious"; "Warmth"; "Incredible beauty"; "Overwhelmed"; "I cried"; "A Holy experience"; "Inspirational"; "Warmth in my heart"; "Transported"; "Felt a more healing, transcendental energy"; "Spiritually higher"; "Brought visions"; "Touched me deeply"; "Combination of color" "Painting and music was very healing and spiritually uplifting"; "Confirms and re-affirms our connection to universal laws"; "Emotional response"; "Power"; "Spiritual experience"; "Fantastic - the most inspiring exhibit I have ever seen"...

DISCUSSION

Four general results emerged:

1. Most people (92%) do report a more relaxed, uplifted and a generally positive response to the experience. It seems that further study in multi-sensory environments would be helpful as the ancillary positive conditions of a darkened room, the color-light baths that the viewer/participants walk into as they view the paintings and the special music (commissioned for its relaxing sound qualities) seemed to enhance the therapeutic effect upon the viewers and all contributed to the totality of the experience.

2. There were some general sex and age differences. More single people and more women seemed to come to the exhibition. Men were twice as likely to report being unaffected by the exhibit and younger viewers were more likely to report being unaffected (Tested by chi-square, $p < .05$).

3. The fact that 66% of the respondents said they would like to be on the mailing list was also an important piece of information.

4. For some people, (approximately 7% of the total respondents) the exhibition seemed to have to

have an extraordinary healing or transformative effect, either physically, emotionally, or spiritually.

CONCLUSION

There is a growing number of artists in the United States, and perhaps around the world, who see their art practice as a healing experience for themselves, others, the culture and the Earth.[1] Diverse in the forms of their art-making, these creators include visual artists and others who are not so easily defined.

Although the style of their art varies, these artists share a commonality of dedication to the interconnectedness of life. They also express a desire for their art to make a difference not only in their own lives, but in the lives of others and the physical world in which they live.

This type of art could be called *transformative art*. This means any visual or performing art that expresses or evokes spiritual truths or higher states of consciousness that lead to a greater understanding of oneself, humanity, nature, the cosmos and their interdependence. Transformative art is intended to directly effect or heal the body, mind and spirit of the artist through the creative process and of the receptive viewer/audience through the experience of the art itself. A presentation of transformative art differs from the usual exhibition one sees in a museum or gallery.

In the transformative art experience, it is important to understand that the artist intentionally creates the art for a healing or therapeutic effect for him/herself and for the viewer. The artist often feels a higher purpose and sees art-making as a path to greater spiritual evolvement. Sometimes the artist sees him/herself as a shaman or healer.

Usually the transformative art experience demands more of the viewers and often challenges them to participate in a new way in an aspect of their inner self. This sort of activity presents a radical change in priorities for both the artist and the viewer.

The original purpose of art, starting with cave painting, was for healing or protection. Siberian shamans who built environments for healing their patients created exquisite costumes and instruments to aid them in their healing work. Once again, artists are cleaning up rivers using ceremony and ritual. They are recycling cast-off machine parts and creating sculpture. They can be found using sound, color and light in hospitals as well as museums, going into cancer centers and creating art with AIDS patients with the intention of raising consciousness of art as a healing force.

The transformation of culture can occur only if we are willing to allow new ways of being together harmoniously to emerge. Artists can be a major force and a peaceful army to help create the wholeness which our culture so sorely needs.

"In America, a number of artists are currently working in a spiritual mode. They hold onto and bear with the art system only to utilize its distribution and communication potential, and its occasional economic largesse. They see art as more than paint on canvas, more than commodity, status object or investment ploy. Art is a quest, a healing and devotional activity that change the artist, the viewer and life as we know it."[2]

REFERENCES

1. Cemblest, R.: The Ecological Explosion. Art News Magazine, Summer, 1991. pp. 97-105.
2. Perreault, J.: Introduction Essay. A Moving Point of Balance catalog, p.8.

CHAPTER 33

Art and the Frail Institutionalized Elderly:
A Multifaceted Approach

Glen Paul

INTRODUCTION

Upon admission to a long-term-care (LTC) health facility, an elderly resident is confronted with the formidable challenge of adapting his or her identity, built up over a lifetime of experience as a healthy and capable person, to circumstances of dependence, increasing physical and cognitive impairment, and an institutional life style.[1] If depression, aggression, and other dysfunctional responses are to be prevented, opportunities must be incorporated into the resident's institutional experience for the maintenance of a positive sense of self and the development of a positive attitude toward living in the LTC facility.[2]

The production and consumption of art (the process of making your own and experiencing someone else's, in both time- and object-based forms) are used to address these needs at University Hospital in Vancouver, Canada. Since 1986, the departments of physiotherapy, occupational therapy, music therapy, and volunteer services, as well as an interdepartmental Art and Environment Committee, have involved the 300 geriatric residents at the University of British Columbia Site Extended Care Unit (UBC ECU) in a comprehensive program of art activities. Our experience is consistent with the generally held view that an interdisciplinary approach to resident treatment, in this case using art, is highly effective.[3] Art, a focus of intellectual, emotional, and spiritual expression, is used to balance the unit's primary focus on physical health so that quality of care and quality of life are fostered equally. Increasingly, this balance between medical and psychosocial concerns is recognized as essential to good long term care.[4]

The term *art therapy* has evolved from the name for a particular psychotherapeutic tool into a title that indicates the broad nexus between psychotherapy and art.[3] Art is not presented to UBC ECU residents as therapy. Rather, their preconceived notions of art as the embodiment of beauty, skill, achievement, and status are acknowledged, and the expressive process is developed in conjunction with those beliefs. Residents are invited to understand art as a process of personal and interpersonal integration, but are not required to abandon traditional academic concepts in order to work with art.

ANCHORING THE PAST

Residents at the UBC ECU have demonstrated that successful adaptation to institutional living is built upon the foundation of an affirmed past. They express the desire that past experiences, values, habits, goals, relationships, and achievements are not negated by institutionalization, but are carried over and respected even if current activities and abilities are greatly diminished. Art is used in several ways to provide this affirmation. If a resident has produced art in any form, as a professional or hobbyist, it is displayed or performed within the unit. For example, film makers have screenings of their work and dancers give demonstrations of their moves. Those who have not produced work of their own but who have studied, collected, or found special meaning in the work of an artist, have it incorporated into their environment and their relationship with that art acknowledged.

Typically, residents have given up a home fashioned over a lifetime into a sanctuary of personal control. By bringing art from that home into UBC ECU, they not only make a statement about who they have been, but make a powerful claim on the hospital room (or part of a room) allotted to them as their personal space. Art is provided for residents who no longer have possessions from their pre-institutional life to rekindle their traditional connections with art. For residents whose cognition is modified by senile dementia into a concern with the past, references to historic art have great meaning.

Acknowledging residents' historic art production and consumption activities has proven not only to strengthen their identity, but also to provide a means of social contact and integration into the UBC ECU community. Art produced by residents in the past makes statements to which others respond. It serves as a catalyst for discussion with residents, staff, and visitors, prompting an exchange that may start with the art at hand, perhaps old photographs or quilting, but invariably develops into other areas of dialogue. Work by artists the resident enjoys is often recognized by others who share their appreciation of it, so that it serves as a bridge of common interest.

MASTERING THE PRESENT

Art is used in the UBC ECU not only to reinforce residents' pasts, but also to address their present concerns. They face four general tasks in successfully adapting to institutional living: finding out how the LTC facility works and how it can be made to work for them, feeling 'at home' in the facility, building new social relationships, and finding meaning and purpose in their lives in the LTC facility.[5] Exposure to the literature and drawings of other residents on the themes of relocation stress and strategies, and the production of their own art about those experiences, are used to assist residents in exploring the structure of the UBC ECU and their place in it. Art production and consumption as a group, as a theater audience or as individual cast members of a theatrical production also foster a sense of community in residents. Involvement in art activities such as attending chamber music recitals or working collaboratively on window paintings is a stimulating yet non-threatening way for residents to get to know each other. The art activity, adapted to compensate for the residents' disabilities, provides a shared experience of normalization and accomplishment.

Finding meaningful ways to spend time in the UBC ECU is reported by residents to be a major challenge. The loss of self-esteem in retirement from former roles as productive workers, a common problem among the elderly, is exacerbated by the limitations imposed by their disabilities and institutionalization on choosing and developing new activities.[3] Boredom and apathy often result. Art production and consumption afford residents meaningful leisure activities and, if pursued more intensively, fulfilling occupations. Activities of art consumption such as listening to a storyteller or watching a dancer usually appeal to even the most apathetic resident, who is then gradually introduced to more demanding forms of art consumption, such as going on a bus tour

of architecture in the local area. Similarly, art production is started with simple exercises such as drawing a family tree, and progresses toward more demanding projects such as making a video.

SEEING THE FUTURE

Perhaps the most difficult issue expressed by residents in the UBC ECU is the contemplation of the future. Their failing health and advanced age make the prospect of death a looming reality and the possibility of afterlife an important question. Often, they conceive of a life after death in terms of traditional religious imagery. Traditional paintings and literary works are used in the unit to stimulate consideration of and discussion about this issue, and art production, e.g. drawing and dance, on this theme is encouraged. The non-linguistic art forms are ideally suited to this subject, which residents find the most difficult topic to articulate in words.

CONCLUSION

In summary, the UBC ECU experience has shown that an interdisciplinary, multifaceted approach to the use of art in an LTC facility can significantly augment the quality of life for its frail elderly residents. Art production and consumption activities can build upon residents' preconceived notions of art as a prestigious vocation into activities of personal expression and growth. Art, the mediated expression of thought and emotion, can be immensely useful to the institutionalized elderly seeking to retain their past, cope with their present, and face their future.

REFERENCES

1. Weiner MB, Brok AJ, Shadowsky AM: Working with the Aged, 2nd ed, 53-61. Norwalk, CT: Appleton, 1987.
2. Zusman J: Some explanations of the changing appearance of psychotic patients. International Journal of Psychiatry 4:216-237, 1967.
3. Valletutti PJ (ed), Christoplos F: Interdisciplinary Approaches to Human Services, 1-11, 13-16, 93-107. Baltimore: University Park, 1977.
4. Anderson BR: What makes excellent nursing homes different from ordinary nursing homes? Danish Medical Bulletin 5:7-11, 1987.
5. Canadian Association on Gerontology. 19th Annual Scientific & Educational Meeting: Victoria, BC, Oct 25-28, 1990. Ottawa: CAG, 1990.

CHAPTER 34

Art Therapy with
Schizophrenic Suicidal Patients

Dalia Merari

A state of depression following an acute schizophrenic phase is well-known in psychiatry and much has been written about its occurrence.[1] On the other hand, depression may also exist during the course of this acute phase, in which case it may assume either of the following two forms: open and explicit or masked.[2,3] The latter is often hard to diagnose as the overwhelming, florid, and global clinical picture masks the depressive symptoms. Thus, lack of proper diagnostic techniques combined with the heavy imprint of the psychotic symptoms denies one the ability to identify this masked depression . An early diagnosis of masked depression is crucial as it enables the therapist to follow the development of this phenomenon and choose the appropriate therapeutic approach especially at the height of the phase.

In this study, the author has concentrated on drawings made by a group of schizophrenic patients who had attempted suicide prior to their hospitalization. It has been indicated that suicide attempts more often committed during the post-psychotic state.[4] The act of suicide was committed at a time when it seemed that the patient's condition had improved yet his inner feelings and the stress of life brought the patient to this fatal decision. It was further suggested that schizoid suicide was not merely an expression of a death wish, but an expression of an unconscious, deep-rooted wish that death could have lead to a rebirth.[5] It was a desire to escape from a situation which the person could not cope with, a wish to return to the womb so as to be reborn with a chance for better life.

The symbols which appeared in our patients' drawings could be associated with those that signal death. These symbols served therefore as the impetus for this study. The author attempted to discover and expose the masked depression in a suicidal patient using the patient's drawings as the analytical medium.

This patient was one of a group of patients which constituted the study group.

SAMPLE

The sample comprised 10 schizophrenic patients who were hospitalized in a psychiatric hospital, all of whom made a suicidal attempt before the hospitalization; and three committed suicide after. All patients were in an acute psychotic state, had a serious difficulty in verbal emotional expression but revealed significant expressive capability using graphic symbols.

CASE STUDY

Uri, 25, was hospitalized following a suicide attempt. He was the elder son of a two-children family. There were persistent conflicts between his parents that he was asked to interfere in and resolve. He graduated from high school as a mediocre student and later served in the army. After discharge, he attended a reception clerk's course. Following graduation, he tried unsuccessfully to get a job in an hotel. He became desperate and later on decided to commit suicide.

Describing this attempt on his life, in the hospital, he said "Now, I would not even scratch myself." In the hospital he felt sheltered and secure. The therapeutic framework was for him a replacement for his family. Uri was active and cooperative. At that period his medical record revealed "improvement in his condition. There is however a conspicuous poverty in expression coupled with increasing 'closeness'. The level of conversations is low. The will and drive for death decreased but apathy became prominent."

Figure 1 is one of a series of drawings in which Uri's helplessness came to the fore. Using Gouache colors the *capsule* and the arrows pointing out were painted red while the incoming, piercing arrows were painted blue. Red is a hot and temperamental color,

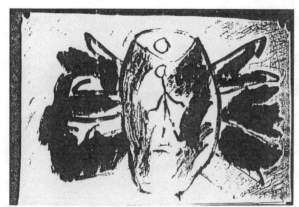

Figure 1: "Capsule and Arrows," illustrating Uri's helplessness.

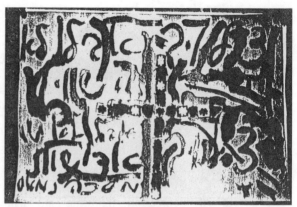

Figure 2: "The Cross," Uri's second drawing.

whereas blue is cool and tempered. The specific fashion of their application well represents Uri's ambivalence in terms of the opposite direction of the arrows. Following the application of the Gouache colors, he chose a more moderate color - green, which for him symbolized hope. The opposite forces acting in this drawing are multi-dimensional:

   a.   the capsule represents both isolation and protection from the hostile external world;
   b.   the arrows symbolize the pressures exerted on him; those that emanate from him and that are attracted to him, which often collide with each other;
   c.   the hope, which is represented by the green background color, and the tempest represented by the arrows in the center also constitute opposing forces.

The clinical description of Uri as an apathetic and poor patient may be explained by the fact that most of his energy was directed at his inner conflicts as revealed by his drawings.

His next drawing (Fig. 2), *The Cross*, was made of various materials. A floral fabric served for the cross which was carefully cut and glued to the paper. This piece was made with utmost concentration. Using a pencil he wrote "a cross may also be a flower if one knows how to make things." At this stage he accelerated the pace of his work. Using a brush and black color Uri filled in the spaces between the flowers and added in writing "apathy, mask." He then continued using green. Being careful about color cleanliness he wrote "crossed, crossed" adding, using red "but not Jesus, but not Jesus" and the word "fed up" (a single word in Hebrew). Finally he covered the drawing in orange. The description of the process of drawing is crucial to the understanding of Uri's psycho-dynamics. Along the course he revealed his ambivalence to life. The cross as a symbol of death

and martyrdom is composed of flowers - the symbol of beauty and vitality and of black lines which express depression and sorrow. Initially the drawing was well planned and organized but slowly Uri lost control of his emotions expressing despair. The various colors have symbolic significance. Following the "fed up" interjection he became scared of the contents of the drawing and tried to conceal and cover his explosive emotions.

The third drawing (Fig 3) may be described as an act of emergency following his former drawing. In it, he calls for help using the word "save me" in various languages and in a very forcefully colorful and desperate manner. The bars serve as if to guard against an uncontrollable emotional explosion.

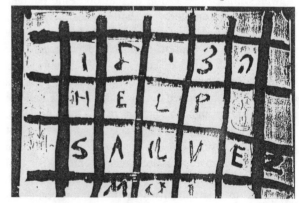

Figure 3: "Save Me," Uri's third and last drawing.

DISCUSSION

Uri's capacity to challenge his condition was very limited. Following his discharge, desperation and depression became increasingly dominant. He was then treated at a day-care center until he had to move to a clinic nearer to his location. The disengagement from the hospital might have resulted in his decision to put an end to his life.[6] Uri viewed death as a savior and redeemer. He had dreams of other worlds and thoughts about reincarnation. He mentioned that the idea of existence after death was initially encouraging but later it has turned into something frightening: "Here, one may finish off with one's life. In the nether world there is an endless continuity."

It should be emphasized that during the period when his drawings were made, Uri consciously denied his wish for death. It is possible that the glimmer of hope shown in his drawings was indeed part of this complex emotional system. On the other hand, his difficulty in fighting the conflicts, the challenges, and the desperation brought him to form an alternative conception of the world and a choice of death as the redeeming solution. Uri committed suicide two months following his discharge from the hospital.

REFERENCES

1. Mayer Gross W. Uber die Stellunosnahme auf Aubgelaufenen Auten Psychose. A Gesamte Neurol Psychiat, 60: 160-212, 1920.

2. Johnson DA. Study of oppressive symptoms in schizophrenia. Br J Psychiat, 139: 89-101, 1981.

3. Planasky K. Psychotropic drugs and depressive syndromes in schizophrenia. Psychiat Quart, 52: 214-220, 1980.

4. Schneidman, Farberow, Litman. The Psychology of Suicide. N Y, Jason & Aronson, 1976.

5. Guntrip H. Schizoid Phenomena: Object Relations and Self. London, Hogarth, 1959.

6. Fromm-Reichman F. Principles of Intensive Psychotherpy. Chicago, The University of Chicago Press, 1950.

CHAPTER 35

Bridge Drawings as a Projective Technique for Assessment with Substance Abusers

Ronald E. Hays • *Sherry Lyons*

Art therapists often seek a focused art-therapy technique to use with a specific population. We know that certain patient populations have characteristics seen in assessment as well as needs seen in treatment that would make a particular art-therapy technique either tailor-made or not at all applicable.

Symptom groups found to open up more on drawings than on other projective techniques are the alcoholics. In psychologically evaluating the personality patterns of alcoholics...drawings, relative to other projective techniques, are receiving increasing attention because they have been found to be ... difficult to falsify, and in its application there is no barrier of education or language ... it also requires little time and is simple to give.[1]

The *bridge-drawing technique* was developed by the authors[2] and used with various populations. The substance abuser seemed to be one that responded particularly well to this technique, in both assessment and treatment.

The professional response to the authors' earlier work suggested further investigation with specific patient populations. The substance-abuse population was selected for various reasons. Outstanding among these are the patients' problems with communication,[3] their use of water in imagery,[4] and their use of denial and resistance in treatment.[5] A review of the literature[6] revealed certain characteristics of substance abusers that were most often addressed in art therapy. They were found to be: (1) a tendency to avoid feelings, (2) communication difficulties, (3) a need for a non-threatening way to express oneself, (4) low self-esteem, (5) loneliness, (6) self-attack, (7) dependency/ autonomy ambivalence, (8) suspicion, (9) control problems, (10) identity problems, and (11) fear.

The authors felt that these issues and needs could be addressed using the bridge-drawing technique. From the projective qualities that were present in the verbal associations to bridges, it was felt that the actual drawing of a bridge would help to concretize the patient's symbolic imagery. Through the results of research on bridges drawn by patients, an appreciation developed for this projective's ability to aid addicted patients in communication. In treatment, the bridge drawing aids the art therapist in assessing the patient's relative position in therapy and predicting the course of treatment.

Bridge drawings by more than 200 substance abusers were examined for similarities of expression with respect to eleven variables. Differences seen in the drawings of the various addictive populations were presented through representative drawings of the specific addictive groups: alcoholics, drug abusers, and eating-disorder patients.

The directions given to the patients in groups were as follows: (1) Draw a picture of a bridge going from some place to some place. After the majority of patients were finished drawing the bridge: (2) Indicate with an arrow the direction of travel; and (3) Place a dot to indicate where you are in the picture.

The eleven variables utilized for assessment are listed below, along with the respective characteristics of the drawings of each substance-abuse group:

1. *Directionality*: An arrow was used to denote the direction of travel when crossing the bridge. Drug (*D*) and alcohol abusers (*A*) indicated movement to the future. Eating-disorder (*ED*) subjects seldom depicted a direction of travel. It was extremely difficult for them to identify a direction toward a treatment goal.

2. *Placement of Self*: This appears to reveal how the person sees himself/herself in relationship to a goal. *D*, self in the past, not in treatment; *A*, self in middle of the bridge (treatment); *ED*, self more often in the past — difficult to see self in recovery.

3. *Places Drawn on Either Side of the Bridge*: This indicates a specific goal to be reached. *D*, future highly idealized; *A*, addiction and recovery on each side of bridge, concretizing it as a metaphor; ED - symbolic, abstract places - denial of reality.

4. *Solidarity of Bridge Attachments*: This indicates the firmness of the connections and the grounding of the bridge. *D*, strong attachments in one-third of patients; *A*, often not attached, but solid when attached; *ED*, attachments solid.

5. *Emphasis by Elaboration*: This shows whether emphasis is placed in the past, future or on the bridge itself. *D*, focus on past or bridge; *A*, no particular emphasis; *ED*, focus on past and future.

6. *Bridge Construction*: This indicates the strength of the bridge and the commitment to maintain the communication. *D*, most were steel, strong therapy commitment — if not steel, materials and commitment tenuous; *A*, stone or steel, but often with no guardrails; *ED*, tenuous construction, often with unidentifiable materials.

7. *Type of Bridge Depicted*: *D* and *A*, excessive and strong supports revealing wish or need for them; *ED*, usually no visible means of support.

8. *Matter Drawn Under the Bridge*: This is perceived as threatening or non-threatening in nature. *D*, water often agitated and divided into good and bad; *A*, calm water; *ED*, often nothing depicted — inability to identify problem to solve.

9. *Vantage Point of the Viewer*: *D*, close, secure and honest, or distant and indirect; *A* and *ED*, close and eye level.

10. *Associations to the Drawings*: *D*, often grandiose, saturated with denial; *A*, guarded, defended and employing great denial; *ED*, highly intellectualized.

11. *Consistency of Gestalt*: Any parts of the picture that do not seem to fit with others indicates an incongruity. *D*, intense color and agitated line quality; *A*, absence of integration, organic line quality, and little or no color used; *ED*, integrated use of color, line quality and form.

REFERENCES

1. Hammer E: The Clinical Application of the Projective Drawings, 603. Springfield, IL: Charles C Thomas, 1980.

2. Hays R, Lyons SJ: The bridge drawing: A projective technique for assessment in art therapy. Arts in Psychotherapy 8(3): 207-217, 1981.

3. Nucho AO: Art therapy. *In* Waldorf GF (ed), Counseling Therapies and the Addictive Client. Baltimore: University of Maryland School of Social Work and Community Planning, 1977.

4. Albert-Puleo N, Osha V: Art therapy as an alcoholism treatment tool. Alcohol Health and Research World 1(2):28-31, 1976-77.

5. Kaufman GH: Art therapy with the addicted. Journal of Psychoactive Drugs 13(4):353-360, 1981.

6. Moore R: Art therapy with Substance Abusers: A review of the literature. Arts in Psychotherapy 10(4):251-260, 1983.

CHAPTER 36

Club Rusk: A Creation of the Wheelchair Accessibles

Laurie Brand • *Hollister Gignoux* • *Lynn Kable* • *Susan Stoltz*

PURPOSE

The video production *Club Rusk*, a work which combines art, music, live action, Super 8 and animated film with video, provided adolescent and young-adult patients with the opportunities to explore psychosocial issues related to their hospitalization. These patients were hospitalized due to spinal cord injury, congenital disabilities, and head trauma. Feelings of anger, fear and frustration were expressed through addressing issues that included social isolation/relationships, loss of body functioning, and cognitive/physical impairment.

METHODS

Film

The young-adult patients formed a production company called the *Wheelchair Accessibles,* and were assigned roles such as director, camera operator, and production manager. During workshops, they were taught technical film and video skills, and created their own script and storyboard around the common theme of the hospital. Super 8 film was used to create the actual video.

In the scenes which could not be shot due to technical, artistic or logistic reasons, stop-motion animation of art materials was used to create the image. The art of animation utilizes frame-by-frame movement of art work or materials.

Art Therapy

Through the use of art materials such as collage, acrylic paints, and construction paper, the patients were able to create a visual work which combined live action, drama, documentary and animation. Animation was chosen by the patients to express the characters' dreams and fantasies, and enabled them to portray feelings experienced during their hospitalization. The patients met weekly to coordinate ideas.

Music Therapy

An electronic keyboard was used which provided many options for the creation of a musical soundtrack. Acoustical instruments such harmonica and percussion (drums, claves, and guiros) were also utilized. The patients composed music and wrote all the lyrics to the songs. They met for music-therapy groups twice weekly for the duration of the production; after the music was completed, the patients performed live and were professionally recorded by a sound engineer.

GROUP PROCESS

The combination of using film, art and art-therapy, and music and music-therapy processes enabled the patients to explore interpersonal as well as individual aspects of their rehabilitation. During the making of the video, the patients, ages 15-22, were living in a communal-like atmosphere. The close proximity and lack of privacy were potential causes of tension and uneasiness. The structured environment that the video production created enhanced positive feelings of belonging among the patients, as well as the various staff members who participated in the project.

The project gave the patients the freedom to be creative and spontaneous in their self-expression, while at the same time addressing vital concerns regarding long-term hospitalization. Significant adolescent issues such as sexuality, body image, and self-esteem are particularly important to adolescents in long-term rehabilitation, as they are compounded by the physical and cognitive impairments these young adults face.

The three different modalities used (film, art and music) each served to further rehabilitation goals. Following is a brief description of each of the processes that took place during the video production:

Film/Process

The *Club Rusk* video was filmed entirely from the perspective of a patient in a wheelchair. This provided a unique visual opportunity for the non-disabled, newly disabled, or congenitally disabled viewer to share in this experience. For the patients, it was an opportunity to share with others their perspective on their environment and personal feelings.

Patients worked together closely as part of a production team; they screened all footage, selected the shots, revised the storyboard plan, and in post-production had the final say in editing. They had the opportunity to be interviewed regarding their feelings about the project; this segment appears at the end of the 11-minute video.

The process of creating a video to be publicly viewed created a sense of responsibility and maturity among the patients. There was a serious yet friendly atmosphere at the production meetings, and this attitude prevailed throughout the project.

Art and Art-Therapy Process

This process enabled the patients to physically construct feelings initiated by the multimedia video process. They gained a sense of empowerment by being able to create a fantasy through the use of art materials. One of these fantasies, the hospital burning down, was created through the animation of paint, cut paper, and collage material.

For some, this control had been lost after their injury and prolonged hospitalization. Anger related to disability could be expressed in the safety of the art studio and peer group. The combined use of collage and animation allowed for a wide scope of experimentation and creative development. For many, this was an introduction to a new technique and design concept.

Music and Music-Therapy Process

Through the group music-making process, patients were able to blend modern and primitive sounds with rhythms and tonalities from their varied ethnic backgrounds. This helped to foster an original musical blend which precisely captured the group's spirit.

Feelings addressed in the original song lyrics were related to anger, frustration, acceptance of disability and loss, self-esteem, camaraderie, humor and togetherness. Participation in the music-therapy group gave the patients an opportunity to be creative, spontaneous, and honest in a structured environment.

The group enabled patients to express feelings regarding hospitalization both verbally, through discussions and lyric-writing, and nonverbally, through playing an instrument. For some, playing an instrument was carried over from their pre-hospitalization, and they were able to share their special talents with peers and reconnect with a positive aspect of their lives. For others, the music group was a time for learning new instruments and techniques. Cognitive as well as physical challenges were met in this way, and new creative skills developed.

SUMMARY

Primary concerns of adolescents in long-term rehabilitation were counterbalanced by the opportunity to participate in a multidimensional creative process. Without such opportunities, patients might become emotionally withdrawn and apathetic, causing problematic interpersonal dynamics which can impede the rehabilitation process.

The multimedia approach of using film, art and music combined with the processes of art therapy and music therapy provided an ongoing opportunity for young-adult rehabilitation patients to explore personal and interpersonal aspects of hospitalization. With the added component of film and video production, the creative process allowed patients to receive validation, positive feedback and recognition from those who viewed the video — other patients, doctors, nurses and staff members, as well as family and friends.

The most enduring benefit of the project, however, is the existence of lasting documentation that will be viewed by others, who will undoubtedly be moved and touched by the powerful experience that is *Club Rusk* — a video that reflects a challenging time in the lives of a group of people who were able to unite, pool their talents, and create a meaningful work of art.

ACKNOWLEDGEMENT

The Club Rusk *project was funded by a grant to Hospital Audiences, Inc. from the New York Council on the Arts/Arts-In-Education program, in collaboration with the Therapeutic Recreation Department of Rusk Institute. It was created during the fourth year of HAI's* Film, Animation and Video with Hospitalized Children *project.*

Club Rusk *is currently in non-commercial distribution through HAI for the purpose of educating therapists, artists and film/video makers in arts and health-care venues.*

PART III

BIOMECHANICS
AND ERGONOMICS

CHAPTER 37

Upper Extremity Biomechanics in Musicians

Kai-Nan An • *Ben M. Hillberry* • *Jaiyoung Ryu* • *Fadi J. Bejjani*

Disorders of the upper limb in performing artists can result from direct or indirect trauma or from overuse. These injuries occur when the objective exceeds the physiologic tolerance. Biomechanical research enables us to estimate the capacities of the body and the load environment encountered by the muscle, bone, and joint during various types of artistic activities. Potential strength and movement of the upper limb depend on the characteristics of muscle contraction and the mechanical advantage of the individual muscles acting at the shoulder, elbow, wrist, and hand joints. Numerous analytic and experimental methods have been employed for establishing the functional strength and load as function of the joint range of motion. In this paper, techniques for such biomechanical study, as well as the available data pertaining to the upper limbs, will be reviewed. The implications of these findings to the prevention, diagnosis and treatment of occupation related disorders will be also be discussed.

KINEMATICS

Kinematics is the study of motion without reference to the forces causing this motion. This fundamental branch of dynamics finds a challenging application in the study of human movement. Joint function is determined primarily by the shape of the contact surfaces and constraints of surrounding soft tissue. In reality, all anatomic joints have six degrees of freedom (DOF) in which six independent parameters must be measured and described if the position, or motion, of the attached limb segments in space are to be defined. However, for the study of function and performance of a joint, very commonly only the rotations are considered. For general joint motion in space, three angles of rotations are required to specify the joint orientation and motion. Unfortunately, for finite spatial rotation, the sequence of rotation is extremely important and must be specified for a unique description of joint motion. The concept of Eulerian angle description, based on a specific sequence of rotation, has been adopted in the field of orthopedic biomechanics to unify the description of finite spatial rotation.

Experimentally, three methods have been commonly used for the measurements of joint orientation and limb position in activities of given tasks. The electromechanical linkage method uses exoskeletal linkage systems containing rotatory potentiometers. The linkages are then attached to the proximal and distal segments of a joint where the relative joint motion is measured. A second method using a stereometric approach for kinematic analysis was developed based on the principle that the position and orientation of a rigid body in space can be defined when three noncolinear points fixed to it are defined. The spatial coordinates of these reference markers could be measured by using any of the stereophotographic systems or ultrasonic transducers. Most recently, a third method based on the magnetic tracking system has been available for the direct measurement of three-dimensional kinematics.

The range of wrist motion required to perform activities of daily living has been studied.[1] To perform all activities in a normal and comfortable manner, a total of 60° of wrist extension, 54° of flexion, 40° of ulnar deviation, and 17° of radial deviation is required. The majority of the hand placement and range of motion tasks could be accomplished with 70% of the maximum range of wrist motion. This converts to 40° each of wrist flexion and extension, and 40° of combined radioulnar deviation.

Although the elbow has a normal arc of flexion-extension of 0° to 150-160° and pronation and supination of 75° to 85°, respectively, the full arc of motion is not generally used for most activities of daily living. A study of the functional arc of motion revealed that 15 activities of daily living could be carried out with an arc of motion of 30° to 130° of flexion-extension.[2] Furthermore, the pronation-supination required for these same activities is 50° each. It should be noted that the activities studied were of a routine and sedentary nature. Special requirements for other activities, including occupational tasks, have not been clearly elucidated at this time.

The range of shoulder complex motion involved in activities of daily living has been examined by using the 3Space Tracker system. Analytically, the amount of arm elevation and circumduction which also define the plane of elevation were used to define the shoulder complex motion. The mean positions assumed by the shoulder complex were ranged from 120° of circumduction anterior to the body to 80° of circumduction posterior to the body; and 20° to 130° of arm elevation. For activities with the joint placed in extreme of its logical range of motion, abnormal loading and injury on the joint and surrounding soft tissue could be expected.

Dexterity

A dexterity testing board which utilizes both the manipulation ability of the thumb and the fingers, as well as the adaptability of the hand in handeling objects of varying sizes has been developed[3]. A dexterity test was found to be a useful tool to document the manipulation ability of the hand with different stages of pathology, surgical, and medical treatments. Dexterity testing with objects of varying sizes is essential. For example, it was observed that patients with finger or thumb joint replacement showed more improvement in the dexterity of handling objects of larger size as compared with that of handling smaller objects. This finding might have some impact on implant design and surgical procedures.

KINETICS

For the assessment of the force and moment encountered by the upper extremity during various activities, dynamometers and transducers have never been used. On certain occasions, direct application of the strain gauge on the equipment involved in the activities has also been attempted. Both static strength under isometric contraction and dynamic strength under isokinetic contraction have been measured to define the potential of the body. In addition, the endurance or fatigue characteristics of the muscle group could also be considered as an important factor for performing arts activities.

Potential strengths of various joints in the hand and wrist in normal subjects have been acquired by using the dynamometers for hand pinch and grasp functions. The normal pinch strengths ranged from 3 to 10 Kg and the grasp strengths ranged from 20 to 40 Kg. Wrist position and grasp size have significant influence on grip strength. The isometric strengths of the isolated finger and thumb functions are also measured and could be useful information for the assessment of the efforts of the hand muscle involvement during various art activities.

The strengths of the wrist joint are in the range of 10 to 20 Nm of flexion, 6 to 10 Nm of extension, 10 to 18 Nm of radial deviation, and 10 to 20 Nm of ulnar deviation. Depending on joint angle, elbow strength ranged from 30 to 70 Nm for flexion and 20 to 40 Nm for extension with maximum strength at 90° of elbow flexion.

Musicians' Strength

The upper extremity muscle strengths of professional musicians, including string players, harpists, guitarists, and pianists, have been evaluated. It was found that all string players were symmetrical in their grip and pinch strength despite their handedness. However, asymmetries were found in pianists for the left and right grip strength and for guitarists in both grip and pinch strengths.[1,4] Since playing music involves both hands almost in equal fashion, it was not surprising to observe the symmetry in musicians upper extremity strength.

Extensive electromyographic studies on violin vibrato showed it to be directly dependent on finger/wrist flexor-extensor alternate firing, with pronator and supinator muscles helping to stabilize the elbow joint.[5] Besides, forces of theses muscles during vibrato were computed, utilizing calibrated surface EMG equations. Forces were greatly variable and ranged from 4 to 8 N for the flexors and almost half for the extensor group.[6-8] Ongoing studies are increasing the EMG resolution and number of separate upper extremity muscles tested for both the vibrato and the bowing sides, and adding video analysis for better understanding of the kinematics involved.

Tendon Excursion

The ability to control movements of an individual digit of the hand or a limb of the arm depend very much on the anatomic arrangement of the musculotendinous complex. Biomechanical functions of the musculotendinous complex have been examined based on the relationship of the tendon excursion and the joint angular displacement. The rate of change in tendon excursion as the joint rotates is equal to the moment arm of the associated muscle or tendon for that specific joint motion. The moment arm defines not only the effectiveness of the tendon in rotating the joint but also the mechanical advantage of the tendon in resisting external loads.[8]

The characteristics of the muscle and tendon moment arms for a given load are achieved through specific anatomic constraints. Pulley structures on the palmar side of the digits, for example, restrain bowstringing of the digital flexors when flexing the joints.[9] Alterations of the pulley system in the hand will disturb the relationship between the tendon excursion and joint angular displacement, and thus joint function. On the dorsal sides of the digits, the extensor mechanisms composed of the extrinsic extensors and intrinsic muscles are even more intricate. Proper balance of the excursion and tension among the various branches of the extensor mechanism is important to the coordinated movement of the joints. On the other hand, any imbalance of the extensor mechanism will result in possible deformity of the digits.

The magnitude of tendon excursion during joint movement for a given task would also be important for assessing possible overuse injury due to cumulative trauma.

Muscle and Joint Force

The magnitude of muscle and joint forces experienced for a given task depends on the externally applied load encountered and the mechanical advantage of the musculotendinous structures at the joint, as well as muscle physiology. The force-generating potentials of the muscles are the ultimate determination of the strength and power of the hand and arm. Physiological cross-sectional area (PCSA), which was defined as the volume of the muscle divided by the fiber length of the muscle at resting, has been used to assess the force generating potential of a given muscle.[10]

Furthermore, the characteristics of muscle force generation depend on the length-tension relationship. Simply, there is a region of optimal muscle for maximum performance of the muscle force.[11] The size of an object held in the hand will determine joint configurations, and thus the moment

arms as well as the involved muscles' lengths. All of these parameters will eventually govern the amount of muscle tension and resultant joint forces. Based on analytic evaluation, the forces involved in the upper extremity are not trivial and should not be overlooked.[12,13]

BIOMECHANICAL MODELING OF A FINGER

Biomechanical models are useful tools for understanding the behavior of physiological structures. These analytically based models provide mathematical representations that describe form, function, strength, and performance of the structure. The model can then be interrogated to provide insight as to function and to evaluate strength and performance. The models can assist in improving performance, providing optimum methods, diagnosing performance related injuries, and improving performance techniques.

Modeling Methods

Free Body Diagrams

For a mechanical structure, of which the upper extremity is a prime example, the first step is to draw an appropriate free body diagram (*fdb*). This *fbd* is a simplified representation of the structure which also shows the forces acting on it. An example is illustrated in Figure 1a. The distal phalanx is schematically represented as being separated at the DIP joint. A force is applied at the fingertip, and the tendon forces and reaction forces in the joint are required to maintain the free body in an equilibrium state.

Equilibrium Equations

For a body in equilibrium, Newton's law states that the sum of the forces acting on the free body must equal the acceleration of the body. For two dimensions this must hold in the x and y directions:

$$\Sigma F_x - ma_x = 0$$
$$\Sigma F_y - ma_y = 0$$
$$\Sigma M - I\alpha$$

equation (*1*) where:

F_x, F_y = x,y components of the force
M = moment at a given point
m = mass of free body
I = moment of inertia
a_x, a_y = x,y components of acceleration
α = angular acceleration

Applying these three equations to the free body diagrams of Figure 1 gives a set of equations from which the tendon and joint forces for a known

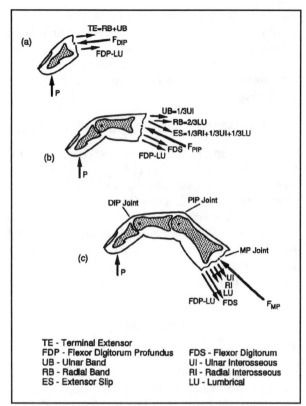

TE - Terminal Extensor
FDP - Flexor Digitorum Profundus
UB - Ulnar Band
RB - Radial Band
ES - Extensor Slip

FDS - Flexor Digitorum
UI - Ulnar Interosseous
RI - Radial Interosseous
LU - Lumbrical

Figure 1: Phalangeal segments in equilibrium

fingertip force, P, and known accelerations can be determined. For static conditions or slow moving conditions, the accelerations are zero or near zero and can be neglected, especially when the mass is small.

Model Evaluation

Representing each of the *fbd*s shown in Figure 1 with equation *(1)* provides a finger model for determining tendon and joint forces. The results depend on the input conditions: 1) fingertip force, 2) finger accelerations, and 3) angular position of the fingers. For the finger model, experimental measurements revealed that the acceleration and finger mass provided only a very small inertia force and, therefore, could be neglected.

Finger Force Model Derivation

The resulting model is similar to that of Weightman and Amis,[14] and was developed to examine finger forces during piano playing. Since the finger inertia forces were found to be negligible, a quasistatic model was developed. It was assumed that the phalangeal segments were rigid bodies, and the motion was two-dimensional and in the sagittal plane. Since the finger joints are synovial fluid joints, the IP

and MCP joints were assumed frictionless. Both the IP and MCP joints have relatively fixed centers of rotation and, therefore, pin joints were assumed. Tendons were assumed to be tight at the time of key impact because of the small inertial force required to accelerate the finger toward the key.

Based on the physiology and anatomy of the finger, the tendons and intrinsic muscles required to balance the fingertip/key force (assumed to be applied normal to the fingertip contact surface) are shown in Figure 1. The long extensor tendon is needed only to raise or extend the finger and can thus be neglected in piano key strike actions. Dorsum palpation of the dorsiflexed wrist during maximum force exertion at keystrike shows this to be true. From anatomic observations by several authors,[15-17] the intrinsic muscle forces and tendon tensions shown in Figure 1 were assumed to be proportional to the physiological cross-sectional area of the muscles.

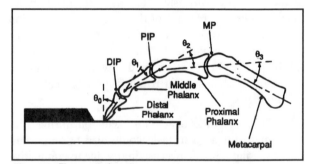

Figure 2: Finger angles, θ_i

The four angular finger segment positions, θ_i, which describe the finger posture at key strike are the key contact angle, and DIP, PIP, and MP flexion angles as shown in Figure 2. Wrist and forearm position are indirectly determined by specifying these four angles, since piano bench height is typically adjusted to position the elbow slightly above the level of the keyboard. Tendon moment arms and angles between the tendons and the more distal phalanges including the effect of the pulleys at each joint are calculated by the model for each finger configuration using the sagittal plane coordinates from the normative model for the hand developed by An, et al.[18] The bowstring model was used to determine the nonlinear relationship between tendon and intrinsic muscle moment arms and joint flexion angles. Because the paths of the tendons are guided by pulleys distal and proximal to the joint centers, flexor tendons on the palmar aspect of the joint move away from the joint centers during flexion (Fig. 3), decreasing the

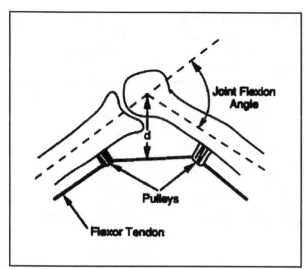

Figure 3: *Tendon bowstring model*

tendon tensions required to balance a given fingertip load. Tendon and intrinsic muscle moment arms were normalized with respect to the distance between the center of rotation of the DIP joint and the center of the concave surface of the PIP joint.

The quasi-static keystrike assumption provides nine equilibrium equations of Newton's second law, neglecting inertial terms, by balancing the moments and forces at each of the three finger joints. Summing moments about the center of rotation (Fig. 1) of each of the joints (DIP, PIP and MP) gives:

$$(FDP - LU) (d_2) - TE (d_1) - P (L_1 \sin \theta_1) = 0 \quad (2)$$

$$(FDS) (d_6) + (FDP-LU) (d_3) - ES (d_7) - RB (d_4) - UB(d_5)$$
$$- P[L_1 \sin\theta_1 + L_2 \sin(\theta_1 + \theta_2)] = 0 \quad (3)$$

$$FDS (d_9) + (FDP - LU) (d_8) + LU(d_{11}) + RI (d_{10}) + UI (d_{12})$$
$$- P[L_1 \sin\theta + L_2 \sin(\theta_1 + \theta_2) + L_3 \sin (\theta_1 + \theta_2 + \theta_3)] = 0 \quad (4)$$

where d_j is the tendon moment arm of tendon j, θ_i is the flexion angle of joints 1, 2, or 3 (DIP, PIP, or MP), and P is the fingertip force.

Assuming a unit fingertip key force, P, the tensions in the tendons and intrinsic muscles (now normalized in terms of the input force, P, can be determined by solving equations *(2)-(4)*. The reaction forces at the articulating surfaces of the joints are determined by balancing forces in the vertical and horizontal directions for each of the phalangeal segments shown in Figure 1, assuming that each joint reaction force passes through the joint's center of rotation.

Average Joint Stress

Average joint stresses for the DIP, PIP, and MP joints were determined by dividing the force by the joint area. This gives an average stress over the contact area for each joint and for each finger position considered. The articulating joint contact areas for the DIP, PIP. and MP joints used in determining the joint stresses were those measured by Moran, et al.[19]

Optimization

An objective function which can be minimized or maximized provides an alternate solution method. As applied in this study, the forces in each joint and in each tendon were selected as objective functions and minimized with respect to the combined angular finger position, i.e. Θ_0, Θ_1, Θ_2, Θ_3. The optimization program uses a numerical search strategy which finds the minimum value of the objective function, or, in this case, a joint or tendon force.

Observations from the Model

The model can provide insight into the influence of fingertip force and finger positions which can reduce forces in the finger. This may lead to improving performance, reducing pain, or alleviating injury. Figure 4 illustrates two representative finger positions and the corresponding DIP joint forces for the two positions. The joint and tendon forces are normalized with respect to the fingertip force. Multiplying the joint or tendon force by the actual fingertip force will give the total joint or tendon force. The results for five increasingly curved finger positions are shown in Figure 5. Comparing the joint stresses with the joint forces shows the influence of the joint area on joint stress.

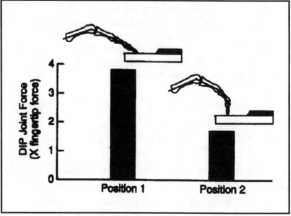

Figure 4: *Normalized DIP joint force for two typical pianist finger positions.*

Using the optimization routine, the finger positions which minimize each of the joint and tendon forces were determined. These results, shown in

Figure 6, illustrate finger position which can reduce finger forces. Table I gives the complete force data for each of the positions of Figure 6. In the optimization study, the minimum position solution surface is relative flat near the maximum and, therefore, slight variation in position from the minimum will show only a small increase in force.

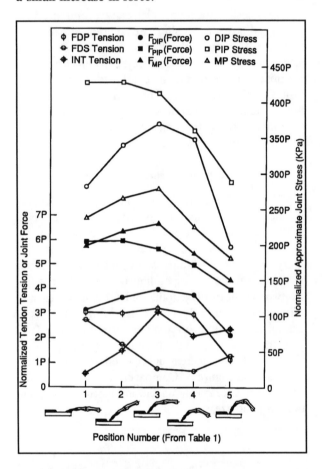

Figure 5: *Normalized finger tendon forces, joint forces, and joint stresses for five finger postures, varying from straight to increasingly curved. These data are also listed in Table I.*

Using video kinematic analysis and mathematical optimization parameters of energy (velocity), force (acceleration), and smoothness of motion (jerk), Bejjani, et al.[20-24] compared three piano techniques utilizing different finger and wrist positions during the performance of various musical tasks. The position found to be optimal kinematically was similar to position number 5 (Fig. 5, Table I). It was also pointed out that professional pianists often switch from one position/technique to another during the course of the same piece of music to fit the demands of the moment, thus rendering optimization somewhat tentative. Video analysis is a non-invasive, non-

obtrusive technique to the musician, not interfering with his/her concentration and focus on the instrument. Moreover, it can usually be performed on location, avoiding laboratory bias.

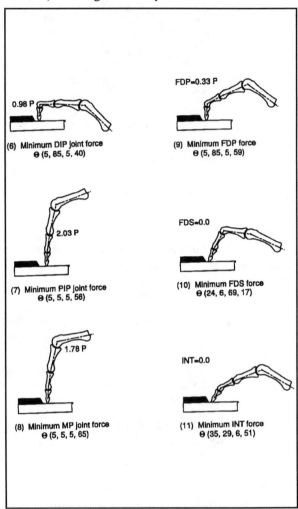

Figure 6: *Finger posture for minimum joint and tendon forces. Complete force data for each position are given in Table I.*

WRIST MOTION ANALYSIS IN PIANISTS

Nine pianists from the department of music at Texas Tech University, in El Paso, were studied: two subjects were concert pianists and professors of music, while the remaining seven were doctoral students majoring in piano. Custom designed electrogoniometers were attached to both wrists of each pianist to monitor wrist motion. Each pianist played slow, medium, and fast exercises, and classical examples in four different categories: trills, arpeggios, octaves, and broken octaves. A digital metronome was used for tempo reference and all performances were recorded audiovisually. Electrogoniometer data were visualized

No.	Objective Function Minimized	Position $\theta_0, \theta_1, \theta_2, \theta_3$ (degrees)	Normalized Forces (X fingertip/key force)												
			Joint Reaction Forces			Tendon Tensions									
			F_{DIP}	F_{PIP}	F_{MP}	INT	FDP	FDS	UI	RI	LU	RB	UB	ES	TE
1	-	80,5,5,20	3.07	5.88	5.72	0.49	2.97	2.65	0.11	0.34	0.04	0.03	0.04	0.16	0.06
2	-	45,5,10,5	3.70	5.93	6.41	1.52	3.02	1.74	0.35	1.05	0.13	0.08	0.12	0.51	0.20
3	-	40,5,35,10	4.04	5.72	6.73	3.17	3.23	0.77	0.73	2.17	0.26	0.18	0.24	1.06	0.42
4	-	40,5,35,35	3.78	5.01	5.46	2.13	3.01	0.67	0.49	1.46	0.18	0.12	0.16	0.71	0.28
5	-	10,25,50,40	2.16	4.00	4.40	2.42	1.15	1.31	0.56	1.66	0.20	0.13	0.19	0.81	0.32
6	F_{DIP}	5,85,5,40	1.00	4.42	4.03	0.16	0.34	4.00	0.04	0.11	0.01	0.01	0.01	0.05	0.02
7	F_{PIP}	5,5,5,56	1.44	2.03	1.87	0.19	0.45	0.53	0.04	0.13	0.02	0.01	0.01	0.06	0.02
8	F_{MP}	5,5,5,65	1.44	2.02	1.78	0.17	0.45	0.53	0.04	0.12	0.01	0.01	0.01	0.06	0.02
9	FDP	5,85,5,59	0.98	4.31	3.91	0.03	0.33	3.96	0.01	0.02	0.00	0.00	0.00	0.01	0.00
10	FDS	24,6,69,17	3.64	4.69	5.67	3.93	2.62	0.00	0.90	2.70	0.33	0.22	0.30	1.31	0.52
11	INT	35,29,6,51	2.55	5.20	4.80	0.00	1.99	2.79	0.00	0.00	0.00	0.00	0.00	0.00	0.00
12	$1/F_{DIP}$	47,5,59,5	4.41	5.74	7.09	4.23	3.63	0.24	0.97	2.90	0.35	0.23	0.32	1.41	0.56
13	$1/F_{PIP}$	58,16,6,5	3.21	6.39	6.64	1.07	2.84	2.90	0.25	0.73	0.09	0.06	0.08	0.36	0.14
14	$1/F_{MP}$	49,5,38,5	4.25	6.13	7.35	3.59	3.54	0.86	0.83	2.47	0.30	0.20	0.28	1.20	0.48
15	1/FDP	56,5,56,5	4.31	5.72	6.93	3.85	3.68	0.45	0.89	2.65	0.32	0.21	0.30	1.28	0.51
16	1/FDS	5,82,5,5	1.15	5.13	5.33	0.96	0.45	4.25	0.22	0.66	0.08	0.05	0.07	0.32	0.13
17	1/INT	8,6,80,5	2.89	4.36	5.84	4.97	1.69	0.00	1.14	3.41	0.41	0.28	0.38	1.66	0.66
18	$F_{DIP}+F_{PIP}+F_{MD}$	5,5,5,85	1.44	2.02	1.78	0.16	0.45	0.52	0.04	0.11	0.01	0.01	0.01	0.05	0.02
19	FDS + FDP + INT	5,5,5,85	1.44	2.02	1.78	0.16	0.45	0.52	0.04	0.11	0.01	0.01	0.01	0.05	0.02

Table I: Normalized resultant joint forces and tendon tensions for various finger positions on the keyboard.

through a monitor, recorded directly by the custom made computer software, and later analyzed using the MathCad software package. Data analysis was done in two groups, because of two distinctly different ways of practicing and playing the piano. Group 1 was a *weight-playing* group, and was represented by one professor and his four students. This group stressed increased usage of intrinsic muscles and forearm rotations and reduced usage of wrist flexors and extensors, in an effort to decrease the chance of occurrence of overuse syndromes, such as tennis elbow. Group 2 was a *traditional* group, and was represented by one professor and his three students.

Trills and arpeggios required wider wrist motion than other tasks, which may explain why these are considered more difficult to play. Group 1 used less wrist motion than Group 2. No close relationship was found between wrist motion and tempo.

REFERENCES

1. An KN, Bejjani FJ: Analysis of upper-extremity performance in athletes and musicians. Hand Clinics 6:393-403, 1990.

2. An KN, Morrey BF: Biomechanics of the elbow. *In* Morrey BF (ed), The Elbow and Its Disorders, 43-61. Philadelphia: WB Saunders Co, 1985.

3. Chao EYS, An KN, Cooney WP, Linscheid RL: Biomechanics of the Hand. A Basic Research Study. Singapore: World Scientific Publishing Co Pte Ltd, 1989.

4. Bejjani FJ, Nilsson G, Kella J: Effect of the instrument on the musician's musculoskeletal system. *In* Atwood DA, McCann D (eds), Proceedings of the 1984 International Conference on Occupational Ergonomics, vol I, 247-241. Toronto, Ontario, Canada: Human Factors Conference, Inc, 1984.

5. Titiloye VM, Bejjani FJ, Xu N, Tomaino CM: Upper extremity force requirements in violin vibrato: A dynamic electromyographic study. *In* Anderson PA, Hobart DJ, Danoff JV (eds), Electromyographical Kinesiology. Amsterdam, Netherlands: Elsevier Science Publishers BV, 1991.

6. Bejjani FJ, Ferrara L, Pavlidis L: A comparative electromyographic and acoustic analysis of violin vibrato. Medical Problems of Performing Artists 4(4):168-175, 1989.

7. Bejjani FJ, Pavlidis L. Kinetics of violin vibrato. J Biomechanics 23(7):730, 1990.

8. An KN, Chao EY, Cooney WP, Linscheid RL: Normative model of the human hand for biomechanical analysis. J Biomechanics 12:775-788, 1979.

9. Lin GT, Amadio PC, An KN, Cooney WP: Functional anatomy of the human digital flexor pulley system. J Hand Surg 14A:949-956, 1989.

10. An KN, Hui FC, Morrey BF, Linscheid RL, Chao EY: Muscles across the elbow joints: A biomechanical analysis. J Biomechanics 14:659-669, 1981.

11. An KN, Kaufman KR, Chao EY: Physiological considerations of muscle force through the elbow joint. J Biomechanics 22:1249-1259, 1989.

12. An KN, Chao EY, Cooney WP, Linscheid RL: Forces in the normal and abnormal hand. J Orthopedic Research 3:202-211, 1985.

13. Morrey BF, An KN: Biomechanics of the shoulder. *In* Rockwood CA, Matsen FA (eds), The Shoulder, Vol 1(6), 208-245. Philadelphia: WB Saunders Co, 1990.

14. Weightman B, Amis AA: Finger joint force predictions related to design of joint replacements. J Biomed Eng 4, 1982.

15. Landsmeer JMF: The coordination of finger joint motions. J Bone and Joint Surg 45-A(8), 1963.

16. Smith RJ: Balance and kinetics of the fingers under normal and pathological conditions. Clin Orthop Rel Res 104, 1974.

17. Chao EY, An KN: Determination of internal forces in the human hand. J of the Eng Mech Div, February 1978.

18. An KN, Takahashi K, Harrigan TP, Chao EY: Determination of muscle orientations and moment arms. J Biomech Eng 106, 1984.

19. Moran JM, Hermann JH, Greewald AS: Finger joint contact areas and pressures. J Orthopaedic Res 3(1), 1985.

20. Bejjani FJ, Xu N, Parnianpour M, Pavlidis L: Optimizing kinematics and kinetics of piano performance. J Biomechanics 23(7):730, 1990.

21. Bejjani FJ, Xu N, Parnianpour M, Pavlidis L: Optimizing kinematics and kinetics of piano performance. Proceedings of the 13th Annual Meeting of the American Society of Biomechanics: 158-159, 1989.

22. Bejjani FJ, Ferrara L, Xu N, Tomaino CM, Pavlidis L, Wu J, Dommerholt J: Synchronized electromyographic, video and sound analysis of piano performance with comparison of three methods. *In* Presperin JJ (ed), Technology of the next Decade. Proceedings of the 12th Annual Resna Conference, 258-259. Washington, DC: Resnapress, 1989.

23. Bejjani FJ, Ferrara L, Tomaino CM, Xu N, Pavlidis L, Wu J, Dommerholt J: Comparison of three piano techniques as an implementation of a proposed experimental design. Medical Problems of Performing Artists 4(3):109-113, 1989.

CHAPTER 38

Quantitative Analysis of the Motion and Balance Function of Artists

Kerong Dai • Chris J. Snijders • Hideo Yano

Posture and motion are two of the main factors that influence performance quality of performing and visual artists. Through their consummate coordination and preeminent balance ability, artists create harmonious, graceful, and attractive performances. The objectives of this paper are to introduce the technique, apparatus, and basic knowledge of quantitative evaluation of the motion, posture, force, and balance function of artists during performance. These would serve as bases for modification of their training program, correction of their performing posture, analyzing the mechanism and improving the management of their acute and chronic occupational injuries and diseases, and evaluating training and management results.

MATERIALS AND METHODS

Body posture can exist without noticeable motion, but motion always involves posture. The latter is at the origin of numerous physical problems of performing and visual artists. To analyze posture and movement, technology has become available for measurements in biomechanics laboratories as well as on stage.

In posture, static muscle forces are of interest, especially to maintain the trunk in an upright position. Postural change has two major aspects: change in the position of the trunk and change in the shape of the spine, the latter being defined by flexion, extension, lateral bending, and torsion. The position of the trunk is measured by an inclinometer placed on a small area of the skin of the thoracic spine.

For change in the shape of the spine, a good approximation can be achieved by using the indirect method of measurement shown in Figure 1, indication points A and B on the back. The change in the distance between them is a measure for the sum of the rotations in several joints. Measured between T8 and L5, the length of the contour of the back

increases if the subject bends forward, and decreases if he bends backward. Lateral bending can be determined by the measurement of the difference in length of the skin surface on each side of the spine. Torsion of the spine as a whole concerns the rotation of the shoulders in relation to the pelvis and can be up to 40° to either side. As the largest part of this rotation takes place in the thoracic spine, measurement thereof can be restricted to that region.

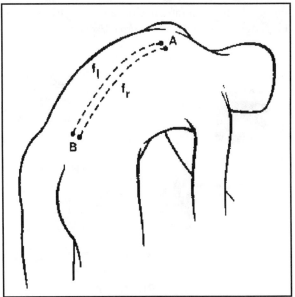

Figure 1: Inclinometer on the thoracic spine. The change of distance between A and B measures lateral bending.

The most important design requirements were that the instruments should be concealed under the subject's clothing, that the subject should suffer no inconvenience in carrying out his normal daily activities, and that the measurements should be continuous.

Data recording is as follows: After attachment of the sensors and a calibration procedure, the transducer signals are either recorded on a modified four-channel cassette recorder (Medilog 4-24, Oxford Medical Systems) or on a digital data storage device (Ramcorder 1), which will be described later. From the signals, various parameters can be calculated.[1]

The analog recorders use a vulnerable audio cassette tape, they have a limited signal-band width (DC-10Hz), a simple take-up mechanism which can cause tape-speed errors, and lastly, they need a separate, costly replay device. With the technique of using semiconductor memories available for portable data storage, the data-recorder Ramcorder 1 was developed.[2] The basic principle is rather simple: Analog signals are digitized by an analog-to-digital converter and the values of the samples are stored in a semiconductor memory (Fig. 2). After data collection, the memory contents are transferred to a personal computer system (PC) and are available for further analyses.

Ramcorder 1 has a 1.2 Mbyte data storage capacity (SRAM) and provides many user programmable settings. There are, for instance, 43 different sampling rates available ranging from 1 sample/hour/channel to 512 samples/second/channel.

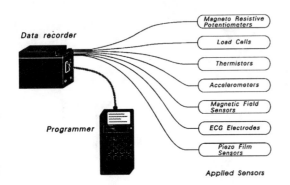

Figure 2: Part of the Ramcorder set and sensors.

RESULTS

Forces

The following distinction is made for measuring forces: 1) forces exerted by the body on instruments; and 2) body-supporting forces. Small sensors were developed to measure the forces exerted on the keys of a piano. Here, the force perpendicular to the key and the shear force can be of interest.

Balance Function

The basic principles of the system of human balance function evaluation lie in the pathway of the center of gravity of the body, sway amplitude and

frequency which are capable of quantitatively reflecting the balance ability of the body.[3] The subject stands on the platform of a dynamometer, maintaining a specific posture. Load and time data are entered through amplifier and A/D converter into the computer. Then, the distance between the instant projection point of the center of gravity of the body and the center of the platform can be calculated, and the balance parameters and dynamic curves within certain period will then be obtained (Appendix). For each of the postures, the following eight parameters were obtained: average and maximun A-P sway amplitude, average and maximum L-R sway amplitude, maximun displacement range of the center of gravity (A-Pand L-R), and frequency of the sway of the center of gravity (A-P and L-R).

The process of the above-mentioned measurements are simple, prompt, and non-invasive. And the data could be used for evaluation and modification of a dancer's training program.

Body Fluctuation

Measurement of body fluctuation is valuable for examining the degree of vertigo, and equilibrium dysfunction. In the last ten years, video development and computerized analysis software have made it possible to examine the fluctuation and micro vibrations of each segment of the body. Motor skill, particularly in dancing, is intimately related to segmental body fluctuation and to respiration.

REFERENCES

1. Groeneveld WH: A solid state recording system for ambulatory monitoring of postural signals. Proc Biotelemetry XI, Yokohama, Japan, in press.
2. Snijders CJ, van Riel MPJM, Nordin M: Continuous measurement of spine movements in normal working situations over a period of 8 hours or more. Ergonomics 30(4):639, 1987.
3. Lichtenstein MJ, Shields SL, Shiavi RG, et al: Exercise and balance in aged women: A pilot controlled clinical trial. Arch Phys Med Rehabil 70:138, 1989.

Appendix. Curve diagrams of balance function of a girl with 2 years artistic gymnastics training, in neutral (a-c), and in single stance on forefoot after 6 rounds of whirling performance (d-f): a,d, pathway of center of gravity; b,e, A-P sway amplitude-time curve; c,f, L-R sway amplitude-time curve; 1,2, maximum range of A-P and L-R direction; SA, sway amplitude.

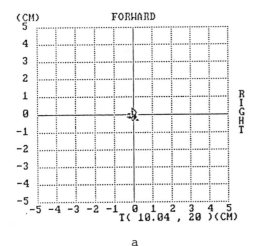

a

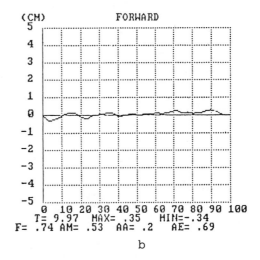

b

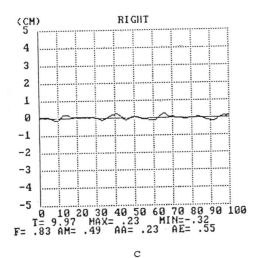

c

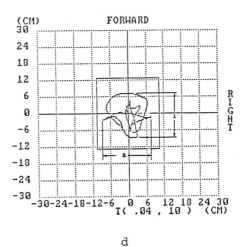

d

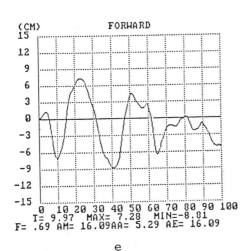

e

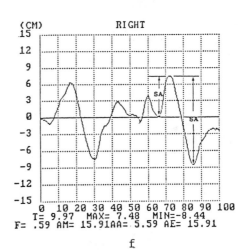

f

CHAPTER 39

Dynamic Loading on the Musculoskeletal System

Arkady S. Voloshin

INTRODUCTION

Everyday physiological activities, such as walking, stair climbing and even bus riding result in severe dynamic loading on the human musculoskeletal system. This loading is a part of the continuous dynamic onslaught on the various parts of the locomotor system. As evident from experimental data,[1] there is a need for a least some dynamic excitation in order to sustain normal bone growth and development. However, there also exists an overwhelming evidence that excessive dynamic loading may be one of the reasons behind osteoarthritis and related chronic degenerative diseases.[2-4] To provide a meaningful degree of protection, one needs a tool capable of evaluating and quantifying the amount of dynamic loading the musculoskeletal system experiences during various activities. Such a tool is presented here together with the results pertinent to walking, running, stair climbing, jumping, and flamenco dancing. Possible ways to reduce the amount of this loading are discussed as well as effect of body fatigue on the ability of the musculoskeletal system to attenuate and dissipate dynamic loading.

METHODOLOGY

An accelerometric technique[5] is employed to obtain the quantitative values necessary to evaluate the amplitude of the shock wave initiated during foot strike and propagating through the entire musculoskeletal system. Here, a novel approach was utilized by which a small low-mass PCB piezoelectric accelerometer (Type 303A02) was placed on the skin surface of the subject's tibial tuberosity. The accelerometer was rigidly connected to a specially built T-shaped aluminum holder, weighting 2 grams, which was attached to the subject with a velcro strap to record the actual bone acceleration in the tibia, at heel strike.

The natural frequency of this lightweight accelerometer attachment is above normal running frequency, thus avoiding inaccuracies due to resonance.[7-9] The comparative evaluation of this setup with an accelerometer attached directly to the tibial tuberosity by screws[10] shows a mere 5% reduction in the signal amplitude with the non-invasive setup. Since variation between different steps can be of the same order of magnitude, this margin of error was deemed acceptable. With the appropriate modelling and calibration procedures, even such negligible discrepancy can be accounted for.[11]

The accelerometer output was fed into a TEAC HR-30 portable analog data recorder. The power packs along with the data recorder were placed in a custom designed casing to protect against shocks and to be worn by the subject while performing various physical activities of interest to this investigation. The assembly was then securely attached to the subject's back to allow for natural motion, without an excess of weight or trailing wires.

After the subjects performed all necessary tests, the tape was removed and played back on a multi-channel analog cassette data recorder. Each analog cassette tape has the capabilities of storing 45 minutes of seven channels of data in a frequency range of DC up to 1250 Hz. These tapes were fed into a personal computer, modified into a high-speed multi-channel data acquisition and storage system. The sampling rate was 1000 samples/sec, thus allowing the accurate acquisition of signals from 0 to 500 Hz.

RESULTS

The initial investigation was aimed to establishing a baseline. A healthy, young population of 40 students were used and signals from their tibial tuberosities were recorded during level walking. The average acceleration was 2.4g (range 0.8 to 4.2g). Typical acceleration and pressure patterns are shown in Figure 1.

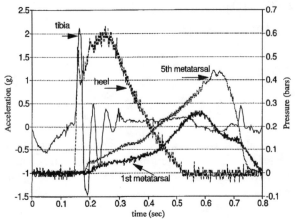

Figure 1: *Typical acceleration and pressure patterns associated with heel strike, during walking.*

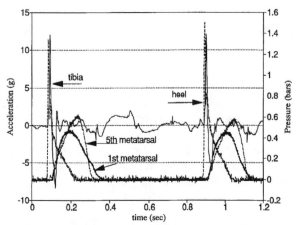

Figure 2: *Typical acceleration and pressure patterns recorded during running on an asphalt surface.*

Running is the other widespread physical activity.[12,13] Statistics show that 40 million Americans will run this year and 60% will suffer some kind of injury.[14] Thus, there is a significant interest in the analysis of dynamic loading while running as well as in the effect of running surfaces.[15-17] Nine subjects (six males and three females) participated in this study. Their average weight was 691±83 N (range 578-809 N). They were running an average of 14.8 km (9.2 miles) a week during the testing period. Their mean age was 21 years. Data collection involved running on each of three surfaces (grass, asphalt and, indoor track) successively. The order of running was different for each subject, and the total time spent on one

surface was 3-5 minutes. Since the total testing procedure involved running a distance of less than 500 meters per surface, the fatigue effect was assumed to be negligible. A typical accelerogram recorded on the left tibial tuberosity while running on asphalt is shown in Figure 2. All subjects were classified as heel strikers, which was confirmed by the pressure patterns acquired.

Results of this investigation clearly show that running generates much higher dynamic loading then walking and that the choice of running surface is of great importance (Table 1).

Table 1: *Dynamic loading on the musculoskeletal system, during running on various surfaces.*

SURFACE	Heel Strike (g) (mean±S.D.)	Difference (%)
Asphalt	13.67±3.12	19.92
Grass	17.07±4.32	--
Polyurethane track	14.36±2.78	15.88

Physical activities such as stair walking and jumping result in increased dynamic loading on the musculoskeletal system. Loy and Voloshin[18] showed that walking down a staircase induced shock waves with an amplitude of 130% of those observed in walking up stairs and 250% of those measured in level walking. The jumping test revealed levels of the shock waves nearly eight times higher than in level walking. It was also shown that the shock waves invading the system may be generated not only by heel strike, but also by a metatarsal strike. In this study an effort was made to moderate the dynamic loading through the use of a specially designed viscoelastic insoles. They caused a significant reduction in shock wave amplitude (9 to 41% depending on insole type and physical activity).

Flamenco dancing

The percussive footwork during dancing generates a series of shock waves which may impose unusual demands on the dancer's musculoskeletal system. The observed shock waves were characterized not only by relatively high magnitudes, but also by a presence of a high frequency component.[19] A viscoelastic in-shoe insole reduced the amplitude of the dynamic loading by 9 to 29%, depending on the dance and performer.

One of the interesting aspects of dynamic loading on the musculoskeletal system is its dependence not only on footwear, surface, physical activity, but also on the state of the body. Recent work has shown that fatigue can significantly increase dynamic loading.[20] An increase of up to 30%, depending on the subject and degree of fatigue, was observed.

CONCLUSIONS

The described technique of acquiring biomechanical data is useful for the evaluation and comparison of different types of motion. Moreover, one may use the described experimental procedure as an important tool for developing and rating new shock absorbing insole and footwear designs.

The greater repetitive impulsive loads experienced during running, jumping and flamenco dancing may tend to accelerate the degenerative processes of joints and bones. Future research will be needed to identify the most significant frequency ranges encountered during such activities, so that the proper surfaces and footwear combination may be determined to reduce dynamic loading on the musculoskeletal system.

REFERENCES

1. Gross, T. S. and Rubin, C.T. Site-Specific Adaptation of the Growing Skeleton to Altered Mechanical Stimuli. Proceedings of the 15th Annual American Society of Biomechanics Meeting, 142-143, October 16-18, 1991.

2. Radin, E. L., Paul, I. L., and Rose, R. M. Role of Mechanical Factors in Pathogenesis of Primary Osteoarthritis. The Lancet, 4, 519-522, 1972.

3. Voloshin, A. S., and Wosk, J. In-Vivo Study of Low Back Pain and Shock Absorption in Human Locomotor System. J. Biomech. 15, 21-27, 1982.

4. Radin, E. L., Orr, R. B., Kelman, J. L., Paul, I. L. and Rose, R.M. Effect of Prolonged Walking on Concrete on the Knees of Sheep. J. Biomechanics 15, 487-492, 1982.

5. Light, L. H., McLellan, G. E., and Klenerman, L. Skeletal Transients on Heel Strike in Normal Walking with Different Footwear. J. Biomechanics, 13, 477-480, 1980.

6. Voloshin, A. S., and Wosk, J. Influence of Artificial Shock Absorbers on Human Gait. Clinical Orthopaedics and Related Research, 160, 52-56, 1981.

7. Saha, S., and Lakes, R. S. The Effect of Soft Tissue on Wave Propagation and Vibration Tests for Determining the In-Vivo Properties of Bone. Journal of Biomechanics, 10, 393-401, 1977.

8. Ziegert, J. C., and Lewis, J. L. The Effect of Soft Tissue on Measurements of Vibrational Bone Motion by Skin-mounted Accelerometers. J. Biomech. Eng. 101, 218-222, 1979.

9. Loy, D. The Biomechanical Evaluation of the Various Modes of Human Locomotion, M.S. Thesis, Lehigh University, 1987.

10. Voloshin, A.S. and Simkin, A. Evaluation of the Skin-Mounted versus Bone-Mounted Accelerometer. Proceedings of the Vth Mediterranean Conference on Medical and Biological Engineering , 32-33, Patras, Greece, 1989.

11. Kim, W. Model of the Heel Strike Effect. Ph.D. thesis, Lehigh University, 1991.

12. Drez, D. Running Footwear, Examination of the Training Shoe, the Foot and Functional Orthotic Devices. Am. J. Sports Med., 8, 140-141, 1980.

13. Gudas, C. J. Patterns of Lower-Extremity Injury in 224 Runners. Compr. Therap. 6, 50-59, 1980.

14. Clancy, W. G. Runners' Injuries. Part Two. Evaluation and Treatment of Specific Injuries. Am. J. Sports Med., 8, 287-289, 1980.

15. Nigg, B.M., Denoth, J., Kerr, B., Luethi, S., Smith, D, and Stacoff, A. Load Sport Shoes and Playing Surfaces in Sport Shoes and Playing Surfaces, Human Kinetics Publishers, Inc., 1-23, 1984.

16. Sheehan, G. Running Wild: Injuries and Biomechanics. Physician Sportsmed. 12, 43, 1984.

17. Slocum, D. B., James, S. L. Biomechanics of Running. Journal of the American Medical Association. 205, 721-728, 1968.

18. Loy, D., and Voloshin, A.S. Biomechanics of stair Walking and Jumping. Journal of Sport Sciences, 9:137-149, 1991.

19. Voloshin, A.S., Bejjani, F.J., Halpern M. and Frankel, V.H. Dynamic Loading on Flamenco Dancers: A Biomechanical Study. Human Movement Science, 8:503-513,1989.

20. Milgrom, C., Finestone, A., Shlamkovitch, N., Wosk, J., Laor, A.,Voloshin A.S. and A. Eldad, Prevention of Overuse Injures of the Foot by Improved Shoe Shock Attenuation: A Randomized Prospective Study. Clinical Orthopaedics and Related Research (in print).

CHAPTER 40

Physically Efficient Cello Playing

Jeffrey Solow

It is often useful to analyze a subject by stripping away the nonessentials and reducing it to its fundamental elements. Applying this procedure to cello playing leads to the question: "What is the goal in playing the cello?" The answer might be summed up as follows: (1) Make it sound good. (2) Don't injure yourself in so doing. While number (1) would seem to be *the* goal, it seems safe to assume that every cellist wants to "make it sound good" for more than just one or two performances. If this is indeed the case, then healthy playing is of equal importance to good-sounding playing. It is reasonable, though, not to stop quite yet but to add one more idea: (3) Try to achieve number (1) as easily as possible.

This last seems not quite as fundamental as the previous ideas, but it is the one that opens up the entire concept of physically efficient cello playing. The author will show what is meant by first explaining playing at its most theoretical level.

To play the cello, the player uses his or her muscles to raise the arms against the earth's gravity, causing them to gain potential energy. Just as the potential energy in the slowly falling weights of a grandfather clock drives the pendulum and the gears of the clock, so the potential energy of the arms is transformed into the kinetic energy of their motion. (Unlike the weights, however, the cellist does not let his arms drop all the way down before he 'rewinds' them. As he plays, his muscles must be continuously raising his arms as they drop to keep them at the same height and replenish their potential energy.) The moving arms then impart their kinetic energy to the cello, which converts it into sound waves — another form of kinetic energy.

The two arms work in essentially the same way. The muscles of each arm hold it in a position so that its weight feels balanced on the cello. The only real difference between the two is that the left arm moves vertically up and down the fingerboard while the right arm moves laterally. (With the right arm, the bow provides a sort of variable extension that enables the arm to remain in constant contact with the string as it [the arm] swings from side to side.)

Physical efficiency is the production of a maximum amount of work output for a minimum energy input. The 'trick' in playing the cello efficiently is finding the position for the arms in which the holding muscles do the least amount of work that will still cause, as well as allow, the cello to produce its sound properly.

Understanding the concept and theory of physically efficient cello playing is important, but intellectual understanding alone is not enough. Playing is an experiential activity; to truly understand physically efficient playing, one must experience what it *feels* like to play efficiently. As a teacher, the author uses experiential exercises to help students find this feeling. Excellent results have been achieved using successive approximation as a teaching technique.

We usually begin with the bow arm (the right arm). First, the student is asked to let his arm hang loosely at his side. This is the position in which the arm 'wants' to be — at its lowest level and totally relaxed. He is then asked to place his hand on his hip and feel the weight of his arm pushing into it. It is pointed out that although this feels very relaxed, it is not totally so — the upper arm muscles are actually holding the arm in such a way that its weight is directed into the hip. When the student is asked to relax these muscles completely, his arm again falls to his side. This notion of directed weight is the basic principle of efficient bowing. The arm's muscles hold it in such a way that its weight, which 'wants' to make it drop down and hang by the side of the body, is instead directed to the point of contact between the arm (extended by the bow) and the string.

The student continues by resting his upper arm on the fingerboard of the cello. In this position, it is virtually assured that he will feel the arm's relaxed weight (particularly the weight of the upper arm) resting on the fingerboard. Next, he is asked to move his arm farther out and rest his forearm on the fingerboard. At this point, the student is told to allow his elbow to drop so that he is resting his forearm on the fingerboard and his upper arm on the body of the cello itself; then to use his upper arm muscles to raise the arm just enough so that it is not touching the body of the cello but resting only on the fingerboard. This way he feels exactly how much his muscles must work in order to direct the arm's weight to the desired spot. He also can distinguish the difference between his upper-arm weight and his forearm weight.

Continuing in the same manner, the student rests his arm on the fingerboard at points progressively closer to his hand and nearer to the end of the fingerboard — always making sure that he feels the minimum amount of muscular exertion necessary to balance in each new position. When he reaches the point where his arm ends and the bow begins (in this exercise, the bow is held in a loose fist), he discovers that the feeling of balance remains exactly the same. Once the bow is balanced on the string, it is simple to imagine that the string is a sort of ball bearing or roller, and the arm easily swings from side to side as it rests upon it. Often, at this point a look of dawning comprehension lights up the student's face, followed by the words, "I never knew it was so easy!"

The left arm functions, to a large extent, by 'walking' on its fingers. In actual walking, torso balance shifts forward, whereupon it is caught on top of the moving legs. Similarly, when the balance of the upper arm shifts, it must be caught by another finger or the arm will fall over. The student can feel this by 'walking' his arm along a tabletop or along the back of a chair. This walking image can be strengthened by imagining that the fingerboard is a staircase and the fingers stand on the horizontal surfaces of the steps. Picturing this helps the student feel that his balance is aligned vertically in the earth's gravity even though his fingers look angled back in relation to the surface of the fingerboard.

Like the bow arm, the left arm, too, 'wants' to fall down and hang by the body's side; however, the muscles of the arm direct its weight to the fingers resting on the fingerboard. This remains true even as one plays in the higher positions; the arm extends horizontally in front but continues to 'want' to fall vertically. These horizontal and vertical components blend to keep the hand and fingers always balanced at the same angle in relation to the fingerboard, just as a funicular railway moves up and down a mountain slope without spilling its passengers.

Physical efficiency enables the cellist to play with the least possible effort and, as a result, his body remains relaxed. Relaxation causes a heightened sensitivity to both the bodily and instrumental sensations of playing. This improves technical and artistic control of the cello and means years of better performances without injury.

CHAPTER 41

Inter-Observer and Intra-Observer Reliability of Postural Examination of Student-Musicians

Willem C.G. Blanken • *Henk van der Rijst* • *Paul G.H. Mulder*
Marjon D.F. van Eijsden-Besseling • *Gustaaf J. Lankhorst*

INTRODUCTION

Postural abnormalities, especially when existing over a long period of time, are generally considered to give rise to painful conditions.[1,2] Among musicians and dancers, musculoskeletal problems are prominent and many of these disorders are thought to arise from faulty alignment.[3] Not only in daily medical practice, but also in various studies, the assessment of posture is still largely by clinical observation and subjective impression.[1,4-6] The aim of this study is to investigate the inter-observer and intra-observer reliability of the clinical observation of 18 different postural features.

MATERIALS AND METHODS

From a group of freshmen of the Rotterdamsch Conservatorium, 24 subjects were randomly selected (11 men, 13 women, mean age 20 years, range 17-29). The instruments played were: piano (3), violin (6), cello (1), bass (1), harp (1), guitar (4), flute (2), clarinet (2), oboe (1), trumpet (2) and trombone (1). A standard examination procedure developed by our department for the physical examination of dancers and musicians was used (Table I) and the results were interpreted according to Peterson Kendall et al.[7]

EXPERIMENTAL DESIGN

Measurements were carried out according to the principle of the repeated latin square design. Subjects were divided into three groups, which differed only in the order in which the three observers made their assessments {1, 2, 3}, {2, 3, 13} and {3, 1, 2}.

INTER-OBSERVER AND INTRA-OBSERVER RELIABILITY

Every subject was examined by an observer who recorded his findings on the above mentioned list. One week later the same procedure was repeated.

Calculation of inter-observer and intra-observer reliability was based both on the method of the relative agreement (Po) between observers, within one observer and on the measure k. Relative agreement is defined as the proportion of the number of concordant assessment pairs on the total number of assessment pairs. According to Behrens and Brambing,[8] relative agreement is considered to be high when Po > 0.80. Kappa is a measure of agreement with correction for chance agreement. Kappa is denoted by k. In case of complete agreement, k = 1. If observed agreement is greater than chance agreement, K > O, and if observed agreement is less than or equal to chance agreement, K ≤ O. According to Landis and Koch,[9] values of k > 0.75 may be taken to represent excellent agreement beyond chance and values < 0.40 poor agreement. Values between 0.40 and 0.75 are judged to represent fair to good agreement beyond chance. As 18 different features are assessed with a kappa calculated for each feature, the weighted average of these kappa values is considered. The interpretation of the magnitude of the overall k is like that of the unweighted kappa.

RESULTS

High relative agreement (Po > 0.80) within one observer was found in 56% of the variables; between observers, relative agreement was over 0.80 in 50%. Excellent agreement beyond chance was found in 25% within one observer and in 13% between observers. Fair to good kappa values were recorded in 44% of variables within one observer and for 47% between observers. Between observers, kappa was not calculable in two cases, but relative agreement was complete. For position of head (variable 1) and postural characteristics of the cervical spine (variables 6 and 9) within one observer, kappa was not calculable for all three observers.   Overall kappa values for observers 1, 2 and 3 were, respectively, 0.59, 0.56 and 0.51. The weighted inter-rater kappa values were 0.48, 0.32 and 0.25. Results are shown in Tables II and III.

Table I: Summary of Examined Variables

1. Head
   posterior view
   - neutral position • anterior tilt • posterior tilt
   - lateral tilt towards left
   - lateral tilt towards right
   - rotation toward   • rotation toward
     left   right

2. Shoulders
   posterior view
   - neutral position, not elevated or depressed
   - left depressed   • right depressed

3. Pelvis
   posterior view
   - level
   - lateral tilt; high on left
   - lateral tilt; high on right

4. Leg length
   - equal
   - left leg longer   • right leg longer
   - amount in centimeters ....

5. Pelvis
   side view
   - level
   - anterior tilt   • posterior tilt
   - rotation towards   • rotation towards
     left   right

6. Cervical spine
   side view
   - normal curve, slightly convex anteriorly
   - accentuation of cervical lordosis
   - diminution of cervical lordosis

7. Thoracic spine
   side view
   - normal curve, slightly convex posteriorly
   - accentuation of thoracic kyphosis
   - diminution of thoracic kyphosis
   - structural   • non-structural

8. Lumbar spine
   side view
   - normal curve; slightly convex anteriorly
   - accentuation of lumbar lordosis
   - diminution of lumbar lordosis
   - structural   • non-structural

9. Cervical spine
   posterior view
   - normal; straight in drawing
   - C-curve; convex towards left
   - C-curve; convex towards right
   - structural curve
   - non-structural curve
   - deviation to plumb line
   - non-deviation to plumb line

10. Thoracic spine
    posterior view
    - normal; straight in drawing
    - C-curve; convex towards left
    - C-curve; convex towards right
    - structural curve
    - non-structural curve
    - deviation to plumb line
    - non-deviation to plumb line

11. Lumbar spine
    posterior view
    - normal; straight in drawing
    - C-curve; convex towards left
    - C-curve; convex towards right
    - structural curve
    - non-structural curve
    - deviation to plumb-line
    - non-deviation to plumbline

12. Cervical spine
    posterior view
    - normal; straight in drawing
    - torsion towards left
    - torsion towards right

13. Thoracic spine
    posterior view
    - normal; straight in drawing
    - torsion towards left
    - torsion towards right

14. Lumbar spine
    posterior view
    - normal; straight in line
    - torsion towards left
    - torsion towards right

15. Hip joints
    posterior and
    side view
    - neutral position: neither flexed nor extended, neither abducted nor adducted
    - flexed left   • flexed right
    - extended left   • extended right
    - abducted left   • abducted right
    - adducted left   • adducted right

16. Knee-joint
    posterior and
    side view
    - neutral position; neither flexed nor hyperextended, neither genu varum nor genu valgum
    - flexed left   • flexed right
    - genu varum   • genu valgum

17. Ankle joints
    posterior and
    side view
    - neutral position; legs vertical and right angle to sole of foot
    - plantar flexion left
    - plantar flexion right
    - valgus position left
    - valgus position right
    - varus position left
    - varus position right

18. Feet
    posterior and
    side view
    - neutral position; parallel or toeing out slightly; no pronation or supination; normal arches
    - abduction left   • abduction right
    - adduction left   • adduction right
    - pes cavus left   • pes cavus right
    - flatfoot left   • flatfoot right
    - splayfoot left   • splayfoot right
    - others

Table II: Inter-Rater Reliability

Variable	Observers 1-2			Observers 2-3			Observers 3-1		
	Po	Kappa	Significance	Po	Kappa	Significance	Po	Kappa	Significance
1.	1.00	(−)		1.00	(−)		1.00	(−)	
2.	0.88	0.78	+	0.35	0.03	−	0.35	0.07	−
3.	0.76	0.60	+	0.77	0.62	+	0.82	0.68	+
4.	0.59	0.41	+	0.59	0.42	+	0.88	0.80	+
5.	0.82	0.68	+	0.94	0.77	+	0.82	0.62	+
6.	1.00	(−)		1.00	(−)		1.00	(−)	
7.	0.88	0.22	−	0.65	0.19	−	0.53	0.18	−
8.	0.71	0.51	+	0.59	0.31	+	0.88	(−)	
9.	1.00	(−)		0.82	−0.09	−	0.47	0.14	−
10.	0.94	0.66	+	0.38	−0.07	−	0.82	0.45	+
11.	0.88	0.77	+	0.88	0.64	+	0.88	(−)	
12.	0.82	0.36	+	0.94	0.64	+	0.71	0.33	+
13.	0.82	0.23	−	0.69	0.11	−	0.71	0.18	−
14.	0.88	(−)		0.71	(−)		0.88	(−)	
15.	0.94	0.64	+	1.00	1.00	+	0.94	0.64	+
16.	0.88	0.43	+	0.82	(−)		0.65	−0.10	−
17.	0.94	(−)		0.82	0.34	+	0.88	(−)	
18.	0.76	0.49	+	0.65	0.20	−	0.76	0.68	+

| K=0.48 | K=0.25 | K=0.32 |

****

K	=	overall kappa value
Po	=	relative agreement (%)
kappa	=	kappa value
(−)	=	kappa value not calculable

DISCUSSION

This study focuses on the inter-observer and intra-observer reliability of physical examination of posture. In general, posture is evaluated in a subjective clinical way.   In order to establish objective methods of examining alignment several investigations have been performed.[1] A number of standardized measurements for certain postural characteristics have been described, but a comprehensive test is not available. The intra-observer reliability in the present study approaches good agreement beyond chance, but only in one case out of three did the inter-observer reliability prove to be fair.   Other values of inter-observer reliability were poor. When considering the reliability of separate variables, such as the level of anterior and posterior iliac spine and iliac crest, findings were good to excellent and consistent with those described by Nelson et al.[10] For all three observers, kappa was not calculable for the position of head and characteristics of the cervical spine in lateral and posterior views, because no abnormalities were established. Measurement of postural characteristics of the thoracic spine proved generally unsatisfactory.

In conclusion, examination of posture as described herein is not to be recommended.   The authors consider it to be important — especially with respect to dancers and musicians, who make high demands upon their physical functioning and for whom correct

Table III: Intra-Rater Reliability

Variable	Observers 1-2			Observers 2-3			Observers 3-1		
	Po	Kappa	Significance	Po	Kappa	Significance	Po	Kappa	Significance
1.	1.00	(−)		1.00	(−)		1.00	(−)	
2.	0.77	0.59	+	0.77	0.57	+	0.88	0.72	+
3.	0.82	0.76	+	0.77	0.67	+	0.77	0.61	+
4.	0.82	0.51	+	0.82	0.62	+	0.77	0.63	+
5.	0.88	0.72	+	0.88	0.77	+	0.94	0.77	+
6.	1.00	(−)		1.00	(−)		1.00	(−)	
7.	1.00	1.00	+	0.94	0.77	+	0.77	0.39	+
8.	0.77	0.61	+	0.72	0.52	+	0.71	0.56	+
9.	1.00	(−)		1.00	(−)		1.00	(−)	
10.	0.77	0.38	−	0.67	0.25	−	0.29	0.11	+
11.	0.82	0.50	+	0.73	0.29	−	0.82	−0.09	−
12.	1.00	(−)		1.00	(−)		0.88	0.22	−
13.	0.88	0.46	+	0.60	0.46	+	0.59	0.36	+
14.	0.94	0.77	+	0.94	0.77	+	0.53	−0.20	−
15.	1.00	1.00	+	1.00	1.00	+	1.00	1.00	+
16.	0.94	0.77	+	1.00	(−)		0.94	0.82	+
17.	1.00	(−)		0.94	(−)		0.77	(−)	
18.	1.00	1.00	+	0.67	0.46	+	0.77	0.19	−

K=0.59   K=0.56   K=0.51

****

K = overall kappa value (see text)
Po = relative agreement (%)
kappa = kappa value (see text)
(−) = kappa value not calculable

posture is described to be essential — to develop standardized methods and well- defined criteria for assessing postural characteristics.

REFERENCES

1. Weinstein SL, Zavala D, Ponsetti IV, et al: Idiopathic scoliosis. Long-term follow up and prognosis in un-treated patients. J Bone Joint Surg 63A:702-712, 1981.

2. Dieck GS, Kelsey JF, Goel VK, et al: An epidemiologic study of the relationship between postural asymmetry in the teen years and subsequent back and neck pain. Spine 10:872-877, 1985.

3. Fischbein M, Middlestat SE, Ottavi V: Medical problems among ICSOM musicians: Overview of a national survey. Medical Problems of Performing Artists 3:1-8, 1988.

4. Loebl WY: Measurement of spinal posture and range of spinal movement. Ann Phys Med 9:103-110, 1967.

5. Viviani GR, Budgell L, Dok C, et al: Assessment of accuracy of the scoliosis school screening examination. Am J Pub Health 7:497-498, 1984.

6. Willner S: A comparative study of the efficiency of different types of school screening for scoliosis. Acta Orthop Scand 53:769-774, 1982.

7. Peterson Kendall F, Kendall McCreary E: Muscle Testing and Function. Baltimore: Williams and Wilkins, 1983.

8. Behrens E, Brambing M: Beurteileruberein-stimmung einer deutschen Version der "International Classification of Impairments, Disabilities and Handicaps (ICIDH)" der Weltgesund-eitsbehorde. Int J Rehab Res 10: 391-404, 1987.

9. Landis JR, Koch GG: A one-way components of variance model for categorical data. Biometrics 33: 671-679, 1977.

10. Nelson R, Nestor DE: Atlas of standardized low-back tests and measures of the National Institute for Occupational Safety and Health. Scand J Work Environ Health 14:82-84, 1988.

CHAPTER 42

Role of the Larynx in
Instrumental Music Performance

Dietrich Balser

The role of the larynx with respect to instrumental music is surprisingly central. During playing several etudes and concert pieces, the electromyogram (EMG) of the larnyx-lowering muscles (L) in cellists, as well as other control parameters (objective: EMG of various trunk muscles, EKG, thoracic and abdominal respiration, sound pressure level; and subjective: expert rating of acoustical and physiological performance specifications) were recorded. Further insight was given by fiberoptic laryngoscopy during violin playing. Results are discussed with regard to optimal psycho-physiological conditions as well as prevention of overuse and performance anxiety symptoms. Didactic conclusions thereby derived are explained.

INTRODUCTION

During instrument-playing, subjective perceptions of the larynx remain nearly always in the periphery of consciousness. Its function will be registered only when it does not function normally. Then, it does becomes noticeable as a "lump in one's throat," an uncontrollable airway resistance due to a negative emotional affect, such as anxiety.

Further indices of a complex relationship between laryngeal function and the whole boy can be found: 1) Muscular: The sphincter activity of the larynx influences the effectiveness of the auxiliary respiratory muscles and the postural muscles of the trunk; 2) Psychoacoustical: The system larynx-ear is impregnated with our primary sound pattern (the vocal tone), which, in the best scenario, acts as a gestalt-like mental concept and reflexively initiates the senso-motory control of each sound production.[1-3] With rhythmical instances, the larynx as breathing valve obviously is correlated to respiration.

A question, therefore, arises: Is the larynx iust a small wheel in the whole works or could a function-hierarchy be discovered whereby this organ takes on the role of the "order parameter" and "slaves" the appertaining subsystems.[4]

In addition to a comprehensive investigation into conditions required for functional (optimal) playing of instruments,[5] it was the aim of one experiment not only to visualize the importance of laryngeal function for instrumental performance but, beyond this, to derive conditions under which the latent potential of laryngeal function can be utilized for both pedagogic and therapeutic (prevention, rehabilitation) applications.

MATERIALS AND METHODS

Six cellists — three students and three teachers — played a concert piece and an etude *son filé* several times. Before each repetition, the cellists had to perform body- or breathing exercises.

The variables of the experimental design were selected with the intention of gathering information in the following areas:

1. Physiological phenomena: electrical activity (EA) of the larynx-lowering muscles (L), abdominal- and dorsal muscles);

2. Psychological phenomena: extroversion;[6]

3. Mental phenomena: based on heart rate variability (HRV) derived from the EKG;

4. Rhythmic phenomena: breathing, vibrato; and

5. Other control values: sound pressure level.

Thus, the objective and subjective measurement methods balanced each other. Of special importance was the expert rating of the different quality aspects of the music performance.

In all testing, subjects were instructed to react as minimally as possible.

To directly film the larynx of two violinists, after local anesthesia, a fibroscope was inserted through the nose to a position just over the vocal cords.

RESULTS AND DISCUSSION

Coincidence of Physiological and Emotional Opening

Larynx-lowering muscles: The EA of L demonstrates that when the larynx is lower in the throat, resulting in a wide opening as a breathing valve, playing is improved. The auxiliary respiratory muscles are unburdened, and so the sensibility and flexibility of the muscular movement is improved.

Stability of the larynx position: Figure 1 shows that a physical opening of the larynx cannot happen without a simultaneous emotional opening. The considerably calmer and more stable behavior of the larynx during better playing can, together with the preceding result, psychologically be considered as freedom from fear, which leads to emotional stability.

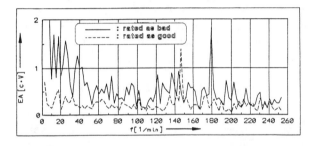

Figure 1: *Spectral power density of the electrical activity (EA) of the larynx-lowering muscles (L). The frequency range corresponds to the up-and-down movements of the larynx in the neck. The upper curve is the averaged spectrum of all the pieces rated as poorest, and the lower dotted curve of all pieces rated as best.*

Breathing and posture pattern: During better playing, the wider emotional opening of the larynx is associated with a more distinct abdominal respiration (correlation of the quotient of thoracic/abdominal respiration with extroversion: $r = 0.70$, $p = 0.14$; without one outlier: $r = 0.97$, $p = 0.01$) and to a typical pattern of trunk muscle contraction.[7, 8]

Rhythmic Interconnection of Functions

Reflexive Muscle Activities: Figure 2 shows how the subject strived for coordination between the rhythm of the musical pieces and his own body's. Reactions of the larynx before entries are as follows: The short muscle activities at the breathing valve initiate reflexively a rhythmic interconnection of all individual functions of the body. This can also be seen in the abdominal musculature (A). Just at the moment

of the reflexive release, there is an activity interruption in A. This short relaxation increases the flexibility and elasticity of the abdomen under the diaphragm.

Rhythm and voluntary motor control: In this connection, an interesting result is highly involuntary control of the complexity of single functions as a mental condition for such reflexive playing: HRV is higher during better playing ($p = 0.05$). According to Luczak,[8] this is to be interpreted as less mental strain.

Larynx in vivo: The results are confirmed by the laryngoscopy film. On the whole, three phenomena can be recognized: 1) reflexive larynx activities upon entry; 2) tension of the vocal cords varying with pitch; and 3) synkinesis: increase in associated laryngeal movements with higher emotional engagement of the musician.

CONCLUSIONS

Latent potential of the larynx: Evidently, the larynx can be termed as being an interface for the connection of emotional and muscular movements. Therefore, this highly differentiated and sensitive region of the body determines, by its degree of opening and movement during playing, the motoric sensibility and flexibility as well as permeability of the body for emotional impulses.

Didactic implications: Although the results suggest that the teacher not bring laryngeal function to the students' consciousness, the potential of the larynx can still be stimulated very effectively by indirect instructions.[5] For intuitive individual instruction, knowing the inseparability of ear-larynx sensomotoricity is essential. Practical consequences are that motoric development of optimal playing is possible only in parallel to voice development, and that the "ear" has to lead optimal playing and pedagogy by means of sound perceptions.

Performance stress and overuse: It becomes clear that the cornerstone of all playing anxiety and overuse was already laid by lessons which forced a general concept upon the student, leading to arbitrary differentiation of "correct" and "incorrect," trying to hide mistakes (doctoring instead of keeping alive the chances of self-awareness and growth through one's mistakes). Over the years, a vicious cycle is established, which begins with guilty, tense concentration on flawless movements, followed by fear of loss of safety and control. This results in an

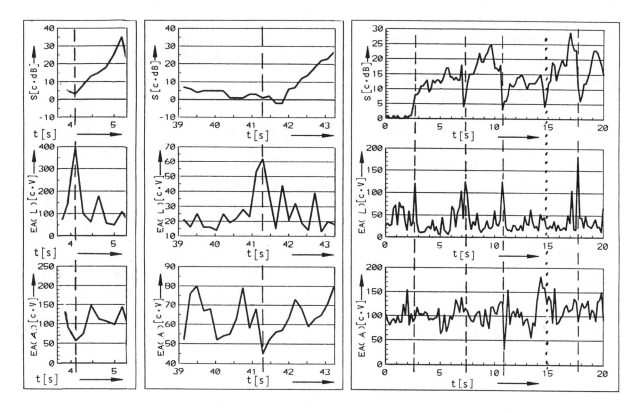

Figure 2: *Sound level S (top) and electrical activity EA of the larynx-lowering-muscles L (middle) and obliquus abdominis externus muscle A (bottom) versus time. The vertical dotted lines indicate attacks or entries at the beginning of a piece or of a new phrase. They become recognizable by a steep rise in the sound level.* Left: *concert piece, entry at the beqinning of the piece.* Middle: *Concert piece, entry at the beginning of a new phrase in the piece.* Right: *étude, entries with the changes of bow; the dotted line indicates an entry without L-reaction; A is very active (unflexible abdomen) and S reaches during the following stroke a maximum ("scrape," too high bow pressure)*

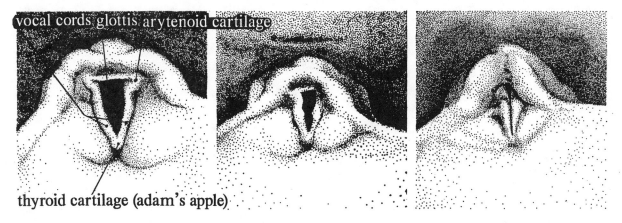

Figure 3: *Glottis opening and tension of the vocal cords of a violinist (seen from above, lower edge is the front).* Left: *without tone production;* middle: *pitch C_4 (one-line C);* right: C_7.

inflexible larynx and, therefore, dysrythmic, cramped movements. Finally, it seems as if only increased concentration can help.

Rehabilitation: An undisturbed function-gestalt manifests in a coincidence of psychophyiological and psychoacoustical optimal conditions. Consequently, an optimal sound can result only from effective movements with minimal effort. Functional playing is the best prevention and the best guarantee of successful rehabilitation. A union of medical and pedagogical endeavor, of arts and medicine, is therefore necessary.

REFERENCES

1. Landzettel: Die Bedeutung der Formantenbildung beim Instrumentalspiel. *In* Rohmert W (Ed): Beiträge zum 2. Kolloquium Praktische Musik-physiologie, 199-208. Köln: Schmidt, 1991.

2. Rohmert G: Der Sänger auf dem Weg zum Klang. Köln: Schmidt, 1991.

3. Tomatis A: L'oreille et la Voix. Paris: Laffont, 1987.

4. Haken H: Information and Self-Organization. Synergetic Series Vol 40. Berlin: Springer, 1988.

5. Balser D: Untersuchung funktionaler Ablauf-beding ungen komplexer sensumotorischer Fertgkeiten am Beispiel des Streichinstrumenten-spiels. Frankfurt: Lang, 1990.

6. Eysenck HJ, Eysenck S: Manual of the Eysenck Personality Inventory. London: University of London Press, 1971.

7. Glaser V: Rehabilitation of efferent spinal tracts by tactile-kinetic stimulation of communicative intentions. International Symposium on Neuro-orthopaedics and Rehabilitation, Prague, 1986.

8. Glaser V: Eutonie. Das Verhaltensmuster menschlichen Wohlbefindens. Heidelberg: Haug, 1990.

9. Luczak H: Fractioned heart rate variability. Ergonomics 11(21):895-911, 1978.

CHAPTER 43

Study of Posture in String Instrumentalists

Lionel Guilbert

Musicians suffer ... violinists, percussionists, violists, organists ... The music flows to soothe the soul, but there is pain behind each melody.

With theatrical flourish and seemingly effortless ease, night after night, year after year, these maestros sway, blow and scratch pure magic from their tubes and valves, their skins and strings; but only they, and, of course, their physiotherapists, know where it hurts — the wear and tear on the players themselves, the pressures, strains and pains of prolonged, repetitive playing.

The problems seen by the author in his clinical practice are usually (1) those linked to posture (reaction of the body against gravity) and (2) those due to contact, (pressure and vibration of the instrument against the hands, mouth, chin, shoulder, sternum, etc.). Pity the harpist, who may have up to five points of contact with the instrument.

The energy expended by the instrumentalist may be compared with that of a high-level sportsman. There is the same routine of coaching, learning, training and practice. Dedication, commitment, time and energy lead eventually, it is hoped, to virtuoso professional performance.

Each sport has its special postures, crouches and movements, and so it is with each instrument.

In musicians, a technical and musical apprenticeship creates a body position which drifts, after a period of years, into a personal playing style, i.e. an integration of all the elements of instrumental technique, enabling the interpretation to take over.

The body cannot stay fixed in a standing or seated position during the hours of rehearsal and performance. As the position of the body changes, the points of contact between the body and the instrument are also altered. A swaying of the body always takes place along an axis which depends on the instrument, the experience of the instrumentalist, and even on his/her gender.

RESTING ON THE CHIN

Among the different music stands observed by the author at the Conservatory of Music of the 10th district of Paris, those of the violinist and the violist present some particularities. Aside from many points of tension in the back as well as the neck and hands, the contact of the mandible against the chin-rest (third contact) often causes local physical problems requiring medical treatment or, sometimes, making it necessary to give up the practice of the instrument altogether.

The violin rests on the internal tip of the clavicle, in contact with the external posterior part of the neck. The head, rotated and inclined to the left, presses the lower edge of the horizontal segment of the mandible against the instrument. The pressure, approximately 350 g, is exerted along an oblique axis from high to low and from outside to inside. Think of it as a downward pressure, with an element of "hacking" at the level of the gingival and dental area. The mandible position depends on the morphology of the violinist, and how he holds his head and rotates and inclines it.

Globally, the lesions seem proportionate to the subject's ability to move in space. The more static and stiff, he or she is, the more serious the mandibular impact, as if the violinist "clung to" this sole point of contact.

EFFECTS OF RESTING THE MANDIBLE

This contact brings about, sooner or later, dermatosis in the upper posterior part of the Malgaigne triangle, under the mandible. Its exact place is between the middle third and the posterior third of the top of the neck, at the level of the superior insertion of the sternocleidomastoid. It covers an area of about 2 to 3 square centimeters and is accompanied by gum- and tooth circulatory problems. In its acute phase gingival pain, gum boils, and tooth-loosening may occur. These disorders do not affect all violinists to the same extent. They are most common and more serious in violists. The viola appears to be a more dangerous instrument. It would seem that the larger size instrument and medium sound frequencies cause more damage.

Dermatosis often occurs in teenagers who practice for long periods of time. It seems to subside and vanish with time.

Pathophysiology

The anatomical points of the mandible where dysfunctions occur are circulatory, lymphatic and dental. Too strong a horizontal strength exerted on the teeth brings about pressure at the level of the socket bottom, which may result in atrophy of the socketbone and loosening of dental fixation.

METHODOLOGY

Our observation focused on a population of 120 string instrumentalists, aged 15 to 19 years (65 girls and 55 boys; 91 violinists and 29 violists). They had been trained in diverse schools. Their posture was often fixed, but not irreversibly. Their past history and their families' were free of any dental pathology.

Postural and Ergonomic Re-Harmonization

Postural re-harmonization calls on sensory elements responding to stimulation of the exteroceptors and proprioceptors. This stimulation results in a re-evaluation of the hand movements starting from the sensory inheritance.

Posture is first the resting of feet on the ground. The base is about 40 cm wide, and looks roughly like an isosceles triangle with its vertex towards the left *foot,* itself turned to the left. Violinists support themselves alternately on one *foot* and the other, on their right and their left, swaying as if going towards their instrument. But the return to the right foot takes place in a vertical plane, perpendicular to the ground, and must not go past it or the subject will be thrown off balance, which would have repercussions on the velocity of the arms. The position of the left arm and the presence of the violin act as a counterbalance.

The pelvis is slightly rotated, the lumbar vertebrae convex forward. This lumbar attitude gives the scapular belt greater mobility. When some of these parameters are disturbed, work *on posture* consists of going back to square *one* in the statics of the subject without his/her instrument.

The aim of this therapeutic approach is to lighten the pressure of the mandible on the chin-rest without loss of stability.

Parallel to this work on posture, gingival and dental lesions must be treated medically, together with the draining of mucous in gingival and dental tissues.

Finally, the instrument can be padded by wearing the chin-rest with a layer of specialized elastomers to dampen the vibration.

RESULTS

Three quarters of the subjects treated showed improvement after about a month-and-a-half of biweekly sessions using manual methods.

The gingival area seemed better vascularized, the dental system more stable. Total disappearance of the lesions was observed in 12 subjects.

The violists did not respond as well to treatment.

CONCLUSIONS

It is difficult to prescribe a preventive and systematic treatment for all young violinists, but one can at least inform teachers and parents and encourage them to watch the gingival and dental state of their children. One should always consider prophylaxis aimed at reducing the damaging effects of the chin-rest.

All musicians are affected in some way, and each section of the band or orchestra has its specific problems. Conservatories of music themselves have an educational role to play in informing young instrumentalists of potential problems and how to alleviate them as much as possible by the use of instrument pads, different playing postures, and lighter *contact* pressure with the instrument.

CHAPTER 44

Joint and Tendon Forces in Pianists' Hands

B.M. Hillberry, F.G. Wolf, S.L. Hiner, M.S. Keane, and K.D. Brandt

INTRODUCTION

Rapid, repeated and precise movements sustained over long periods of time are likely to predispose accomplished instrumentalists to injuries resulting from overuse. These injuries include tendinitis and nerve entrapments, such as carpal tunnel syndrome. The purpose of this study was to gain an understanding of how tendons, joints, ligaments, and muscles interact in a performing pianist's hand and how this understanding may elucidate modifications in performance technique that would prevent or alleviate musculoskeletal injuries. In addition the variation in tendon and joint forces are investigated.

METHODS

In this study the performance technique of 8 injury-free accomplished pianists (Table 1) was biomechanically evaluated to provide a quantitative database for future comparisons between healthy musicians and those with performance-related injuries. Finger tip forces during playing were measured using a digital Yamaha CLP-300 Clavinova electronic piano which we calibrated to provide keystrike force. This piano has been designed to sound and feel much like a grand piano with damped, weighted keys and realistic action. Hand and finger positions were recorded with two video cameras (Figure 1) to determine key contact angle and finger joint angles for the right index finger at the position of maximum keystrike force (fully depressed key). The keystrike force, key contact angle, joint angles (Figure 2) and hand size provide the necessary inputs to a two dimensional, quasi-static mathematical model of the finger developed by Harding et al.[1] This model calculates the joint and tendon forces at each of the three joints of the digit. Experimental measurements of finger accelerations showed that inertia forces were less than 3 percent of the muscle forces and therefore a quasi-static model could be used. Finger joint and

Table 1: *Subjects Participating in the Study.*

Subject	Gender	Experience (yrs)	Right index finger length (mm)
1	M	12	95
2	M	33	94
3	M	59	97
4	M	50	97
5	M	33	110
6	M	50	93
7	M	20	106
8	M	34	95

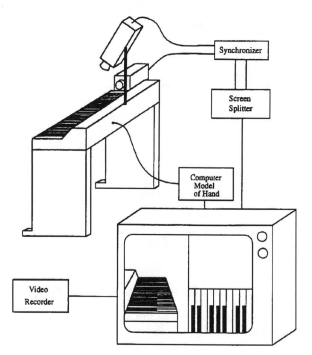

Figure 1: *Laboratory Test Facility.*

tendon forces were determined for each subject for ten specific notes struck with the right index finger while playing the same selected piece of music. The

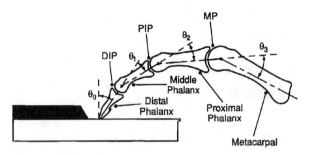

Figure 2: Finger Nomenclature.

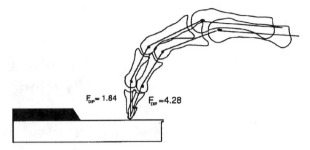

Figure 3: Minimum and Maximum DIP Force Coefficients for Subject 3.

Table 2: Joint and Tendon Forces (lbs) for Subject 3.

Joint or tendon	Notes struck									
	1	2	3	4	5	6	7	8	9	10
DIP	0.36	0.91	0.30	4.36	0.44	0.61	3.21	2.31	1.31	1.22
PIP	1.01	2.04	0.86	6.69	1.22	1.61	8.42	5.46	3.58	2.91
MP	1.22	2.61	1.07	8.17	1.50	2.03	11.23	6.08	4.41	3.31
INT	0.63	1.67	0.64	4.16	0.82	1.09	7.10	2.37	2.40	1.25
FDP	0.17	0.49	0.11	3.30	0.19	0.36	1.72	1.20	0.56	0.68
FDS	0.48	0.65	0.38	1.09	0.55	0.71	3.20	2.51	1.60	1.35
Keystrike Force	0.17	0.35	0.16	1.02	0.23	0.23	1.25	1.02	0.66	0.52

pianist was unaware of the notes to be analyzed, which were contained within a page of Mendelssohn's *Midsummer Night's Dream*. The dynamic level of the notes analyzed varied from pianissimo to forte.

For each of the selected ten notes, finger tip force, finger tip/key angle and finger joint angles were measured. From the finger angle data, normalized joint force and tendon tension coefficients were determined using the finger model. These were determined for the metacarpophalangeal joint (MP), proximal interphalangeal joint (PIP), distal interphalangeal joint (DIP), flexor digitorium profundus tendon (FDP), flexor digitorium sublimis tendon (FDS) and intrinsic muscle tendon (INT). The actual joint or tendon force was obtained by multiplying the corresponding force coefficient by the measured finger tip force.

Two-way analysis of variance methods were used to quantify the differences between subjects and notes. Statistical Analysis Software, SAS, was used to perform all statistical computations. Variance component estimation was used to estimate the variability in data between subjects and between notes. The variance component estimation also quantified the amount of variability in the data due to experiment error and random effects. Correlation coefficients and P-values were calculated to check for linear relationships between groups of data. Nonlinear behavior was not checked because the sample size was small.

RESULTS AND DISCUSSION

Typical results are shown for Subject 3 in Table 2 and Figure 3. Figure 3 illustrates the finger positions for the minimum and maximum values of the force coefficient for the DIP joint from among the ten notes analyzed. The difference in DIP joint force shown is due to finger position only. Table 2 lists the total joint and tendon forces and the keystrike force.

The average and standard deviation of the keystrike force is presented in Table 3 for the subjects and in Table 4 for the notes. The different dynamic levels of the music where the notes were selected are also indicated in Table 4. This variability in dynamic level is observed in the variability of the keystrike force (Table 3). The keystrike force inverserly correlated with number of years of experi-ence (r = 0.78, p $\langle$ 0.03).

Table 3: Keystroke Force Values for each Subject.

Subject	Minimum (lbs)	Maximum (lbs)	Mean (lbs)	Standard Deviation (lbs)
1	0.61	1.91	1.25	0.40
2	0.16	0.77	0.45	0.20
3	0.16	1.25	0.56	0.41
4	0.16	1.33	0.54	0.41
5	0.24	2.27	0.87	0.61
6	0.35	1.60	0.75	0.42
7	0.33	2.27	1.22	0.67
8	0.19	2.27	0.99	0.54

The mean joint and tendon force coefficients for each subject were highly variable. The joint and tendon force coefficients are related to the finger position and are independent of the keystrike force. For example the mean force coefficient for the INT tendon varied from 3.79 to 7.7, an 86.5% difference. Within subject variation was also significant, e.g., the INT force coefficient standard deviation was 2.40 lbs for subject 1. These results indicate a large variation in finger position both within and between subjects. The mean total joint and tendon forces were also highly variable. For example the mean value of the MP joint force varied from 3.87 to 11.58 lbs between subjects, a 200% difference.

No correlation was observed between the force coefficients and the keystrike force. This means that the finger position did not correlate with the keystrike force. No correlation between subjects was observed for keystrike force (p < 0.05) or for joint and tendon force coefficients (p < 0.05). This may be due to the large variation in dynamic level of the music.

Table 4: Mean Joint and Tendon Forces (lbs) and Dynamic Level for Each Note.

Note struck	DIP	PIP	MP	INT	FDP	FDS	Dynamic level
			Joint or tendon				
1	2.30	4.60	5.35	2.38	1.53	1.65	p
2	3.40	6.09	7.35	3.71	2.46	1.64	p
3	2.19	4.12	4.83	2.08	1.60	1.36	p
4	2.51	4.40	5.59	3.10	1.87	1.00	p*
5	2.43	4.39	5.54	3.13	1.70	1.05	p
6	3.36	6.91	8.84	5.05	2.27	2.13	f
7	2.46	5.19	6.86	4.33	1.52	1.48	f
8	4.02	7.39	8.86	4.62	2.61	2.07	mf*
9	1.94	4.79	6.17	3.56	1.08	1.84	pp
10	1.82	4.45	5.47	2.68	1.06	1.92	pp

p*: Note 4 occurs 3 measures after a sforzando. The pianist may have returned to piano or mezzo forte depending on his interpretation of the music.

mf*: Note 8 occurs on the second beat between a sforzando and a piano. The piano and sforzando are seperated by 4 beats. The music is 3/8 time and should be played andante expressivo.

CONCLUSIONS

A method for determining finger joint and tendon forces during piano playing has been demonstrated. The results from eight subjects shows a wide variation in keystrike forces and finger forces with no correlation between subjects. Correlation between notes was inconclusive. The lack of correlation could be attributed to the personalized presentation of the music by each of the subjects and the large variation in dynamic level of the music. The keystrike force was found to inversely correlate with subject experience.

REFERENCES

1. Harding, D.C.; Brandt, K.D.; and Hillberry, B.M. Minimization of Finger and Joint Forces and Tendon Tensions in Pianists. J. Medical Problems of Performing Artists, 1989, pp. 103-108.

ACKNOWLEDGEMENT

This research was supported in part by the National Institute of Health Grant AR 20582 through the Indiana University Multipurpose Arthritis Center.

CHAPTER 45

Effect of Strap Design
on Back Muscle Activity in Guitarists

Fadi J. Bejjani • *Michelle Chin*

Much has been written about back- and neck pain in general, especially in occupations prone to sustained and distorted postures as well as cumulative trauma. Guitar playing falls into this category. Significant prevalence of back- and neck disorders was found in guitarists as compared to other musicians.[1] Conventional guitar straps attach at both ends of the guitar and go over the musician's head, resting on his/her left shoulder. The average electric guitar weights 8 lbs., while the electric bass weighs approximately 12 lbs. It is not uncommon, therefore, to find guitarists who are suffering from trapezius-, shoulder- and/or lower back pain. Answers to these disorders have been varied and sporadic, ranging from redesigning stands, cushions, stools, or straps to establishing specific preventive and curative exercise programs for this at-risk group.

A few years ago, the SPINStrap was designed by a professional jazz bassist in Williamsport, Pennsylvania, with the ambitious goal of drastically reducing muscle tension and fatigue in professional guitarists. It was expected to fulfill this goal because of the following outstanding ergonomic features: (1) breadth of strap (almost double the breadth of

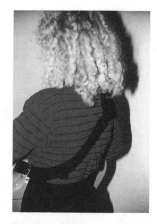

Figure 1c: SPINStrap — left side view. Note attachment to guitar and adjustability.

ordinary straps), likely to decrease pressure on the shoulder by increasing the contact area; (2) nature and thickness of the strap material, likely to further decrease pressure by absorbing some of the weight of the guitar; (3) right shoulder position (instead of the usual left shoulder position), increasing the mechanical advantage of the neck muscles in counteracting the torque created by the weight of the guitar by enhancing the respective lever-arms ratio; and (4) direct attachment to the center-of-gravity area of the guitar (instead of the usual two-point attachment), better balancing the instrument and dividing its weight evenly between the two sides of the strap (Figs. 1a-c).

Recently, physiological and biomechanical evaluation of the strap was undertaken at the Noll Laboratory for Human Performance Research of Penn State University.[2] The study compared the SPINStrap to conventional guitar straps with regard to force and pressure distribution on the shoulder and back, electromyograph activity of selected muscles, and even heart rate. Overall improvement in all of these parameters was noted when using the SPINStrap.[2]

This pilot study planned to carry further the Noll research regarding electromyographic muscle activity of the entire spine, with an attempt to statistically validate the results. The senior author had used the strap clinically with guitarist-patients with significant success.[3]

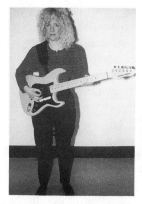

Figure 1a: Using the SPIN-Strap — front view. Note right shoulder position and breadth of strap.

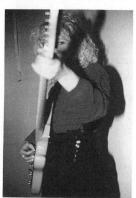

Figure 1b: SPINStrap — rear view.

MATERIALS

Four male professional rock- and jazz guitarists from different bands participated in the study (Table I). They all performed 100% standing, except G.S. (70%). Surface EMG electrodes, mounted on differential preamplifiers (average gain x 350), were placed on the back of each subject, symmetrically at 4 cm, at the C7, T6, T10, L3, and S1 levels on each side of the spinous processes. These electrodes were connected to the Ariel Performance Analysis System (APAS) via a 32-channel A/D board. Data were sampled in real time at a sampling rate of 1000 Hz. Each data sampling lasted for 3 seconds.

Table I: Demographic Data

	Age	Age Started Playing Guitar	Years of Performing Experience
J.C.	29	11	14
R.G.	43	14	23
G.S.	27	13	9
M.W.	31	14	15
Mean	32.50	13	15.25
± *SD*	7.19	± 1.4	5.81

METHOD

The experiment was performed in two phases:

Phase 1: After placement of the electrodes as above (Fig. 2), the first sample was taken in neutral posture without the guitar, followed by a second sample with the guitar but not playing. The latter served as baseline activity readings for the EMG channels. The subjects were then instructed to perform three pieces of music of no more than 3 minutes each with their custom-

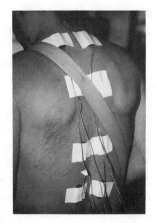

Figure 2: Electrodes placed at C7, T6, T10, L3 and S1 levels on each side of spinous processes.

ary guitar and strap, at slow (60/min.), medium (110/min.) and fast (160/min.) tempos. The order of the pieces was randomly assigned. During each piece, a minimum of three 3-second samples of data were collected at 1-minute intervals. At the end of the first phase, the SPINStrap was mounted on each subject's guitar (Figs. 3a, 3b). The subjects were instructed to

actively use the guitar with its new strap for the three weeks to follow.

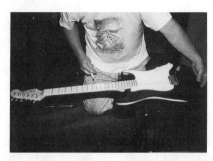

Figure 3a: Determining center of gravity by balancing guitar.

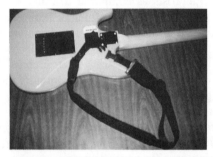

Figure 3b: Mounted strap. Note custom-applied attachment plate in the center-of-gravity area of guitar, and thickness of strap material.

Phase 2: Subjects were retested exactly as in Phase 1, this time playing the same pieces of music with their customary guitar and the SPINStrap.

Data were analyzed with the APAS. Maximum EMG RMS values, across trials, were obtained for each of the 3-second data samples in each of the channels, after rectification. Muscle data while playing was then normalized to baseline readings, thus minimizing data scatter. A multiple analysis of variance with repeated measures was performed, taking into account the trial, tempo, and strap effects. Each subject was used as his own control.

RESULTS

The MANOVA procedure was performed twice — first with the data organized by side (left and right), then with the data organized by spinal level (T6, T10, and L3; C7 and S1 data were found to be unreliable and were eliminated). Tables II and III, respectively, show the means and standard deviations of these two sets of data.

Table II: Mean ± SD of Maximum, Normalized RMS EMG Data by Side

	SLOW		MEDIUM		FAST	
	Right	Left	Right	Left	Right	Left
Conventional Strap	1.711 ± .455	2.067 ± .775	2.014 ± .420	2.354 ± 1.044	2.161 ± 1.067	2.354 ± .760
SPINStrap	1.086 ± .363	.945 ± .207	1.483 ± .426	1.235 ± .255	1.551 ± .505	1.373 ± .462

Table III: Mean ± SD of Maximum Normalized RMS EMG Data by Spinal Level (C.S. = Conventional Strap)

	SLOW		MEDIUM		FAST	
	C.S.	SPINS	C.S.	SPINS	C.S.	SPINS
T6	2.111 ± .630	1.085 ± .556	2.607 ± 1.121	1.732 ± .494	2.956 ± 1.226	2.079 ± .762
T10	1.732 ± .488	1.080 ± .202	1.654 ± .250	1.226 ± .250	1.883 ± .502	1.249 ± .441
L3	1.824 ± .639	.882 ± .142	1.884 ± .588	1.119 ± .343	1.932 ± .379	1.059 ± .203

Table IV represents the statistical analysis of the various effects. The side effect was not significant, suggesting a tendency to symmetric playing of rock/jazz guitar with regard to lumbar spinal musculature. The speed effect was significant, suggesting that the faster the tempo, the more muscle activity. Spinal level effect was also significant, suggesting decreased muscular activity from top to bottom in the thoracic and lumbar spine while playing the guitar. Indeed, the highest muscle activity levels were recorded at the T6 level (Table III). Finally, the strap effect was borderline significant, with the data clearly showing lower EMG readings with the SPINStrap as compared to conventional straps (Tables II and III).

Table IV: Multivariate (Pillais Test) and Averaged (F Test) Analysis of Variance Results By Effect

EFFECT	PILLAIS TEST		F TEST	
			.00	p = .966
Speed	.87165	p = .046	5.36	p = .033
Spinal Level	.96872	p = .006	12.17	p = .004
Strap			6.55	p = .063

CONCLUSION

Because of the small number of subjects, these results are still tentative and cannot be generalized as yet. In this pilot study, however, there is enough evidence to support the usefulness of the SPINStrap for decreasing muscle activity, and hence fatigue, in the spinal musculature during guitar playing. It is strongly recommended that the study be carried further, increasing the number of subjects and including both genders, to further quantify and ascertain the effect of the SPINStrap on spinal muscle activity. Longitudinal studies would also help assess the long-term effect of the strap and the reversibility thereof.

The experimental design proved valid, reproducible, and easy to use. It can be performed in a clinical setting to map abnormal muscle tension in guitarists and other musicians.

REFERENCES

1. Bejjani FJ: The biomechanical profile: Its use in performing arts medicine. Annual Meetings Course Supplements of the AAPMR and the ACRM 3:1371-1378, 1989.

2. Loomis J: Use of the SPINS strap and conventional straps while exercising with a guitar: A physiological and biomechanical evaluation. Unpublished final report, May 1992.

3. Bejjani FJ: Occupational disorders of performing artists: Diagnosis and treatment. *In* DeLisa J, et al (eds.): Rehabilitation Medicine: Principles and Practice. Philadelphia, PA: JB Lippincott Co (in press).

ACKNOWLEDGEMENT

This project was supported by a grant from the Pennsylvania Ben Franklin Partnership Program.

CHAPTER 46

Static and Dynamic Operation of Coxal Joints in Ballet Dancers

L. Y. Kirienko • *S.N. Vlasenko*

There are a number of problems in choreography connected with the development of coxal joint mobility. It is difficult to increase their range of motion, as these joints are surrounded by large ligaments and muscles, and their bones surfaces are highly congruent.[1,2]

In practice, we sometimes encouter ranges of motion that exceed 180° on the coxal amplitude scale. To study the mechanism of such extreme motions, radiographs and videofluoroscopy of the coxal joints[3] of dancers, enrolled in choreography and calisthenics, were taken during the performance of static and dynamic figures of large amplitude.

Thirty-seven radiographs of active and passive bendings, sideway drivings and straightenings, and sagittal and frontal splits, with the imprints of joint surfaces were obtained.

While analyzing the radiographs obtained, the following tasks have been put to solve:

1) What do the limits of joint mobility depend on?

2) How can the amplitude of joint motion be increased?

3) What changes take place in the coxal joint surface during motion?

Skeletal mobility, as delineated by the contiguity of the edges of joint surfaces (usually separated by a distance of 1.2 to 2 cm), is usually considered to determine the limits of joint mobility. However the radiographs obtained show a discrepancy between joint surface edges of about 1.5 to 2 cm. Hence the structural features of coxal joints must make it possible to perform motions beyond *skeletal mobility*.[4]

The amplitude of sideway driving depends on the amount of leg supination.[5-7] However, in practice, there are situations when it is necessary to perform motions of large amplitude with the leg pronated. Related radiographs showed that these motions were only possible when the flexion angle of the pelvis is increased, i.e., when the greater trochanter is kept posterior to the iliac bone so that it doesn't hinder the motion.

On videofluoroscopy, the greater trochanter was seen from beneath when the leg was supinated, and from above when the leg was pronated (Figure 1). It is worth mentioning that the subjects were not given any special instructions as to positioning of the leg.

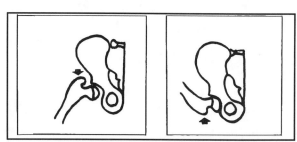

Figure 1: *Greater trochanter position in supination (left) and in pronation (right).*

CONCLUSIONS

1. The limits of joint mobility depend on skeletal muscles mobility, which is activated upon contiguity of the edges of joint surface.

2. There are two possible ways to increase the amplitude of coxal joint motion:

    a) by means of leg supination;

    b) by means of pelvis bending forward with the leg pronated.

3.   Certain changes in the position of the greater trochanter are determined by the character of the coxal joint motion. In turn, the position of the greater trochanter is a determining factor of coxal joint motion amplitude.

4.   In order to decrease pain and prevent joint injury, it is necessary to be aware of the relationships between joint surfaces and apophyses.

REFERENCES

1.   Fick R. Handbuch der Anatomic and Mechanik der Gelenke. 1(3):651, 1901.
2.   Hyrtl E. Handbuch der topographischen Anatomie 2:488, 1882.
3.   Ivanitski, M.F. Essays on Plastic Anatomy of Man. Moscow, Art, 80, 1955.
4.   Kurachenkov, A.I. Changes in Bone Joints Apparatus in Young Sports men. Moscow, Physical Culture, and Sports, 230, 1958.
5.   Ivanitski, M,F. Anatomy of man. Physical Culture and Sports, 520, 1965.
6.   Kopeikin N.G., Sermeev B.V., to the Problem of Coxal Joints Mobility. Materials of the IXth World Conference on Physiology, Morthology, Biochemistry and Biomechanics of Muscles Activity, Moscow, 37, 1966.
7.   Maikova-Stroganova V.S., Bones and Joints on X-Ray Photographs. Leningrad, MedGiz, 482, 1957.

CHAPTER 47

Biomechanical Muscle Stimulation in Performing Arts and Sports

Vladimir Nasarov

The author's muscle stimulation technique (B.M.S.) consists of the mechanical stimulation of human muscles, using a vibration of definite shape, amplitude and frequency, for a certain period of time. The special training apparatus used in B.M.S. differs from an ordinary vibrational massage because it is carried out lengthwise, along the muscle fiber, in its dynamic or static state, allowing the muscle to perform as in any physical exercise. However, the time needed in B.M.S. for reaching a muscle's peak performance is much shorter than in traditional methods of training in remedial gymnastics.

At present, B.M.S. is successfully being applied to training in classical ballet and sports, and in medical rehabilitation and cosmetics.

PHYSIOLOGICAL BASIS

It is known that, during their normal activity, muscle fibers always vibrate with different frequencies. These frequencies accumulate in the tendons and ligaments, producing a complete wide-spectrum oscillatory process, which can then take a random character when the muscle is in a relaxed state. When muscle tension increases, the amplitude of such oscillations increases in parallel (sometimes up to tenfold) and the spectrum of their frequency becomes narrower. At maximum tension, the spectrum of the oscillations traveling through the muscle and tendon becomes practically monochromatic.

It is also known that various receptors in the body are sensitive to stimulations of variable amplitudes and frequencies. The mechanoreceptors located in the muscles, tendons and fasciae are no exception. Natural vibrations of the working muscle are, to a certain extent, a manifestation of their biomechanics, which play an essential role in the stimulation of mechano-receptors, allowing a direct signal connection between the peripheral motor apparatus and the central nervous system. This connection is the link through which artificial stimulation of the oscillatory regime of muscles by means of special devices (B.M.S.) would convert normal vibrations into longitudinal muscle oscillations. To achieve a positive effect, it is recommended to set parameters of stimulation as close as possible to the natural maximum or submaximum of the working muscle. Thus, by using a medium muscle tension and volitional effort, a physiological response can be achieved, comparable to that obtained with the maximum regime of a working muscle.

Physiological experiments have shown that, in perfect human muscles, biomechanical stimulations increase blood flow. The same effect is visually demonstrated on an isolated animal muscle where, after connecting a clear perithelium tube to the vein artery of the muscle, thus destroying the *rami musculares,* stimulation with B.M.S produced a one-way flow of the blood, as in the heart. Thus, with B.M.S application, one can, through the muscles, regulate blood flow, creating hyperemia not only locally but also in other organs. Intensive stimulation of the mechanoreceptors with B.M.S allows dominant excitation in different parts of the central nervous system, producing reflex connections.

CONCLUSIONS

Appropriate implementation of these mechanisms would give us a whole new spectrum of training and rehabilitation possibilities for enhancing the development of joint mobility, muscle strength, and movement coordination. A clear application exists in the fields of performing arts and sports medicine (Figure 1). Biomechanical stimulators were designed for all basic groups of muscles, the most widely used being: the hands, arms-legs-abdomen, shoulder girdle, and face-neck-head devices.

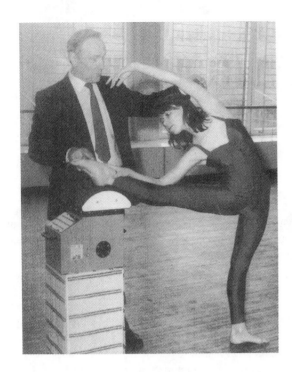

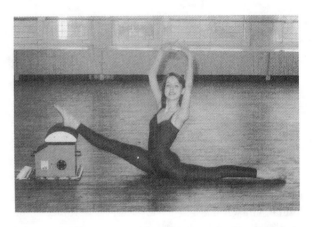

Figure 1: *Dancer training with the B.M.S. device, under Dr. Nasarov's supervision. Left: the dancer is performing a simple stretching exercise, à la seconde. Above: the dancer is in a split position.*

CHAPTER 48

Body and Movement Awareness Education for Musicians: A Case Study Illustrating Basic Exercises and Principles

Paul Linden

INTRODUCTION

Body- and movement-awareness education can help musicians make dramatic improvements in their ability to perform. Difficulties which musicians often experience fall into three broad overlapping categories — physical strain, performance anxiety, and the general feeling of not performing up to full potential. Rather than focusing specifically on the performance problems or working on mastery of instruments or technique, the author concentrates on mastery of the performer's *self*, using an approach centering on fundamental principles of mind/body coordination.[1,2] These principles apply in all performance situations, and provide a framework for analyzing and improving performance.

The approach begins with the idea that the various forms of difficulties musicians face are interconnected. Mind, body, and spirit are linked; thoughts, feelings, beliefs and intentions shape and are shaped by muscle tone, breathing, body alignment, energy flow and movement. A person's overall habits of posture and movement are intimately connected to his or her choices about what to be, how to act in the world, and what to believe the world is. Improving the specifics of a performer's way of making music, therefore, involves working with everything from the body mechanics of the action, to the emotional and interpersonal feelings involved, to the world view which underlies the sense of self.

Body awareness is an effective and convenient tool for addressing and learning about the *whole self*. Music is as much an emotional and spiritual as a physical endeavor, but it is helpful to focus on the body aspect of music because that is solid and easily observable. Changing body use directly changes the physical pattern of performance, but it is also a direct means of changing the underlying emotional and spiritual elements of performance.

As a general rule, physical and emotional performance difficulties always involve some form of tension, constriction, limpness, twisting or imbalance in breathing, muscle tone and posture. Examining the places and patterns of such body blockages is a way of discovering and understanding inappropriate movement patterns and hidden feelings and thoughts. Freeing up the blockages is a way of working out the difficulties.

Freeing blockages means finding the fundamental state of wholeness and balance which is the opposite of and solution to any particular mental and physical imbalance. In this balanced state, mind, body, and spirit are integrated. The self is free and open. It is calm and alert, powerful and loving, sensitive, fluid and stable. This is as much a description of a musculoskeletal configuration as it is of a psychospiritual state, and working with body processes is a way of accessing the total process.

CASE STUDY

A jazz pianist who experienced disabling pain in his upper right arm when he played came for lessons to explore whether he was doing anything as he played which caused the pain.

Body Mechanics

At the beginning of the first lesson, the pianist was observed sitting, standing and walking, and some interesting imbalances in his body use were noticed. Rather than using his body as an evenly balanced, unified whole, he seemed to use it as a collection of mismatched parts. When he stood, his right shoulder was lower, and his right pectoral muscle was softer and stood out less. When his left hip was held immobile while pushing back on his left shoulder, he stood firm without bending, but when the same was done on his right, his torso was weak and he flopped back. As he breathed while lying on his back, there was noticeably more movement in his chest than in his abdomen. When he tried to breathe from his diaphragm, his chest didn't move. It was difficult for him to get his chest and abdomen moving evenly and together.

Specific performance difficulties are usually part of a general underlying dysfunctional movement pattern. Improving the general pattern as well as the specific performance pattern gives the best chance of resolving these difficulties. Because of the overall lack of body integration seen in the pianist, it was decided to start by focusing on the general theme of stability and power, and particularly on how the pelvis operates as a foundation for the torso.

Since excess tension in the muscles of the abdomen and pelvic floor interferes with the free, powerful and balanced use of the whole body, work was begun on pelvic relaxation. Alternately tightening and releasing his abdominal muscles, enabled him to feel how to keep his abdomen released, soften his breath, and breathe diaphragmatically, gently expanding both his abdomen and lower back as he inhaled.

Once the pianist could relax the core of his body, he had to learn to use it in a stable and efficient manner. Sitting on a firm, flat chair without touching the back support, he experimented with the movements of slumping down and sitting up straight. He realized that when his pelvis tipped too far forward or backward, his spinal column did not have a level foundation on which to rest and his back curved too much and assumed either a slumped (Fig. 1) or a swaybacked (Fig. 2) position. He could feel that this destroyed the architectural integrity of his body structure — his musculoskeletal system was not positioned to support weight and deliver power effectively.   He could also feel that the correct alignment of the pelvis (Fig. 3) allowed stable positioning of the torso.

In moving from a slumped to an erect position, however, the pianist experienced some discomfort. He also needed to find the right way to move the pelvis into the correct position. He was using the muscles along his spinal column to rotate the pelvis by pulling up on the back edge of the pelvic bowl, and this created tension in his back.   Rather, he was shown how using the psoas (a deep core muscle) to rotate the pelvis in effect pulls the front edge of the pelvis down, and he felt how this allowed him to assume an erect posture without any strain.

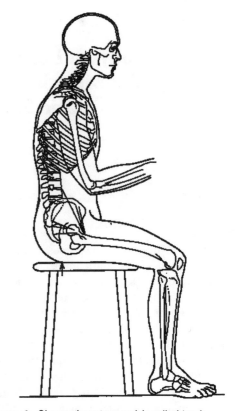

Figure 1: *Slumped posture, pelvis rolled back.*

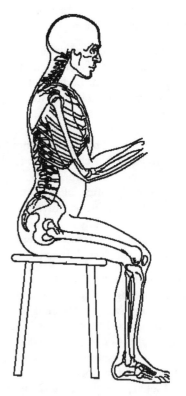

Figure 2:   *Swaybacked posture, pelvis rotated forward.*

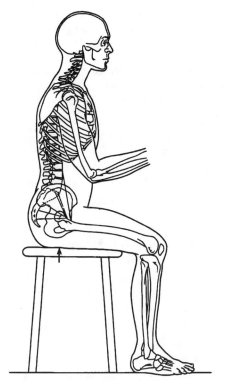

Figure 3: Well-supported posture, pelvis centered.

Using his body in a relaxed, balanced, and stable manner was then practiced in various actions such as sitting down, standing up, walking, pushing, pulling and lifting. These actions involved some effort, and when he exerted strength, he hardened and constricted his movements. When asked about it, he realized that trying *hard* was part of his image of what strength was, and that created excess tension in many of his movements. The idea that strength is tough and hard is, of course, very common in our culture.

Building on the foundation of relaxed breathing, the pianist was shown how to focus the power of his breath. Using imagery direct breathing movements, he was asked to inhale into his pelvis/abdomen and then exhale outward through his arms, legs and head — the feeling a starfish might have breathing *radiantly* outward through its star limbs. In order to incorporate that imagery process into practice of large movements involving application of strength, he pushed on the instructor with various body parts, lengthening and releasing his muscles while creating outward pressure.

Strategies of Action

Work was then directed toward applying this body awareness in his piano playing. The breathing

exercises generated a relaxed strength. He began to understand that when he played the piano, he was forcing his muscles to move against internal resistance, creating strain just when he needed to move in the freest possible manner. The pianist had been injured a number of times on his right side and realized that he had been attempting to protect his arm by stiffening it. This was another source of strain and actually made the arm feel worse.

The pianist often engaged muscles in his back and elevated and stiffened his chest. This tension in the back and chest spread into his arms and increased their tension. By softening and dropping his chest, he became able to open his whole body in a relaxed manner.

At this point (the fourth lesson), it was time to go to the piano and use what he had learned in touching the keyboard. As he sat in front of the piano, however, rather than releasing his weight onto the piano bench, he still carried a lot of tension high in his back. He practiced pushing his left foot down into the floor and toward the left to initiate a rotation and lean of his torso to the right, and then take that into a back-and-forth movement using each foot in turn. That brought his awareness into the lower half of his body and helped him feel how his feet, legs and hips acted to help support and move his torso and, consequently, his arms.

He realized that since he had not been using the lower half of his body enough, the upper half had been forced to work too hard, and this was another source of back tension and arm strain. As the pianist learned to include in his awareness his legs and the sensations of his feet touching the floor or the pedals, he began to feel a new support and freedom of movement in his arms.

Up to this point, he had played just a few notes at a time, not actually playing *music*. As soon as he began to play, however, he lost his awareness of his pelvis and breathing and shifted into what seemed to be primarily a "head-and-hands" state of existence. He appeared to feel that eyes to see, ears to hear and hands to play contained all of his musical being.

The pianist was instructed to stand up, touch the piano with no idea of playing, and feel how just touching the piano led to his assuming his habitual muscular/energetic state.

Work then focused on generating the state of ease and balance and not interrupting it when he touched the piano. He felt that in his habitual strategy for playing, when he lifted his hands, he initiated the movements by tensing his shoulders. He was shown that it was possible instead to relax his arm and to activate movement from a graceful lengthening of the whole arm. The feeling was that movement of the arm was initiated from the pelvis and the fingertips, with everything in between participating in a released way. That way of moving the arm drastically reduced the strain he felt and increased his strength.

At the beginning of the next lesson, the pianist said that in practicing at home he had felt that his arm worked better when he used it the way he had been shown. As he played and really began to get into the music, however, he rolled his pelvis back and hunched himself down over the keys. He explained that he didn't like playing with his head upright and his body open because, as a jazz pianist, he often played in bars. People in the audience were frequently not listening. They were often drunk and unpleasant, and his overwhelming desire was to go into himself, the piano and the music and create a barrier between himself and his audience.

He recalled that early in his career, one day he had accidentally fallen into that posture, and an older musician said, "Now you look like a jazz pianist!" He explained that it had to do with the essential process of jazz improvisation, noting that a jazz musician has no written, preordained piece of music to play. Jazz focuses on self-expression, and the player is the point, not the piece.

There were personal, interpersonal, social, and artistic reasons for his habitual strategies of body use. Lessons had started with considerations of relaxation and body mechanics, and had proceeded to examining his beliefs about strength and effective action. Now, they moved on to focus on examination of the structure of the self that creates the music. Then they had proceeded to examining his beliefs about strength and effective action. And now we moved onto focus on issues of vulnerability and boundary protection and on an examination of the structure of the self that creates the music.

It was pointed out that the pianist's thoughts actually came from deep within himself, though he had created a complex feedback loop between himself and his instrument in which each exerted influence over the other. He was really talking about a fundamental element of the creative process that, like breathing, had both an inward and outward beat. He had to go inward to feel his musical impulse, and he had to go outward to the piano and the sound to execute the musical thought and gain further musical inspiration.

In locating the source of musical thought in the instrument, however, he actually to some extent lost his experience of his inward self. He had to remold his *self* into a new, more symmetrical and expansive shape in order to achieve a balance between the inward and outward functions of creativity. That new shape allowed him to access new power and sensitivity in the creative process, and it also acted to reduce the strain on his arm.

In the end, the pianist reported that his arm was ninety-five per cent better. He said he didn't feel that he had learned a static formula which dictated the *right way* to play, but that he had increased his awareness so he was better at reading the cues his body and the sound of the music were giving him. He had learned how to adjust himself when things were not working together optimally, and he even valued the occasional twinge in his arm because it notified him that he had started to forget himself.

CONCLUSION

The body- and movement-awareness exercises described here are some of the basics of the process of developing a strain-free and effective way of creating music, but they are just the beginning. There are many other exercises and topics to be addressed in working with musicians. Exercises such as feeling the sound vibrations of the music in every part of the body or projecting the body-sense into the physical material of the instrument have a lot to offer musicians. Further topics could involve feeling the nonverbal spatial pressures that connect members of a group as they play together or learning to mold the audience's attention with the musician's breath.

Body awareness is the key to the process of investigation described herein. Whatever habits of body image, self-image and movement performers have, it is on the basis of those habits that they will sing or play their instruments. Tense, unbalanced patterns of action get in the way of the ability to play freely, with power and sensitivity and feeling. Remembering to observe, interpret and control their physical responses gives performers powerful tools for creating a state in which they can concentrate well, move freely, perceive sensitively, and exert efficient power.

PART IV

DANCE MEDICINE

CHAPTER 49

Relationship Between Technical Faults
and Dance Injuries: Correction and Prevention

Luana Poggini • *Anna Paola Pace* • *Donatella Di Mastromatteo*

Dance technique, in every type of professional dance, represents the highest expression of the elegance and harmony of human movement. To achieve this constant fusion of grace, strength, and energy, the dancer has to firmly train his body to perform very complex exercises with the greatest accuracy. This accuracy is the basic principle of dance style.

As Natalia Dudinskayn wrote in her reminiscences of her instructor, Madame Vaganova: *It is not necessary to be a special connoisseur in the field of ballet to attend the performances of our theater and of everyone — from the girls in the corps to the leading ballerinas. They have something in common in their manner of execution. A single style, a single handwriting...*[1] A good dance style, therefore, develops through hard daily work during classes and rehearsals.

In this context, the dance teacher and the teaching method are very important in directing the students' efforts towards the learning of dance technique secrets. Since dance in our time is technically more complex than in the past, it has become almost impossible to develop technique safely without a thorough understanding of biomechanical principles. For this reason, today's dancers demand explanation and logic from their teachers as they analyze and correct movements.

To meet those demands, dance teachers began to cooperate with medical doctors and physiotherapists, creating a new branch of medicine, *dance medicine*. In the past several years, many authors described the dangers of poor or incorrect training.[2-6]

Technical errors and incorrect body posture are certainly the most important risk factors for dance-related injuries. Since the authors believe that preventing dance injuries is one of the most important tasks for all involved in teaching young dancers, in 1988 an affiliation was established among the National Dance Academy, the First Department of Orthopaedic Surgery, and the Department of Physical Therapy and Rehabilitation at the University of Rome "La Sapienza."

The National Dance Academy of Rome is the only public dance school in Italy. Students of both sexes begin their courses at the age of 11 years, and they take their first degree after eight years. During this period, they study classical and modern dance daily, as well as many theoretical subjects, in order to improve their artistic education. After the first degree, dancers can take a Ph.D. in dance choreography, while working with renowned international teachers.

This school, with its 400 students, can be a continuing source of data about the incidence of dance injuries occurring among dance students as compared to professional dancers.

In order to identify the most frequent dance-related injuries, a survey of 458 dancers was performed, using a simple questionnaire modified from Washington.[7] One hundred seventy-six were students at the National Dance Academy of Rome (oldest students only), and the other 282 were professional dancers from such Italian theaters as La Scala, the San Carlo, the Opera, and other noted Italian ballet and modern dance companies. Demographic distribution, physical characteristics, and work load are described in Tables I, II, and III, respectively.

Table I: Description of Sample (n = 158)

Age	Sex	Dance Level
Min. 15 years	F = 330 (72.05%)	Professional: 282
Max. 57 years	M = 126 (27.95%)	Students: 176

Table IV represents the summary of distribution of dance injuries. Most suffered ailments in more than one part of the body, and only 13 dancers of 458 (9 students and 4 professionals) did not report any dance-related physical problem.

Table II: *Physical Characteristics by Sex*

Females (n = 330)	Males (n = 128)
Weight = mean 49.5 Kg	Weight = mean 66.9 Kg
Height = mean 164 cm	Height = mean 175 cm

Table III: *Daily Work Load and Dance Type*

Students		Professional Dancers	
Classical: 2-4 hrs.	= 0	Classical: 3-7 hrs.	= 154
Modern: 2 hrs.	= 18	Modern: 2-4 hrs.	= 39
Classical + Modern	= 158	Classical + Modern	= 89

The authors' approach to treatment and prevention of these injuries is a global one: (1) The dance teacher, the physiotherapist, and the orthopaedist work together closely in an effort to help the young dancer have a long and safe career; (2) The dance teacher must check the accuracy of the dancer's movements and correct technical errors as early as possible; and (3) The physiotherapy treatment for each ailment takes into account posture and movement, the real problem often being far from the painful area. Traditional physiotherapy focuses primarily on muscle strengthening, on the basis that gravity is counteracted by extensor muscles, which are themselves too strong and short. Thus, most of the physiotherapy work has to focus on balancing strong and weak muscles, hypo- and hypermobile joints.

Table IV: *Dance-Related Injuries by Site and Dance Level*

Site	Total #	Students n = 176		Professionals n = 282	
Cervical spine	216	59	(33.5%)	157	(55.6%)
Dorsal spine	49	9	(9.1%)	40	(14.2%)
Lumbar spine	212	61	(34.5%)	151	(53.5%)
Shoulder	96	18	(10.2%)	78	(27.6%)
Elbow	12	4	(2.2%)	8	(2.8%)
Wrist	52	14	(7.9%)	38	(13.4%)
Hand	20	5	(2.8%)	15	(5.3%)
Hip	225	92	(52.2%)	133	(47.1%)
Knee	252	80	(45.4%)	172	(60.9%)
Leg	48	15	(8.5%)	33	(11.7%)
Ankle	298	92	(52.2%)	206	(73.0%)
Foot	186	58	(32.9%)	128	(45.3%)

The high incidence of cervical spine injuries in this survey (157 dancers, 55.6%) does not correspond to previously published surveys.[7-9] This is probably inflated by reversal of the cervical lordosis that is, in many cases, less pronounced than in the general population. This stiffness is due to a muscular imbalance around the neck; the continuous tension of the trapezius can produce a reduction of cervical lordosis until it becomes straight. At this point, the sternocleidomastoid inverts its action, changing the cervical curve in kyphosis. In most of the professional dancers, there were early signs of cervical osteoarthritis, probably related to poor posture and alignment.

In all cases of chronic cervical pain, the authors suggest a careful evaluation of the entire body alignment, including the dorsal spine, lumbar spine, and upper- and lower extremities.

Low back pain is certainly one of the most frequent spinal disorders encountered in dancers (34.6% of students, 38.9% of professionals).

As Kostrovitskaya said in describing the basic position of the trunk, *The body should be erect, with the stomach tightly pulled up, the buttocks muscles pulled up and tense, the shoulders lowered, and the thorax open.*[10]

According to Micheli,[11] there are three categories of lumbar spine problems in dancers: mechanical low back pain, discogenic pain and spondylolysis. Low back pain was present in 61 students. In most, physical examination showed only a dynamic hyperlordosis during dance work and sometimes poor *en dehors* at the hip joint. This condition is usually associated with mechanical low back pain without any sign of discal suffering. Among professional dancers, a high incidence of discogenic back pain was found. Low back pain was found in 110 dancers, and 41 had associated sciatica. A young male dancer presented an acute disc herniation after an incorrect lift and needed surgery. Spondylolysis was observed in only 10 subjects. This low incidence is probably due to the design of the study, whereby dancers reported only injuries previously diagnosed.

A good turnout involves complete external rotation at each hip without any other rotation at the knee and foot.[12] This optimal condition, as described in traditional textbooks, is fairly rare. In practice, dancers use up the 60°-70° of external rotation at the hip and reach the final position only by recruiting external rotation at the knee, tibial torsion, and forefoot. If the turnout at the hip is very poor (significant anteversion of the femoral neck), they tend to increase the lumbar lordosis, quickly flexing and *screwing* the knees, rotating the feet out farther than the hips (overturning).[13] In addition, the weak abductors do not control the turnout at the hip, aggravating any overturning at the knee. All these common tricks can cause damage to the medial meniscus, as well as patellar tendinitis and many foot problems.

Pain around the front of the knees is a very common complaint in dancers. In fact, many pathological conditions present as anterior knee pain. Certain anatomical variations of the knee, such as swayback knee, increased Q angle, and external tibial torsion, can represent risk factors. In this survey, there were 11 cases of patellar dislocation (1 male, 10 female). Since ballet training does not cause hyperextension of the knees, it is important to point out that a poor teaching method may aggravate and increase the amount of swayback by allowing the dancer to push the knee back on the supporting leg. A student with hyperextension of the knees must be instructed to pull up with the thighs and then keep the knees in neutral position as much as possible. The therapist can help the dancer with a global rearrangement of posture.

Abnormal foot positions are quite frequent among young dancers of both sexes. The most common is rolling. In this condition, all the weight is borne over the medial part of the foot, flattening the medial longitudinal arch. Over the years, a dancer with rolling feet can develop lordotic posture, tibialis posterior tendinitis, severe hallux valgus, and Achilles tendinitis. Almost all Italian female dancers present a hallux valgus deformity, but it is symptomatic in only 10% of students and 13% of professionals. Peritendinitis of the Achilles tendon is present in 24% of students and 34% of professionals. There were 2 total subcutaneous ruptures of the Achilles tendon, both in professional female modern dancers (one with a long history of peritendinitis). They both were able to return to dance 12 months after surgical repair of the tendon.

Correct position of the foot is very important also during pointe work. If the young dancer does not control foot position on pointe and carries all the weight over the lateral aspect of the feet (sickling), he/she can frequently sustain an acute ankle sprain.

The ankle is the most common site of dance-related injuries. Ankle sprains were found in 41 students (23.2%) and 125 professional dancers (44.3%).

According to other surveys,[7-9] the upper limbs are not frequently involved in dance-related injuries. Poor teaching methods can cause tension around the neck and shoulders. Novice dancers tend to place the arms too far back, thus requiring many postural compensations in order to maintain the center of gravity over the base (hyperlordosis, overturning). In this case, the technical error has to be corrected as soon as possible, relieving the muscle spasm, particularly in the pectoralis.

REFERENCES

1. Vaganova A: Basic Principles of Classical Ballet: Russian Ballet Technique. New York: Dover Publications, 1969.
2. Clarkson PM, Skrinar M: Science of Dance Training. Champaign, IL: Human Kinetics Books, 1988.
3. Gelabert R: Preventing dancers' injuries. Phys Sports Med 8(4):69-76, 1980.
4. Howse J, Hancok S: Dance Technique and Injury Prevention. London: A & C Black, 1983.
5. Ryan AJ, Stephens RR: Dance Medicine: A Comprehensive Guide. Chicago: Pluribus Press, 1987.
6. Sammarco GJ: Diagnosis and treatment in dancers. Clin Orthop 18(7):176-187, 1984.
7. Washington EL: Musculoskeletal injuries in theatrical dancers: Site, frequency and severity. Am J Sports Med 6(2):75-98, 1976.
8. Rovere GD, et al: Musculoskeletal injuries in theatrical dance students. Am J Sports Med 11 (4):195-198, 1983.
9. Quirk R: Ballet injuries: The Australian experience. Clin Sports Med 2(3):507-514, 1963.
10. Kostrovitskaya V, Pisarev A: School of Classical Dance. Moscow: Progress Publishers, 1978.
11. Micheli LJ: Back injuries in dancers. Clin Sports Med 2(3):473-484, 1983.
12. Pappacena F: Tecnica della Danza Classica: l'Impostazione. Roma: Gremese Ed, 1986.
13. Sammarco GJ: The dancer's hip. Clin Sports Med 2(3):485-505, 1983.

SUGGESTED READING

1. Fitt SS: Dance Kinesiology. New York: Schirmer Books, 1988.

2. Nixon JE: Injuries to the neck and upper extremities of dancers. Clin Sports Med 2(3): 459-472, 1983.

3. Perugia L, Postacchini F, Ippolito E: The Tendons: Biology, Pathology, Clinical Aspects. Milano: Kurtis Ed, 1986.

4. Poggini L, Martini G: Controllo posturale e dansa classica: Una indicazione fisiatrica. Il Fisiatra 1: 11-13 1989.

5. Reid DC, et al: Lower extremity flexibility patterns in classical ballet dancers and their correlation to lateral hip and knee injuries. Am J Sports Med 15(4):347-352, 1987.

CHAPTER 50

Strategies and Approach to Treatment of Dancers with Psychiatric Disorders

Judith R. F. Kupersmith

OBJECTIVES

- To address the psychiatric problems of dancers.

- To provide effective treatment for this population.

OVERVIEW

- Understanding stress as experienced by dancers.

- Linking psychological issues to specific stress experience (derail distress).

- Choosing a treatment modality that is most effective.

- Clinical examples to demonstrate the process.

STRESS

- Stress of Ordinary Living
  - Dancer as a whole person
  - Vicissitudes of life and growing up
    - Family dysfunction
    - Peer pressure
    - Illness and death
    - Dating and romantic involvements
    - Substance abuse

- Stress Specific for Dancers
  - Orthopedic
    - Body as instrument
    - Maintain optimal function despite excessive demands
    - Injuries — vulnerability, overuse phenomena, accident prone
    - Debilitation and chronic illness, e.g. arthritis
  - Nutritional
    - Maintenance of low body weight
    - Maintenance of strength and endurance
    - Incidence and prevalence of eating disorders
  - Gynecological
    - Low body weight and delayed menarche
    - Low body weight and amenorrhea
  - Social
    - Limited social experiences due to:
      - Long hours in training
      - Competition for few coveted places
      - Prevailing attitudes in dance world
    - Adult decision-making in preadolescent and adolescent age group:
      - Relocation due to training
      - Independent living
      - Jobs, resumes, agents, etc.

- Stress by Developmental Stages
  - Students
    - Body type and changes during puberty
    - Emphasis on intense competition/ classes, auditions, performance
    - Parental authority and development of artistic talent
  - Performers
    - Maintenance of professional status vs. striving for higher goals
    - Performance anxiety
    - Competition and success — effect on relationships
  - Dancers in Transition
    - Mid-life crisis and career change
    - Retraining
    - Absence of economic stability
    - Loss of friends
    - Loss of livelihood
    - Loss of identity

PSYCHOLOGICAL ISSUES

Table I: *Symptom Formation*

	Professional Dancers	Performing Artists Seeking Treatment	Louisville PACH*
Depression	72%	84%	95%
Difficulty sleeping	59%	52%	55%
Loneliness	45%	72%	65%
Divorce or break-up with significant other	35%	40%	55%
Loss of job	25%	40%	55%
Travel-related stress	36%	-----	-----
Severe anxiety	-----	62%	85%
Family problems	-----	48%	40%
Getting along with others	-----	26%	20%
Death of significant other	-----	14%	15%

*   Performing Arts Center for Health

Table II: *Diagnostic Categories*

	Performing Artists Seeking Treatment	Louisville PACH
Adjustment disorders	24.0 %	35%
Dysthymia	33.0 %	35%
Major depression	15.0 %	20%
Eating disorders	8.8 %	10%
Panic disorder	-----	5%
Bipolar affective disorder	8.0%	5%
Schizophrenia	2.2%	-----
Substance abuse	1.1%	5%

- Strengths and Development of Character Traits
  - Intelligence
  - Perseverance
  - Dedication
  - Responsibility
  - Attention to detail
  - Motivation
  - Ability to problem-solve
  - Single-mindedness
  - Concentration
  - Internalization of work role/self-image

- Conflict and Resolution
  - Student
  - Body image
  - Self-esteem
  - Sexuality
  - Sibling rivalry
  - Inspiration to dance
  - Motivation to become a dancer
  - Traditional values, i.e. discipline, obedience, and conformity leads to mastery

□ Performer

  · Career vs. artistry
  · Narcissism vs. altruism
  · Exhibitionism
  · Activity supersedes passivity
  · Maturation as an artist vs. as an adult

□ Dancer in Transition

  · Identity and self-image
  · Loss and abandonment
  · Denial and acceptance
  · Retraining and supports

TREATMENT MODALITY

■ Psychopharmacotherapy

  □ Usefulness in specific conditions, e.g. depression, anorexia/bulimia
  □ Objections due to side-effect profile, sensitivity to physiological changes

■ Psychotherapy

  □ Individual vs. group
  □ Crisis intervention
  □ Short- and long-term therapies
  □ Dynamic vs. cognitive

■ Combination

CLINICAL EXAMPLES

■ A 25-year-old white, married female dancer with diagnoses of major depression and dysthymia.

■ An 18- year-old white, single female ballet dancer with diagnoses of adjustment disorder with mixed emotional features.

■ A 30-year-old white, single male dancer with alcohol dependence and abuse.

CHAPTER 51

Physical and Psychological Aspects of Dance Medicine

William G. Hamilton • *Michelle P. Warren* • *Linda Hamilton*

Classical ballet is uniquely different from all other disciplines in the performing arts. In addition to aesthetic concerns, its physical demands are comparable to those found in professional football. To meet these standards, the dancer must display a tremendous amount of strength in a thin, aesthetically proportioned body. Research suggests that balancing ballet's dual demands of artistry and athleticism can be costly. Problems include physical injuries, disability, and menstrual dysfunctions. Serious eating disorders also are prevalent, due to the low weight required in dance. To provide appropriate services for dancers, a comprehensive treatment approach encompassing the structural, hormonal, and mental aspects of dance medicine must be considered.

COMMON ORTHOPEDIC PROBLEMS

The professional ballet dancer is the product of a demanding selection process beginning with the first ballet class and continuing through his/her entire career. This 'Darwinism' produces a 'thoroughbred racehorse' with unique features: flexibility, strength, and an extreme range of motion of the joints of the lower extremity. The dancer's *instrument* is based on a combination of selectivity and early training that occurs before skeletal maturity, when the musculoskeletal system is pliable. One should keep this in mind when treating dancers — not infrequently, their problems are related to the fact that they may not have the right body. Proper turnout is especially important, and turning out from the floor up rather than from the hip down can cause a multitude of problems.

Because of the rigid technical requirements of classical ballet, dancers must conform to certain orthopedic dimensions or else be weeded out of the system. Many of the following problems occur when the dancer pushes his/her anatomy beyond its physical limits. Others include the strenuous athletic demands which place dancers at risk for certain injuries, particularly as they grow older.

SPECIFIC CONDITIONS

Foot/Ankle

■ *First Metatarsophalangeal (MP) Joint*: Ninety degrees of dorsiflexion is necessary for a complete relevé. In older dancers, impingement spurs frequently build up on the dorsum of the joint, limiting motion and forcing the dancer to *sickle* the foot in relevé.

■ *Lesser Metatarsophalangeal Joints*: Metatarsalgia is rare in dancers. When seen, one should look for something unusual, such as:

  □ *Freiberg's Disease*: Symptoms may precede the x-ray appearance by as long as six months).
  □ *MP Joint Instability*: Positive "Lachman test" of the MP joint; the "dancer's fracture" of the 5th metatarsal in the distal diaphysis.

■ *Stress Fracture of the Base of the 2nd Metatarsal*: The most common stress fracture in the dancer's foot.

■ *Cuboid Subluxation*: Difficult to diagnose, often overlooked.

■ *Anterior Impingement of the Ankle*: Common in older male dancers who have done a lot of jumping.

■ *Posterior Ankle Pain*:

  □ Posterolateral; the os trigonum; positive "plantarflexion sign."
  □ Posteromedial: flexor hallucis longus tendinitis — "dancer's tendinitis."

■ *Achilles Tendinitis and Rupture*: Tightness is a predisposition, surgery must restore physiological length.

- *Stress Fracture of the Distal Fibula*: Occurs where the toeshoe ribbons pass over the Achilles tendon.

- *Stress Fracture of the Tibia*: The "dreaded black line." Difficult to treat.

The Knee

- *Infrapatellar Tendinitis*: "Jumper's knee," a common condition, hard to treat; surgery may be necessary.

- *Meniscal Tears*: Arthroscopy usually needed.

- *Anterior Cruciate Ligament Tears*: A complex problem; reconstruction is usually, but not always, necessary.

The Hip

- *Acetabular Dysplasia*: A subtle condition, it may be a precursor to osteoarthritis.

- *Osteoarthritis*: Is it more common in dancers than in non-dancers?

The Spine

- *Scoliosis*: Very common in dancers, but usually it is mild.

- *Spondylolysis*: It presents with a painful arabesque.

- *Spondylolisthesis*: A more severe version of spondylolysis.

MEDICAL AND ENDOCRINE PROBLEMS

The dancer, especially the female ballet dancer, is exposed at a young age to a number of environmental factors which affect the reproductive system. Students who start training for ballet as a profession usually start classes at an early age (8 years or younger) and continue training through adolescence. The ideal form for this art is thin, usually 10-20% below ideal body weight. Nutrition may be compromised as students diet to conform to this ideal. This may be a particularly difficult time, as weight gain is normal during puberty. All of these factors, including poor nutrition and dieting, low weight, high exercise load, training in adolescence and stress, may affect normal pubertal development as well as reproductive cycles.

Our studies have shown a high incidence of delayed menarche, occurring in almost 70%. Ballet dancers, however, are well below their peers in weight.

Dancers did achieve a body weight and a body fat appropriate for menarche four to six months before menarche occurred. Observations over a two-year period showed that the advancement of pubertal stages occurred during times of rest, an association that was particularly marked in thinner individuals. Dancers, when injured, showed advancement of pubertal stages during these times of enforced rest, with some dancers exhibiting a "catch-up" puberty, going through all the stages of puberty in four to six months instead of the usual two years. Thus, pubertal development appears to be affected by the low weight of dancers, as well as the large amount of activity necessary for training and performing.

Another common problem in more mature dancers is the occurrence of secondary amenorrhea, or absence of periods. This problem occurs with varying frequency — 30 to 70%, depending on the report. Here also, there is a strong interaction between activity and body weight, with the incidence of reproductive dysfunction increasing with hours of exercise per week. The problem is easily reversed, usually with a small amount of exercise and an increase in weight.

Our studies have revealed another important causal factor: The majority of dancers with amenorrhea report an eating disorder — usually, anorexia nervosa. There is increasing evidence that the reproductive dysfunction seen in dancers may be related to dieting and eating disorders, particularly in disciplines where a low body weight is an advantage.

The mechanism for the reproductive dysfunction appears to occur at the level of the hypothalamus in the brain. An area called the *arcuate nucleus* contains neurons which manufacture gonadotropin releasing hormone (GnRH). This hormone travels down the axon and is secreted into the medial central area of the hypothalamus, where it is picked up by a venous plexus and taken to the anterior pituitary. There, it stimulates the secretion of luteinizing hormone (LH) and follicle stimulating hormone (FSH), which, in turn, stimulate ovarian hormones. The pulses of GnRH are key to menstrual cyclicity. It has been well shown that in the nutritionally deprived, the pulses of LH slow or may be completely absent, regressing to a prepubertal pattern. This problem occurs as well in amenorrheic athletes. Thus, the pulse generator in the arcuate nucleus is very sensitive to environmental factors such as dieting, low weight, and exercise.

The effects of these hormonal problems were thought, until recently, to be of little consequence because of their reversibility. Recent evidence shows that stress fractures, which occur in 30% of dancers, are related to the delay in puberty. Scoliosis, or curvature of the spine, is also directly related to a delay in menarche. Both of these problems are also more frequent in dancers who report secondary amenorrhea. More serious problems are occasionally seen, including one dancer who developed complete collapse of the femoral head. Thus, the skeletal problems seen in dancers, including injuries, may be related to lack of sex hormone — in particular, estrogen.

The majority of bone mass is accumulated during adolescence, and the delay in hormone secretion and absence with amenorrheic intervals appears to prevent the important accretion of bone and the attainment of peak bone mass. This leaves a weaker bone which is subject to injury, particularly with overuse syndromes. Our studies also show that bone in hypoestrogenic dancers does not show adequate reaction to stress and does not accumulate bone mass in a normal manner. A two-year follow-up shows that bone mass remains well below what is observed in normal dancers. Thus, hormonal deficiencies can have serious medical consequences, and if the problem persists, hormonal replacement is offered.

PSYCHOLOGICAL STRESSES

The unique stresses and strains in ballet often set up poorly equipped dancers for problems during their careers. This is particularly evident in females who attempt to conform to ballet's physical ideal through excessive food restriction. The consequences of dieting on body weight and metabolism can lead to a number of nutrition-related health problems, the most serious of which are anorexia nervosa and bulimia. This section concentrates on the onset of eating disorders in this select group of performing artists.

The etiology of eating disorders is multi-determined, involving cultural, psychological, and biological variables. The degree of vulnerability depends on the mix between the individual and her environment. Biological factors are extremely important in ballet because this form of dancing is not aerobic. Only 200 kcal are typically expended by women in a one-hour ballet class. A low weight cannot be achieved through exercise alone; thus,

dieting often becomes the vehicle through which the aesthetic demands of this profession are met.

Research on the physiological mechanisms associated with dieting suggests that tampering with weight can lead to a number of adverse reactions. These effects, though variable depending on the person, are thought to be due to the body's attempt to defend its preferred weight in the face of powerful efforts to restrict food intake. It has been hypothesized that a genetic *set-point* for weight exists which determines the amount of fat stored in the body by regulating perceptions of hunger, activity level, and metabolic rate. Although a person's set-point is complexly determined, genetic endowment is significant. Up to 69% of the variance in body-mass index can be explained by family-line resemblances, even when members are separated at birth.

The consequences of dieting have been demonstrated in studies of starvation, where bingeing, depression and, in some cases, psychotic levels of disorganization, are common. These results, which are unrelated to prior psychological adjustment, are attributed to the individual's attempts to overpower the body's natural level of fatness by resisting its set-point. In light of these findings, restrained eaters would then face certain inevitable hazards, as dieting would comprise a counter-regulatory behavior accompanied by severe psychological stress.

In ballet, dancers who are not naturally thin are at a distinct disadvantage. The aesthetic ideal requires that they conform to a weight that is considerably below the norm. Yet, genetic endowment and the hazards of dieting place them at risk in trying to achieve this goal weight. In contrast, dancers who undergo a strict selection process during their formative years are weeded out of the system if their bodies stray from a prepubescent shape. Those who survive this process appear to be more naturally suited to the demands of this profession. In a survey of four national ballet companies, the authors found that dancers chosen from general auditions reported a higher incidence of familial obesity (42% vs 5%) and eating disorders (46% vs 11%) than those who had been selected from company schools. Both groups were equally thin, suggesting that the less selected dancers were achieving their low weight through deviant eating behaviors.

Treating dancers with eating disorders is often difficult because there is a realistic component to their preoccupation with weight. A combination of individual therapy and nutritional counseling often works best. Changing unhealthy eating patterns is an arduous process. As the dancer begins to learn healthy ways to eat, a certain amount of weight gain may occur until the body adjusts. This can be extremely disconcerting. Successful treatment may mean achieving a more realistic weight goal, as well as including low-impact aerobics and appropriate food choices in their regime. Schools can help in this process by paying even greater attention to selection factors. Dancers who are not naturally thin would do better to choose an athletic discipline where the caloric expenditure is higher and a thin ideal body is not a particular requirement.

SUMMARY

The dancer's body is a complex instrument that is affected by structural, hormonal, and mental factors. It is recommended that services be available at schools and companies to help dancers cope with the physical and psychological consequences of ballet. We have found that the best approach involves a multidisciplinary team comprised of an orthopedist, physical therapist, nurse, nutritionist, and clinical psychologist. Dance-medicine specialists who are aware of the particular needs of these artists have the opportunity to help them cope with the inherent stresses of this profession.

CHAPTER 52

Achilles and Patellar Tendinitis in Ballet Dancers

Federico Fernandez-Palazzi, and Salvador Rivas

Overuse injuries of tendons are well known to occur in persons that due to their activity submit the tendon to excessive stress. This is the case of classical ballet dancers who, upon getting "en pointe," "demie-pointe" or "plié" exert forces that although being normal in magnitude, are increased in frequency thus giving overuse lesions to the Achilles tendon, and upon hyperextending the knee in lifting or jumping or lacking of spring mechanism in falling from a jump, exert these deleterious forces on the patellar tendon giving rise to symptoms of the so called Jumper's Knee. The causes of these tendinopathies are either abnormal tension or incorrect use. Their development and progression to chronic tendinopathy, as well as measures preventing this are analyzed. The different methods of treatment, conservative with rest and refraining from dancing, local means such as ice and adhesive strapping, antiinflamatory drugs, local injections, thermotherapy and laser therapy are dicussed. Surgical techniques are described both for Achilles and Patellar tendinitis. Roentgenographic diagnosis of status and progression of the tendinopathy is stressed as a very valuable accessory tool. Lesion similarities between Achilles and patellar tendons are noted.

INTRODUCTION

Tendinitis is a primary inflammation of the tendon with a secondary involvement of the peritendon. It is due to a devitalization and disruption of tendon fascicles pursuing repetitive microtrauma by overuse of the tendon, accompanied by an inflammation of the peritendon (peritendinitis).[2] It is well known[1,2,7,8] that the tensile load required for the proper dynamic use of the tendon added to the gravitational elongation creates microtears of tendon fascicles and a secondary inflammatory reaction that, upon continuing dancing, produces an overload irnmature scar, thus worsening the lesion. Repeated microtrauma causes local inflammatory degeneration with central necrosis that may lead to rupture.[1,2,7]

ACHILLES TENDINITIS

The Achilles tendon is for the dancer the most vulnerable part of the body. The Achilles gets involved in classical ballet because the dancer spends most of his/her time in the demie-pointe position or relevé, which is on the metatarsal heads, whereas the Achilles tendon is tightened or stretched on plié (dorsiflexed ankle).

Almost every classical ballet movement begins in demi-plié. Upon demi-plié depends the ability to jump or land steadily. Demi-plié ensures that the Achilles tendon is supple, pliant and in working order. There are some factors that, when existing in the ballet dancer, may facilitate the Achilles tendinitis to appear. These are: Tight heel cord, valgus heel, and pronated feet.

The above conditions, compounded by a poor gastrocnemius-soleus flexibility and an improper exercise routine with unscheduled periods of rest (90% of dancers, mostly those belonging to "corps de ballet") and shoe wear may alter the physiologic requirements of the working strength of the Achilles tendon developing an overuse tendinitis. Dancing surface also plays an important role. In a previous paper, Achilles tendinitis started when dancing on wood surfaces in 4 %, on linoleum in 23 %, and on cement in 45 %.[3] This means that the shock-absorbing quality of the dancing floor is of great importance. The harder and stiffer the floor, the easier for Achilles tendinitis to develop. Dancers accustomed to dance on a certain surface may get injured when dancing on a different one, as usually happens when on tour or as a visiting dancer.

PATELLAR TENDINITIS

The Patellar tendon is also exerted in many ballet positions that require hyperextemsion of the knee. The that the laxity required for a good leg figure irnplies hyperextension of the standing knee in most "en-pointe" positions, such as in an arabesque (Figure 1) or attitude; hyperextension of the moving knee, such as in a pirouette en dehors à la seconde; or hyperextension in both moving knees in the entrechat. Hyperextension is also required to enhance support in males dancers preparing to lift their partner. All these positions require a tight knee hyperextension that, in: relation to the commonly seen patella alta, gives repetitive abnormal movements at tendon level which, if not properly controlled, can generate tendinitis.

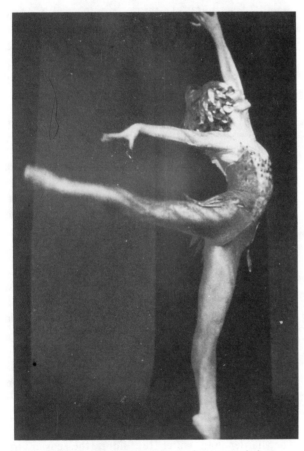

Figure 1: Stravinski's Firebird. Note the hyperextended position of the knee.

There are two different causes of this abnormal stress on the patellar tendon: 1) in cases of hyperextension, repetitive continuous traction is exerted on the tendon fibers, especially proximally at the distal pole of the patella (where an osteophyte appears in chronic cases); 2) in dancers lacking spring movement, this traction is exerted abruptly and can affect the entire length of the tendon, sometimes even acutely avulsing its distal insertion from the tuberositas tibialis.

SYMPTOMS AND DIAGNOSIS

In both cases of tendinitis, the symptoms are those of any inflammatory process: swelling, tenderness, pain, induration, with occasional presence of nodules and crepitus.[1,2,5,7] These symptoms appear in sequence, depending on the stage of the disease when the patient is seen. In the Achilles tendinitis, these may appear at the muscle-tendon joint, at the body of the tendon (the most frequent site due to characteristic anatomic features), or at the insertion of the tendon on the calcaneus, with different sites for symptoms depending on the localization.[2,5] In the Patellar tendon, the pathology can be located on insertion on lower pole of patella (the most common), along the tendon or at its insertion on the tibia.

In some cases, a roentgenogram of the ankle can help evaluate the intensity of the affection, as well as monitor progress of the tendinitis. If a lateral soft roentgenogram is taken of the affected ankle an alteration of the triangular shadow between the posterior surface of the tibia and the deep aspect of the Achilles tendon can be seen (Figure 2). These roentgenographic signs have not been found at the knee, where only a calcification or a spike osteophyte at the lower pole of patella can be seen. At this level, xerographies are usually more helpful.

CLASSIFICATION

It is important to treat any type of tendinitis as soon as it appears in order to diminish the time the dancer is off dancing. Also, as the tendinitis gets worse, the treatment takes longer to be effective.

Based on these facts, the authors propose a new four-phase classification for Achilles and patellar tendinitis, based on the presence of pain during dancing[3]:

- *Phase I:* pain only after dancing;
- *Phase II:* pain upon starting dancing that decreases once warmed up, only to reappear after dancing;
- *Phase III:* pain during and after dancing; and
- *Phase IV:* when rupture occurs.

Regarding duration of symptoms, Achilles or

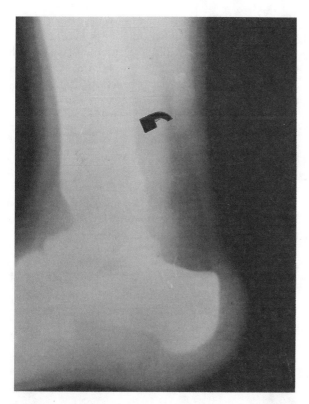

Figure 2: Lateral x-ray of an ankle with Achilles tendinitis. Note the soft-tissue swelling indicated by the arrow.

patellar tendinitis classically follow a three-stage classification:

- *Acute:* less than three weeks duration;
- *Subacute:* less than six months duration; and
- *Chronic:* more than six months duration.

If not properly treated by trained and health professionals, the symptoms and phases progress from bad to worse. In professional dancers, most tendinitis are "worked through" on their own, with different methods of self-care and treatment. This condition is so common that almost every dancer has it at one time or another and only when the condition becomes persistent will the dancer see the physician. If the tendinitis is treated in stage acute and phase I the results are much better with a shorter treatment time than in a chronic phase III.

OCCURRENCE PER DANCE LEVEL

In classical ballet there are three stages or categories of dancers. The Soloist or principal, being the star, has a more elaborate routine and steps and is the most demanding role. Coryphee is the dancer

that acts in small groups and is a future star. The Corps de ballet are those who make the accompaniment and dance in large groups.

Taking into consideration the total numbers of dancers studied by the authors, the corps de ballet dancers presented with the most injuries (56.6%). In the group of the front-line dancers and soloists, two out of three coryphees and two out of seven soloists had some type of tendinitis (Achilles more frequent in females, and patellar more frequent in males).

TREATMENT

Achilles Tendinitis

The treatment of Achilles tendinitis in ballet dancers is similar to that in other types of athletes with some specific differences related to the proper art of dancing. A ballet dancer can not be kept from dancing for a long period, because he or she not only gets out of training but looses flexibility and ability to continue in the same dancing level.

Treatment consists mainly of rest and activity modification. Practices are reduced in intensity and duration. Local measures required are, hot and cold contrast baths, nonsteroidal antiinflamatory drugs, and specific adhesive bandages that diminish some of the tension forces on the tendon. Cortisone injections must be used very seldom and carefully due to the possibility of producing a more dangerous lesion with weakness and rupture; should be used only as a last recourse and with a period of rest after the injection. In this point, the opinions of different authors differ, but there is no doubt that if properly indicated and used this type of injections have its place in treatment of tendinitis if used only once or twice with an interval of two to three weeks and only in acute cases, in which the dancer is required to perform by necessity. Shortwave laser beams are used not only as an antiinflamatory but also as a mean of improving cell metabolism as well. The use of a laser beam in medicine was introduce in the 60s, with Maiman,[4] who obtained the "light amplification by stimulated emission of radiation" but it is not until 1965 that a proper and useful adaption of the laser to medicine was done. The low-intensity laser beam obtains a normalization of the bioenergetics condition of the body, accelerates the metabolic processes, thus generating fine changes of function without causing major organic damages. The medical laser beam emits a radiation intensity that does not permit a destructive caloric effect. Thus, its therapeutic effect is not based as much on its thermal effect - practically minimal in relation to other sort of electrothermotherapy and with a typical local antiinflamatory action- but on its deep biostimulant effect.[1,7] In our center, a dosage of 4 - 6 watts and 6 and 10 Joules in ten sessions, is used. In our hands this method of treatment gives better results in chronic cases with fifteen sessions in four different areas of the tendon.

A heel rise in an ordinary street shoes to release the tendon during walking and a correct controlled stretching program increase range are most useful.

Very few cases do not subside with this treatment and will require surgery. An exploration of the diseased tendon may be performed, the degenerated fibers are resected together with any necrotic tissue and the tendon is reinforced with sutures. When necessary a bony prominence from the calcaneous, such as in Haglund's deformity is excised. Surgical treatment should be left as the final and last recourse, the excision of affected tissue taken to a minimum and when a large defect is to be removed a graft or other type of plastic reconstruction should be performed, having in mind in these cases that the future career of the dancer can be jeopardized.

Most important are the exercises during the recovery phase, these being gastrocnemius-soleus stretching:

a.   leaning against the wall with knees fully straightened and the feet separated from the wall 40 cm, and then obtaining 30-45 of ankle dorsiflexion, trying not to raise the heels; or

b.   standing on the forefoot on a step of a shir with the heel out, making a toe raise and a heel drop.

After every session, ice must be applied to decrease any inflammation that may have arisen.

The patient may return to dance only when pain on palpation and tenderness have subsided. The return to dance must start progressively with classes and avoid any abrupt movement.

Patellar tendinitis

All of the has its place in the treatment of patellar tendinitis as well.

Since the dancer should be kept off dancing for the shortest period possible, the authors have developed a conservative treatment that has yielded very good results. The patient is treated for four weeks with daily sessions of cryotheraphy for 12 minutes followed immediately by ultrasound for 10 minutes and refrain from dancing, *not* using any type

of bandage. With this treatment we have been able to treat 50 cases of patellar tendinitis - of them 16 recurrences treated by different methods - with only 4 surgeries required due to failure. Once the symptoms subside, the patient restarts training using adhesive strapping to lessen traction forces on the tendon until s/he is fully fit again (Figure 3).

In order to localize the actual spot affected in the tendon, the dancer is asked to perform a jump, then point out the tender spot. At that site, a local injection of 1 c.c. of anaesthetic is given and the jump repeated. If pain is not present in the second jump, this would be the site to treat. This method helps focusing the treatment, especially when it involves an injection.

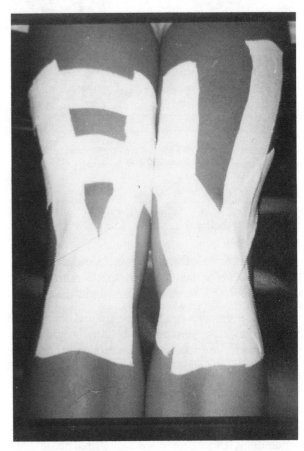

Figure 3: *Protective adhesive bandages for patellar tendinitis.*

If surgery is required and the lesion is in the length of the tendon we use the procedure described by Thomasen from Denmark. Under local anaesthesia a transverse incision is made over the tendon, this is exposed and split longitudinally and the degenerated tissue found within the tendon excised, and the tendon reinforced.

If the lesion is in the insertion of the tendon on the lower pole of patella then an extended procedure is required with resection of the apex of the patella and performing longitudinal scarifications on the Sharpey fibers of the anterior aspect of the patella continuing distally in longitudinal parallel superficial cuts in the tendon in order to produce strong scar tissue, reinforcing the area.

DISCUSSION

Several studies performed on the Achilles tendon demonstrated that the weakest part of the tendon corresponds to the lower middle third, this being due to its special vascularization, which presents a relatively avascular zone of 2 to 6 cm from its insertion.[4,7,8] This corresponds to the most frequent clinical site of Achilles tendinitis, as per the authors' experience and others.[2,3,5]

The lesions found in the tendons showed tendinitis with or without associated pathologies such as peritendinitis; and were histologically similar in both the Achilles and patellar tendons.

Achilles tendinitis is the most frequent lesion in ballet dancers appearing in 30.9 % of dancers, and it is caused hy repetitive microtrauma and overuse. There are some important predisposing factors such as improper muscle flexibility, improper exercise routine and excessive work. Dancing surface also plays an important part in the development of this pathology (45% of cases developed while dancing on hard surfaces). The appearance of Achilles tendinitis is not influenced by the dancer's level but by an improper dance technique. The best results are obtained with correct treatment in acute cases. The more long standing the symptoms, the more difficult to obtain an excellent result. Laser short wave is very useful in recovery of chronic cases. Surgery may relieve the symptoms. It unfortunately means quite often that the dancer will have to abandon active dancing.

Patellar tendinitis a little less frequent (23%), and is also an overuse lesion produced by the repetitive

traction on the tendon fibers that happens during the characteristic "hyperextended" knee position so often required in ballet, aggravated by jumping or landing without a proper spring movement. It is seen most often in male dancers. Improper muscular training or flexibility, change of choreography or intensive training and performance and above all fatigue inducing loss of control during movements are aggravating conditions.

Symptoms should be treated as soon as possible before a chronic condition develops. The conservative treatment used by the authors, of alternative cryotherapy and ultrasound has given promising results. As with Achilles tendinitis, surgery should be left as a last recourse, because very often implies the impossibility of returning to same dancing level.

REFERENCES

1. Camara Anguita, R., Guillen Garcia, P., Galves Failde, J.M., Valls Cabrera, M. and Miranda Mayordomo, M.: Rodilla del Salhdor. Tratamiento rehabilihdor. Rehabilitacion 19 (3): 341, 1985.
2. Clement, D.B., Taunton, J.E. and Smart, G.W.: Achilles tendinitis and peritendinitis: Etiology and treatment. Am. J. Sports Medicine. 12 (3): 179, 1984.
3. Fernandez-Palazzi, F., Rivas, S. Achilles Tendinitis in ballet dancers. Clin. Orthop. and Relat. Res. 257: 257, 1990.
4. Gonzalez Ittirre, J.J. and Severio, F.: El Laser en el deporte. Rehabilitacion. 19 (3): 365, 1985
5. Hashd, K.,Larson, LG.and Lindholm, A.: Clearance of radiosodium after local deposit in the Achilles tendon. Ach Chir. Scand. 116 :251, 1959.
6. Hamilton, W. Personal communication, 1981.
7. Krahl, H.: Jumper's knee - atiologie, diferentialdiagnose und therapeutische Moglickeiten. Orthopade 9: 193, 1980.
8. Langergen, C.and Lindholm, A.: Vascular distribution in the Achilles tendon- an angiographic and microangiographic study. Ach Chir Scand 116: 491, 1959.

CHAPTER 53

Soft Tissue Lesions of the Foot and Ankle: Evaluation and Treatment

Russell Woodman

INTRODUCTION

Soft tissue lesions are frequently treated by the physical therapist. Two major problems in treating these types of lesions are identifying the tissue causing the pain and selecting the appropriate modality to diminish the pain. In recent years, physicians and physical therapists have become increasingly interested in the evaluation and treatment methods of soft tissue lesions developed by the late Dr. James Cyriax. His method employs a systematic approach for identifying the exact location of the soft tissue lesion. His non-surgical treatment options include manipulation, deep friction massage, orthotics, exercise, patient education, and the injection of various drugs. If these methods fail, then surgery is considered. The purpose of this chapter is to introduce the clinician to the Cyriax approach to the examination and treatment of soft tissue lesions at the ankle and foot. This approach is particularly applicable for injuries which occur in industry, sports, and dancing.

HISTORY and INSPECTION

The examination procedure starts with a careful patient history, inspecting the patient's posture, testing selective tissue tension, and palpating the suspect area. Diagnostic tests such as the local injection of an anesthetic, taking x-rays, and performing other sophisticated procedures can also be employed.

History

The examiner asks as many questions as deemed necessary regarding the patient's symptoms, including what may have initially caused the symptoms and what, at the present time, alters the symptoms. A knowledge of how tissues refer pain and parasthesias is important; the clinician must keep in mind that a lesion of the low back, hip, and knee can refer symptoms to the lower leg.[1] As the dancer describes those activities which increase the lower leg, ankle or foot pain, the examiner begins to develop an idea of where the problem may lie drawing on their knowledge of applied anatomy as well as dance. Specific examples will be cited under the heading of differential diagnosis.

Inspection

This includes noting any abnormalities in superficial tissue such as bruising, swelling or callousing, as well as gait and postural analysis. Ballet dancers who wear tightly fitting shoes often develop skin lesions and hyperkeratoses at the medial aspect of the first metatarsal head, fifth metatarsal head, interphalangeal joints and adjacent to the toenails.[2] Dancers with acutely painful ankle disorders will exhibit an antalgic gait; typically, one in which heel-strike or push off are diminished. This results in a shortened swing phase which becomes more obvious as the pace is increased. Gait and postural analysis may also reveal a supinated or pronated ankle. The methodology for identifying these abnormalities is not within the scope of this paper. Examples of the types of soft tissue lesions these abnormalities can lead to are listed under the differential diagnosis section.

PHYSICAL EXAMINATION

Selective tissue tension testing is the foundation of Cyriax's physical examination. This form of testing aids in identifying the tissue or joint responsible for the patient's complaints. It is imperative that the patient understands that the examiner needs clear answers to which movements alter the symptoms as described in the historical portion of the examination. Negative findings are as important as positive ones since they also help to clarify the diagnosis. Active, passive, and mid-range isometric muscle testing are used to examine each anatomical region. Active movement is used as a functional test for mobility and symptom reproduction. At the ankle, standing active plantarflexion is used as a resistive test. Passive range of motion testing is used to test the state of non-contractile tissue. This test determines if the movement causes the patient's pain, if the joint has normal range of motion, and if the joint has a normal end feel. Seven different end feels are possible:

1. A bone to bone end feel is the normal end feel for elbow extension and various other motions. It can also occur in a joint that has ankylosed or that has a mal-united fracture.

2. Tissue approximation occurs on passive plantarflexion as the heel engages the tendon Achilles against the distal tibia. This end feel can also be felt on such movements as elbow and knee flexion.

3. Capsular end feel is elicited at a synovial joint as the slack is taken up in the joint's capsule. This is the normal end feel at the talocalcaneal, mid-tarsal joints and first metatarsophalangeal joint.

4. A springy end feel occurs at the talocalcaneal joint when a fragment of cartilage (loose body) is compressed between the two bony surfaces.

5. Spasm is a protective mechanism. When a joint is in acute arthritis or when a fracture is present, the muscles around the joint will contract to prevent further motion and more pain.

6. An empty end feel indicates that a very painful pathology, such as a fracture, is present. Like spasm, it is elicited by pain and is a protective mechanism. As the examiner starts to reach the anticipated normal end feel, the patient either pushes the examiner away or warns the examiner not to go any further due to increased pain. The examiner perceives no tissue tension, he is simply not allowed by the patient to move the limb any further.

7. Neurogenic hypertonus indicates psychological involvement. The examiner initially perceives a strong resistance to movement caused by muscle contraction. As the examiner applies sustained pressure, the muscle relaxes and discloses full joint range of motion. Resistive isometric muscle testing with the joint held at mid-range assesses the state of the contractile tissue, innervation, and bony attachments.

The response to muscle testing will fall into one of the following categories:

1. A strong and painless response is normal.
2. A strong and painful response is indicative of a minor lesion, such as tendinitis or muscle strain.
3. A weak and painful response reflects severe tendinitis, muscle strain, fracture at the muscle's bony attachment, or serious disease.

4. A weak and painless response is a sign of a neurological deficit or a total breach in a muscle.

5. Pain due to repetitions of muscle testing suggests a minor tendinitis, a muscle strain or an irritation of a bursa.

When examining the dancer, it may be necessary to ask him/her to perform repetitive muscle testing in order to bring on the pain.[3] Table 1 lists from proximal to distal, the passive and resistive movements in the Cyriax examination of the dancer's ankle and foot.

Table 1: *Cyriax Evaluation of the Dancer's Ankle and Foot.*

Movement	Tissue Tested
Passive dorsiflexion	Capsule and articular surface of ankle joint
Passive plantar flexion	Capsule and articular surface of ankle joint
Resistive dorsiflexion	Dorsiflexor muscle group
Resisitive plantarflexion	Plantarflexor muscle group
Passive varus	Capsule of talocalcanean joint and middle fasciculus of lateral ligament
Passive Valgus	Capsule of talocalcanean joint
Sprung mortice test	Inferior tibiofibular ligaments
Passive inversion combined with plantarflexion	Anterior fasciculus of lateral ligament
Passive eversion combined with plantarflexion	Deltoid ligament and posterior fasciculus of lateral ligament
Passive adduction of sub-talar joint	Subtalar joint capsule Middle fasciculus of lateral ligament
Passive abduction of subtalar joint	Subtalar joint capsule
Passive dorsiflexion of midtarsal joint	Midtarsal capsule and ligaments
Passive plantarflexion of midtarsal joint	Midtarsal capsule and ligaments Tibiotalar ligament
Passive abduction of midtarsal joint	Midtarsal capsule and ligaments calcaneocuboid ligament
Passive adduction of midtarsal joint	Midtarsal capsule and ligaments
Passive lateral rotation of midtarsal joint	Midtarsal capsule and ligaments
Passive medial rotation of midtarsal joint	Midtarsal capsule and ligaments
Passive extension of first metatarso-phalangeal joint	First metatarso-phalangeal joint capsule
Passive flexion of first metatarso-phalangeal joint	First metatarso-phalangeal joint capsule
Resistive flexion of first metatarso-phalangeal joint	Flexor Hallicus Longus

DIFFERENTIAL DIAGNOSIS

Anterior Leg

a- Anterior Compartment Syndrome: The patient complains that she loses the ability to dorsiflex the ankle following periods of lower extremity exertion. This condition is caused by an abnormally tight fascia in the anterior compartment of the lower leg which is compartment become engorged with blood during activity. Consequently, the engorged muscles occlude the lumen of the anterior tibial artery, temporarily paralyzing the dorsiflexors.[4] This condition requires a surgical fasciotomy.

b- *Myosynovitis of the Tibialis Anterior*: The dancer complains of pain over the anterior aspect of the ankle joint which can be increased by isometric dorsiflexion. The muscle has become irritated by tying ballet shoes too tightly.

c- *Sprained Anterior Tibiotalar Ligament*: "Over pointe" sprains the ligament. Passive plantarflexion is full but painful. The ligament is palpated by pushing the tendons of the anterior compartment aside. In this case, deep friction massage is curative. If the dancer rolls over the anterior aspect of the ankle and foot, the joint capsule can be partly ruptured or the toe extensors can become inflamed. Treatment consists of resting, icing, and elevating the ankle as well as teaching the dancer a more stable point stance.

d- *Anterior Periostitis*: The ballet dancer lands flat on her foot feeling immediate pain at the front of the ankle. Passive dorsiflexion is full but painful. A steroid injection is curative. A small heel lift on the ballet shoe will prevent recurrence.[5]

Posterior Leg:

a- *Partial Rupture of the Gastrocnemius*: The lesion is most frequently in the medial head of the muscle. It is sometimes seen in tap dancers or those engaged in vigorous ankle plantarflexion. The patient experiences immediate calf pain and is unable to painlessly push off when walking. During the acute stage, treatment consists of daily deep friction massage (Fig. 1), electrical stimulation and a heel lift to ease the stress on the muscle during ambulation.[6]

b- *Tendinitis of the Tendo Achilles*: Overuse of the gastrocnemius, such as in ballet or aerobic dancing, can cause a tendinitis. This condition is particularly prevelant in individuals with excessive pronation due to a forefoot varus deformity.[7,8] Repetitive standing plantarflexion brings on the pain. Treatment consists of deep friction massage (Fig.2), stretching and eccentric exercises as suggested by Stanish.[9] An aerobic dancer may benefit from an orthotic device.[10]

c- *Flexor Hallucis Longus Tendinitis*: This muscle's tendon is inflamed by pointe dance activity. The symptoms are pain on muscle testing and crepitus. Treatment includes the prescription of oral anti-inflammatory drugs, rest, and ice.[11]

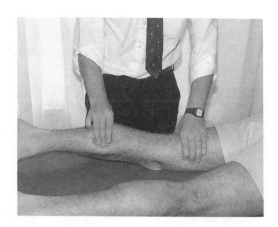

Figure 1: Deep Friction Massage to the Medial Belly of the Gastrocnemius: Horizontal to and fro motion.

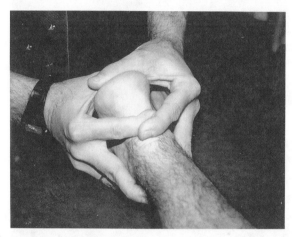

Figure 2: Deep Friction Massage of the Distal Fibers of the Tendo Achilles, by alternate shoulder abduction-adduction.

d- *Traumatic Periostitis of the Lower Tibia (Dancer's Heel)*: The distal tibia can be bruised by the the upper edge of the posterior surface of the calcaneus during pointe. The pain is felt at the back of the heel and is reproduced by passive plantarflexion. Treatment consists of injecting a steroid and educating the dancer as to the mechanism of the injure. Repetitive over-pointing must be avoided.[12]

Lateral Leg

a- *Lateral Ankle Sprain*: Ballroom dancers who wear spike heels and ballerinas may sprain the anterior or middle fasciculus of the lateral collateral ligament or the calcaneocuboid ligament.[13] Sometimes the peroneal muscle is overstretched. Treatment during the acute phase consists of rest, ice, compression, elevation and daily deep friction massage. Rarely are these patients subjected to plaster of paris casting. If so, they will need more extensive physical therapy, consisting of therapeutic exercise to increase muscle and joint function. If adhesions form, deep friction massage and manipulation are curative (Fig. 3 and 4).

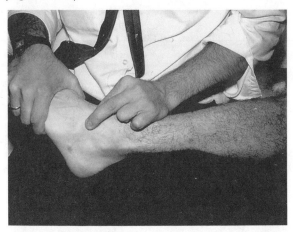

Figure 3: *DFM of Anterior Fasciculus of the Lateral Collateral Ligament (ankle in dorsiflexion/inversion).*

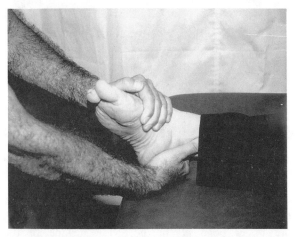

Figure 4: *Manipulation for Anterior Fasciculus Adhesion (ankle plantarflexed, hindfoot in varus, forefoot inverted).*

b- Peroneal Tenosynoviitis: Shin splints is the general name given to lower leg pain.[14] It does not, however, name the specific tissue at fault. One cause of shin splints is peroneal tendinitis. It is an overuse phenomenon. Isometric eversion is strong but painful. This lesion responds well to deep friction massage (Fig.5).

Medial Leg

According to Schafle, forcing turnout is the most common technical error made by ballet dancers.[15] This motion causes pronation and a myriad of overuse syndromes. Forcing turnout occurs when one places

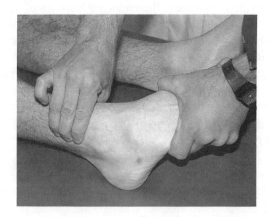

Figure 5: *DFM of the Proximal Fibers of the Peroneals, ankle maintained in inversion.*

the foot in an abducted position beyond that which can occur at the hip joint. One possible cause of forced turn out is inadequate flexibility of the hip joint capsule, and/or the iliacus and psoas muscles.[16] Forced turnout subjects the tissues on the medial side of the ankle and forefoot to abnormal stress leading to problems such as tibialis posterior tenosynovitis and a sprained deltoid ligament:

a- Tibialis Posterior Tenosynovitis: Tenosynovitis of the tibialis posterior is another cause of shin splints. Isometric inversion combined with plantarflexion is strong but painful. Tenosynovitis of the leg must be differentiated from a stress fracture of the tibia. If finger tapping the tibial crest is more painful than isometric muscle testing then a stress fracture should be suspected. Tibialis posterior tenosynovitis responds well to deep friction massage.[17] If physical examination reveals excessive pronation, an orthotic device can be placed in the patient's walking shoes.

b- Sprained Deltoid Ligament: The deltoid ligament is sometimes sprained by sudden excessive turnout, but the onset is usually gradual. It typically occurs in an aerobic dancer who has excessive pronation. Treatment consists of a local steroid injection and an orthotic device to control pronation.

Foot

a- Plantar Fasciitis: The most characteristic symptom of plantar fasciitis is severe pain at the heel on getting up to walk after sitting. Activities such as prolonged walking and aerobic dancing are also painful. Examination is negative except for tenderness at the medial plantar surface of the heel, and in some cases, postural examination reveals excessive pronation. In these situations, the appropriate orthotic is indicated[18]; otherwise a heel lift thick enough to relieve the pain is added to the shoes. If these measures do not provide total relief then a localized corticosteroid injection is indicated.

b- Hallux Abductus: When performing pointe, dancers may pronate the foot to obtain greater stability. This allows the forefoot to evert and greater stress is placed on the medial aspect of the first metatarsal head and hallux. Interdigital spacers of lambswool, felt or foam can be used to decrease the tendency of hallux malalignment. The dancer may need stretching exercises to improve hip external rotation and to prevent the damaging effects of incorrect turnout.

c- Traumatic Arthritis of the First Metatarso-phalangeal Joint: Ballet dancing places tremendous stress on the great toe. Clinical signs of first metatarsophalangeal arthritis are pain on weight bearing, painful limitation of passive toe extension, and full flexion with slight discomfort. Treatment consists of joint mobilization exercises and traction to increase range and decrease pain.

DEEP FRICTION MASSAGE (DFM)

The purpose of this section is to briefly explain the theoretical rationale for DFM and its clinical application (Table 2). The four major uses of DFM are in the treatment of tendinitis, tenosynovitis, strained muscle belly and sprained ligament. Minor breaches in tendon can heal by scarring. When the muscle contracts an inflammatory process (tendinitis) is created at the junction between normal tendon and the scar. The DFM breaks up or softens the scar allowing for equal stress along the tendon during muscle contraction. In tendons with a synovial sheath, breaking up or softening the scar eliminates it as a source of irritation to the inner lining of the synovial sheath. Tendinous lesions usually require rest and 6-12 twenty minute sessions of DFM performed every other day. while tendinitis causes symptoms after scarring occurs, muscle strains and ligamentous lesions cause immediate pain. Therefore, the patient may be seen within a couple of days of the injury to prevent painful adhesions or a few weeks later when an adhesion has occurred.

a- Recent Muscle Strain: Daily treatment consists of five minutes of DFM and electrical stimulation to prevent adhesions.

b- Muscle Belly Adhesion: If proper initial care is not administered, painful adhesions can develop in a muscle belly requiring rest and 6-12 20min. sessions.

c- Recent Ligamentous Sprain: Passive or active joint movements work in conjunction with DFM to prevent adhesions at the site of ligamentous sprains.

d- Ligamentous Adhesion: Sprained ankles are still occasionally treated by immobilization. This is unfortunate because painful adhesions are likely to occur. Fortunately, they respond well to one or two twenty minute sessions of DFM and manipulation to break the adhesions.

Table I: *The Eight Rules of Deep Friction Massage*

1. Diagnostic movements and palpation must single out the tissue at fault and the exact spot on that tissue.

2. The physical therapist's fingers and patient's skin must move simultaneously to avoid injury to the skin.

3. The friction must be given perpendicular to the tendon's fiber to smooth it down.

4. The friction must be given with sufficient sweep to assure that the whole scar is treated.

5. The friction must be given deeply. It must be administered within the patient's pain tolerance. The pain will gradually diminish during the massage.

6. If the lesion lies in the belly of the muscle, the muscle must be put on slack. This will aid in the separation of the muscle fibers during the massage.

7. The patient must adopt a posture which will adequately expose the tissue.

8. Tendons with a sheath must be put on stretch to assure maximum success of the massage.

REFERENCES

1. Cyriax J: Textbook of Orthopaedic Medicine Vol. 1 (8th ed.). London, Bailliere Tindall, 1982, pp. 22-42.

2. Kravitz, SR: Dance medicine. Clin Podiatry 1(2):417-430,1984.

3. Cyriax J: Textbook Of Orthopaedic Medicine Volume One ed. 8. London, Bailliere Tindall, 1982, pp. 43-69.

4. Horn, CE: Acute ischemia of anterior tibial muscle. J.Bone Joint Surg. 27: 615-617, 1945.

5. Cyriax J: Textbook Of Orthopaedic Medicine Vol. 1(8th ed.). London, Bailliere Tindall, 1982, p. 427.

6. Cyriax J: Textbook Of Orthopaedic Medicine Vol. 1(8th ed.). London, Bailliere Tindall, 1982, p. 418.

7. Rivas, S. Achilles tendinitis in ballet dancers. Clin Orthop. 257: 257261, 1990

8. Clement DB, et al: Achilles tendinitis and peritendonitis: etiology and treatment. Journal of Orthopaedic medicine. 12: 45-49, 1990.

9. Stanish, WD, et al: Eccentric exercise in chronic tendinitis. Clinical Orthopaedics and Related Research. 208: 65-68, 1986.

10. Riddle, DL, Freeman, DB: Management of a patient with the diagnosis of bilateral fasciitis and achilles tendinitis. Phys. Ther.68(12):1913-16 1988.

11. Bachrach, RM: Team physician #3. The relationship of low back/pelvic somatic dysfunction to dance injuries. Orthop Rev. 17(10): 1037-1043, 1988.

12. Cyriax J: Textbook of Orthopaedic Medicine, Vol. 1(8th ed.). London, Bailliere Tindall, 1982, p. 435.

13. Quirk, R: Ballet injuries. the Australian experience. Clin Sports Med. 2(3): 507-514, 1983.

14. Gans, A: The relationship of heel contact in ascent and descent from jumps to the incidence of shin splints in ballet dancers. Phys. Ther. 65(8): 1192-1196, 1985.

15. Schafle, M: The child dancer. Medical considerations. Pediatr Clin North Am. 37 (5): 1211-1221, 1990.

16. Reid, D: Prevention of hip and knee injuries in ballet dancers. Sports Med. 6 (5) : 295-307, 1988.

17. Woodman, RX, Pare L: Evaluation and treatment of soft tissue lesions of the ankle and forefoot using the Cyriax approach. Phys. Ther. 62 (8): 1144-1147, 1982.

18. Riddle DL, Freeman, DB: Management of a patient with a diagnosis of bilateral plantar fasciitis and achilles tendinitis. Phys. Ther. 68(12): 1913-1916, 1988.

ACKNOWLEDGEMENT

Special thanks for the professional assistance of Miss Judy and her dance students of Wallingford, Connecticut in the publication of this chapter.

CHAPTER 54

Retrocalcaneal Bursitis in Ballet Dancers: Sonographic Diagnosis and Treatment

Anders Wykman

BACKGROUND

Irritation at the posterosuperior aspect of the heel is common in ballet dancers of both sexes. The symptoms may have various causes and have been variously referred to in the literature.[1] Two bursal structures can anatomically be distinguished at the insertion of the Achilles tendon, the superficial subcutaneous, and the deep subfascial bursa. An inflamed superficial bursa is palpable at the tendon insertion, directly over the Tuber calcanei. This condition is supposedly related to mechanical causes; that is, friction between the shoe and the posterosuperior aspect of the calcaneus.

If the deep subfascial, retrocalcaneal bursa is inflamed, tenderness is less well located, but is usually palpable anterior to the tendon. It presents as posterior pain when the Achilles tendon rolls over the Tuber calcanei, as in the grand plié.

Treatment begins with rest, physiotherapy, and/or nonsteroidal anti-inflammatory drugs (NSAIDs). If this proves ineffective, instillation of steroids into the bursa often provides relief. The retrocalcaneal bursa, however, is a dangerous place to inject steroids, as it can weaken the Achilles insertion.[2] If injected into tendons, steroids may cause tendon ruptures.

Sonography has previously been used to diagnose pathology of the Achilles tendon in runners. Maffulli et al. could distinguish between paratendinitis, tendinitis, and enthesopathy.[3]

METHODS

Acuson 128, an ultrasound equipment with a linear transducer 5.0 MHz, was used to diagnose retrocalcanear bursitis in 6 male and 3 female professional ballet dancers, mean age 24 years. The dancers were members of the Royal Swedish Ballet in Stockholm.

RESULTS

In all cases, an enlarged, fluid-filled cyst was identified between the posterosuperior part of the calcaneus and the Achilles tendon. The patients were treated by heel elevation, NSAIDs, and physiotherapy including stretching, eccentric exercises and coordination training. Four dancers healed ,in 2-4 weeks and they returned to full activity. In 5 dancers, 4 male and 1 female, there was no improvement with conservative treatment alone. In these cases, sonography revealed a still enlarged and fluid-filled retrocalcanear bursa. Under sonographic guidance, a cannula of 0.8 mm diameter was introduced percutaneously into the bursa. The aperture of the cannula was easily identified by sonography. The thick, semi-fluid content of the bursa was aspirated, and through the same cannula 0.1-0.3 ml of Depomedrone (Methylprednisolon Acetate) was instilled. Following a few days' rest, the patients began training. All 5 dancers returned to full-time dancing activity within 14 days.

CONCLUSION

Sonography is an easy, non-invasive method of diagnosing retrocalcanear bursitis. Steroids have proven to be effective in the treatment of this condition. Steroids may cause considerable damage, however, when deposed close to, or into, tendons. To ensure an optimal and safe instillation of steroids, sonography has been used to identify the injection cannula.

REFERENCES

1. Martin BF: Posterior triangle.   J Foot Surg 28(4):312-317, 1989.
2. Hamilton WG: Foot and ankle in dancers. Clin Sports Med 7(1):143-173, 1988.
3. Maffulli et al: Ultrasound diagnosis of Achilles tendon pathology in runners. Brit J Sports Med 21(4):158-162, 1987.

CHAPTER 55

Postural Stability in Classical Ballet Dancers

Johan Leanderson • *Anders Wykman* • *Charlotte Nilsson*

INTRODUCTION

A classical ballet dancer is a combined artist and high-performance athlete.[1-3] Previous studies have shown that the foot-and-ankle region is the most frequent location of injury in many sport activities as well as in classical ballet.[4-7] A sprained ankle is the most common traumatic injury. Many individuals (18-48%) develop late symptoms after such an injury.[8, 9] The symptoms are either a subjective feeling of instability or repeated sprains, i.e. functional instability. Such instability may be caused by mechanical instability, peroneal muscle weakness, tibiofibular sprain, or a proprioceptional defect.[10, 11]

Postural stability requires adequate proprioception from the ankle joint. The purpose of this study was to register and analyze postural stability in a group of classical ballet dancers. The influence of an ankle joint injury on postural stability was also demonstrated.

SUBJECTS AND METHODS

Forty-nine dancers at the Royal Swedish Ballet, 25 female and 24 male, who had been dancing since they were 10 years old, participated in the investigation. Mean age was 26.2 years. Previous injuries to the lower extremity were registered. A control group of 23 normally active young men and women (ages 20-29) were also examined.

During the investigation, 3 dancers sustained an ankle sprain, which caused absence from classes and performances for at least one week. In these dancers, multiple recordings of postural stability were made during 12 weeks following the injury.

Stabilometry

The individual to be examined stood on a Statometer, which is a specially designed, portable, computer-assisted force platform. It gives continuous reading of the load. The signals are amplified, digitalized, and analyzed by a personal computer.

Recording

The recordings were made in a separate room. Subjects were asked to stand with one foot lifted and in contact with the standing leg. Arms were held to the chest and the subjects were asked to look at a spot on the wall four meters in front of them. After an adaption period of 30-60 seconds, recordings of 60 seconds were made for each foot.

Data Analysis

Variations in the electric potentials caused by the sway of the subject were transformed into the following variables: (1) mean sway amplitude in sagittal and lateral direction (mean sway) and (2) sway area. Student's T-test was used for statistical analysis.

RESULTS

The dancers demonstrated a smaller mean sway on the left foot than on the right foot ($p < 0.001$). Male dancers displayed a smaller sway area than female dancers ($p < 0.01$). These differences could not be seen in the control group. Mean sway and sway area did not differ significantly between dancers and controls.

Eight dancers had suffered from an ankle sprain during the year prior to this investigation. The injured dancers had impaired postural control compared to the non-injured dancers ($p < 0.01$).

Three dancers sustained an ankle sprain after our initial recordings. These dancers demonstrated impaired postural stability for several weeks, compared to the condition before the injury. During rehabilitation, postural stability gradually improved, and full-time dancing resumed. After 12 weeks, however, two of three dancers had not regained the Stabilometry result observed before the injury.

DISCUSSION

The present study could not demonstrate differences in postural stability between classical ballet dancers and a control group. When individuals within the group of dancers were compared, however, significant differences were noted concerning stability of the left and right feet. Also, sway area was greater for female than for male dancers.

Dancers usually rotate standing on the left foot. This could be a contributing factor to the differences between left- and right-foot stabilometry results.

The present investigation demonstrates that there is an impaired postural stability following ankle sprain. The authors have also shown that stability improves during rehabilitation. This study, however, is still inconclusive regarding whether postural instability leads to ankle sprain or vice-versa.

Considering the observations of improved postural stability in this group of dancers following active rehabilitation, the authors suggest that this analysis serve as an assessment tool following ankle joint injuries.

REFERENCES

1. Kirkendall D, Calabrese LH: Physiologic aspects of dance. Clin Sports Med 2:525, 1983.
2. Mickeli LJ, Gillespie WJ, Walafsek RA: Physiologic profiles of female professional ballerinas. Clin Sports Med 3:199, 1984.
3. Schantz P, Astrand PO: Physiologic characteristics of classical ballet. Med Sci Sports Exercise 5:472-476, 1984.
4. Bowling A: Injuries to dancers: Prevalence, treatment, and perceptions of causes. Br Med J 298:731-734, 1989.
5. Colliander E, Eriksson E: Injuries in Swedish elite basketball. Orthopaedics 9(2):225-227, 1986.
6. Hardaker WT, Margello S, Goldner JL: Foot and ankle injuries in theatrical dancers. Foot Ankle 6:59-69, 1985.
7. Teitz C: Sports medicine concerns in dance and gymnastics. Clin Sports Med 2:571, 1983.
8. Freeman MAR: Instability of the foot after injuries to the lateral ligament of the ankle. J Bone Joint Surg 47B:669-677, 1965.
9. Freeman MAR, Dean MRE, Hanham IWF: The etiology and prevention of functional instability of the foot. J Bone Joint Surg 47B:678-685, 1965.
10. Gauffin H, Tropp H, Odenrick P: Effect of ankle disc training on postural control in patients with functional instability of the ankle joint. Int J Sports Med 9:141-144, 1988.
11. Tropp H: Functional instability of the ankle joint, Thesis. University of Linkoping, Medical Dissertation, Linkoping, Sweden, 1985.

SUGGESTED READING

Wykman A, Goldie I: Postural stability after total hip replacement. Int Orthop 13:235-238, 1989.

CHAPTER 56

Study of the Nature and Characteristics of Dance Injuries

Tianxiang He • *Junzhi He* • *Lin Yang*

Abstract

Through direct observation and combining the characteristics of traditional Chinese medicine with the art of dance in the senior author's practice for several decades, the nature and characteristics of injuries caused by improper dance movements have been uncovered. Incidence of injuries is directly proportional to dance movements and length of dance education. In the five-year school system, the incidence of injuries is low at the two ends (among junior and senior students; high among intermediate students). Incidence is higher in boys and in lower limbs. Ankle-joint injuries make up the highest incidence (30%); waist the second highest (16.9%) and knee-joint the third (16.6%). Joints are the most often injured overall (61.83%), muscles and tendons are second (29.02%), and bone injuries third (9.5%). The measurements performed for correction and prevention not only help prevent the vicious cycle of training-injuring-treating-injuring, but also promote dance medicine as a field in its own right.

The main tool of dance performance is the human body, and it is rare that the body is naturally entirely fit for this task. In both training and performance, the skills of jumping, turning, looping, spinning, circling, bending, twisting, and leaning greatly influence the body's natural attitude and balance. Sometimes a new complex movement is repeated so many times that it causes stress beyond physical limitations; hence, the importance of using traditional Chinese medicine combined with the characteristics of dance training to improve teaching and skill and to prevent injuries.

MATERIALS

The authors have analyzed the nature and characteristics of dance injuries and established a scientific system of prevention and treatment based on 3,204 persons with dance injuries among students in all four grades, admitted from 1977 to 1985.

RESULTS

The usual characteristics of dance injuries were as follows:

1. *Low at both ends and high in the middle.* An example is the students admitted in 1980. The length of schooling for them was five years, which were divided into three main periods: elementary, middle, and senior. During the elementary period, which consisted of three semesters, the total number of injuries was 192.5 (27.4% of the total number of students); during the senior period, also three semesters, the number of injuries was 131.5 (18.7%); and during the middle period, which consisted of four semesters, the number of injuries reached 378 (53.9%). This was because at the elementary stage, students received training which involved mainly the primary movements, slow rhythms and little intensity, strength and speed, resulting in fewer injuries. At the senior level, students had more experience and were skilled in acrobatic gymnastics, thus reducing the possibility of injury. At the middle level, however, students were offered more varied and intensive training, but had failed to grasp the major points of skilled movements. As a result, they were injured more frequently and seriously.

2. Among those injured in training, *males were more often affected than females* (2,091 or 62.45% vs. 1,203 or 37.55%). This was because the amount of training for male students was usually much greater than for female students.

3. *The number of injuries was directly proportional to the age of the students.* For the students admitted in 1977, the average age was 13.6 years, each being injured 10.3 times per year; but the average age of students admitted in 1985 was 11.5 years, with each injured only 7.2 times per year.

4. *Occurrence of injuries was indirectly proportional to the duration of schooling.* If the school duration was short with extensive curricula and intensive training, there was an increased chance for the student to be injured. Indeed, among students

admitted in 1977 (three-year curriculum), 103 were injured, while among students admitted in 1985, only 7.2 were injured, probably because of the extension to a five-year school system.

5.   *There was a close association between dance injuries, training intensity, and level of artistry.*   By analyzing the education and training schedules, training intensity and levels of artistry, it was shown that the injured cases in the middle level of training gradually increased: e.g. the incidence in first-grade students was 33.3%, but in the fifth grade it rose to 77.8%; injuries due to jumping increased from 9.99% to 27.23%, its occurrence reaching as much as 56.36%.

6.   The rate of injuries of the lower extremities was much greater than of the upper. It was estimated that among students of the four grades, there were 3,204 persons injured,   covering 24 sites and areas. Among these cases, joint injuries were most frequent (61.83%); muscle injuries were second (29.02%); and bony injuries third (9.15%).   Among joint injuries, ankle injuries were first (30%); lumbar second (16.9%); knee third (16.6%); and toe fourth (5.2%).

7.   Because of the new theory and concept that prevention and protection of dance injuries should involve treatment of the body as a whole, injuries among students admitted in 1985 decreased by 31% in comparison with those among students admitted in 1977. The new therapy considers the vital energy, blood, and physique as a whole.   Treatment and dancing are integrated.   As a result, injuries among students admitted in 1985 decreased by 31% in comparison with students admitted in 1977.

DISCUSSION

The main points of this new concept are:

1.   Physicians should know the principles and the processes of dancing in order to determine the causes of injuries, make clinical diagnoses, and prevent the cycle of training-injury-treatment and retraining-reinjury-retreatment. On this basis, a cure is obtained more rapidly, the effects are much more satisfactory, and return to full function occurs more quickly.

2.   Based on physical characters such as little eruption of muscles and instability of joints in young students, the authors changed the previous method of dredging the stagnation of blood and regulating the flow of vital energy into a therapy that includes removal of blood stasis, promotion of blood circulation, acceleration of healing of injuries or

wounds, and reinforcement of the student's physique. The principle of combining treatment with dance movements as an approach to restoring function not only improves muscle capacity, but may keep the dancer's figure slender and improve dance skills.

3.   According to the degree, sites, and nature of injuries, the authors emphasized a combination of active and passive motion and persisted in appropriate scientific training, so that injured muscle fibers could recover by repeated stretch and contraction, fostering circulation of blood and vital energy.   This was an improvement over the previous method, which consisted of stopping training while treating an injury.

4.   It is essential that prevention and protection keep pace with training, physiology, and education. Preventive treatment should be carried on in male students age 12-14 and female students age 10-12, at the elementary stage. At the middle level, since male students of age 14 and female students of age 12 are in   puberty   and   injures   brought   about   in comprehensive training are usually more severe, the treatment should be more intensive.

Because of great energy consumption and high risk of severe injury, treatment for senior students should be focused on avoidance of over-fatigue and recovery from it if it does occur. As far as medication, the authors prefer local application because of greater effectiveness and less undesirable side effects.   In the process of treatment, the physician should press the points with his fingers and at the same time massage with the appropriate medication, coordinating his shoulders, elbows, wrists and fingers, to relieve pain.

5.   Prevention   is   of   paramount   importance. Active prevention entails careful selection of top students.   It is not only dependent upon sight and touch, but, in particular, upon the scientific means of examining the balance of the organs, age, and changes in formation of the bones, such as recessive spinal column fissures, width of the hip joint, size of the buttocks associated with the slant angle of the front neck of femur and the angle of the pubis.

CONCLUSION

It is necessary to provide teachers with feedback and data about the sites, degree, and nature of injuries so that they may provide training scientifically and artistically.   The new method of coordination and combination of treatment with dancing, using the principles of traditional Chinese medicine, will help to enhance the development of dance medicine.

CHAPTER 57

Work Conditions and Musculoskeletal Disorders in Ballet Dancers at Three Theaters in Sweden

Eva Ramel • *Ulrich Moritz*

Abstract

Ballet dancers' experiences in their work environment often include pain and discomfort in the locomotive system. Of 147 professional dancers from three major Swedish companies who were given a questionnaire for this study, 128 responded; 121 had experienced symptoms in the locomotive system during the previous 12 months. Pain and discomfort were primarily in the low back, ankles/feet, and neck. Results showed that lack of self-control was significantly associated with neck disorders, while incidence of ankle and foot disorders correlated with age and number of hours per week spent dancing.

The high prevalence of pain and discomfort in ballet dancers could be interpreted to be a result of an imbalance between their work demands and their resources. This study suggests reasons for this imbalance and offers eleven proposals for changes in the routines at the theaters. Further investigations are necessary, however, to test the impact of these proposals.

This study was carried out at The Royal Theater in Stockholm, Stora Theater in Gothenburg, and Malmö Theater during the fall of 1989. It is part of a project called "The Theater's Working Environment" initiated by the Swedish Theater Union and the Actors Trade Union, in cooperation with Lund University.

BACKGROUND

Many studies have discussed the etiology of dancers' injuries. Earlier studies focused primarily on orthopedic disorders.[1, 2] More recently, authors have been addressing psychological and other factors involved in this complex problem.[3, 4] A few studies were based on dancers' self-reported problems, thus assessing the prevalence in this population.[5, 6] The so-called overuse injury is shown in most studies to be more common than the acute injury,[1-3, 5, 7-9] but the distinction may sometimes be confusing. An acute injury such as a common ankle sprain may well be the result of a tired, *overused* artist due to an overloaded work situation.

In a study of the Swedish theater's working environment, 17% of the total artist work force had reported work-related injuries in 1980-84.[10] A few years later (1984-88), this number had doubled to 33% of the 932 artists studied. Most injuries had been reported among ballet dancers; 156 dancers reported 168 injuries.[11] A closer look, however, revealed that the 168 reported injuries were, in fact, divided among 98 dancers and that some dancers had not reported any injuries at all.

Artists work under a great deal of psychological stress, and dancers are no exception.[3] This stress, which can be divided into *positive* or *negative*, has been shown to play a part in the development of illness.[12] Self-control, influence in the work situation, and social support[13] have also recently been shown to have an impact on the development of musculoskeletal disorders.[14]

AIM OF THE STUDY

The aim of the study was to shed light on how the dancers experienced their work situations and the extent to which they experienced disorders in the musculoskeletal system. "Disorders" was defined as "pain, ache, discomfort," in accordance with the standardized Nordic questionnaire for the analysis of musculoskeletal symptoms.[15] This questionnaire assesses associations between musculoskeletal symptoms and perceived work situation, as well as the imbalance between dancers' professional demands and their own resources as a possible stress factor.

METHODS AND MATERIALS

Of the five theaters in Sweden with a ballet company, three were chosen to participate in this study because they had more than 10 dancers in the company and they had a *home* scene. Together, these theaters in Stockholm, Gothenburg, and Malmö had 147 dancers who were asked to complete a questionnaire in the presence of the senior author during the 1989 fall season. Two of the dancers were temporarily abroad and had the forms mailed to them, but neither responded. The survey consisted of the above-mentioned standardized Nordic questionnaire and 22 other questions concerning background, stress, general training, and their own ideas of reasons for symptoms and ways to prevent musculoskeletal problems.

The Nordic questionnaire consists of three different question levels: (A) Symptoms any time during the last 12 months; (B) Symptoms any time during the last 7 days; and (C) If existent, have these symptoms prevented the subject from doing his/her daily work any time during the last 12 months. The questions cover the neck, shoulders, elbows, wrists/hands, upper back, low back, hips/thighs, knees and ankles/feet.

The 74 dancers of The Royal Theater in Stockholm answered 12 additional questions about their psychological and social working conditions.[16-18]

A total of 128 dancers (87%) answered the questionnaire. Ten men and nine women did not respond.

SAMPLE CHARACTERISTICS

The group consisted of 128 dancers (75 female, 53 male). General starting age, present age, height and weight, and hours per week spent dancing are shown in the table below.

Background Data for Subjects

	MEAN VALUES AND RANGE	
	Female	*Male*
Age when starting*	9 yrs (4-16)	12 yrs (7-22)
Present Age	27 yrs (18-43)	28 yrs (17-47)
Weight	51 kg (42-62)	70 kg (58-85)
Height	166 cm (157-176)	179 cm (169-188)

*Dancing 3 times/week or more.

TIME SPENT DANCING PER WEEK			
	<30 hrs	31-40 hrs	>40 hrs
Number of Dancers	10 (8%)	92 (72%)	26 (20%)

To be able to interpret the answers from the questionnaire and obtain a better understanding of the dancers' unique work situation, it was necessary to observe daily classes and rehearsals. During this time, several dancers and teachers, as well as therapists and orthopedic surgeons connected with the dance companies, were interviewed.

This study is part of a larger project concerning the theater's working environment, in which the method used was the so-called research circle.[10] This meant that there was much cooperation between the authors and the two professional elite dancers in the research circle.

The Chi-square test, variance analysis, multiple regression and Kruskal-Wallis test were used in the statistical analysis of the results, and a probability level of p<0.05 was considered statistically significant.

RESULTS

Almost all of the dancers (95%) experienced musculoskeletal problems at some time during the previous 12 months. Most problems were in the lower back (70%), ankles/feet (63%), and neck (54%) (Fig. 1). Regional differences showed that the dancers in Gothenburg had significantly more problems with their feet (p<0.05), while the dancers in Malmö had fewer problems in their upper backs and their feet (both p<0.05).

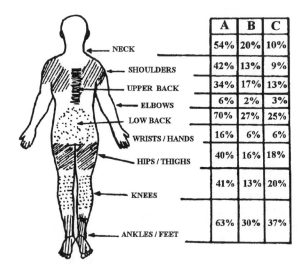

	A	B	C
NECK	54%	20%	10%
SHOULDERS	42%	13%	9%
UPPER BACK	34%	17%	13%
ELBOWS	6%	2%	3%
LOW BACK	70%	27%	25%
WRISTS / HANDS	16%	6%	6%
HIPS / THIGHS	40%	16%	18%
KNEES	41%	13%	20%
ANKLES / FEET	63%	30%	37%

Figure 1:   *A.   Musculoskeletal symptoms during last 12 months;   B.   Symptoms during last 7 days;   C.   Symptoms had impaired daily work during last 12 months.   Relative prevalence for 128 dancers.*

Looking back only seven days, 30% of the dancers had experienced symptoms in the ankles/feet, 27% in the low back, and 20% in the neck.

Dancers were kept from work by 37% of the ankle/foot problems, while 25% of the low back problems had been a hindrance at some time.

Although over half of the dancers experienced neck problems, this seldom prevented them from working. In total, 168 of the 472 problems had been a hindrance (36%), and 47 of the 128 dancers had been kept from work (37%) because of these problems. The regional comparison showed that the dancers in Stockholm had been kept from work because of problems with their ankles/feet more than other groups (p<0.01), and the dancers in Malmö had been kept from work less often (p<0.05).

Of the 128 dancers who answered, only seven had not had problems of any kind; four of these dancers were in Stockholm, three in Malmö. Five of them were men with many years of professional experience, while the remaining two were very young women with less than a year of experience.

The problems were evenly distributed between genders, but taller dancers had more problems with their wrists/hands, knees, and ankles/feet (p<0.05); heavier dancers had more problems with their knees (p<0.05). Dancers older than 25 years had more shoulder- (p<0.01) and ankle/foot problems (p<0.05). Number of years at work was correlated in this study only with shoulder problems. Dancing both classical and modern ballet generated more shoulder problems (p<0.05), and dancers who felt their psychological stress was "insignificant" had fewer shoulder problems. Dancers with neck trouble stated more often that they felt completely governed by others, and those without had more often come in contact with Tai Chi (both p<0.05).

As for the 64 dancers in Stockholm who answered the 12 additional questions about their psychological and social work conditions, almost all liked their work (Fig. 2). When answering the questions about how much influence they had at work, they scored an average of 1.4 out of 4. Only 21% of the Stockholm dancers felt they had any influence at all.

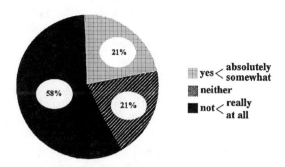

Figure 3: Relative division between "yes" and "no" answers about influence at work.

On a scale of 0 to 4, the dancers felt that the social support was lowest from the chief of the ballet (2.0), while other people at work gave them more support (2.8), but most was from family and friends (3.5).

A multiple regression analysis performed on the variables "how well do you like your work," "influence at work," and "social support" showed that the group of questions about influence at work explained musculo-skeletal problems to some degree, but the other variables did not. This means that dancers with problems did not feel they could influence their work as much as dancers with no problems did.

DISCUSSION

This study, which is based on the dancers' self-reported experiences, shows a very high prevalence of musculoskeletal disorders. These 'aches and pains' could be attributed to a combination of hard work — both physically and mentally — tough competition, and a stiff routine training program with little understanding of individual differences. Poor environmental conditions — with hard floors, cold rooms or tilted floors — as well as poorly planned schedules, were also pointed out.

The study shows that about 60% of the dancers feel completely governed by others in their training. This is alarming, since no one but the dancer should be able to decide how much training his/her body and mind can take. The Stockholm dancers also showed that occurrence of musculoskeletal disorders correlated with less influence at work. This strengthens the idea that dancers should instead be encouraged to take more responsibility for themselves and be given the time and opportunity to do so. The situation today is still very much that of an old-fashioned parent-and-child (theater-and-dancer) relationship which the dancers feel is unsatisfactory.

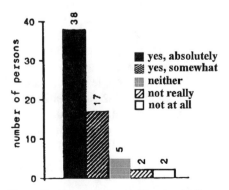

Figure 2: How well do you like your job?

The imbalance between the dancers' resources and the demands of ballet could be due to the fact that dancers are not permitted to take the responsibility to practice their own body knowledge.

CONCLUSION

Changing routines in the world of ballet is not accomplished easily, but there seems to be a growing interest in trying new ideas. The following eleven points could be used as grounds for discussion about what could be done in the different theaters:

1. More encouragement in the educational system to enhance dancers' body awareness and make them take a greater responsibility for themselves.

2. *Transition* class in the theater for novice newly employed dancers.

3. Greater training variety with warm-up before class, aerobic and mental training, and emphasis on long-range goals.

4. Special mental training for artists.

5. Better organization of class schedules and rehearsal work.

6. Individual assessment for each dancer every year.

7. A planned routine for rehabilitation.

8. Divided artistic and administrative leadership.

9. Organization of older dancers helping the younger.

10. Greater opportunities for dancers to influence their work.

11. A plan for voluntary assistance before retirement or at other times when a dancer must give up his/her career.

REFERENCES

1. Thomasen E: Diseases and injuries of ballet dancers. Universitetsforlaget i Århus, 1982.
2. Hamilton WG: Foot and ankle injuries in dancers. Clinics in Sports Medicine, January 1988.
3. Stephens RE: The etiology of injuries in ballet. *In* Ryan AJ, Stephens RE (eds), Dance Medicine. Chicago: Pluribus Press, 1987.
4. Bejjani FJ: Occupational biomechanics of athletes and dancers: A comparative approach. Clinics in Podiatric Medicine and Surgery 4:671-711, 1987.
5. Perreault M: Preventing injuries in theatrical dance: The Quebec dancers' and producers' viewpoints. Paper presented at International Conference on Medicine for the Performing Arts, Jerusalem, Israel, 1989.
6. Bowling A: Injuries to dancers: Prevalence, treatment, and perception of causes. British Medical Journal 298:731-734, 1989.
7. McNeal AP, Watkins A, Clarkson PM, Tremblay I:. Lower extremity alignment and injury in young, preprofessional, college and professional ballet dancers: Dancer-reported injuries. Medical Problems of Performing Artists 5:83-88, 1990.
8. Sammarco GJ: Diagnosis and treatment in dancers. Clinical Orthopedics and Related Research 187:176-187, 1984.
9. Howse J, Hancock S: Dance Technique and Injury Prevention. London: A & C Black, 1988.
10. Lindström KG, Persson LI, Ruth W, Svenstam Å: The theatre's working environment and its future development. Report of a research circle working in cooperation with the Swedish Theatre Federation and Lund University. Pedagogiskt utvecklingsarbete vid Lunds Universitet nr. 89:172, 1989.
11. Persson L: Arbetsskaderapporter: Artister 1984-1988. Personal communication, 1989 (in Swedish).
12. Frankenheuser M: Stress en del av livet. Brombergs, Värnamo, 1983 (in Swedish).
13. Frankenheuser M: Stress, hälsa, arbetsglädje. Arbetsmiljöfondens Informationsskrifter best. nr 60-10-44, Stockholm 1987 (in Swedish).
14. Theorell T, Harms-Ringdahl K, Ahlberg-Hultén G, Westin B: Psychosocial job factors and symptoms from the locomotor system — a multicausal analysis. Scand J Rehab Med, 1991 (in press).
15. Kourinka I, Jonsson B, Kilbom Å, et al. Standardized Nordic Questionnaires for the analysis of musculoskeletal symptoms. Appl Ergonomics, 3:233-237, 1987.
16. Gardell B: Arbetsinnehåll och livskvalité. Prisma, Lund, 1976 (in Swedish).
17. Lindell J. Mätning av upplevelser i arbetsmiljön. Management Media, 1982 (in Swedish).
18. Caplan RD, et al: Job demands and worker health. Main effects and occupational differences. US Department of Health, Education and Welfare, 1975.

CHAPTER 58

A Database of Isoinertial Trunk Strength Tests in Three Planes of Action Among Dance Students

L. Poggini • *P. Di Marco* • *L. Vitangeli* • *G. Martini*

The strength and mobility of the torso are critical for all types of dance (classical, modern, ethnic, etc.). In classical ballet, dancers learn in their first years of training to stabilize the spine during some movements, such as pirouettes and jumps, but they also need a wide spinal range of motion in order to correctly perform the big positions backward (attitude and arabesque).

Despite these observations, many dance students do not take care of their trunk muscles and very often develop different types of muscular imbalances that can represent important risk factors for spinal dance-related injuries. In a recent survey among 176 students of the National Dance Academy in Rome, 61 subjects were found to be suffering from low back injuries (34.6%).

Since there is no isoinertial database available for trunk strength in young dancers, this study attempts to establish normative data in a group of dance students of both sexes using the B200-Isostation. This is a triaxial system that measures the torque, angular position, and velocity of trunk movements for all axes simultaneously. The mode of muscular contraction in this system is isoinertial, as the resistance against which the trunk is moved remains constant throughout the range of motion.

MATERIALS AND METHODS

The sample comprised 18 students of the National Dance Academy (14 females and 4 males) with no history of low back pain.

For females, mean age was 15.7 years, mean weight 46.9 Kg, and mean height 162.9 cm. For males, mean age was 16.7 years, mean weight 69.2 Kg, and mean height 180 cm.

All of the subjects performed daily classical and modern dance for 2.5-4 hours.

Each dancer was positioned on the B200-Isostation in neutral with the flexion-extension axis aligned with their L5-S1 spinal level. All subjects were instructed to perform two different tests: First, after a short period of warm-up, they performed an isometric test, and then three dynamic tests (one for each plane of action) of 10 repetitions each against resistance equal to 50% of the maximum isometric strength of the trunk muscles, calculated in the first step. The young dancers also answered a simple questionnaire to identify their habits regarding warm-up, strengthening exercises, and stretching exercises, and the possible spinal symptomology.

RESULTS

The parameters were selected in correlation with the spinal movements (flexion-extension, lateral flexion, and rotation).

For the isometric test, the difference between $T+$ (flexion, right lateral flexion, right rotation) and $T-$ (extension, left lateral flexion, left rotation) was computed, in order to identify the stronger side of the body (Delta T) (Table I). Mean moments were also computed for the three planes (Table II).

For the dynamic tests, the difference between $T+$ and $T-$ (d T, indicating the muscular effort) and between $V+$ and $V-$ (d V, indicating the muscular facilitation) were calculated. Work and power were also considered to evaluate the 'productivity' of the subject (Table III). The endpoint position data and the ROM data were used to evaluate the D-ROM, indicating possible restrictions of the movements (Table IV).

Table I: *Isometric Test: Individual Values of Delta T = Flexion-Extension or Right-Left (Rotation and Lateral Flexion)*

N	Sex	Rotation Delta T	Flex-Ext Delta T	Lat Flex Delta T
1	F	8.5	8.2	8.5
2	F	21.2	22.2	8.5
3	F	23.3	69.9	17.0
4	F	3.0	15.9	12.7
5	M	19.0	12.7	6.4
6	M	12.7	143.0	44.5
7	F	-8.5	22.3	-4.2
8	F	0.0	12.7	23.3
9	F	14.9	47.7	6.4
10	F	19.1	6.4	8.5
11	M	6.3	60.4	-4.3
12	M	25.4	-44.5	36.0
13	F	4.2	-22.2	-6.4
14	F	8.5	-41.3	21.2
15	F	-2.2	15.9	2.1
16	F	8.5	-25.8	8.5
17	F	8.5	12.7	2.1
18	F	-2.2	3.2	10.6

Table II: *Mean (m) Isometric Moments, with Standard Deviation (sd) and Confidence Interval (ci)*

	FlexExt.	Lat. Flex.	Rotation
m	66.76	52.80	21.99
sd	42.61	26.84	21.13
ci	66.70 ± 21.20	62.8 ± 13.3	21.00 ± 10.50

Table III: *Individual Muscular Effort (d T) and Facilitation (d V) Values for All Three Planes, During Dynamic Testing*

N	Sex	Rotation d T	Rotation d V	Flex.-Ext. d T	Flex.-Ext. d V	Lat. Flex. d T	Lat. Flex. d V
1	F	-0.6	3.9	0.6	2.4	8.0	2.3
2	F	0.5	3.9	7.2	7.1	2.1	4.8
3	F	-0.5	7.8	12.7	-14.3	6.3	2.3
4	F	-1.1	-11.6	0.8	-4.7	2.1	9.5
5	M	-1.6	-16.8	1.6	2.4	8.5	2.4
6	M	2.1	0.0	28.6	64.1	0.0	9.5
7	F	-2.1	5.8	2.4	-59.4	2.1	7.1
8	F	-1.6	-5.8	7.1	-19.0	2.1	9.5
9	F	2.1	-3.8	8.0	-11.9	2.1	7.2
10	F	1.6	-3.9	6.8	-21.4	2.2	2.3
11	M	-9.0	11.6	19.0	-40.3	-2.1	19.0
12	M	2.1	5.8	-15.9	21.3	2.1	19.0
13	F	-2.1	17.4	4.0	19.0	4.2	0.0
14	F	-2.1	3.8	4.7	-47.5	2.1	4.8
15	F	-2.1	0.0	4.0	2.4	2.1	19.0
16	F	-2.6	2.0	3.1	-40.3	4.3	14.3
17	F	-2.2	-2.0	2.4	4.8	2.1	11.9
18	F	-2.1	13.5	3.2	-16.7	2.1	9.5

Table IV: *Mean (m) Moment (Rm), Velocity (Vm), Work (W)), Power (P), Range of Motion (ROM), Right/Flexion Endpoint (ROM+), Left/Extension Endpoint (ROM-), with Respective Standard Deviation (sd) and Confidence Interval (ci) Values for All Spinal Planes of Motion During Dynamic Testing*

	Tm	Vm	W	P	ROM	ROM+	ROM-
			Flexion/Extension				
m	54.89	61.52	825.81	76.97	83.97	51.42	31.07
sd	32.22	14.27	649.52	57.77	17.45	13.57	6.53
ci	54.90	61.50	825.80	76.80	84.00	51.42	31.10
	±16.00	±7.10	±328.10	±8.70	±6.70	±6.70	±3.20
			Lateral Flexion				
m	39.62	65.58	455.90	58.63	65.21	32.20	33.01
sd	14.94	25.57	330.37	49.59	18.65	10.25	9.03
ci	39.60	65.60	456.00	58.60	65.20	32.20	33.00
	±7.40	±12.70	±164.30	±24.70	±9.80	±5.10	±4.50
			Rotation				
m	21.53	58.67	322.39	28.42	85.53	43.37	42.16
sd	14.00	17.48	252.62	26.18	15.20	7.48	8.16
ci	21.50	58.70	322.40	28.40	85.50	43.40	42.20
	±7.00	±8.70	±125.60	±13.00	±7.60	±3.70	±4.10

DISCUSSION

The results obtained through the isometric test indicate that most dance students utilize more muscular strength during extension (78%), right lateral flexion (72%) and right rotation (78%) (Tables I and II).

The isodynamic tests reveal a higher muscular effort in flexion than in extension. During lateral flexion, movement is more comfortable to the right, while during rotation, movement is easier to the left. The mean values of the Tm, Work and Power are higher for flexion/extension, lower for rotation and intermediate for lateral flexion (Tables III and IV).

Range of motion, as expected, is wider in flexion, but many dancers complained because the B200-Isostation stopped their spinal extension short; lateral flexion and rotation are wider to the right. In any case, range of motion in dance students was wider than in the general population.[1-4]

As expected, male dancers are stronger and faster than females. Mean work and power values of the males are three times larger than of the females.

REFERENCES

1. Nelson JK, Johnston JW: B200 sample population data. Isotechnologies Inc, 1988.

2. Bejjani FJ, Halpern N, Nordin M, Pavlidis L, Pio A, Dominguez R, Greenidge N, Frankel V: Spinal motion and strength measurements of Flamenco dancers, using 3D motion analyzer and Cybex II Dynamometer. *In* de Groot G, Hollander AP, Huijing PA, van Ingen Schenau GJ (eds): Biomechanics XI-B, 925-930. Amsterdam, Netherlands: Free University Press, 1988.

3. Bejjani FJ, Halpern N, Tomaino CM: Spinal motion and strength in flamenco dancers. Proceedings of the 7th Conference on Medical Problems of Musicians and Dancers, 1989.

4. Parnianpour M, et al: A database of isoinertial trunk strength tests against three resistance levels in sagittal, frontal and transverse planes in normal male subjects. Spine 14(4):409-411, 1989.

CHAPTER 59

Analysis of Isokinetic Characteristics and Jump Ability in a Group of Professional Dancers

Luana Poggini • Cesare A. Pistara • Andrea Ferretti

In daily classical ballet training, the class begins with the barre exercises, and then, as the movements are mastered, is taken to the center of the room. Since the barre exercises are used for muscular development and the study of the basic principles of dance technique (turnout, plié-relevé, organization and coordination of all movements), they are quite similar for dancers of both sexes. During the center exercises, however, female dancers perform pointe work and male dancers study the various types of jumps. The purpose in conducting this study was to analyze the correlations between the muscular strength, fly time, and the height of different kinds of jumps.

MATERIALS AND METHODS

Thirteen professional dancers of both sexes, without any knee- or ankle pathology, were studied. There were 8 females and 5 males; ages ranged from 17 to 31 years (mean age 25 years) (Table I).

Table I: *Physical Characteristics of Subjects*

N	Sex	Age	Type of Dance	Height (cm)	Weight (Kg)	Weekly Workload (hours)	Dom. Side
1	M	26	C/M	170	64	24	R
2	M	17	C	187	70	28	R
3	M	28	C	180	69	40	R
4	M	26	C/M	175	66	36	R
5	M	30	C/M	176	72	40	R
6	F	24	C	174	59	36	L
7	F	23	C	171	50	14	R
8	F	29	C/M	165	52	18	R
9	F	31	C	160	47	18	R
10	F	17	C	172	50	28	R
11	F	30	C	167	50	24	R
12	F	25	C/M	171	57	16	R
13	F	18	C/M	180	47	18	R

The study was divided into two sessions: Using a Cybex II Dynamometer, knee (flexion/extension) and ankle (dorsiflexion/plantarflexion) torques were measured. All of the dancers were requested to perform six consecutive repetitions of the flexion/extension movements, after a variable period of warm-up, according to their personal demands.

In the second session, fly time and height of different jumps were measured, using the Ergo Jump. All dancers performed four types of jumps: (1) a squat jump on both legs to analyze the explosive strength, (2) an elastic jump on both legs to analyze the resilient strength, (3) two short series of three jumps on one leg alternately to evaluate any bilateral strength difference between, and (4) a long series of ten jumps with both legs trying to reach the maximal raise in all jumps.

RESULTS

Data obtained during the Cybex II test are shown in Tables II and III; results of the Ergo Jump test are shown in Table IV. Results obtained with the Cybex II were compared with those obtained by Nisonson and Liederbach[1] (Table V).

DISCUSSION

The Italian male dancers present less quadricep- and hamstring-muscle strength than U.S. dancers; the data are quite similar for the females. Regarding ankle data in dancers of both sexes, the authors found the dorsiflexors to be stronger in the Italian dancers, but the plantarflexors are less powerful (Table V). This lesser global strength of Italian dancers is due to the type of dance training they undergo, including a different weekly workload and, too often, very poor conditioning.

Table II: Cybex II — Knee Data

N	Sex	Ext./BW		Ext. Torque		Flex. Torque		Work Est.		Work Flex.	
		R	L	R	L	R	L	R	L	R	L
1	M	145%	141%	93	90	47	40	346	362	756	638
2	M	304%	291%	212	203	97	94	1395	1318	704	664
3	M	171%	146%	119	101	45	57	862	843	387	328
4	M	155%	152%	102	100	57	73	762	737	421	417
5	M	196%	179%	141	129	71	82	1013	741	588	598
6	F	119%	126%	69	73	38	43	646	593	307	355
7	F	241%	268%	120	134	51	58	872	847	244	447
8	F	148%	182%	77	95	49	43	719	809	438	304
9	F	106%	136%	50	64	34	44	450	754	251	471
10	F	233%	268%	116	134	66	47	824	787	304	354
11	F	180%	192%	90	96	49	49	731	670	433	477
12	F	172%	163%	98	93	37	40	714	628	356	319
13	F	136%	136%	64	64	44	35	458	409	231	187
MEAN		177	183	104	106	58	54	755	730	417	427
S.D.		±55	±56	±41	±37	±17	±18	±269	±233	±170	±141

Table III: Cybex II — Ankle Data

N	Sex	Torque P - Flex.		Torque D - Flex.		Work P - Flex.		Work D - Flex.	
		R	L	R	L	R	L	R	L
1	M	49	54	24	25	283	274	171	165
2	M	77	65	28	29	262	222	131	125
3	M	55	62	30	29	251	323	182	200
4	M	44	45	23	23	193	164	131	117
5	M	50	38	27	26	129	122	88	106
6	F	40	33	20	19	179	163	122	141
7	F	20	21	40	39	115	103	211	181
8	F	40	38	21	19	222	192	152	121
9	F	30	25	27	19	175	157	110	127
10	F	42	48	23	21	146	218	123	97
11	F	39	41	24	26	218	201	130	125
12	F	38	33	21	20	214	156	140	97
13	F	21	23	17	17	133	114	92	100
MEAN		42	40	25	24	194	193	137	131
S.D.		±14	±14	±6	±6	±53	±60	±35	±32

Table IV: Ergo Jump Data

N	Sex	Squat Jump m.	Elastic Jump m.	3 Jumps Right m.	3 Jumps Left m.	10 Jumps m.
1	M	0.295	0.372	0.139	0.141	0.250
2	M	0.522	0.508	0.217	0.201	0.437
3	M	0.457	0.486	0.207	0.193	0.378
4	M	0.377	0.356	0.164	0.146	0.224
5	M	0.425	0.481	0.235	0.245	0.346
6	F	0.312	0.273	0.143	0.136	0.210
7	F	0.207	0.270	0.167	0.166	0.228
8	F	0.346	0.320	0.198	0.193	0.286
9	F	0.271	0.357	0.177	0.184	0.199
10	F	0.201	0.291	0.122	0.114	0.235
11	F	0.249	0.290	0.187	0.209	0.165
12	F	0.222	0.372	0.116	0.115	0.160
13	F	0.162	0.339	0.111	0.102	0.150

The data regarding ankle movements are not easily explained; the differences are probably due to the type of dance training and environmental factors such as the type of dance floor.

Chmelar et al. found that 63% of 37 female dancers studied demonstrated specific weaknesses in the force decay rate of the quadricep curves.[2] The authors found it in only two dancers, one male and one female, and for this reason do not consider this particular shape of the curve significant.

Since volleyball and dance exercises are classified as non-endurance type of physical activity,[3] the Ergo Jump test data indicated that dancers of both sexes have significantly less explosive and resilient strength than volleyball players.[4] This is due to the particular biomechanical characteristics of jumps in classical ballet, and — especially for female dancers — to the physical characteristics of the dancers (Table I).

Dancers, in fact, have particular nutritional practices and are too often excessively lean; females are not used to the modifications of their bodies.

Finally, these data show that correct dance training produces the proper balance in muscular strength between the lower extremities.

Table V: Data Comparison

	Males (ft. - lbs.)	Females (ft. - lbs.)
A.		
Knee Extension	140.6	76.5
Knee Flexion	92.7	50.6
Ankle Plantarflexion	63.2	42.7
Ankle Dorsiflexion	13.5	9.0
B.		
Knee Extension	129.3	90.1
Knee Flexion	66.6	45.5
Ankle Plantarflexion	53.9	33.4
Ankle Dorsiflexion	26.4	23.3

A = *Nisonson and Liederbach data (1989)*
B = *Poggini, et al. data (1993)*

Regarding the biomechanical characteristics of the jump in classical ballet, the authors found that, paradoxically, explosive jumps are higher than resilient jumps. This is due to the fact that jumps start and end in precisely codified positions, while the body must be maintained in another position during the fly time. In order to achieve accuracy of movements, most classical dancers sacrifice jump height.

Analyzing the Ergo Jump data, the authors found that among male dancers, there is a direct correlation between height of the explosive jump and the quadricep torque/weight ratio (for example, subject #2 in Tables II and IV). Among female dancers, the same type of correlation was not found (for example, subject #7 in Tables II and IV); rather, a correlation between the height of the resilient jumps and plantarflexors torque/weight ratio was found. These data could suggest that female dancers jump using more calf- than quadricep-muscle strength.

REFERENCES

1. Nisonson B, Liederbach M: Normative Cybex data on professional ballet dancers. Abstracts of the Seventh Annual Symposium on Medical Problems of Musicians and Dancers, 32-33. Snowmass, CO, 1989.

2. Chmelar RD, et al: Isokinetic characteristics of the knee and trunk in ballet and modern dancers. Abstracts of the Seventh Annual Symposium on Medical Problems of Musicians and Dancers, 34. Snowmass, CO, 1989.

3. Cohen JL, et al: Cardiorespiratory responses to ballet exercise and the VO2max of elite ballet dancers. Med Sc Sports Ex 14(3):212-217, 1982.

4. Bosco C: Elasticita muscolare e torxe esplosiva nell attivitá fisico-sportiva. Societá Stampa Sportiva, 1985.

SUGGESTED READING

1. Kirkendall DT, et al: Isokinetic characteristics of ballet dancers and the response to a season of ballet training. J Orthop Sports Phys Ther 5(4): 207-211, 1984.

2. Mostardi RA: Musculoskeletal and cardiopulmonary evaluation of professional ballet dancers. *In*: The Dancer as Athlete: The 1984 Olympic Scientific Congress Proceedings, Vol 8, 101-107. Champaign, IL: Human Kinetics, 1986.

CHAPTER 60

Occupational Ballet Injuries:
A Four-Year Study of Venezuelan Dancers

Federico Fernandez-Palazzi • *Salvador Rivas*
Berenice Espejo • *Yngrid Perez*

INTRODUCTION

In order to evaluate the possible injuries substained by a professional classical ballet dancer, a retrospective study was performed analyzing the clinical records of the dancers of the Teresa Carreño Ballet Company during the period 1984 to 1988. The parameters evaluated were age, sex, body area affected, diagnosis and type of lesion, frequency of lesions, and an analysis of the form of progression of the lesion (starting point and affected side in relation to time), as well as percentage of lesion in relation to hemibody and/or lower limb mostly affected or susceptible.

MATERIAL

Forty-two dancers were reviewed — 19 males and 23 females. Age ranged from 16 to 25 years. Data emanated from the clinical records of the dancers.

RESULTS

Of a total of 390 lesions, 220 were in the ankle and foot (57.41%), 38 in the knee (9.74%), 38 in the trunk (9.74%), 27 in the hip (6.92%), 27 in the upper limb (6.92%), 21 in the thigh (5.38%), and 19 in the leg (4.87%).

Ankle and Foot

Of the 220 lesions, 140 were in females (35.89%) and 80 in males (20.51%). The 5 most frequent lesions were:

- hallux metatarsophalangeal sprain (53 cases);
- ankle sprain (46 cases);
- Achilles tendinitis (39 cases) (Fig. 1);
- peroneal muscle distention (31 cases); and
- flexor hallucis longus tendinitis (18 cases).

In males, the most frequent lesion was ankle sprain (25 cases), followed by Achilles tendinitis (20 cases) and peroneal distention (15 cases). Fracture of the 5th metatarsal occured in 3 cases (Fig. 2). Nine different types of lesion were seen in male dancers.

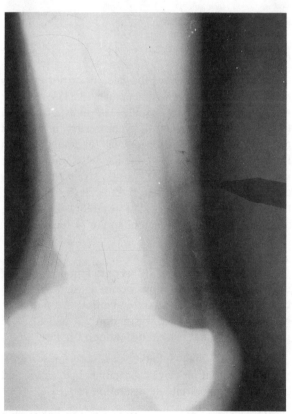

Figure 1: *Achilles tendinitis low penetration x-ray (notice arrow pointed to soft tissue swelling).*

In females, the most frequent lesion was hallux meta-tarsophalangeal sprain (41 cases), followed by ankle sprain (21 cases) and Achilles tendinitis (19 cases). Females suffered of 12 types of lesions besides the 5 mentioned above: metatarsophalangeal capsular distentions of the other 4 toes (12 dancers); 5th metatarsal fracture (3); ingrown toenail (5); tarsal sprain (3); plantar fasciitis (2); sesamoiditis (3); and bunion bursitis (1).

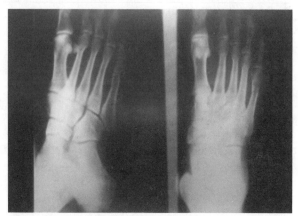

Figure 2: Fifth metatarsal fracture.

Knee

The 38 lesions about the knee occurred twice as often in females (6.41%) as in males (3.33%). There were 7 types of lesions: patellar lateral hyperpression (16 cases — pure lateral hyperpresion in 12 and patellar subluxation in 4); patellar tendinitis (only in females) in 8 cases (Fig. 3); medial collateral ligament sprain (4 cases); posterior capsule strain (4), usually related to a ligament lesion; Baker cyst (3 — 2 males), treated conservatively; patellar instability (2 females); and lateral collateral ligament sprain (1 female).

Leg

Of the 19 leg lesions, 12 were in females and 7 in males. Four types of lesions occured: shin splint (13 cases); tibialis anterior tendinitis (3 females); gastrocnemius proximal distention (2 males); and proximal peroneal muscle distention (1 male).

In males, shin splints were seen in 4 cases, proximal distention of gastrocnemius in 2 cases, and proximal peroneal muscle distention in 1 case.

Only 2 types of lesions were seen in females: shin splint (9 cases) and tibialis anterior tendinitis (3).

Thigh

Total lesions at thigh level were 21 (5.38% of total lesions), more frequent in males (33.33%) than in females (2.05%). Four types of lesions were

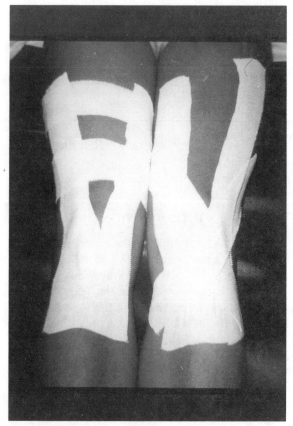

Figure 3: Strapping for bilateral patellar tendinitis.

present: hamstring distention (13 cases); quadriceps tear or distention (5 cases, all males); vastus lateralis rupture (2 cases); and quadriceps wound (1 male).

In males, there were 6 hamstring distentions, 5 quadriceps tears, 1 vastus lateralis rupture and 1 thigh wound.

In females, only 2 types of lesions were present: hamstring distention (7 cases) and vastus lateralis rupture (1 case).

Hip

Twenty-seven lesions occured, of which 17 were in females (4.35% of total body lesions) and 10 in males (2.56%). Nine types of lesions were seen: rectus femoris tendinitis/distention (12); sacroiliac sprain (3); snapping hip — only in females (2); thigh weakness — only in males (2); adductor distention (2); hip external rotator distention (2); gluteus medialis distention (2); sciatic nerve irritation (1); and gluteal abscess (1).

In males, rectus femoris tendinitis was seen in 3 cases, followed by sacroiliac sprain (2) and thigh weakness (2).

In females, rectus femoris tendinitis occurred in 9 cases, followed by snapping hip (2). There was no thigh weakness in females.

Trunk

Eighteen lesions occurred — 21 in females (5.38% of total body lesions) and 17 in males (4.35%). Seven types of lesions were found: back pain (10 cases); neck pain (5 cases); paravertebral muscle contractures (4 cases); acute torticolis (1 case); lumbar sprain (1 male); serratus major distention (1 female); and spondylolistesis, treated conservatively (1 male).

In males, back pain (12 cases) was more frequent due to the lifting of the partner in dancing, followed by para-vertebral muscular contracture (2); cervical pain (1); lumbar sprain (1); and spondylolistesis (1).

Upper Limb

The total number of lesions was 27, with 17 in males (4.35% of total body lesions) and 10 in females (2.56%).

Six different types of lesions were reported: rotator cuff lesion (10); stress pain in upper limb — only in males (7); trapezius myositis — only in females (6); wrist sprain (2); metacarpophalangeal sprain of thumb (1 male), with proximal epiphyseal fracture of distal phalanx due to abnormal lifting (Fig.4); and acromioclavicular sprain in 1 male, also due to abnormal lifting.

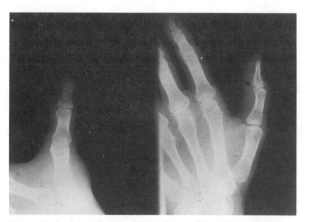

Figure 4: *Avulsion fracture of the thumb IP joint (see arrow).*

In males, there was equal incidence of rotator cuff lesions and stress pain of upper limb (7 cases each). All other lesions were seen in one case each. Males suffered 5 different types of lesions.

Females presented 3 types of lesions: trapezium myositis (6 cases), rotator cuff lesions (3), and wrist sprain (1).

DISCUSSION

In reviewing the lesions reported above, one can see that some lesions are more common in females, such as MTP joint sprain at the hallux or the other 4 digits, tibialis anterior tendinitis, shin splints, patella subluxation, and rectus femoris sprain, all related to the positions *en point* and *en dehors*, and occurring in the lower limb.

In males, lesions of the trunk and upper limb occured more frequently due to the requirements of lifting the partner.

Issues to be considered include poor training, tiredness, excessive training, resuming dancing before a lesion has completely healed, dancing on different types of floors, etc.

In studying the appearance of the aforementioned lesions and the progression of some of them, the authors noticed a repeated pattern that can be summarized as follows:

● If the original lesion is at the spine or hip level, it will progress affecting the strongest lower limb and upon reaching the foot will affect the other limb starting at the knee or foot level.

● If the lesion is present equally at hip or thigh levels, it will progress to both lower limbs, but upon reaching the foot will affect primarily and more intensely the weakest foot, which is usually the left.

● If the lesion is at knee level, it will descend to the foot on the same side or give rise to lesions such as tendinitis or sprains of the contralateral foot.

● If the lesion starts at foot level, there are three possibilities: (1) it will recur and worsen in the same foot; (2) it will affect the spine and then contralateral foot; or (3) it will affect the contralateral foot, then ipsilateral knee.

● When a lesion becomes recurrent, every new occurrence is more severe.

● The interval for recurrence of a lesion is from 15 days to 2 months.

● Lower limb injuries occur more frequently in the weakest limb (left), but lesions are more severe in the dominant limb (right).

● The right hemibody was affected in 41.66% of cases and left hemibody in 58.33%.

SUGGESTED READING

1. Fernandez-Palazzi F: La otra cara de la danza. Aspectos ortopedicos del ballet.   Caracas: Monteavila, 1990.

2. Ryan AJ, Stephens RE: Dance Medicine. A Comprehensive Guide. Chicago: Pluribus Press, 1987.

3. Sammarco GJ: Injuries to dancers. Clinics in Sports Medicine. Philadelphia: WB Saunders, 1983.

4. Thomasen E.: Diseases and Injuries of Ballet Dancers. Arhus: Universitetsforlaget, 1982.

CHAPTER 61

The Cause of Medial Pain After Inversion Trauma of the Ankle

C. N. van Dijk

Ballet is a physically demanding art. As in many strenuous physical activities, the incidence of supination trauma of the ankle joint is the highest among all traumatic injuries. The author performed a prospective study of patients age 18-40 years who presented with a painful ankle after supination trauma. In all patients, arthrography was performed within 24 hours of injury. Extensive physical examination of the ankle joint was performed within four to seven days.

All patients who had a positive arthrogram and/or positive physical examination and who visited the hospital in an even week were operated on. All patients with a positive arthrogram who visited the hospital in an uneven week were treated with a bandage. Physical examination appeared to be more reliable than arthrography in diagnosis.[1]

A total of 400 patients in the study had a rupture of one or more of the lateral ankle ligaments, confirmed either by surgery (50%) or by arthrography. In this group of 400 patients, 65% had pain on palpation of the medial aspect of the ankle joint, four to seven days after trauma.

At the six-month follow-up, 28% still complained of their ankle joint medially (26% in the operative treatment group and 29% in the conservative treatment group). This was independent of the form of treatment.

Many authors have reported a high incidence of residual complaints after treatment of lateral ligament ruptures. This seems to be independent of the form of treatment.[2-8]

Real instability for which operative reconstruction is necessary is rare. Complaints usually consist of functional instability, pain on activity, and swelling.[3, 6, 8-10] Pain and swelling are usually located on the medial aspect of the ankle joint.

The etiology of this medial pain varies among different authors: haemarthros,[11] partial rupture of the deltoid ligament[4, 5, 12] soft tissue impingement,[9] osteochondral fracture of the talus,[13] or arthrosis.[14] In an attempt to identify the cause of this medial pain, a consecutive series of 30 patients were studied. They all underwent surgical repair of the acutely ruptured lateral ankle ligament. Most had only a rupture of the anterior tibiofibular ligament. Some had a combined rupture of anterior tibiofibular ligament and fibulocalcaneal ligament.

During the surgical procedure, arthroscopy of the ankle joint was performed, whereby the medial aspect of the ankle joint was visualized. The tip of the medial malleolus, the cartilage of the medial malleolus, and the facies medialis of the talus could thereby be inspected, as well as the synovium and deltoid ligament.

In 19 patients, there was a fresh injury of the cartilage. Most typically, the injury was located at the tip and/or anterior distal part of the medial malleolus (13), as well as on the facies medialis of the talus (8). In five patients, there was damage to the cartilage of the anteromedial aspect of the distal tibia. Only one patient showed a cartilage defect on the medial edge of the talus. In five patients, the cartilage destruction was such that a loose body had formed. In most cases, the cartilage defect was combined with some synovitis or formation of fibrous bands. Macroscopic damage to the subchondral bone was present only in the patient with the cartilage damage on the medial edge of the talus. In one patient, there was a partial rupture of the deltoid ligament. Four patients showed only signs of synovitis or formation of fibrous bands. In five patients, there was no abnormality found on the medial aspect of the ankle joint.

In conclusion, two-thirds of these 30 consecutive patients with a rupture of one or more of the lateral ankle ligaments suffered macroscopic damage to the cartilage on the medial aspect of the joint. The reason seems to be that when the talus supinates, an impingement occurs between the tip of the medial malleolus and the facies medialis of the talus. When there is axial compression, the edge of the talus can impinge on the anteromedial distal tibia as well.

As previously stated, a significant number of patients have long-term ankle complaints after inversion trauma, especially those involved in strenuous activities such as ballet. In a minority, the complaint is instability; but more often, pain and swelling on the medial aspect of the ankle joint cause functional limitation. The cartilage damage on the medial aspect of the ankle joint could easily explain these complaints.

REFERENCES

1. Van Dijk CN: Unpublished data.
2. Schaap GR, DeKeizer G, Marti RK: Inversion trauma of the ankle. Arch Orthop Trauma Surg 108:273-75, 1989.
3. Staples OS: Result study of ruptures of lateral ligaments of the ankle. Clin Orthop 85:50-58, 1972.
4. Staples OS: Injuries to the medial ligaments of the ankle. J Bone Joint Surg 42A:1287, 1960.
5. Pankorrich AM, Shivaram MS: Anatomical basis for variability in injuries of the medial malleolus and the deltoid ligament. Acta Orthop Scand 50:225-236, 1979.
6. Borien WR, Staples OS, Russel SW: Residual disability following acute ankle sprains. J Bone Joint Surg 37:1237-1243, 1955.
7. Klein J, et al: Operative oder konservative Behandlung der frischen aussenbendruptur am oberen Sprunggelenk. Unfallchirurg 91:154-160, 1988.
8. Freeman MAR: Treatment of ruptures of the lateral ligament of the ankle. J Bone Joint Surg 47B:661-668, 1965.
9. Wohn I, Glassman F, Sideman S, Levinthal DM: Internal derangement of the talofibular component of the ankle. Surg Gynec Obstet 91:193-200, 1950.
10. Hoogenband CR, Moppes vd FI: Die behandlung der lateralen ligamentrupturen des oberen sprunggelenkes mit der Coumansiandage und direkte mobilisation. Hefte Unfallheilk 198:1030, 1987.
11. Hackenbruch W, Karpf PM: Kapselband-verletzungen des Sprunggelenkes. Forschr Med 95:1599-1605, 1977.
12. Goldstein IA: Tear of the lateral ligament of the ankle. New York State J Med 48:199-201, 1948.
13. Rettine KA, Morrey BF: Osteochondral fractures of the talus. J Bone Joint Surg 69Bl:89-92, 1987.
14. Zingher E, Gianella G, Vogt B: Spatfolgen und invaliditat bei bandverletzungen der Sprunggelenke. Zeitschrift fur Unfallmedizin und Berufskrankheit 74:91-95, 1981.

CHAPTER 62

Hip Range of Motion: A Comparison Between Ballerinas and Non-Dancers

Lynne A. LiGreci-Mangini

INTRODUCTION

The five basic positions of ballet require that the hip joints be externally rotated to maintain the alignment referred to as *turnout*. In order for this movement to be considered correct from a technical as well as mechanical standpoint, the rotation should originate at the hips.[1, 2] Range of motion of the hip joint is naturally limited by ligaments, soft tissue, and bony configuration.[3-6] The dancer whose external rotation is limited by these anatomical considerations must compensate to attain the correct ballet posture.[7,8] These compensations have been cited as a causative factor leading to the high incidence of injury to the back, knees, and feet.[9-15] This evidently occurs because of the habitual pattern of the dancer to force the motion lacking at the hips through other joints in the kinetic chain.[1, 8, 12, 16, 17]

The main purpose of this study was to describe and compare the hip range of motion of professional ballerinas and non-dancers. It was also hoped that by comparing two age- and sex-matched groups, conclusions could be made as to whether the differences in range of motion between the groups resulted from training or innate hypermobility.

MATERIALS AND METHODS

The subjects for this study included 15 female New York City Ballet Company dancers and 15 female physical-therapy students. They were age-matched, with a mean age of 24.4 ± 4.45 years for the dancers, and 24.4 ± 2.64 years for the non-dancers. The dancers averaged 15.66 ± 4.97 years of dance training, and 5.9 ± 4.41 years of professional dance experience. The non-dancers were accepted as participants only if they had never had any dance or gymnastic training. All of the subjects tested were in a non-warmed physiological state as defined by no

exercising, dancing, or stretching for at least one hour prior to testing. All subjects read and signed a consent form approved by the Institutional Review Board at Touro College prior to being measured. The subjects also completed a brief questionnaire pertaining to their dance experience, and their injury profile. The questions were designed to screen individuals not suited for the study because of hip, knee, or back pain that could limit their natural end range of hip movements.

Two standard goniometers, one plastic 18", and one metal 21" locking type, were used for the purpose of measuring hip range of motion. A Skan-a-Graf@ (Reedco Research, Auburn, N.Y.) and carpenter's level were used to ensure a vertical plumb line when measuring hip rotations. The measurements were performed on a portable treatment table, and a stabilization strap was used when measuring in the prone position. One examiner performed all measurements to prevent inter-tester error, as intra-tester reliability has been found to be higher than inter-tester reliability.[18-21] Hip joint measurements were performed according to the guidelines of the American Academy of Orthopaedic Surgeons, and standard orthopaedic texts.[22, 23] All measurements were performed bilaterally, at the passive end range of the motion being tested. Measurements were performed in the following sequence:

Subject supine:

1. Hip flexion with the contralateral leg extended (R/LFLEXCE).

2. Hip flexion with the contralateral leg flexed (RILFLEXCF).

3. Hip abduction with the legs neutral (R/LABDN).

4. Hip abduction with the legs in external rotation or turnout (R/LABDT).

5. Hip adduction (R/LADD).

Subject prone:
> 6. ip extension (R/LEXTN).
> 7. ip internal rotation (R/LIRP).
> 8. Hip external rotation (R/LERP).

Subject sitting:
> 9. Hip internal rotation (R/LIRSIT).
> 10. Hip external rotation (R/LERSIT).

The collected data were then entered into the SPSS/ PC+ statistical computer software system and a one-way analysis of variance (ANOVA) between the two groups was performed for each variable. Statistical significance was indicated by a probability quotient less than 0.001 ($p < 0.001$). The mean range of motion and the standard deviation from the mean for each variable were also calculated using the SPSS/PC+ system.

RESULTS

The hip range of motions determined in this study are presented in Tables I and II. The information collected was separated by group, and the means and standard deviations for each motion measured are presented. The average range of motion for each parameter for both groups combined are also presented in Tables I and II. The right and left hips were analyzed as separate entities, with the right hip being presented in Table I and the left hip in Table II. Graphical representation of Tables I and II are shown in Figures 1 and 2, respectively.

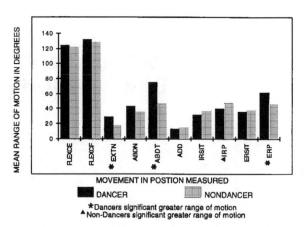

Figure 1: Right hip range of motion comparison.

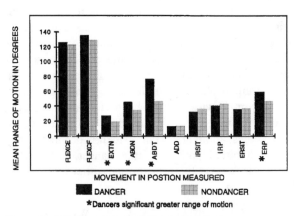

Figure 2: Left hip range of motion comparison.

Table III presents the results of the one-way analysis of variance between the two groups. Significant differences at the 0.001 confidence level were found in the following measurements: right and left hip extension, right and left hip abduction in turnout, left hip abduction in neutral, right and left hip external rotation in prone, and right hip internal rotation in prone.

No significant differences at the 0.001 confidence level were found in right and left hip flexion with either the contralateral leg flexed or extended, right hip abduction in neutral, right and left hip adduction, right and left hip internal rotation in sitting, left hip internal rotation in prone, and right and left hip external rotation in sitting. The dancers had the greater range of motion in all values of significance except for right hip internal rotation in prone. Non-dancers showed a greater range in the latter.

TABLE I						
Mean Range of Motion						
RIGHT MOVEMENT IN POSITION MEAUSRED	BALLERINA'S RANGE OF MOTION IN DEGREES		NONDANCER'S RANGE OF MOTION IN DEGREES		AVERAGE RANGE OF MOTION FOR BOTH GROUPS	
	MEAN	S.D. ±	MEAN	S.D. ±	MEAN	S.D. ±
RFLEXCE	124	±5.0	121	7.1	122	±6.0
RFLEXCF	132	5.2	128	6.9	130	6.5
REXTN	28	5.1	18	3.3	23	6.3
RABDN	43	6.3	35	5.5	39	7.0
RABDT	75	10.1	45	4.4	60	17.1
RADD	12	3.1	14	3.5	13	3.3
RIRSIT	31	6.1	37	5.7	34	6.4
RIRP	39	6.2	47	5.3	43	7.0
RERSIT	35	4.6	37	4.0	36	4.3
RERP	61	6.1	45	5.5	53	10.1

TABLE II						
Mean Range of Motion						
LEFT MOVEMENT IN POSITION MEAUSRED	BALLERINA'S RANGE OF MOTION IN DEGREES		NONDANCER'S RANGE OF MOTION IN DEGREES		AVERAGE RANGE OF MOTION FOR BOTH GROUPS	
	MEAN	S.D. ±	MEAN	S.D. ±	MEAN	S.D. ±
LFLEXCE	126	±6.0	122	8.8	124	±6.5
LFLEXCF	135	5.2	129	8.4	132	8.3
LEXTN	27	4.0	18	4.6	22	5.4
LABDN	45	6.4	35	7.0	40	8.3
LABDT	77	10.5	46	8.0	61	18.1
LADD	12	3.4	14	4.3	13	4.0
LIRSIT	32	6.1	36	5.8	34	6.1
LIRP	40	7.3	44	3.7	42	6.1
LERSIT	35	4.9	37	5.4	36	5.1
LERP	59	4.8	46	5.2	53	8.3

TABLE III

ONEWAY ANALYSIS OF VARIANCE (ANOVA)

VARIABLE	$F_{1, 28}$ RATIO	F PROBABILITY
RFLEXCE	1.4913	0.2322
RFLEXCF	4.3784	0.0456
REXTN	42.1953	*0.0000
RABDN	12.5358	0.0014
RABDT	118.9577	*0.0000
RADD	3.6951	0.0648
RIRSIT	8.1588	0.0080
RIRP	13.8764	*0.0009
RERSIT	1.5184	0.2281
RERP	55.7074	*0.0000
LFLEXCE	3.4115	0.0753
LFLEXCF	6.4988	0.0166
LEXTN	37.1800	*0.0000
LABDN	16.8287	*0.0003
LABDT	101.5763	*0.0000
LADD	3.3746	0.0768
LIRSIT	3.0133	0.0936
LIRP	3.1463	0.0870
LERSIT	0.5532	0.4632
LERP	52.1925	*0.0000

* Significance $p < 0.001$

DISCUSSION

An often debated question is whether joint flexibility is acquired through training or is inherited. The results of this study suggest that the greater range of hip motion exhibited by the dancers was more the result of training than innate hypermobility. This is because of the significantly greater range of motion the dancers possessed in hip extension, abduction and external rotation, the motions most commonly associated with ballet technique.[1, 2] This reasoning does not rule out, however, the possibility that ballet self-selects these traits rather than endows them. In order to safely suggest training as a self-inclusive factor, hip range of motion measurements would have to be taken of the dancers in their early training years.

Even so, if the greater range of motion exhibited by the dancers was merely the result of hereditary hypermobility, then dancers would be expected to have a significantly greater range of motion in most or all movements measured. This summation is consistent with the findings of several authors.[24-28] It contradicts the findings of a study which concluded that ballet dancers had a higher incidence of hypermobility than non-dancers because they exhibited increased mobility in joints that were not the object of training.[29]

The dancers exhibited no significantly different degree of hip internal and external rotation in the sitting position, whereas hip external rotation was significantly greater in dancers in the prone position and hip internal rotation was significantly greater in

the non-dancers on the right side in the prone position. These findings were consistent with those of Jacobs and Young,[30] who also found significant differences in external rotation in dancers with the hip extended, but no differences in the sitting position when the hip was flexed. Kravitz et al.[11] and Kapandji[31] offer the explanation that when the hip is flexed, the anterior ligaments slacken so that the osseous limitations of movements are evident. Thus normal hip biomechanics would dictate that there be more movement in the flexed position.[4, 6, 31, 32] This was not the case with the dancers, where the prone position (hip extended) afforded a greater range of external rotation. This could indicate that the dancers ligamentous laxity from training allows a greater range of external rotation where it would normally be limited by soft tissues, but that when they are tested in a position where actual osseous anatomy dictates motion, they have the same degree of motion as their non-dancing counterparts.

Hip adduction did not show significant differences between the two groups. This result is inconsistent with Reid et al.[28] who found that the dancers had significantly less adduction than the comparison group, but is in agreement with the findings of Micheli et al.[33]

Hip internal rotation was found to be significantly less for the dancers in the right hip prone. This absence of bilateral pattern makes it difficult to determine whether femoral retroversion was present in the dancers studied. If femoral retroversion was a factor then increased external rotation would directly correlate to decreased internal rotation.[34-38] Though the dancers did have greater external rotation, decreased internal rotation was present only on the right. This may reflect a clinical tendency, since both Micheli et al.[33] and Miller[13] found no evidence of femoral retroversion in the dancers they studied.

A direct comparison of range of motion among this and other studies is difficult because testing positions and conditions were often varied. In general, hip flexion and internal rotation measurements were consistent with those reported by other authors,[28, 32, 39-42] except Svenningsen et. al.[43] and Johnston,[3] who both reported higher scores in the subjects they studied.

Hip adduction range was much smaller in this study as compared to others, and could be attributed to differences in measuring technique.[3, 22, 23, 31-33, 41, 43, 44] Hip internal and external rotation in sitting were generally consistent with other authors, while hip extension measurements were so varied between authors that direct comparison was not possible.[22,27,32,38,40,41,44]   Kushner et al.[45] measured hip abduction in 0°, 45°, 60°, 70°, 80°, 90° and maximal range of external rotation. The amount of abduction in turnout found in this study most closely resembled that found by Kushner et al.,[45] at 45° of external rotation. Abduction ranges, measured in neutral, were consistent with other studies[22, 31, 40, 41, 44]

CONCLUSIONS

Within the limitations of this study, the following conclusions were drawn:

1.   Professional ballerinas possessed a significantly greater range of hip motion than non-dancers in external rotation, abduction, and extension.

2.   There were no significant differences between ballerinas and female non-dancers in hip adduction and flexion range of motion.

3.   Hip rotations were found to be greater when measured with the hip extended than with the hip flexed to 90°.

4.   Flexibility in the ballet dancer appears to be influenced by training rather than innate hypermobility.

REFERENCES

1. Clippinger-Robertson K.: Biomechanical considerations in turnout. J Physical Education, Recreation and Dance 58(5):37-40, 1987.

2. Gelabert R: Turning out. Dance Magazine 51(2): 86-87, 1977.

3. Johnston RC: Mechanical considerations of the hip joint. Arch Surg 107:411-417, 1973.

4. Matles AL: Motions of the hip hoint. Bulletin of the Hospital for Joint Diseases 36(2):170-176, 1975.

5. Radin EL: Biomecahanics of the human hip. Clin Orthop Rel Res 152:28-34, 1980.

6. Singleton MC, LeVeau BF: The hip joint: Structure, stability, and stress. Phys Therapy 55(9):957-973,1975.

7. Fry RM: Dance and orthopaedics. Orthop Review 12(11):49-56, 1983.

8. Howse AJG, Silver D: L.A. dance clinic: Hip problems. Dance Magazine 59(5):99, 1985.

9. Andersson S, Nilsson B, Hessel T, Saraste M, Noren A, Stevens-Andersson A, Rydholm D: Degenerative joint disease in ballet dancers. Clin Orthop Rel Res 238: 233-236, 1989.

10. Ende LS, Wickstrom J: Ballet injuries. The Physician and Sports Med 10(7):101-108, 1982.

11. Kravitz SR, Huber S, Ruziskey JA, Murgia CJ: Biomechanical analysis of maximal pedal stress during ballet stance. J Amer Pod Med Assoc 77(9):484-489, 1987.

12. Micheli LJ: Prevention of dance injuries. In Cantu R, Gillespie J, Sports Science: Bridging the Gap, 137-141. Lexington, MA: Collamore Press, 1982.

13. Miller EH, Schneider HJ, Bronson JL, McLain D: A new consideration in athletic injuries: The classical ballet dancer. Clin Orthop Rel Res 111: 181-191, 1975.

14. Quirk R: Injuries in classical ballet. Australian Family Physician 13(11):802-804, 1984.

15. Washington EL: Musculoskeletal injuries in theatrical dancers: Site, frequency, and severity. Amer J Sports Med 6(2):75-98,1975.

16. Reid DC: Preventing injuries to the young ballet dancer. Physiotherapy Canada 39(4):231-236, 1987.

17. Ryan AJ, Stephens RE: Dance Medicine: A Comprehensive Guide (1st ed), 115-116. Chicago, IL: Pluribus Press, 1987.

18. Boone DC, Azen SP, Lin CM, Spence C, Baron, C, Lee L: Reliability of goniometric measurements. Phys Therapy 58(11):1355-1360, 1978.

19. Ekstrand J, Wiktorsson M, Oberg B, Gillquist J: Lower extermity goniometric measurements: A study to determine their reliability. Arch Phys Med Rehabil 63:171-175,1982.

20. Mayerson NH, Milano RA: Goniometric measurement reliability in physical medicine. Arch Phys Med Rehabil 65:92-94, 1984.

21. Mitchell WS, Millar J, Surrock RD: An evaluation of goniometry as an objective parameter for measuring joint motion. Scottish Med J 20:57-59, 1975.

22. American Academy of Orthopaedic Surgeons: Joint Motion: Method of Measuring and Recording, 56-65. New York: Churchill Livingstone, 1965.

23. Norkin CC, White DJ: Measurement of Joint Motion: A Guide to Goniomety (3rd ed), 76-87. Philadelphia, PA: FA Davis Co, 1986.

24. Claessens A: Body structure, somatotype, maturation and motor performance. J Sports Med 27:312-317, 1987.

25. Klemp P, Learmonth ID: Hypermobility and injuries in a professional ballet company. Br J Sports Med 18(3):143-148, 1984.

26. Klemp P, Stevens JE, Isaacs S: A hypermobility study in ballet dancers. J Rheumatol 11(5): 692-696, 1984.

27. Nelson JK, Johnson BL, Smith GC: Physical characteristics, hip flexibility, and arm strength of female gymnasts classified by intensity of training across three age levels. J Sports Med 23:95-101, 1983.

28. Reid DC, Burnham RS, Saboe LA, Kushner SF: Lower extremity flexibility patterns in classical ballet dancers and their correlation to lateral hip and knee injuries. Amer J Sports Med 15(4): 347-352, 1987.

29. Grahame R, Jenkins JM: Joint mobility: Asset or liability? A study of joint mobility in ballet dancers. Ann Rheum Diseases 31:109-111, 1972.

30. Jacobs M, Young R: Snapping hip phenomenon among dancers. Amer Corrective Therapy J 32(3): 92-97, 1978.

31. Kapandji IA: The Physiology of the Joints: Vol II Lower Limb (2nd ed), 12-21. New York: Churchill Livingston, 1971.

32. Ellis MI, Stowe J: The Hip. Clin Rheumatic Diseases 8(3):655-675, 1982.

33. Micheli LJ, Gillespie WJ, Walaszek A: Physiologic profiles of female professional ballerinas. Clin Sports Med 3(1):199-209, 1984.

34. Fabry G, MacEwen GD, Shands AR: Torsion of the femur. J Bone Joint Surg 55A(8):1726-1738, 1973.

35. Giladi M, Milgrom C, Stein M, Kashtan H, Margulies J, Chisin R, Steinberg R, Kedem R, Aharonson Z, Simkin A: External rotation of the hip: A predictor of risk for stress fractures. Clin Orthop Rel Res 216:131-134, 1987.

36. McSweeny A: A study of femoral torsion in children. J Bone Joint Surg 53B(1):90-95, 1971.

37. Merrifield HH: Influence of gait patterns on hip rotation and foot deviation. J Amer Pod Assoc 60(9):345-351, 1970.

38. Staheli LT, Corbett BS, Wyss C, King H: Lower extremity rotational problems in children. J Bone Joint Surg 67A(1):39-47, 1985.

39. Ahlback S, Lindahl O: Sagittal mobility of the hip joint. Acta Orthop Scand 34:310-322, 1964.

40. Allander E, Bjornsson OJ, Olafsson O, Sigfusson N, Thorsteinsson J: Normal range of joint movements in shoulder, hip, wrist and thumb with special reference to side: A comparison between two populations. Int J Epidemiology 3(3):253-261, 1974.

41. Boone DC, Azen SP: Normal range of motion of joints in male subjects. J Bone Joint Surg 61A(5):756-759, 1979.

42. Troup JDG, Hood CA, Chapman AE: Measurements of the sagittal mobility of the lumbar spine and hips. Ann Phys Med 9(8): 308-321, 1968.

43. Svenningsen S, Terjesen T, Auflem M, Berg V: Hip motion related to age and xex. Acta Orthop Scand 60(1):97-100, 1989.

44. Roaas A, Andersson BJ: Normal range of motion of the hip, knee and ankle joints in male subjects, 30-40 years of age. Acta Orthop Scand 53:205-208, 1982.

45. Kushner S, Saboe L, Reid D, Penrose T, Grace M: Relationship of turnout to hip abduction in professional ballet dancers. Amer J Sports Med 18(3):286-291, 1990.

CHAPTER 63

Dancers' Professional Training
for Prevention of Tissue Wear and Tear

Marguerite Papadimitriou-Boulenger

In Greece, any graduate dancer has the right to open a school and teach dancing. Our concern is whether he or she has the proficiency for such an important responsibility — not only from the artistic perspective, but also from the physiologic and anatomic perspectives. In other words, does the teacher have sufficient knowledge of the human body, its different stages of growth, and its possible malformations so as to be able to recognize warning signs that an adolescent's body might display while dancing?

As osteopaths, we often see in our practice the injuries which occur to both student dancers and professional dancers. Our observations focus on accidents and problems resulting from ignorance and incorrect performance of the body. Consequently, at school, the aim is to teach, in a practical way, how to avoid tissue injuries to the student's body and, in the event he or she becomes a teacher, to those of his/her pupils.

GLOBAL APPROACH TO
THE HUMAN BODY

We consider the body from a *global* approach, following the principles of osteopathic medicine. This approach was first developed by Dr Andrew Taylor Still[1] a century ago. "The structure rules the function," said Dr. Still. The skeletal formation of the body is the determining factor of good or bad functioning of a dancer's body in his professional life. Moreover, the dance teacher is responsible for the correct formation of the skeleton of the child attending his lessons.

In the application of these principles, we note that the body is able to meet the great requirements and techniques of artistic dancing only if it is free from stress and its physiology and mechanism are well perceived.

TISSUE-WEAR PREVENTION PROGRAM

At the Greek State School of Dance, the dancer's professional training program in this field is carried out on two levels:

1. Each applicant undergoes an *osteopathic and kinesiologic examination.* Following our observations, if required, further exams by an orthopedist, psychologist, general practitioner, etc., are suggested.

2. A course is offered on *basic principles of anatomy and physiology,* adapted to the dancer's art. The lectures aim to provide a local anatomical insight within a global anatomical concept. They cover osseous anatomy, articular anatomy, and muscular and visceral anatomy. We teach how to evaluate the contraction and tonus of a muscle, and explain the shapes of the bones according to the tensions they are subject to (muscles, ligaments, aponeuroses, articulations. The student is given the opportunity to study x-rays in order to understand his skeleton, particularly if there is a specific problem. The idea is not to give a medical diagnosis, but to understand the positioning of the skeleton and explain possible muscular tensions applied to the skeleton.

AN EXCEPTIONAL TOOL:
BODY SCHEMES AND MUSCULAR CHAINS

The student then gets acquainted with the outstanding studies of the Belgian osteopath Godelieve Struyf-Denys on *Body Schemes* and *Muscular Chains.* These concepts contribute to the understanding of the body's musculoskeletal structure. They are used to teach anatomy in its dynamic functions in order to show the difficulties of movements. The teaching of functional anatomy allows a physiological approach for the preparation of the dancer's body so that he can meet the requirements of choreographic art and technique. We consider that the prime factor is to obtain elasticity of the tissues, which, in turn, is the determining factor in the absorption of tensions, shocks and extreme movements required of the dancer.

We proceed from the principle that everything moves in the human body, and try to have the student understand and feel this in his own body. The student must see and feel the correspondence between his movement and the joints in motion, and simultaneously insert this movement in the basic body scheme. This leads to understanding how, in order to avoid tissue damage, the dancer must master the antigravity forces the body develops in each position. It further leads to the notion of the interrelation between the functioning of a joint and the working of the surrounding tissues such as ligaments, aponeuroses, muscles, etc.

The dancer must learn how to free and release each part of the body at each instant. He must be able to feel the difference between the state of contraction and the relaxation of his musculoskeletal chains. He must learn how to feel the excesses which spread and settle through the following mechanism.

A bone lever on which is inserted a taut muscle changes its position, and other muscles, which are inserted directly or by an aponeurosis on this same bone lever, are liable to be stretched and react to this stimulation. This, in turn, entails the moving of other segments and the stretching of muscular structures, thus forming a chain of tensions which will influence the whole static of the affected individual.

Therefore, this mechanism determines in a successive way a musculoaponeurotic chain and shifting of joints, which we designate by the words 'articular sequence.'

This process, which progresses gradually through a group of muscles, determines in a way tensional bands which appear on the body, from head to toe, or, inversely, from bottom to top, forming longitudinal structures losing gradually their elasticity.[2]

Indeed, a problem or a situation in the locomotor system never remains isolated, but concerns the whole body. Thus, we gradually determine the *physiological* muscular chains which are shaped according to the characteristics of the student's body type, as well as the vicious musculoaponeurotic chains which take form due to the hurtful tensions to which the professional dancer is exposed in his work. These hurtful contractions eventually will influence his physiology, his psyche, and his behavior, and possibly result in irreparable damage such as osteophytes, for example.

THE AXES OF THE BODY

We consider the human body as moving according to two fundamental axes (Fig. 1):

☐   The *vertical* axis, which is made up by the interrelation between the spine joints and the surrounding muscles. This is the basic axis, a functional unit incorporating the trunk and the head.

☐   The *horizontal* axis, or intercourse axis, which is made up by the functional units of the four members. On this axis depend our intercourse activities and our contacts with the surrounding world. Each member determines an articular chain from the shoulders to the phalanges of the fingers and from the hips to the phalanges of the toes.

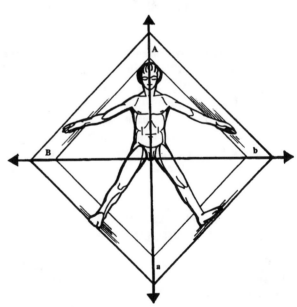

Figure 1:   *Vertical axis of the human body; the functional unit trunk plus head.*

Around these two main axes, the physiological spiral movements take form and combine in order to coordinate and form a *synchronous* action between a muscular chain and an articular chain. The joints are interdependent and constitute a mechanical unit. This suggests that the shape of the articular surfaces and the arrangement of the muscles help the twist of the osseous segments in their mutual relationship within a joint during their movement. This spiral movement generates a tension which forms the *structure* and the *shape* of the osseous segment (Fig. 2).

The foundations of the anatomical assessment of a dancer are based on the above analysis, helping us understand the way the human body works. It is a tool that enables one to feel how to liberate one's own body and use the resources of one's structures. In this way, we hope, the body will be best protected from the strong requirements of the dancer's art.

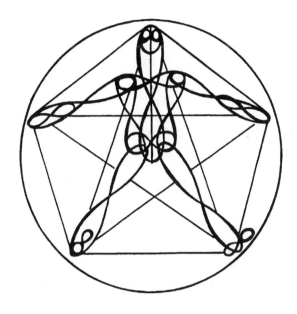

Figure 2: *The spiral movement is used physiologically to bind the muscular chains around or the articular chain in a synchronous action. Diagram drawn from an illustration characterizing the book* La Coordination Motrice *(The Motory Coordination).*[3]

REFERENCES

1. Andrew Taylor Still, 1828-1917. Considered as the founder of the osteopathic medicine. Founded a school in 1892 in Kirksville, Missouri.
2. Struyf-Denys G: Introduction à la Méthode des Chaînes GDS, 10-11. Brussels, Belgium: Institut des Chaînes Musculaires et des lechniques GDS, 1984.
3. Piret S, Béziers MM: La Coordination Motrice. Masson & Cie, 1971.

SUGGESTED READING

1. Struyf-Denys G: Les Chaînes musculaires et articulaires. Société Belge d'Ostéopathie et de Recherche en Thérapie Manuelle, Brussels, Belgium, 1978.
2. Clauzade MA, Darraillans B: Concept ostéopathique de l'Occlusion. Perpignan, France: SEOO, 1989.

CHAPTER 64

Short Gastrocnemius Syndrome

Casimir M. Kowalski

It is necessary, not in only in sports or artistic activities, but also in daily life, to be able to perform about 15° of ankle dorsiflexion, without needing any compensation at the subtalar joint level.

In a series of 2,000 feet, seen by the author, loss of dorsiflexion occurred, with the knee extended, in 40%, suggesting the presence of too short a gastrocnemius muscle.

In order to compensate for this dorsiflexion lag, a torsion movement occurs in the subtalar joint, bringing the foot into maximal eversion and the heel into pronation, in order to allow the upright standing position.

This situation can mainly be observed around puberty. During the growth spurt, the gastrocnemius muscles, which are white muscles with reserve potential, are not solicited during gait, and therefore do not go proportionally to other leg tissues. Thus, the child can present a short gastrocnemius syndrome over a period of one year, sometimes even less.

Children age 8 to 10 years who were diagnosed with short gastrocnemius muscles and flat feet, in absence of therapy, still have short gastrocnemii, but develop cavus feet at the lateral border one year later. A short gastrocnemius and a calcaneus deformity compensating for pronation are the the the only common features between these two foot deformities: In the flat foot phase, there is a ligamentous weakness which strengthens at puberty, leading to the cavus deformity.

One can then hypothesize that a short gastrocnemius is the cause of the common flat foot (*pes valgus planus supinatus*), and the valgus cavus foot (*pes valgus cavus*).

The external valgus cavus foot, or its clinical variants, occur in a much larger proportion than the common flat foot in early childhood. It is the most frequent and pathognomonic clinical expression of short gastrocnemius syndrome. It is characterized by a valgus heel and a medial submalleolar protrusion (Fig. 1).

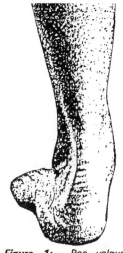

Figure 1: *Pes valgus cavus.*

Finally, valgus cavus foot is also accompanied by a *skiff* great toe. The calcaneus valgus drags the center of gravity medially causing a great-toe reaction to maintain balance by the reflex activity of the intrinsic sole muscles. This puts the great toe into a *skiff* position (proximal phalanx in flexion, distal in extension), increasing stress at the metatarsophalangeal joint, potentially causing a hallux rigidus (Fig. 2).

COMPLICATIONS

The pathological consequences of the short gastrocnemius syndrome are seen both at the foot level and proximally in the lower extremity:

■ calf pain secondary to excessive effort in children who may be considered as bad walkers or even lazy;
■ Achilles tenosynovitis and calcaneal apophysitis in teenagers;
■ intrinsic sole muscles tenosynovitis, at their os calcis insertion (calcaneal spur);
■ metatarsalgia, most constant symptom;
■ ankle sprains;
■ hallux rigidus;
■ fatigue fracture of the lower third of the fibula, due to valgus overload;
■ squinting patellae secondary to valgus cavus foot;
■ hyperlordosis, secondary to lower limb internal rotation, with possible facet syndrome and kissing spine, arrow-headed L1 vertebra (mainly in cases of slow growth), and fatigue fracture of the lumbosacral pars interarticularis.

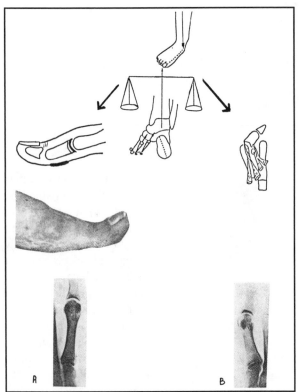

Figure 2: *Complications of the short gastrocnemius syndrome. A, skiff great toe; B, hallux valgus.*

TREATMENT

Surgical stretching of the gastrocnemius, by the Vulpius technique, is now abandonned in favor of phyiotherapy. This consists of proprioceptive exercises in the sagittal plane, on a Freeman platform, for a two-month period, in thirty-minute sessions, three times a week. The gastrocnemius muscle can be stretched this way at any age, except in spastics.

The calf cramps, sometimes nocturnal, which used to occur after sports or artistic activities, gradually disappear. Physical performances such as jumping or running are improved. A maintenance treatment program is necessary through the growth spurt.

SUGGESTED READING

1. De Doncker E, Kowalski C: Le pied normal et pathologique. Acta Medica Belgica, 183, 1970.
2. De Doncker, E, Kowalski C: Kinésiologie et rééducation du pied. Paris: Masson, 1979.
3. Kowalski C: Biomécanique du pied. VIIIème journées de rééducation, IFCS, 13-34. Bordeaux: Pellegrin, 1985.

CHAPTER 65

Occupational Disorders of Dancers

Fadi J. Bejjani

EPIDEMIOLOGY

Patterns of injury in dance, particularly in ballet, tend to be related to age and skill, with knee or hip problems more characteristic of the young and novice, and leg, ankle and foot problems more frequently encountered in the older or professional dancer. There are, however, many exceptions to this rule. Back injuries, for example, may occur at any age or level of skill. They occur in both male and female dancers with a somewhat higher prevalence in the former.[1] Because male dancers are taller and heavier than their female counterparts and leap higher, osteoarthritis of the hip can be a significant problem for the dancer in his fourth or fifth decade. These factors contribute to making the male dancer retire about ten years earlier than the female. The man's career is also made shorter by a later start (about age 16) than that of the woman (about age 6). Ongoing studies on aging dancers (mean age 56), performed at the Corps de Ballet in Oslo, Stockholm, Gothenburg and Malmo, are showing a much higher incidence of first metatarsophalangeal joint (MTP), hip, and knee osteoarthrosis in this group than in the general population.

The career of a ballet dancer, male or female, can end even much sooner. It is virtually impossible, for instance, to return to major dancing after an Achilles tendon rupture. A progressing hallux rigidus spells an end to a career, particularly if first MTP dorsiflexion is already less than 45° at about the age of 18. When a hallux valgus develops later in a dancer's life, no surgery should be undertaken before retirement. Any major operation — that is, a Keller arthroplasty — is not compatible with the continuation of a career as a dancer.

Musculoskeletal injuries represent 85% of ballet dancers' occupational diseases. The injury rate is 25% lower in female ballet dancers than in males. Over a 15-year period of experience with the Australian Ballet, Quirk reported an injury rate of about 3.5 per dancer, all ages included.

The most common hip, thigh, and groin injuries in dancers are clicking hip and iliopsoas tendinitis. Muscle strains constitute more than a third of all injuries. In dancers' lower extremities, hamstring strains top the list, along with calf muscle and foot intrinsics.

Among knee injuries, the most common are patellar chondromalacia, followed by jumper's knee, internal derangement, and subluxating patella. Meniscal tears are relatively rare. As far as leg injuries, calf muscle strains and shin splints are the most common. Shin splints of the lower leg are usually posteromedial in runners and anterolateral in dancers.

Among ankle injuries, sprains and Achilles tendinitis are the most common in dancers. In an early study, osteoarthrosis of the tibiotalar joint was observed in all ballet dancers who had been dancing for more than eight years. Posterior impingement syndrome and damage to the flexor hallucis longus are frequent. Flexor hallucis longus tendinitis is often mistaken for Achilles tendinitis. Partial as well as bilateral tears can be encountered.

Pathologic foot conditions are numerous. Deformities such as hallux valgus, hammer toes, and claw toes are most common. In a Bulgarian study, talonavicular arthrosis was found in 29% of ballet dancers, peritendinous calcium deposits in 25%, and various aseptic necroses of the foot in 14% of female dancers.

Although muscle (29%), tendon (17%), and ligament (15%) together account for 61% of all injuries in ballet dancers, stress fractures are also seen and account for 1.1% of all injuries. The most common sites for stress fractures in dancers are the femoral neck and the tibia. March and Jones fractures are uncommon in this population.

Spondylolysis is an intriguing pathologic entity in terms of occupational biomechanics.   Although its incidence ranges from 25% to 41% in certain ethnic groups such as Eskimos and Aino Japanese, its relationship to certain occupations is undeniable. The incidence in ballet dancers, for instance, is about four times (11%) the incidence in the general Caucasian population.

FUNCTIONAL ANATOMY AND KINEMATICS

In all five foot positions of ballet, the feet are turned out 180° to each other.   Turnout is the very foundation of ballet. Three major factors at the hip determine the external rotation possible for each dancer: anteversion angle, neck-shaft angle, and degree of tightness of the Y ligament of Bigelow. At age 8, femoral anteversion has reduced to about 15°, allowing for about 80° of external rotation at the hip. The child who is unable to externally rotate the hips beyond 45° should not plan to become a ballet dancer.   In the ideal turnout position, the weight should fall from the body to the thigh and directly through the center of rotation of the knee and ankle. Following the kinematic chain theory, this distribution of weight can be achieved only if external rotation of the lower extremities occurs at the hip.

Following the same theory, alignment of the toes without *breaking* at the MTPs, as a straight line through the ankle to the knee, provides the best support for pointe work. There also is more skeletal stability on pointe than on demi-pointe. Approximately 3 to 3½ years of dancing in ballet shoes (soft-toed dance slippers) is required to develop the strength, balance and style that permit a dancer to dance on pointe.   No child nowadays is permitted to dance on pointe until she is at least 11½ years old. Also, because the female pelvis is cylindrical and wider than the male pelvis, a slightly knock-kneed shape is not uncommon in young ballet students, and subluxation of the patella can occur.

Anatomic variations play an often overlooked but very important role in the etiology of injuries; that is, of muscle and tendon strains.   It is known, for instance, that a *peasant* foot, with a squared ankle, a sturdy arch, a broad forefoot, and the first three toes of nearly equal length, is best fit for dancing in toe shoes. On the other hand, a short first ray, whether the shortening is in the first metatarsal or the great toe itself, poses great problems with stability. If the first metatarsal is short, it is not effective for weight transmission, and the dancer must try to maintain stability over the second and third metatarsals. Sickling will occur if the weight is carried too medially in an attempt to get the first metatarsal head satisfactorily down to the ground, and damage will follow — sometimes as proximally as in the trunk.

MUSCULOSKELETAL CHANGES

Hypertrophic changes of the osseous system observed in the growing ballet dancer are most stable. These changes have been described by several Eastern European authors.   About 50% of ballet dancers show hypertrophy of the femur, tibia, and foot bones.   This figure goes up to 79% in another survey.   In the foot, these changes consist primarily of endosteal and periosteal hypertrophy in the second and third metatarsal diaphyses, with narrowing of the medullary canal.   A German study pointed out that unlike ballet dancers, modern dancers all presented flat feet, splay feet, and even hallux valgus.   This was thought to be related to the absence of forefoot support in the shoe, which does not occur in ballet.

FLEXIBILITY AND RANGE OF MOTION

Flexibility of the spine, hips and ankles is, of course, the hallmark of the ballet dancer, and the presence of hypermobility of these joints could be attributable, at least in part, to training. Training is not usually directed to hyperextending knees, elbows and fingers because this leads to unaesthetic postures which are carefully avoided by dancers. The presence of hypermobility in these joints, therefore, is likely to be hereditary rather than acquired.   In the same study, ballet students did show generalized joint hypermobility as compared to a control group of nurses.

Range-of-motion data on the spine and lower extremities, measured by regular goniometer, three-dimensional electromagnetic motion analyzer, Leighton flexometer, or two inclinometers, was compared among female ballet dancers, flamenco dancers, and a control group.   Ballerinas have the widest range of spine flexion-extension, and flamencas a slightly wider range of lateral bending. All ranges of hip and knee motion are wider in ballerinas. Ankle range of motion is wider in ballerinas and flamencas than in controls.   In over 100 dancers with plantar fascia strain and Achilles tendinitis, 60% lacked full ankle dorsiflexion in the first exercise at the barre, demiplié (bending the knee without moving the heel from the floor). Flamencas had a wider range of subtalar and first MTP motion than did controls.

BACK STRENGTH

Loads on the lumbosacral disc of male ballet dancers while lifting their female partners are considerable. They can reach a ratio of 15:1, with regard to the body weight of the lifted dancer. Besides these acute overexertions, dancing involves lighter but repetitive spinal loads due to posture or technique. These are particularly obvious in flamenco dancing.

KNEE STRENGTH

Development of inner thigh muscles and stretching of the hamstrings play an important role in lifting the body off the toes in pointe work. Failure to do so can cause hamstring strains. Strength imbalance in knee muscles has also been proposed as a leading cause of hamstring strains in athletes. A typical proportional ratio (hamstring/quadriceps) is thought to be 2:3.

In order to verify these theories, a comparative knee isokinetic study was performed. Data were compiled from the literature for athletes, ballet dancers, and a control group, and were collected with the Biodex dynamometer for flamenco dancers. In women, knee extension was strongest in athletes and weakest in non-athletes. Dancers fell in between, with flamenco dancers being stronger than ballerinas. Proportional flexion/extension ratios increased as the speed increased in all groups. They were slightly weaker for non-athletes.

In men, knee extension was strongest in athletes and at low speeds. A similar pattern was seen in knee flexion. Proportional ratios increased at higher speeds. Ballet dancers had the highest ratio at low speed.

At peak season, the relative strength ratio (quadriceps/body weight) is 98% for male ballet dancers and 70% for female dancers. Values for male dancers are comparable to male athletes, whereas female dancers are weaker than female athletes.

The balance ratio (right/left quadriceps) is usually close to 1 in athletes, ballet dancers, and flamenco dancers.

ANKLE STRENGTH

The strength required to dance on pointe in ballet makes maximum demands on all intrinsic and extrinsic foot and ankle muscles. Isokinetic ankle torques are, in general, much higher in plantarflexion than dorsiflexion. They are also much higher in men than in women and at lower speeds than at higher speeds. Female ballet dancers and female jumpers have comparable plantarflexion torques.

FLAMENCO DANCING

Using the electrodynogram and skin-mounted accelerometers, foot pressure as well as hip and knee vibrations were recorded in 10 female dancers after a thorough clinical evaluation. A health questionnaire was also distributed to 29 dancers.[1-3]

Foot-pressure and acceleration data reveal the unique percussive nature of the dance form. Some clinical findings such as calluses are related to pressure distribution. Urogenital disorders were unusually frequent in this population. These disorders, as well as the back and neck pain encountered, may be vibration-related. Indeed, the vibration frequencies measured were well within the resonance frequency range of the abdominal viscera and the spine. Nonetheless, the hip joint seems to absorb most of the impact during dancing.[4]

"Vibration-pressure" diagrams were obtained, plotting foot pressure in parallel with accelerometry data. A walking test displayed an obvious slow periodic pattern for all signals. In a relatively slow Allegria step and fast Escudero Redoble step, vibration-pressure relationships were not as clearly defined but highly reproducible in this format, making this a useful tool for evaluating a dancer's biomechanical behavior as well as the effect of floors and footwear on this behavior.

Isometric and isokinetic spinal torques were measured seated in the same group, using the Cybex II dynamometer.[4] Discrete spinal range of motion was also measured with an electromagnetic 3D motion analyzer and compared to the continuous range of motion during dancing. A larger-than-normal spinal extension range and larger isometric extension torques suggest an adaptation to the task. Sustained spinal position close to the functional limits during dancing backsteps such as Zambra may be responsible for the back symptoms reported.

PART V

DANCE THERAPY

CHAPTER 66

The Aesthetics of Healing:
Reflections on the Inner Dance

Miriam Roskin Berger • *Marcia B. Leventhal*

Throughout the history of humankind, dance movement has been as basic to our total well-being and survival as breathing. Dance, our expressive, physicalized action as celebration, preparation, and centering, was integrated into the fabric of our societies and into the very fabric of our alive, breathing cellular state.[1] Dance was, and is, a reflection of all human movement and its meaning. We acknowledge these sources often; so often that at times we may forget their deepest importance to us, and that these sources are connected to intrinsic human needs and aspirations which are also at the core of psychotherapeutic goals.

The artist's process and vision within a therapeutic relationship is a valid means to embody and elicit deep psycho-dynamic insight and resolution that connect to both a personal and universal aesthetic. The therapist, with this perspective, allows the intuitive, psychic, healing, creative internal forces to emerge, and trusts them to provide form and meaning to the transformational processes in therapy.

The world consists of many elements at all levels and dimensions of experience, and the process of creativity can be seen as combining old elements together in new ways. "A new painting, poem, scientific achievement or philosophical understanding increases the number of the ions visible in the ocean of the unknown."[2] Thus, the ocean of the unknown is always with us, and the creative process takes the elements in that ocean, renders them visible, and forms them in new ways. In therapy, the therapist facilitates the same process: seeing the elements, suggesting alternatives, helping to frame and reform the elements.

The whole unfolding of the therapeutic journey is a creative process for the client who, in essence, is developing a new sense of self. He is creating a new person, but not changing the old one totally; it is be-

ing expanded, transformed, transcended. That is the creative process. The human being is the work of art.

Dance as an art form has contributed several elements to dance as therapy beyond its expressive attributes. In performance, one goal is to achieve a balance between spontaneity and control. So it is, also, that a balance is sought within a psychotherapeutic context. No matter what the area of conflict or disturbance, the principles of psychotherapy mandate working towards the goal of developing one's autonomy, balanced within the context of realistic, daily life functioning.

Another element shared by both the art and the therapy processes is that of the blending of the experience of reality with that of the symbolic. One of the most powerful realities of the human condition occurs when feeling and the symbolic expression of this feeling find a match in the forming of the *felt thought* into the expression/reaction. There is a heightened moment of attunement, illumination and insight, and a deep sense of having achieved control of one's internal and external worlds. In dance, there is a unique possibility to achieve such a heightened state of perception. Through the body we have the opportunity to apprehend experience directly, utilizing all of our senses; ultimately organizing impression into perception and symbol. The body is simultaneously the working instrument and the symbol.[3]

The tendency of the human being in creating is to make order and form out of seemingly chaotic and disordered perceptual processes; this can be intensely manifested through dance movement. Within the dance, inherent in its basic tools and elements, exist the capacity to create, to shape, to illuminate patterns of expression and impression; patterns in the body, in space, and in time and rhythm. Behavior and feelings cannot be transformed without insight and understanding of the parameters of one's patterns of behavior, of existence. Dance movement offers a direct and immediate expression of our beliefs, attitudes, and our overall patterns of perception and organization. When patterns are apprehended they can be extended, shaped, and transformed. With force, time, space, and flow as available elements, range may be developed and enlarged, and thus the human being's condition developed and extended. Previous research has correlated range of movement expression to functional behavior; namely, the ability to cope and to make choices.[4]

A final element shared by the client in his therapeutic journey and the artist in his creative journey is that of performing in front of or for a *witness*, an audience — displaying one's journey of discovery in the presence of a significant other, a therapist. In either situation, the artist/client is communicating to and for an objective/subjective observer. Expectations by and of the witness differ, whether audience or therapist, thus the relationship of the artist 'working' or 'working through' also changes. Eventually, though, the energy bond of witness to performer (client to therapist) is decidedly shaped, experienced and expressed within the boundaries of this *holding environment*.

These shared elements of dance as art and as therapy illuminate other crucial core concepts: aesthetics and healing, matrix and pattern, and metaphor and the body as the basis of symbolic language.

The intuitive, creative, psychic, and healing powers of human beings are all contained in the same aspect of the human psyche. The aesthetic urge is also contained herein, and shares in the rational search within the psyche. Healing is an integrative, multidimensional bringing together of disparate, disowned parts of all aspects or qualities of the self. There is a bringing back into alignment, returning the psyche or the organism to harmony, balance, synchrony and attunement within itself.[1]

The aesthetic is a guiding concept which creates an imprint or a pattern, and eventually creates a longing in us to fulfill the dimensions of that pattern. The aesthetic experience is grounded in man's need to identify with the structural components of the natural laws and movement evident in the universe; to bring himself into harmony with the natural polarities of nature. The Greek concept is that reason, the logos, is nature steering all things from within. Man is not outside nature, but within it, and the aesthetic imperative is the link between intuition and rationality, and the primary channel back to the universal consciousness.

According to David Bohm, the physicist who has been investigating the mysteries of mind and behavior relative to the mysteries of the universe, there is no model which can be equal to the whole universe because the only thing equal to the whole universe *is* the whole universe; no one thought can grasp the whole, because thought itself is only a part, not the whole. He suggests that there is a whole coherent space/place concept, encompassing all matter and life, the "implicate order," out of which any current reality becomes shaped into the "explicate order."[5] Joseph Chilton Pearce, influenced by Bohm's thoughts, speaks of the power of an original matrix which affects us throughout our lives. Matrix, which means 'womb' and which becomes 'matter,' 'materiel,' 'mater,' and 'mother,' is a pattern we seek to model throughout our lives because of the power of the initial imprint. The three major characteristics of the womb, all contributing to survival and growth, are: a source of possibility, a source of energy to explore that possibility, and a safe place in which that exploration may be manifested.

To shift from the womb, or a matrix, is to be 'born of it' into another one. The nature of our growth is such that each matrix is larger and less constricting, or more abstract, less concrete than the previous one — each successive one encompasses more possibility and power.[6]

So, it appears that to seek a model is natural and even life-giving, but when we become blocked in our attempt to replicate, over and over, a model or imprint towards which we gravitate (dependent upon our initial experience), growth stops and dysfunction erupts.

How does dance movement contribute to a release from those patterns which prevent expansion and the discovery of new forms which are possibly more appropriate for our development? Can dance movement help us to move ever more freely into and of the implicate order and, if so, how does it support an apprehension of a larger vision of reality, and extensions of our soul-self?

The origin of all art is found in man's use of the elements and processes of nature to serve as a means of foreseeing the future and controlling one's fate. Man observed nature and its changes, and certain changes as signs or omens, and then imposed symbolic significance on these phenomena — divination. He then attempted to control the forces of external nature and his own internal forces by creating his own symbols graphically and through other concrete ways, including sound and movement. Religion and ritual arose from this journey, as did all art and science. And the root of all this extended symbolic language is the human body, and we can return to it, trusting it as the source of universal knowledge.

The steps beyond divination propelled humankind into the expanded realm of metaphor which could encompass larger schemata aimed at explaining, controlling and illuminating the world. Throughout all cultures, the various contents of all mythology and ritual are rooted in a universal human source of both spiritual and real experiences; manifested in balancing the ambiguities of space and time, separation and fusion, life and death.

This urge of man to form, to create patterns mirroring his existence, stems both from the emotional and biological need for harmony, and from the rational need for the imposition of order on existence.

The aesthetic experience emerges from participation in this source and structure. It moves toward a reorientation on a complex present reality in which each of the coordinates of orientation — time, place and person — bears an ambiguous aspect, reflecting the different ways in which the mind functions...the need to keep oriented in a fluid, expanding reality lies at the heart of aesthetic form. Or, to put it the other way around, the significance of aesthetic form is rooted in our biological nature.[7]

In dance therapy, the client and the therapist have direct access to both the individual and universal pool of motor imagery. On an individual level, movement impulse and action will release content and pattern from deep levels of consciousness, which will be performed and expressed once again on a motor level, releasing further kinetic memories. These symbolic forms and patterns experienced on the physical level, in the present, offer immediate information for the formulation of insight and further re-patterning. We hypothesize that certain essences within each movement experience will emerge which will be found to encompass a coherent whole — a coherent whole

in the sense of connected information forming a story and a pattern.

On a universal level, these core patterns and forms will also embrace human archetypes and themes of polarities beyond content. In the experience and the analysis of these pools of information, we also have direct access to the aesthetic impulse or imperative possible within each human being. This urge, as has been stated, is to experience and identify with the laws of nature and the universe and, in doing so, to balance our matrix of dualities and achieve a balanced fluidity. In this journey, the client and the therapist use the movement information to search for meaningful material. They then can mutually create, transforming this material from an implicitly aesthetic source into a fresh perspective, new feeling states, and realigned patterns of behavioral initiation.

This metaphorical, or even mythical, approach within a dance-movement experience is, in the life of an individual, a mature, evolved way of thought or perspective. It is an early scheme of approaching experience in the life of the human race, however, and allows us to return to the universal aesthetic imperative, or the *inner dance*.

REFERENCES

1. Leventhal MB: Healing through rhythm and movement. Keynote Speech, 10th Annual Body-Mind-Spirit Festival, London, England, May 1987.
2. Arieti S: Creativity, The Magic Synthesis, 5. New York: Basic Books, 1976.
3. Berger MR: Towards unity: The arts and creative arts therapies in rehabilitation and healing. International Conference on The Healing Role of the Arts, Rockefeller Center, Bellagio, Italy, 1984.
4. Hunt V: Movement Behavior, A Model for Action, Quest Monograph 2. Tucson, AZ: 1964.
5. Bohm D: Wholeness and the Implicate Order. London: Rutledge and Kegan Paul.
6. Pearce JC: The Bond of Power, 73-74. New York: EP Dutton, 1981.
7. Rose GJ: The Power of Form, 15. New York: International Universities Press, Inc, 1980.

CHAPTER 67

Moving Towards Health: Stages of Therapeutic Unfolding in Dance Movement

Marcia B. Leventhal

Dance movement causes subtle shifts of energy which may be understood through exploration of certain psychodynamic correlates, ancient healing practices, and certain of the newer paradigms affecting our understanding of consciousness and human behavior. Five discrete stages, or levels, of an unfolding process have been distinguished by the author, and serve to aid a client in reaching a more realized integrated potential. How this model of increased awareness fits into a scheme or context of dance as psychotherapy is the focus of this report. The connection dance has to the healing arts is discussed, in conjunction with the relationship dance has to ancient and modern traditions of change and transformation. Thus, the model presented examines dance as a creative art activity, as an ancient, basic, healing model, and as an important therapeutic modality in its current form.

The concept of *unfolding* is used in the context of simultaneously enlarging and deepening a perceptual frame of reference.[1] Each of the stages discussed moves sequentially towards increasing complexity of clients' involvement, and each allows clients to build and to extend their changing views of themselves and their environment.

Though it might be assumed that any or all movement expression of an individual is an authentic moment of self-revelation or discourse, and could therefore be considered *authentic* (as is the current practice of teaching individuals to explore authentic movement as an end in itself in many U.S.A.-based workshops), not all movement expression will support us in our growth and subsequent change. We must go beyond the authentic expressive action/ movement/dance to a place where decision, forming, and clear expression are at the forefront. In this model, finding the authentic moment of expression provides the foundation for building an extended reality or boundary for the client. Selecting and/or creating the movement frames or experiences that can support the individual to grow, to gain insight, to move towards a greater sense of self and individuation, involves a process beyond mere spontaneous expression or an initial felt-level exploration.

Dance-movement events have the potential to alter an individual's perceptual frame of reference, thereby allowing maladaptive patterns to be released and new behavior to be developed. The author supports the concept of dance movement as a primary psychotherapy, with the potential for allowing life's goals to be clarified, restrictive mind-sets to be released and more functional behavioral patterns accessed. Dance therapy is, at its most developed, a primary treatment modality. The trained dance-movement therapist may make interpretations and interventions and help to support the emerging aspects of the ego and the self. The nonverbal language shared between client and therapist develops from the expressive moving body of the individual coping or forming with the natural elements of movement and dance — namely, force, time, space, and flow. Methods and techniques unique to dance-therapy treatment can be and often are population-specific, serving to reach individuals engaged in the struggle towards clarity, self-sufficiency, and insight.

This model offers several levels and stages of participation from the point of view of the therapist as well as the client. It is a model which attempts to aid the client in deepening his or her own process of learning, creating, becoming, and unfolding. Each stage or level allows for a greater sense of mastery and increased control, encouraging a natural growth process to develop.

In order to appreciate the connection of this model with the field of psychotherapy in general and dance therapy specifically, a discussion of dance as a healing art is presented as prelude to the details of the model.

Dance, in its therapeutic and healing capacities, is one of the oldest forms of healing interventions and experiences known to humankind.   Century upon century, in ancient and pre-industrial cultures, the powers of ritualistic movement, trance excitation, and community exultation and release were forms generated and integrated into a culture's social organization. A survey of the dance-history literature points out how dance was integrally woven into the fabric of ancient society; that it both expressed and defined ritual/symbolic processes[2] and ceremonial life. "... dance was not diversion or entertainment, but was a serious part of living. Power was gained from the rhythmic interaction of sound and movement, from the collective expression of emotion, and the cooperating members of the group had a strength greater than any of the group."[3]

Throughout history, we have danced through life's joyous and painful transitions. Celebration, communication, and clarity are the descriptions we glean from our historical documentation. Through the reaching, running, embracing, and shaping of form in space, from the beating and the chanting and the stamping of expressive rhythm, expressive body movement was a basic communicative form shared by all individuals in their various societies.   "Dance metaphorically enacts and communicates status transformations in rites of passage, death ceremonies, curative and preventative rites."[4]

Though moving is the basis of all dance, not all movement is dance. Indeed, our popular, collective perceptions of dance imply an experience outside the boundaries of a particular form or style, such as ballet, folk, or jazz dance.   This basic dance is distinguished from stylized and representational replicas: "...the dance works to present an emotional concept, creating its own vocabulary in the process."[5]

Dance movement, the basic dance/expressive gesture, is the direct apprehension of experience through and by the senses. It is core in creating and sustaining the body image and all subsequent perceptual forming.[6] As a current psychotherapeutic modality, dance therapy involves the engagement of a client at a preverbal level, helping the client deal with issues long buried in the psyche, and possibly not available through the analytic, verbal, sequential mode of processing.

The use of the body in psychotherapy can probably trace its genesis to Freud's early discussion of the importance of body movement in the development of the ego. "The ego is first and foremost a body ego; it is not merely a surface entity, but it is itself the projection of a surface...the ego is ultimately derived from bodily sensations, chiefly from those springing from the surface of the body. It may thus be regarded as a mental projection of the surface of the body."[7]

Later supporters and developers of Freud's theories treated the body manifestations of feelings or unconscious processes as a tool to enhance or deepen the therapist-patient observation.[8-10] As various systems and models of the psychotherapies developed, individual elements of the personality's function emerged as key.[11-13]   Any or all of these therapeutic theories and methodologies help us understand and honor the importance of a dynamic, body-mind therapy, but none quite explains the fundamental essence of dance therapy.

Movement is life. In generating and supporting energy manifestation, individuals seemingly devoid of a conscious will to live re-experience the body's power and thus reconnect with their own sense of self. In dance movement, we begin to recognize space, shapes, size, weight, and contrasts through the first, direct experiences in the body. These are originally stimulated and facilitated by natural body movement in interaction with our environment, and with the forces of gravity. Expression and symbolic forming have a direct link to body movement because of the immediacy of the physical self. From an array of studies in kinesiology, physiology and anthropology, we have learned that dance-movement expression is basic to symbolic formation, creativity, communication, and learning. The tools are immediate, present, and always available, and are simply the macrocosm of the 'tools' available in all of nature in its purest state; before perception of form. That is, force (energy), time, space, and flow. These elements of dance movement are inherent in all of nature, thus in all of life and experience.[14]

Since all development proceeds through a complex chain of sensory-motoric organization, we are able within the dance-movement context to offer a safe place/space in which developmental exploration can be facilitated.   The *dance* helps to both uncover and own the enlarging pattern, and the *movement* helps to identify the primary exploration of self-discovery and awareness.

How, then, might dance combine with a more modern therapeutic model? There seem to be clear parallels between the functions described herein and some of the purposes of therapeutic intervention in general. The broad view places therapeutic intervention as a method serving a variety of human needs, mostly about making the unknown, or the unconscious, clearer. Psychotherapy, like dance, appears to facilitate a sense of self-help or responsibility for oneself, which entails an activation and recognition, at least, of the will, and a strengthening and developing of the ego.

Dance movement transcends pure exercise or pedestrian movement, for it blends rhythm, expression, and flow to help create a transforming experience for the individual in treatment. Being able to directly access patterned behavior and relate it to its concomitant body correlates is key in dance-therapy treatment and essential to this unfolding model. Since there is always a direct relationship between a client's psychodynamic issues and patterned movement responses, being able to work on the body manifestations often directly affects the daily-life issues.

It is not only that the body-mind-spiritual correlates interrelate, but that because early patterns of object relations and self-esteem are initially created through the nonverbal or body-based experiences, beginning probably in utero, the unfolding process offers us a means to access these patterns, evaluate them, decide what we need to release in order to achieve greater functioning, and extend our perceptual awareness, or our own levels of consciousness.

It is suggested that because we are surrounded by patterns, beginning to discern the common elements in these patterns of reaction and relationships helps us discover what we are repeating from habit. This in itself implies a possibility for change, as habits and patterns can be altered, expanded, dissolved. Patterns are inherently linked to growth and development, and we are biologically programmed to develop and grow according to a schedule, or pattern. We could probably say that most of our patterns are indeed our maps — maps which help us make sense of, relate to, and interact with our personal and collective environments. These patterns assist us in negotiating our daily lives, rituals of the mundane but necessary daily events, right through to more abstract life plan/goal-setting, dreaming, creating, etc.

The five-level model of therapeutic unfolding is a map which helps guide the therapist through each potential three-dimensional developmental stage of the client (whether presenting issues are manifest more on body, mind, or spiritual level). In utilizing the unfolding model, we are honoring and calling into service the elements of dance that are connected to the creative processes of the dance experience. Form is actually being facilitated so that gradually, the psyche is realigned with the expressive, natural, creative self. Forming as a concept appears to be fundamental to a comprehensive growth or healing model such as dance-movement therapy. "Form is present throughout nature, in all the forces of the universe, in all the stages of life. The laws which govern natural patterns are not arbitrary; they have a function — to keep life together — and they do so with supreme artistry, coordinating all of life and matter, from the simplest to the most complex."[15]

Healing and forming appear to be closely aligned, since healing per se seems to be an integrative, multidimensional joining of disparate, disowned parts of all aspects or qualities of the self. When there is disharmony, a lack of synchrony, an out-of-phase reaction or behavior, disease, illness, or dysfunction occurs. When consciousness is fragmented, it starts a war in the mind-body system.[16] Cancer has been characterized as unregulated, or out-of-phase, growth of cells in the body. In research in kinesics and nonverbal communication, a lack of synchrony between speech and gestures among various members in schizophrenic families was found.[17] Thus, healing must involve the whole person, in all of his or her complex dimensions. Understanding that we tend to form patterns which, in turn, give our lives shape, certainty, and boundaries, helps us place into perspective a therapy utilizing many systems of perception and expression simultaneously, such as dance-movement therapy.

This model allows the individual to extend his or her boundaries, while making actual decisions on the steps in the process. But since the structure comes from abstract expressive movement, and is still 'meaningless,' the import ordinarily associated with strong aspects of a personal pattern is not yet activated. Thus, the therapist and client are able to create a structure or form for the client as a more comprehensive or extended pattern of evolvement; the client can actually bypass restricting patterns and move into a possibly healthier self-space.

Listed below are five stages and their primary functions. Each stage utilizes a more developed ability of clients to choose, to cope, to draw upon and thus eliminate personally perceived, no-longer-functioning aspects of their patterns. Though the parameters of the unfolding, five-level sequence are concrete, the process remains accessible in the realms of abstract experiencing. Yet there is a clear and direct blending of psychodynamic principles with the creative-process elements most usually associated with dance movement. The name for each stage is at this point descriptive, and serves as a marker for the therapist in helping in the creation of an inviting, holding environment, enabling clients to be more readily stimulated towards their ability to choose, to direct, to express, and to re-form.

1. *Authentic movement.* This level is one of preparation, helping clients to focus inwardly and begin to uncover an inherent pulse/action stimulated by their current state of awareness. This is a time of warming up and heightened awareness of sensation, feelings, thoughts, kinesthetic-body, etc., and the client's associated resonating action.

2. *Expressive movement.* This is a time of uncovering patterned, concrete movement forms. In certain ways it is as if there were a stimulus (i.e. the initial awareness) to which the response is a 'coalesced action.' These are gestures with import, such as a stomp, a punch, a slash, a kick, etc.

3. *Unfolding movement.* This stage is one in which the client is urged to take exploration beyond the coalesced action, letting the expressive gesture lead her into a sensorium of possible explorations. This is a time of stream-of-movement consciousness and increasing readiness, where the client is immersed in ongoing, spontaneous, exploratory dance movement.

4. *Dance movement.* This is a time of heightened mastery, clarification of potential choices for action, and selecting new options for chosen behavior. The client is encouraged to build a phrase from his highlighted or foreground awareness of his previous expressive movement explorations. It is a time for deepening awareness and understanding of one's own particular style, aesthetic, trend, or theme. It is also a time of heightened creativity, where building the dance is encouraged from the elements uncovered during the previously less structured stages of exploration. 'Rehearsal' and 'performance' are encouraged, until the discovered dance moves the client on a 'felt' level.[2]

5. *Integrated movement.* This is the period in which the 'dance' formed in the fourth stage is further abstracted and distilled until what is expressed is a summary or essence of the longer initially formed experience. This final coalesced action becomes stimulus for verbal associations, and foundation for further exploration and dance-building. It serves as conclusion, leading towards insight and possible interpretation, and as stimulus to begin the entire process anew.

Each stage evolves and develops during the course of a client's treatment. The descriptions offered present an outline of key aspects of the stages, but in actuality, very rarely would the therapist use them as a formula or technique/map to elicit response. They serve instead as guideposts for helping a client move into deepening realms of exploration, hopefully moving beyond restricting body-mind patterns.

Beginning at a felt level of sensing and awareness, and working towards a final stage of selecting and forming, five discrete stages or levels can be distinguished. Each of the stages appears to support an individual in her ability to become released from patterned behavior, and move more easily into the experience of self. Further, at each of the stages there appears to be a direct body/mind/spirit correlate, offering insight, clarity, and meaning; thereby affecting the individual's understanding of boundaries, levels of consciousness, transformation, change, and healing. Each of the stages has clear parameters described via dance-movement-therapy concepts. Each stage can lead to a greater ability to discern one's own capacity to explore, eliminate, and rebuild towards a more appropriate life-goal mastery.

It has been posited that dance-movement therapy is a primary psychotherapy with potential for healing or integrating. Beyond mere spontaneous movement, clients are guided toward ever increased ability to express, create, and determine their future.

REFERENCES

1. Bohm D: Wholeness and the Implicate Order, 25. London: Ark Paperbacks, 1980.
2. Langer S: Feeling and Form. New York: Charles Scribner & Sons, 1953.
3. Ellfeldt L: Dance from Magic to Art, 38-39. London: Priory Press Ltd, 1973.
4. Hanna JL: To Dance Is Human, 112. Austin, TX/London: University of Texas Press, 1979.
5. Martin J: The Modern Dance, 8-9. New York: Dance Horizons, 1965. Originally published: AS Barnes & Co, 1933.

6. Leventhal M: Movement and Growth: Dance Therapy for the Special Child, 4. New York: New York University, 1980.

7. Freud S: The ego and the id. *In* Richmond J (ed), A General Selection from the Works of Sigmund Freud, 216. New York: Doubleday & Co, 1957. Originally published: 1923.

8. Reich W: Character Analysis. New York: Farrar, Strauss & Giroux, 1972.

9. Deutsch F: Analytic posturology. Psychoanalytic Quarterly 21:196-214, 1952.

10. Mittleman B: Motility in infants, children and adults: Patterns and psychodynamics. Psychoanalytic Study of the Child 9:142-177, 1954.

11. Mahler M: Thoughts about development and individuation. *In* The Psychoanalytic Study of the Child, Vol XVIII, 307-323. New York: International Universities Press, 1963.

12. Winnicott DW: Mother and Child, A Primer of First Relationships. New York: Basic Books, 1957.

13. Guntrip H: Schizoid Phenomena, Object Relations and the Self. New York: International Universities Press, 1969.

14. Leventhal M: The ancient healing art of dance. *In* Kinesis. Melbourne: Australian Association of Dance Education, 1987.

15. Blom L, Chaplin L: The Intimate Act of Choreography, 83. Pittsburgh, PA: University of Pittsburgh Press, 1982.

16. Chopra D: Quantum Healing, Exploring the Frontiers of Mind/Body Medicine. New York: Bantam Books, 1989.

17. Condon W: Linguistic-kinesic research and dance therapy. Proceedings, American Dance Therapy Association, 21-42, 1968.

CHAPTER 68

The Dance that Heals the Self

Kate T. Donohue • *Nurit Mussen*

Through the rhythms of our body, life is created. Our body and its rhythms are linked to our creativity and to the definition of our souls and self. It is through the body that we first learn to communicate our existence, what we want, who we want near us, who we are, and thus create our own unique world. Through gesture and body expression, we create and share our lives.[1] Developmentally, our body is our means of communicating the expression of self and our ability to create. Historically, preverbal communication was a necessity, for there were yet no words or language. In primitive tribal life, dance and bodily expression were the means to communicate with one's soul, with others, and with the gods and goddesses. Tribal dance was an expression of the whole person and was a means of affirming social and spiritual unity. It was an inextricable part of worship and prayer that "attempted to both structure and explaining life."[2] Shamans and healers used the body as a tool to express and heal the self and to commune with the spiritual and the creative in life. It is the first, most natural, and most immediate tool of our creative powers that assist healing, integration and transcendence.[2]

As primitive cultures moved away from nature, the healing arts and the spiritual became less integrated. The body and mind were split apart. In both the East and West, religion and philosophy separated the spirit from the body. The body and its rhythms were seen as evil, sinful, or to be transcended. Consequently, dance ceased to be a part of religious worship and healing.[1, 5] With the emergence of modern psychotherapies, thought and the mind were seen as portals to the unconscious, to the discovery of the self, and to healing. With these dual forces of religious belief and modern psychotherapy, the body and its rhythms and expression were no longer viewed as a means to express our natural creative and healing powers.[3] Yet, the mind-spirit-body cannot be divided into separate entities. Creative-arts therapists and those interested in creativity know that to express the self, all parts must be explored. Through the integration of the body, mind,

and spirit, there can come healing, definition, and development of the authentic, creative self.

Expressive-arts dance therapists feel that dance is a direct link to the self and is our most basic creative tool. Dance is a language that uses the "totality of body-mind-spirit to relate the most profound experiences, painful and joyous."[2] "The dance can cross the boundary and distinction of the body and soul and reach into the whole person. The dance can be the very release of experience, the sharing of the very depths of emotions and the inspiration of hopes and ideals."[5] Dance keeps us linked to our first source of creativity — the body — and helps us explore our inner-most self and creative potential. It is truly a healing art, not solely a means of appreciative art.[7]

Dance uses the challenge of creativity to move beyond boundaries and delve into our innermost depths. Moustakas discussed the challenge of creativity to which dance directly links us: "To be creative means to experience life in one's own way, to perceive from one's own person, to draw upon one's own resources, capacities, and roots. It means facing life directly and honestly; courageously searching for and discovering grief, joy, pain, struggle, conflict, and finally inner solitude. Only from the search into one's self can the creative emerge.[8] He sees the exploration of the self and the discovery of one's creativity as integrally connected like a circle, a feedback loop in which one heals and expands the other. May concurred with this: "One's creativity is the most basic manifestation of a man or woman's fulfilling his or her own being in the world."[9]

When we explore the innermost self and the creative, a process emerges. This process is sometimes called the journey of the soul/self on the creative process.[10] Many have theorized about it and most agree that this journey has certain stages. The theorized stages of the creative process are:

· *Preparation*: the idea, insight, preparation for the exploration;

· *Frustration*: the retreat from preparation;

· *Incubation*: the submergence into the unconscious;

· *Illumination*: the insight, the inspiration; and

· *Verification/Elaboration*: the production of the original/authentic.[5, 11]

Each person must try to discover his/her own creative process and the sequence that leads to the self and the creative.[12] Dance provides the means to develop this process directly and communicate this journey to one's world.[13] The expressive-arts dance-therapy techniques help patients evolve their own process by paralleling that hypothesized creative process:

· *Preparation*: Introduction through movement.

· *Frustration*: Diverse musical pieces will help awaken the body.

· *Incubation*: So that it can explore aspects of the self and emotions will emerge.

· *Illumination*: The body movement relates to emotions and images. Images also help link us to the creative[14] and the images expand one's knowledge of the self.

· *Verification*: Participants will then explore the movement.

· *Elaboration*: Feelings and images as they relate to the emergence of the self.

Kuettel states that they elicit feelings on a more deep, basic level as compared to traditional verbal therapies.[15] Chodorow felt that the body is a most direct symbol of the unconscious and the mother of the arts.[16] She compares it to sandplay in its potential to move into the inner-most self. Schmais investigated the healing aspects of dance therapy. She identified these nonverbal healing processes: "synchrony, expression, rhythm, vitalization, integration, cohesion, education, and symbolism.[17]

DISCUSSION

Dance therapy has been compared to traditional verbal therapies,[18, 19] thus raising the following challenging questions:

· Can dance therapy reach a deeper level of feeling more immediately?[19]

· Does it help the self emerge more directly?[13]

· Does it stimulate one's creative process and creativity?[16]

· Most importantly, does it heal the self?[17]

REFERENCES

1. Brown NO: Love's Body. New York: Vintage Books, 1966.
2. Chaiklin S: Focus on dance. Journal of the American Association for Health, Physical Education and Recreation (7):701-719, 1974.
3. McNiff S: The Arts and Psychotherapy. New York: Charles C Thomas, 1981.
4. Rank O: Art and the Artist. New York: WW Norton & Company, 1989.
5. Robbins LB: Waking Up in the Age of Creativity. Santa Fe, NM: Bear & Company, 1985.
6. Schmais C, White EQ: Introduction to dance therapy. American Journal of Dance Therapy 9:23-30, 1986.
7. Mettler B.: Creative dance — Art on therapy. American Journal of Dance Therapy 12(2):95-100, 1990.
8. Moustakas C.: Creativity and Conformity. New York: Van Nostrand Reinhold Company, 1967.
9. May R: The Courage to Create. New York: Bantam Books, 1975.
10. Hyde L: The Gift: Imagination and the Erotic Life of Property. New York: Vintage Books, 1983.
11. Edwards B: Drawing on the Artist Within. New York: Simon and Schuster, 1986.
12. Rothenberg A: The Creative Process of Psychotherapy. New York: WW Norton & Company, 1988.
13. Avstreih AK: The emerging self: Psychoanalytic concepts of self development and their implications for dance therapy. American Journal of Dance Therapy 4(2):21-32, 1981.
14. Arietti S: Creativity: The Magic Synthesis. New York: Basic Books; 1976.
15. Kuettel T: Affective change in dance therapy. American Journal of Dance Therapy 5:56-64, 1982.
16. Chodorow J: The Body as Symbol: Dance Movement in Analysis. *In* Schwartz-Salant N, Stein M (eds), The Body in Analysis, 87-106. Wilmette, IL: Chiron Publications, 1986.
17. Schmais C.: Healing Processes in Group Dance Therapy. American Journal of Dance Therapy (8):17-36, 1985.
18. Stark A: The use of verbalization in dance/movement therapy. Arts in Psychotherapy 16: 105-113, 1989.
19. Zwerling I: The creative arts therapies as "real therapies." American Journal of Dance Therapy 11(1):19-26, 1989.

CHAPTER 69

A Nonverbal Intervention for the Severely Language-Disordered Young Child: An Intensive Approach

Diane Lynch Fraser

Daily life, regrettably, is often full of "talk" but bereft of communication. What language-disordered young children need is help in communicating — not simply in talking. Indeed, these children may have more trouble with the social communication features of language than with words or speech. Thus, when designing therapeutic approaches for language-disordered young children, we need to focus on the normal coordination of communication skill across three developmental pathways: motor, social-emotional, and language-cognitive.

We must remember, especially when working with young children, that nonverbal signals — gestures, eye movements, and facial expressions — are crucial to early communication exchange. Severely language-disordered children are limited in the use of nonverbal as well as verbal communication.[1] Non-speech skills can often emerge through intensive nonverbal intervention, including dance-movement therapy. The case study that follows examines the effectiveness of a dance-movement-therapy intervention conducted over a two-year period with one severely language-disordered young child. He was, and remains, enrolled in a therapeutic nursery for young language-disordered children.

Dance-movement therapy is the use of movement as a primary modality to enhance cognitive, emotional or social development. In the treatment of children with language disorders, movement is used to develop social communication skills. When the child can recognize and respond appropriately to the nonverbal signals that accompany language, meaningful verbal interaction is more likely to follow.

Dance-movement therapy is rooted in two theoretical models: developmental and psychodynamic. Principles of growth and maturation guide developmental treatment, directed to remediating specific developmental deficits to stimulate more functional patterns of movement and behavior. A psychodynamic focus, on the other hand, emphasizes the emotional and social aspects of communication and interaction.[2] To address both the developmental and social deficits characteristic of language disorders, it becomes useful to synthesize these two approaches.

A third theoretical model often applied in dance-movement therapy is Jerome Bruner's social/pragmatic theory.[3] Bruner suggests that children learn to communicate by observing how others respond to their communication-like behaviors. For example, if a child points to a spoon and a parent then gives the spoon to the child, and this pattern is repeated consistently, the child comes to understand that pointing at a spoon results in being given a spoon — this connection will be made whether or not the child originally pointed at the spoon because she wanted it.

Children who exhibit syndromes associated with language disorder may withdraw; present a constellation of bizarre, highly stylized and idiosyncratic mannerisms; and seem to live in an intensely personal world cut off from normal means of communication. The dance-movement therapist uses the child's symptoms themselves to draw the child into a therapeutic relationship. Frequently, she imitates the child's movements, to establish rapport with his "movement language." She moves with the child and explores space, distance and direction in harmony with the child.

Children learn how to request, protest, call attention, and regulate the behavior of other people in part through the responses of others. Some of the communication failures of language-disordered children may arise from the difficulty they have picking up social cues. Normally, children learn from the responses of others that talking loudly, laughing, or masturbation is tolerated in certain contexts but not others. Language-disordered children, in contrast, flip their fingers, rock, and talk nonsense despite clear signs of social disapproval. By accepting the language-disordered child's movements, whatever they are, as appropriate, and by responding to them in a reciprocal fashion, the dance-movement therapist gives meaning to the child's gestures. If the child is rocking, the therapist rocks with the child. She may add music — the rocking becomes a dance. In other words, the child's once totally self-absorbed behavior is imbued by the therapist with communicative intent.

CASE STUDY

When Alex S. was 18 months old, he was diagnosed as having infantile autism, a severe language disorder. At that time Alex began play therapy, a psychological intervention. His parents were dissatisfied with this approach, however, and searched for an alternative treatment. At 2 years 5 months, Alex was referred by a neurologist to the School for Language and Communication Development (SCLD) for an initial speech/language evaluation. Alex was accompanied to this evaluation by his mother, a registered nurse, and his father, a physician.

As Dr. and Mrs. S. were talking with the interviewer, Alex responded to his name several times by turning his head in the direction of the speaker. This behavior suggested that he could hear language presented at the level of conversational speech. A complete audiological evaluation conducted subsequent to this interview indicated that Alex's hearing was within normal range.

Language Evaluation

Alex came willingly to the diagnostic room with his parents, but was unavailable for formal diagnostic language procedure. He would not sit and look at pictures with the examiner, listen to stories, or engage in any conversation with the examiner. Observing Alex during play gave the examiner some sense of his language functioning. She was also able to administer the *Receptive-Expressive Language Emergent Scale*[5] (REEL) a parent-report instrument that helped to interpret some of the play in which Alex was engaged during the evaluation.

Throughout the evaluation, Alex would look directly at objects but not at people. He communicated by using gestures and vocalizations such as pointing to a blue ball and saying "bou-bou."

Although Alex's vocalizations during the session were entirely nonlinguistic, his parents said that at home he used gestures and single words such as "kay-kay," "ju" and "bubbie" to get his parents to give cookies or juice and to blow up balloons, a favorite activity.

Cognitively, Alex demonstrated knowledge of object permanence by looking for a ball that had been hidden, and exhibited problem-solving skills by reconstructing a stack of rings. He was able to code and demonstrated the spatial concepts of *in*, *on*, and *under*. When asked to place a ring in a large box, Alex complied, as he did when requested to sit on a chair and crawl under his mother's legs. When the examiner asked him to give her a ball, he did not respond, but his parents said that at home Alex would comply with similar requests.

The examiner described Alex as a child with a severe comprehension- and production-language disorder of unknown etiology, characterized by a limited sound production and a primarily gestural means of communication. Alex's intellectual development seemed far ahead of his social skill. The examiner felt that Alex could be helped by an experience in SLCD's therapeutic nursery and also recommended a complete dance-movement-therapy evaluation to ascertain Alex's need for this kind of individual therapy.

Dance-Movement Therapy Evaluation

One month after the speech/language assessment, SLCD's dance-movement therapist observed Alex during several unstructured play activities. Her observations added a new dimension to the evaluation, especially concerning the impact of physical mobility upon social communication.

The dance-movement therapist described Alex as a child with severe social difficulties. He did not respond to verbal requests, communication was poor and he did not talk at all. The examiner observed nonverbal cues such as eye contact and gesturing, but these were infrequent and often inappropriate. Alex's body was extremely tense during the evaluation, as evidenced by unusual stiffness in his hands and arms. This stiffness appeared to interfere with his movement in and around objects and people. Without the natural arm swing essential to walking, Alex's equilibrium seemed disturbed; he frequently bumped into the examiner and into objects in the room. Alex did not respond to his mirror image and was unable to identify parts of his body for the therapist.

With the initial goal of increasing Alex's body awareness and reducing body tension in the service of communication, the examiner recommended beginning individual dance-movement therapy for Alex twice a week.

First Six Months of Treatment

Alex was wait-listed for the SLCD program and accepted two months later, at 2 years 8 months of age. He was placed with five other language-impaired children in a classroom staffed by a certified speech-language pathologist and two teaching aides. He attended the nursery five days each week for three hours each day. In addition, Alex began individual dance-movement therapy twice a week with the same therapist who had conducted his dance-movement evaluation.

At the same time, Alex's parents were involved in a comprehensive parent-education and peer-support program at SLCD. At home, they implemented therapy techniques such as "narrating" many of the activities in which Alex engaged. For example, if Alex threw pillows, Dr. S. would say "Alex is throwing pillows."

Nonetheless, Alex made little progress during the next six months. In the classroom, he explored objects at a level that remained unchanged from earlier observations. In dance-movement therapy, Alex remained fixated on exploring bubbles. He refused to engage in any other activity.

Six months into treatment, a multidisciplinary team of professionals from SLCD met to discuss Alex and other children who had made limited progress in the program and to consider possible intervention alternatives. The team reviewed a videotape of Alex, then 3 years 2 months, in a small group with his therapist, classroom aide and two classmates. Alex's lack of interactive eye contact, vocalization gesture or proximity and his inappropriate facial expression were noted. Both adults and children were directing their attention to everyone except the self-absorbed Alex. Another way of describing this would be to say that the non-interactive Alex had shaped his environment to be non-interactive as well.

A New Approach

After the team reviewed a number of similar tapes and Alex's parents had made informal observations of these same tapes, a new intervention approach was proposed, with dance-movement therapy as the primary vehicle. In addition to continuing in the therapeutic nursery, Alex would be involved in both in individual and dyadic (two children) dance-movement therapy. It was felt that the dyad as the primary social unit of communication could best facilitate functional nonverbal communication. Thus, during the individual sessions with Alex, the therapist would facilitate adult-child nonverbal interactions. In the dyadic sessions the therapist would facilitate nonverbal interaction between the two children. It was hypothesized that once these nonverbal concomitants of spoken language were in place, functional speech would follow.

The plan was to offer Alex three dance-movement therapy sessions per week for the next year. Each session would be 30 minutes long. One session would be individual; two, dyadic. The same dance-movement therapist would conduct all three sessions. (For Alex this meant a change in therapists, as his initial therapist was leaving SLCD for a new position.) Alex's partner in the dyadic sessions would be a classmate from the nursery with a communication disorder quite different from Alex's. This child was selected as Alex's partner because his communicative behavior was intrusive and demanding. Alex would have difficulty avoiding paying attention to him.

The initial goal of this new strategy was a simple, direct one: to increase both the frequency and duration of nonverbal interactive behavior. Quite naturally, play activities involving climbing and sliding on platforms and crawling in and out of tunnels in "peek-a-boo" style evolved in the individual and dyadic sessions. The dance-movement therapist was able to translate interactions observed in her individual sessions with Alex directly to the dyadic work. For example, if she played peek-a-boo one-on-one, she repeated this kind of nonverbal interaction with the dyad. Due to the severity of Alex's communication disorder, even the small group setting of the therapeutic nursery was still too complex socially to allow him to initiate these interactions there.

After three months of therapy, Alex began to look at people, tolerate people being physically close to him, increase his communicative behavior and vocalizations, and use single words like "ball" and "up" frequently to express his desires.

During the second three months of combined intervention, Alex experienced a tremendous leap in development. At 3½ years, he was able to establish and maintain eye contact during interpersonal exchanges and participate in nonverbal turn-taking routines like waiting for his turn to use bubbles. He used sounds, gestures, and words with some consistency to make requests, call attention, and protest.   Occasionally, Alex would respond appropriately in words to "what" and "who" questions. With adults, he was also responding more appropriately to "yes/no" questions.

During the ensuing four months, Alex continued to progress, although more gradually. Though most of his interaction with his partner in the dyadic sessions could be described as parallel play, he was beginning to request clay and crayons from his partner by extending his hand and saying "cay" or "cayon."

At the conclusion of his second year of combined therapy, Alex continues to be severely impaired in both the comprehension and production of language. He still needs intensive support from adults to participate consistently in play and other activities with children. Yet expectations for him are vastly different than would be the case if he still carried the diagnosis of infantile autism.   The members of the SLCD multidisciplinary team recommend continuation of his therapeutic special education placement as well as dyadic dance-movement therapy to translate the gains he has made in adult-child interaction to communication with other children.

DISCUSSION

Child-development researchers have suggested that children with disabilities may fail to develop fully not because of the disability itself but because of the failure of the environment to provide appropriate experiences and special patterns of care.[6]

The child with a communication disorder cannot be expected to develop language through normal facilitating experiences that most parents and caregivers provide. The child with a language disorder needs a special level of social interaction experiences at both the nonverbal and verbal levels to develop appropriate communication skills.   The ordinary preverbal social exchanges that parents provide for their young children (e.g. rocking back and forth while singing, tickling toes, "peek-a-boo," hide and seek) serve most children well. But language-disordered children cannot absorb these learning experiences

"incidentally." Rather, these experiences need to be presented directly to the language-disordered child as a kind of instruction. By reinforcing and repeating these early nonverbal developmental games, the dance-movement therapist sets the occasion for interaction. She does deliberately what the sensitive parent of a typically developing infant does casually, almost instinctively.

CONCLUSION

Communication is the major goal in dance-movement therapy. Since all communication, whether verbal or gestural, is directed toward someone, movement can have among its other aims the goal of making contact with another human being. One of the major functions of dance historically has been to create unity among people. We need to recognize the relationship-maintaining function of language. We cannot and should not isolate verbal from nonverbal experience.   When we realize that children may benefit from learning to use the language of movement to establish human contact before they are ready to establish contact through words, we can use dance and movement to help children like Alex communicate and connect.

REFERENCES

1. Ricks D, Wing L: Language, communication and the use of symbols in normal autistic children. Journal of Autism and Childhood Schizophrenia 5:191-222, 1975.

2. Whitehouse M: (1979) C.G. Jung and danse therapy: Two major principles. *In* Bernstein PL (ed), Eight Theoretical Approaches in Danse Movement Therapy. Iowa: Kendall/Hunt, 1979.

3. Bruner J: The ontogenesis of speech acts. Journal of Child Language 2:1-19, 1975.

4. Espenak L: Danse Therapy. Springfield, IL: Charles Thomas Publishers, 1981.

5. Bzoch K, League R: Receptive-Expressive Emergent Language Scale. Gainesville, FL: Language   Education   Division,   Computer Management Corporation, 1971.

6. Greenspan SI: Fostering emotional and social development in infants with disabilities. Zero to Three 9(1), 1988.

CHAPTER 70

Treating Scoliosis
with Therapeutic Gymnastics

Lilita Branka-Bakajeva

About 2% of young people in the world suffer from scoliosis.[1] Present day methods of treatment, including manipulative and operative procedures and corrective gymnastics, have resulted in partial correction or stabilization of the condition, but have failed to restore the symmetry of psychosomatic function.

Ballet exercises can be regarded as an act of symmetry.[2] Studies have been undertaken on the use of dance therapy for various musculoskeletal and other disorders.[3-8]

It has been stressed that muscular forces, when incorrectly applied to the spinal column, are the major contributing factors in the aetiology and pathogenesis of scoliosis. Muscles responsible for both flexion and rotation of the vertebral column are involved, but those of rotation override those of flexion by about 200%.[9] Based on the aforesaid and on the principles of symmetry, a method was designed of static-dynamic exercises using classical ballet postures and movements.

The basic static ballet posture regimen was supplemented by a maximal number of movement units. As the holding of a correct ballet posture for a scoliosis sufferer requires extreme concentration initially, a training apparatus (Australian patent #57,189/90) for the fixation of the patients body in the required standing posture was designed and used.

MATERIALS and METHODS

To test the efficiency of the method an experimental Study was conducted with students suffering from 1st to 3rd degree scoliosis at the special High School in Riga. The subjects were divided into an experimental and control group of 10 students each. The experimental group was subjected to ballet exercises and the control group to conventional therapeutic exercises. The one-hour exercises were repeated four times weekly for eight months.

Anthropometric measurements, photography, myotonometry, and radiography were used for the evaluation of this method. Radiography was found to be the most objective indicator. Various other tests were used to monitor the response of the cardio-vascular and respiratory systems.

Various radiographic indices were assessed at the greatest points of the spinal curvature using the following methods:

a. Ferguson's method[10] to determine the angle of the curvature in the horizontal plane;

b. Zausis and James' method[11] to determine the torsion percentage of the vertebrae.

RESULTS

The results of radiographic analysis as measured by the change in spinal curvature and torsion after 8 months of corrective therapy are given in Figures 1 and 2 respectively. For the experimental group, both the pathological spinal curvature and torsion significantly decreased in 7 to 8 months. Markedly less improvement was recorded in the control group.

After one month of ballet exercises, the patients developed the necessary skills for correct muscular activity. A natural *muscle corset* developed after two months and the patients no longer needed to wear a brace.

DISCUSSION

At the conclusion of the eight-month experimental period, the symmetrical interaction of homolateral and antagonist muscles was fully restored and a maximal convsrgence was achieved of the symmetrical, vertebral and gravitational axes of the spine.

One stydy assumed that dissymmetry was the lack of some symmetry-related elements which, however,

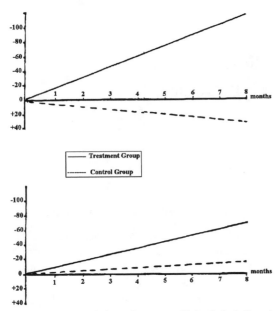

Figure 1: *Increase (+) or Decrease (-) in Spinal Curvature, Standing (above) and recumbent (below), over 8 months.*

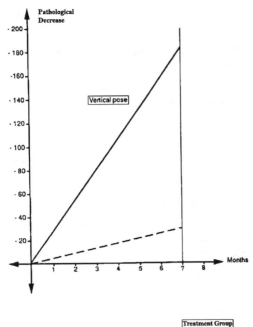

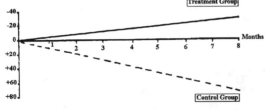

Figure 2: *Increase (+) or Decrease (-) in Spinal Torsion, in standing (above) and recumbent (below), over 8 months.*

exist in a hidden form and may reappear under favorable conditions.

To sustain a classical ballet posture, four times more muscles are involved than to maintain a natural posture. Classical ballet exercises also use a maximal number of movement units. All this may activate the latent neurogenic elements necessary for the restoration of symmetrical muscle function.

The patients in the experimental group also recorded a significant improvement in secondary pathological changes associated with scoliosis. Rib cage expansion increased by an average of 2 cm; lung volume by 100 ml, both due to an increase in intercostal muscle function. Secondar.y kyphosis, bow-legs and knock-knees also improved when using ballet exercises.

REFERENCES

1. Ziporyn, T. Scoliosis management, new subject of numerous questions Journal of the American Medical Association, 254: 3009-3091.

2. Seneshal, M., Flack. Symmetrical Signs Mir, Moscow, 1980.

3. Sparger, C. Anatomy and Ballet. Adam and Charles Black, London, 1970.

4. Lukjanova, E. Breathing Choreography. Iskustvo, Moscow, 1979.

5. Kalinina, I. Age changes in some motor and vegetative functions in professional ballet teaching. Dissertation, Moscow, 1970.

6. Gunter, H. Jazz Dance. Berlin: Henschelverlag, 1980.

7. Bakajeva, L. Bases of classical ballet exercise effectiveness. Med Ref. J. (Moscow), 10: part l, Mscrpt. D9722, 1985.

8. Bordier, G. Anatomie appliquée à la danse. Paris: Amphor, 1975.

9. Civjans, J. Aksenovich, I. Orthopedics, Traumatology and Prothesis, 6: 35-38 1985.

10. Ferguson, A.D. Roentgen Diagnosis of Extremities and Spine. New York: Paul B. Hoeber, 1949.

11. Kazmin, A., Kon, I., Belenky, V. Scoliosis Medicina, Moscow 1981.

12. Kopciks,V., Subnikovs, A. Symmetry in Science and Art. Moscow: Nauka, 1972.

CHAPTER 71

Holistic Neuromuscular Facilitation

Bella Abramowitz Fisher

A party! How can a party be therapy? That depends on who runs it and how. The author is referring to a modified party directed by a physical therapist, which enables him/her to treat, educate, motivate, spark self-expression, revive joy and self-confidence, and accelerate with ease the patient's reentry into the community.

This kind of party is the format for *holistic neuromuscular facilitation* (HNF), a unique, complex physical therapy group treatment to facilitate neuromuscular responses. Based on holism, which is nature's tendency to produce wholes from the ordered grouping of units, HNF uses a guided, integrated, multifaceted approach to help release the body's natural healing forces toward wholeness.

Some of these approaches were begun in 1945, when the author worked as a physical therapist in World War II. While the Battle of Okinawa was raging, many experiences precipitated unorthodox approaches. One such instance involved a patient in the 76th Field Hospital who refused treatment. He was sad, frightened, and withdrawn. After learning that he was spending his wedding anniversary alone, surrounded by gunfire, the author obtained cups of juice as make-believe liquor, and suggested he imagine he was in a nightclub surrounded instead by music and dancing. After a toast to the couple, their favorite song was sung. His response was a flood of tears, followed by heartwarming smiles. Successful participation in the physical therapy process resulted!

Throughout the war, contributions toward what would later become HNF included the use of song, drama, imagery, and humor to help free the patient's ability to utilize the P.T. being offered. Wartime experiences had created an acute need to treat the condition via "the person." Later, hospital confinement and the accompanying "4-wall syndrome" required the same approach.

The next contribution came after the war in 1946, when the author used dance for patients with traumatic injuries in veterans' hospitals. The strengthening, general conditioning, and fun resulting from music stimulation were obvious short-term goals. But the learning of substitutions and/or accommodations to bypass irreparable musculo-skeletal deficits was challenging and especially satisfying as an important long-term goal.

In 1970, after a 24-year hiatus from P.T., exposure to neuromuscular conditions and new treatment approaches at the Rusk Institute of Rehabilitation Medicine piqued the author's curiosity. Proprioceptive neuromuscular facilitation, for instance, emulated natural patterns so that the weaker components could come into play. Proprioceptors are also stimulated; therefore, wouldn't other neuro-muscular responses be facilitated? Since music evokes past spontaneous movement combinations, would not the repeated elicited combinations strengthen the weaker muscles, which, in turn, might be more receptive to voluntary initiation?

These thoughts prompted the author to create a special set-up which would contribute to using dance, not only as an end in itself, but as part of a technique to elicit and improve neuromuscular deficits, as well as to improve the musculoskeletal conditions.

Having long been aware that pain and fatigue often disappear while dancing, the question arose: "What physiological resources are tapped when the psyche is making its wholehearted contribution toward activity?" There were some answers then; there are more today (i.e. endogenous opiates). But did we have all the answers? It seemed that we should provide patients with the most favorable climate possible in order to tap still other unknown psyche/soma connections, and to allow internal processes of the brain to function uninhibitedly during the active state, to promote recovery as well as reduce pain.

Thus evolved the concept of *dynamic relaxation*, which is a process to achieve relaxation for and during activity. It is aimed at getting the patient to feel so totally accepted and comfortable, physically and emotionally, that s/he can function in the most accessible mental and emotional state, and is free enough to actively participate physically as instinctively as possible.

HNF crystallized in 1970. It incorporated natural activities and functional socialization. It used the direct effects of pleasant visual, auditory, gustatory, tactile, olfactory, proprioceptive, vestibular, and kinesthetic stimulation, plus their associated senses of recall (sense-memory). These would also influence emotional tone, which might itself also pull the present deficit into a revoked total functional pattern from the pre-morbid state associated with that emotional tone.

HNF is best implemented in a separate room or area that has no negative association with other treatments, and where the surroundings of music, decorations, and camaraderie will trigger good feelings upon each reentry.

One component of HNF which cultivates receptivity needs reemphasis: sparking fun and humor. We must exercise the ability to enjoy living or it will atrophy.   The party atmosphere enables one to recapture the elusive instinct toward the joy of living and to increase the drive toward the peak of motivation.

The present format of HNF has been used by the author for 17 years at three hospitals and six stroke clubs, for a wide range of conditions. Results have been positive and sometimes dramatic.

The HNF session in the hospital starts as the patients enter the special area and are welcomed to a party-like atmosphere. While establishing the state of *dynamic relaxation*, spontaneous reactions to music are stimulated. This is followed by simple structured movements to music, and builds with progressively more complex coordinated movements, ending with some popular dance and/or song forms. Hands-on for passive- and active assistive range of motion and facilitative techniques can be helpful. Real and/or imaginary props and games are used for change of pace. Refreshments are served as each individual receives transfer training, standing-balance and weight-shift exercises, and ambulation training — all in the guise of ballroom dancing. The session ends with the singing of a popular song which continues as the patients exit.

Progressive dance training is quite an effective technique for progressive ambulation training. Social dancing, after all, is ambulating to music in all directions, using various rhythms. And, of course, the premorbid dance recall for most people is very strong.

The social dance position (modified to each patient's needs) fosters a more normal gait. Inhibiting and distorting effects of assistive devices are minimized. Length of steps becomes more equal and posture improves. The steady beat also promotes equal length as well as equal timing of steps.

As the patient improves, the normal dance position is assumed and advanced dancing is implemented. Gait refinement is promoted. A dance skill is learned.

The session in the post-hospital stroke club is similar, but with additional emphasis on ambulatory and social skills in the form of line-, circle-, square-, folk- and disco dancing. All benefit from these, but especially those with cognitive, perceptual, and aphasic problems.

It has been found that a slow, strong, steady beat, as in tango, slow-rock and Greek dancing, helps patients to develop increased joint stability, increased duration, and smoother movements. This is especially helpful to patients with ataxia. It also improves balance and timing of steps, and increases length of steps.

A fast 3/4 tempo, as in Viennese waltz, facilitates swinging movements and midline crossing in the upper extremities. The fast downward momentum on the first beat propels the next upward rise to the peak of the anti-gravity position, which is sustained by the second and third beats. This helps improve range of motion and muscle strength.

The beat can control, direct, and sustain movement, and therefore needs to be respected. Rhythm and music alone, or even rhythm by itself, can facilitate neuromuscular responses.[1]   When inspired by a physical therapist into dance reactions, this can be even more effective. When incorporated in a happy, accepting, social environment, and augmented by other pleasant sensory stimuli, responses are even further enhanced. The evoked pleasant sense memories and emotional recall can then intensify those good feelings, hastening the creation of an optimal receptive state.

Any one of these elements, when taken alone, could foster improvements. When taken as a whole, however, with overlapping sensory systems, the sum of this integrated approach reaching maximal input has the greatest impact. Potential neuromuscular responses are more easily triggered and more optimal results realized.

Holistic neuromuscular facilitation! A party!! What a wonderfully joyous way to provide treatment for those who need it so much!!!

REFERENCE

Safranek MG, Koshland GF, Raymond G: Effect of auditory rhythm on musical activity. Physical Therapy 62(2):161-168, 1982.

CHAPTER 72

Authentic Movement and Performance

Andrea J. Olsen

In 1979, after seven years performing and teaching professionally as a dancer, the author began writing a book on dance choreography. Thirteen chapters (on rehearsal process, partnering, the use of space...) were written before the section on "movement." At that point, the author realized that she had nothing to say. She had trained in modern dance with Martha Graham, Jose Limon, Erick Hawkins, and had a heritage in ballet, but she had no idea how her own movement was sourced. Then the author met movement therapist Janet Adler, who was interested in working with dancers and choreographers because she felt that much of what she saw in her studio was more compelling than what she saw on stage. Hence the author began working in Authentic Movement and for over a decade has remained fascinated by its richness as a catalyst for creative work and for healing.

Authentic Movement was initially developed by Mary Starks Whitehouse in the mid-years of this century in a process which she called "movement in depth." A student of Mary Wigman and of Martha Graham, Mary was schooled in formal dance training which invited unconscious energies. In the 1950's she shifted her focus from artistic to therapeutic aspects of dance, and began her lifework experiencing and describing the process of "moving and being moved."[1] Since that time, Authentic Movement has been further developed and articulated, most specifically by movement therapists Joan Chodorow and Janet Adler, and is currently employed by various practitioners across the United States and Europe.

The form for Authentic Movement, as refined by Janet Adler, is simple: There is a mover and a witness. The mover closes her/his eyes and waits for movement impulses in the body--the process of being moved. The witness holds the consciousness and observes. After a period of time, the witness calls the movement session to a close, and there is a verbal exchange about what occurred. The witness reflects

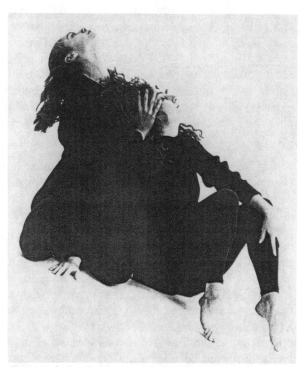

Figure 1: Authentic Movement in Performance

back what was seen, modeling nonjudgmental language, and most importantly, speaking from her/his own experience. Ultimately, the goal is to internalize a nonjudgmental but discerning witness so that we can observe without interrupting our movement life. In this approach to Authentic Movement, the form provides a container in which to practice entering unconscious material, returning to consciousness, and reflecting on or shaping the experience through speaking or creative work.

Our history is stored in our body: evolutionary movement patterns, human developmental reflexes, and personal history. As we close our eyes and allow ourselves to be moved, endless variety and diversity emerge. Much of what we correct in a dance technique class, for example, can be a resource in creative work. A lifted shoulder or a consistently twisted spines are indications of personal story. Our imperfection is our gift. As we learn to listen to the language of the body, we have choice about when and how to use a particular movement. Part of injury and illness is the conflict between what we tell our bodies to do and what they need to do for healing or expression. Part of healing is allowing the unexpressed to be expressed. Authentic Movement facilitates this expression because it integrates our emotional life with our physical selves and promotes consciousness. As we begin Authentic Movement we may face basic fears: hatred of our body, fear of being empty inside, fear of being alone. We may also face self-judgments such as: "I'm too fat"; I'm too thin"; "If I'm not moving, I don't exist"; "If I don't do something good, nobody will love me." As we close our eyes and listen to our bodies, there is also the potential of accepting ourselves just as we are. When fear is replaced with openness, we can learn how rich our inner world really is.

As we use Authentic Movement as a resource for choreography and performance, we are developing a dialogue with our unconscious. Basically, there are different levels of movement which occur from the personal unconscious, the collective unconscious, or the superconscious.[2] These include impulses based purely in sensation (such as stretching or attending to an injury), in disorienting our consciousness (such as spinning, walking backwards), in journeying (such as unfolding a movement story), or in connecting to highly charged material in which we are clearly "being moved" by energies from the unconscious. All of these levels are valuable and necessary aspects of our movement life, and part of the range of Authentic Movement. Within the experience of "connected" movement, where the unconscious is speaking directly through the body, some motions or positions will feel raw (particularly vulnerable or unformed, hard to remember), some unfolding, and others ready for consciousness. Movement which is "ready" returns again and again, is easy to remember and is available, for creative forming. Movement which is raw and unfolding needs time to develop. Part of our responsibility as artists is to know we will be dancing for a lifetime, and that we are not strip mining our unconscious (using every movement which emerges and putting it on stage) or devouring the vital resources of our body (burn out now because we have only so many years to dance). Our body and our unconscious develop a dialogue with our conscious self--a pact of trust which is constantly being negotiated. It has to trust that we will take care of it if it opens. For example, in an injury of the spine or

the ankle the muscles go into spasm to protect us from movement. (If we didn't hurt, we would move!) As the body trusts that we will rest, the spasm can release. That is the negotiation. Can we trust ourself? By internalizing a supportive, nonjudgmental but discerning inner witness, we develop self-trust at a deep level.

The relationship between the mover and the witness parallels that of performer and audience. The multiplicity of the human experience lives in each of us, and the stage provides an opportunity to embody our inner selves in movement as performer, or by empathy or projection as witness. Some people journey deeper in Authentic Movement when they are being witnessed with heightened consciousness as by an audience. Transference between the audience and the performer enables transformation for both.[3] At first the collective mind of the audience supports the surrender of the performer to unconscious energies, but soon the audience surrenders its awareness of self and goes with the performer towards transformation as well. In this context, transformation becomes an inclusive experience. For example, in China during a solo concert when I dropped my head, I noticed that the audience heads would drop; when I lifted my focus, the audience focus would move. I recognized that I was holding the consciousness as they allowed themselves to be moved. I was witnessing a moving audience. In these moments, dance is a vehicle for energies beyond the self which can be invited, or invoked, but certainly not forced. They exist as an aspect of "being moved" available to each of us.

Within the spectrum of collective experience, there is a tremendous relief both as a mover and as a watcher as we realize that our personal movement is part of a larger whole. Group work in Authentic Movement includes experiences of synchronicity, simultaneity, cross-cultural motifs, feats of endurance or strength, interactions with other people and other energies in the room, extraordinary lifts, levels of endurance or dynamics that could never be planned or practiced. Injuries are rare; if the body and psyche are working as one, anything seems possible. If each person is following his/her own impulses, form is inherent in the unfolding of the work. When I first worked with a drummer in Authentic Movement, he paused after an hour of energetic work to let me know that he was just warming up. Two hours of continual improvisation taught me that within my body there is a full range of energy possibilities: an organic need for humor, for dynamic change, for lightness, for weight, and that the full spectrum would unfold if I would take a ride on my inner impulses. We long to be seen for who we are in our totality, not for the limited view of who others think we are or want us to be. Often students ask why their first experience with Authentic Movement is so serious, their first dances so sad. Generally we push into the unconscious what we consider to be negative--our sadness, our meanness, our fear. But below that layer of unexpressed movement is the wealth of human experience. That is the resource from which we draw in Authentic Movement and which we hope to bring to the stage.

As Authentic Movement informs performance, the nature of performance changes. At a mature level, a performer has an articulate, discerning inner witness which allows authentic connections to occur on stage. There are years in performance when we may be driven by our need to be seen, when the ego seeks validation, when we must shape and control, when we desire to transform and know other parts of ourselves, or when we are compelled to create rituals of experience for others. These motivations change during our lives as performers. Dancing at twenty is different than dancing at forty or sixty. As we internalize our own witness and lose in effect our need to be seen by others, new performance motivations occur. What might these be? The practice of being seen being authentic, in an era where the superficial takes precedence. The practice of connecting to energies beyond the self, in an era where spirituality is shapeless. The practice of participating in a community of exchange between dancers and watchers, in an era where dance has been removed from most peoples' lives.

Authentic Movement in performance, both as mover and as witness, allows a process of recognition. As we feel seen, we can see. As we feel heard, we can begin to hear others. As we develop a discerning and supportive inner witness, we can allow others to move and be moved. Then as we dance, we heal; as we heal we dance. The process of listening to the movement stories of our body encourages us to know ourselves and to bring this consciousness to performance.

REFERENCES

1. Whitehouse, M.S. The Tao of the Body. Lecture presented at the Analytical Psychology Club of Los Angeles, 1958. *In* the Library of the C.G. Jung Institute, Los Angeles.

2. Adler, Janet. Who Is The Witness? A Description of Authentic Movement. Contact Quarterly, XII(1): 20-29, 1987.

3. Chodorow, Joan. Dance Therapy and Depth Psychology--The Moving Imagination. London: Routledger Press, 1991.

SUGGESTED READING

1. Bartenieff, Irmgard. Body Movement: Coping With The Environment. New York: Gordon and Breach, 1980.

2. Chodorow, Joan. Dance Therapy and the Transcendent Function. American Journal of Dance Therapy, 2(1): 16-23, 1978.

3. Cohen, Bonnie Bainbridge. Moving From Within. Naropa Magazine: 17-19, 1987.

4. Cohen, B.B. The Alphabet of Movement, Primitive Reflexes, Righting Reactions, and Equilibrium Responses Contact Quarterly, XIV(2): 20-38, 1989.

5. Frantz, Gilda. An Approach to the Center: An Interview With Mary Whitehouse. Psychological Perspectives 3(1):37-46, 1972.

6. Halifax, Joan. Shaman. New York: Thames and Hudson, 1988.

7. Levy, Fran. Dance Movement Therapy: A Healing Art. National Dance Association, 1988.

8. Olsen, Andrea. Bodystories, A Guide to Experiential Anatomy. Barrytown, NY: Station Hill Press, 1991.

9. Whitehouse, Mary Starks. Physical Movement and Personality. Contact Quarterly, XII(1): 16-19, 1987.

10. Whitehouse, M.S. The Transference and Dance Therapy. American Journal of Dance Therapy, 1(1): 3-7, 1977.

11. Whitehouse, M.S. C.G. Jung and Dance Therapy. Eight Theoretical Approaches *In*: Bernstein, P.L. Dance/Movement Therapy. Dubuque: Kendall/ Hunt, 1979.

12. Wigman, Mary. The Language of Dance. Connecticut Wesleyan University Press, 1966.

ACKNOWLEDGEMENTS

This paper is presented in grateful acknowlegment of Daphne Lowell, Joan Miller, Mary Ramsey, Susan Waltner, and Alton Wasson with whom the author worked in Authentic Movement during the last decade.

CHAPTER 73

Dance Therapy with the Orthopedic Patient

Ginger Perowsky

The techniques of dance therapy were developed within psychiatric settings and have had their primary application to the treatment of mental disorders. With patients who are not highly verbal, or as a means of supplementing verbal treatment, dance therapy has proven its worth as a component of the multidisciplinary mental-health system. There is, however, nothing about dance therapy that necessarily limits its application to mental-health settings. Human beings are unified organisms whose minds and emotions are integrated into a moving body.[1] Through movement work with a trained therapist, patients can holistically overcome both chronic and situational difficulties. Both the dance-therapy profession and entire health-care system can benefit by exploring the full range of possible uses of dance therapy techniques outside of traditional settings.[2]

These possibilities were raised for the author while confined to bed for ten days after knee surgery.[3] The experience of immobility was physically very trying; muscles atrophied, her back became stiff, and sores developed from using the elbows, hips and heels as leverage in moving. Trying to stretch while in a cast resulted in tendinitis. Even professional training had not resulted in the ability to accurately determine what movements might cause injury. The physical problems were compounded by the emotional anxiety, tension, and depression that resulted from immobility. Body image is a critical element in the maintenance of a strong and resilient ego and the inability to move impaired this image. Inability to interact with the environment resulted in feelings of powerlessness and utter passivity. It became apparent that the injury the author caused while lying in the hospital bed resulted from these feelings and a desire to affirm herself as a whole person who was in control of her life.

Upon reflecting on this experience, it appeared that the opportunity to engage in an appropriate movement program with an objective professional could have helped to alleviate many of the physical

and emotional problems. Appropriate exercises could have been devised for the non-injured portions of the body. This would have been helpful adjusting to partial immobility and thus would have enabled more effective participation in the orthopedic recovery and rehabilitation process.

Although these problems were probably exacerbated by the fact that, as a dancer, the author has high emotional investment in her self-image as a moving person, it seemed likely that most patients experience similar difficulties. Dance therapy demonstrates that movement is a critical aspect of everyone's self-image; thus, orthopedic patients might benefit physically and emotionally from movement work.[4] As these sorts of problems are not addressed in orthopedic treatment, it seemed it might be desirable for dance therapists to work in cooperation with orthopedic teams as they have long worked with mental-health professionals. By addressing emotional problems, dance therapists might enhance patient comfort and make an important contribution to recovery.[5]

When the idea was presented of applying dance therapy to orthopedics at the large hospital at which the author is employed, her clinical supervisor was very supportive, but it took careful diplomacy to gain the cooperation of the orthopedic staff. Proposals to transgress traditional departmental boundaries generally meet with a degree of distrust; when first approaching the orthopedics department, questions were raised about the author's qualifications to engage in rehabilitation work and whether the clinical role of the physical therapist would be usurped. This distrust was partially based on responsibility to patients and a fear of the further injuries that might be caused by a non-medical professional. Quite rightly, the orthopedic department needed strict assurance that patients' conditions would not exacerbated. Their skepticism was also influenced by an unrealistic image of dance therapy: The thought of patients on crutches dancing across the floor to music seemed foolhardy and grotesque. Only after it was made clear that this work would involve movements that had no impact on injured parts of the body was access to the patients allowed. With a professional practice based on a strict medical model, staff members had difficulty seeing the benefits of holistic patient care that extends beyond the technical treatment of problems localized at a specific portion of the body.

Thus, any dance therapist who wishes to expand her practice outside traditional areas must be willing to deal with problems that are as much political as technical. One must present oneself and one's proposal in a highly professional manner that clearly defines both the goals and limitations of the program, and must demonstrate one's expertise by being willing to confidently answer tough questions. If one merely has a vague idea that dance therapy might be helpful with a particular patient population, the traditional caretakers for that population — quite justifiably — will not look favorably on providing access to the patients. In particular, one must clearly differentiate the goals of the proposed dance therapy from the goals of the work of other disciplines. Thus, it was shown that there was no overlap between the proposed work and that of the physical therapist. Whereas the physical therapist strictly treats the injured part of the body, a dance therapist would treat the whole person and would avoid all movements that might affect the injured part. By making this differentiation, both professional anxieties and fear for the patients were alleviated. The role of the dance therapist is presented as facilitating and complementing the work of the physical therapist, allowing the development of a cooperative professional relationship that benefits both the patients and the orthopedic staff that treats them.

After gaining provisional support from the orthopedic staff, it was necessary to adopt much the same approach with patients as with the orthopedic staff. Like the staff, patients saw their medical problems in a purely technical way and did not quite see the point of engaging in movements not directly tied to their treatment. Someone walking in with a tape recorder and music cassettes did not fit in with the standard medical picture, but overcoming resistance often was possible by asking simple questions about stiffness, pain, and anger stemming from immobility and boredom. The patients acknowledged these discomforts and many were willing to try dance therapy once it was clear that a service was being provided that might be helpful in sup-

plementing, and did not duplicate, their rehabilitation work. The service was offered without pressure and almost in a spirit of fun; this somewhat lighthearted approach was appreciated. Techniques used with each patient varied in accordance with the nature and severity of patient's injury and emotional state.[6] Care was taken not to strain the injured area of the body and to make certain to isolate the movements used from that area. In essence, a program had to be devised for each patient that would exercise the body without injuring it and that would address emotional states and issues.

Dance therapy in orthopedics provides patients with the means of acknowledging negative feelings about themselves and their bodies so that positive healing can occur. This is analogous to the process in group therapy where anger is first expressed, and then more loving feelings.[7] Physical injury often impairs not only a particular part of the body but the patient's entire self-image, and dance therapy provides the means of holistically treating the patient's entire situation. As ballet master David Howard once noted, if a dancer has one leg shorter than the other he will not come walking out on stage slowly, making the problem obvious to everyone; he will come out with a hop and a skip and a jump so that no one will know that one leg is shorter than the other. In the same way, the patient can gain a holistic sense of self through the movements he or she *can* engage in effectively.

An informal process of evaluation has indicated that this dance-therapy program has been beneficial and is appreciated. After the sessions, patients have reported feeling less tense and less stiff; also, more hopeful, energized, and happier. Several have said that they looked forward to the sessions as the only bright part of their hospital stay. This seems to indicate that this service is needed and that it does provide benefits to the patients.

Although the techniques of dance therapy were formulated for psychiatric settings, the project of using dance therapy to treat orthopedic patients provides an example of the ways that dance therapy techniques can be used in settings out of their original contexts. Illness is not without its emotional dimensions, and dance therapy provides a proper way of dealing with those emotions in a nonverbal, and thus non threatening, way. It is recommended, therefore, that we explore placing dance or other creative-arts therapists on consultation liaison teams so that patients who could benefit from dance therapy can be identified and treated.

REFERENCES

1. Siegel EV: Dance-Movement Therapy: Mirror of Our Selves. New York: Human Sciences Press, 1984.
2. Mitchell JD: Dance/movement therapy in a changing health care system. Amer J Dance Therapy 10:4-10, 1987.
3. Perowsky G: Working with pain: a self study. Amer J Dance Therapy 13(1):49-58, 1991.
4. Schilder, P: The Image and Appearance of the Human Body. New York: International Universities Press, 1950.
5. Regelson W, West B: The kinesthetic room: visual and other supportive therapy for confined patients. The Arts in Psychotherapy, 18(1):69-72, 1991.
6. Robbins A, Strauss A: Expressive Therapy: A Creative Arts Approach to Depth Oriented Treatment. New York: Human Sciences Press, 1980.
7. Yalom TD: The Theory and Practice of Group Psychotherapy, 3rd ed. New York: Basic Books, 1985.

SUGGESTED READING

Lamb W: Preserving Mental Heath: the Power of Movement. Columbia, MD: American Dance Therapy Association, 1988.

CHAPTER 74

Working with Dionysus: Dance-Movement Therapy with Recovering Substance Abusers in a Therapeutic Community Setting

Marcia Plevin

Dionysus, the androgynous god of wine and ecstasy, embodies the divine but tragic child — abandoned, dismembered, persecuted, and yet reborn. Many of the recovering substance abusers in the San Carlo therapeutic community come from families or environments in which they, too, experienced abandonment, physical and mental abuse, rape, and incest. They arrive in the therapeutic community looking for support, a new way to live, to be reborn themselves — yet with the terror that they also may fail.

The myth of Dionysus has guided the author toward seeing more clearly how the body-mind-spirit connection can be rewoven through the intervention of a dance-movement therapist. This refers to not only restoring the body symbolically, but actually putting it back together again. In doing so, one is also *putting back* the mind.

The myth informs us that Dionysus is a *chthonic* god, which means descent, subterranean, the world of the unconscious. His myth and presence at the worship of the Elusinian Mysteries, a ritual held every year during the harvest, sheds light on the ultimate transformation process of death and rebirth, making us look more clearly and with awe at the inevitability of these two poles in our lives.[1]

The inevitability of choosing which part of the Dionysus myth to emphasize herein led to recognition of his central core, which can be none other than his duality.

Clinically, Dionysus reveals himself in two predominant movement styles belonging to this population: passive dependent dances which initially are most likely to manifest in sleep, juxtaposed with raucous, unbounded aggressiveness and frenzy. It is also paradoxically seen in the form of ambivalence which causes paralysis between two poles. 'Do I go forward or back, right or left ... if each way is too

frightening ... I'd better not do anything.' Movement here can be holding the body in bound, frozen positions or scattered unfocused attempts to move in any direction.

The 'coming' of Dionysus heralds a need for nourishment, ecstasy, sensual fulfillment, and abandon. Central to his ritual and myth is the vine and drinking the 'sweet nectar,' wine. Irrational rage and madness ensue, as seen in the frenzy of his female followers called maenads, who tear apart, kill, and devour animals and even their own children. The mask, always used in his rituals, confronts us with his duality and makes evident the paradox of his presence; although known as the *liberator*, he is also the *tormentor*.[2] Violence, terror, and destruction move hand in hand with this god who speaks to us of transformation through death and rebirth.

In the ecstatic first phases of drug taking, a person is vulnerable to an energy greater than his/her ability to control it. Fascination but also confusion results, with the craving becoming more and more acute; and, as seen in the myth, one can become mad.

Connected with mystery, spirit, and divinity, he touches powerful sources of the self. Yet, continuing to abuse the body, addicts instead lose touch until the body becomes an unfelt and unknown vehicle. Caught in this archetype, the addict rides a roller coaster from joy to madness, from tragedy to death.

The body is needed to take the drug in; the effect is to lose it. The body is the first source of knowledge of ourselves and the world. Sensing the presence of this archetype and with awareness of his glaring duality, the dance-movement therapist moves and guides the recovering person to remember and rediscover the self through dances that may be entitled *Like Cures Like*. "The deep emotion with which this madness announces itself finds its expression in music and dance."[2]

We begin to open and close ourselves to the world in the first phase of life outside the womb, known psychodynamically as the oral phase. If the star of this choreography is the baby's mouth, then the background is as significant, being the body — of the baby and of the mother, or primary caretaker. They move together in satisfying or unsatisfying rhythms, theirs being a fusional duet in which the baby can not as yet distinguish *self* from other. The baby's body sensations and impulses register in energy pathways which are called *tension flow*.[4] Satisfied with being held or fed, the baby will have a soft, gentle, free-flow rhythm. A look of ecstasy will *flow* across his face. Hungry, the infant tenses; body, arms and legs jab into space, while the held energy build,s until it bursts into a cry. Hunger and gratification become dances that form patterns which, later in life, will emerge as the ability to feel satisfied. Relational attitudes, which have to do with touch, the pleasure or displeasure of contact, will develop from this primary duet.

Dionysus gave the world the vine from which wine flows. In the way milk is nourishment and ecstasy for the infant, wine becomes a substitute 'comforter' or ecstasy for the teenager or adult, masking intoxication with contentment. Entrance of this archetype fills a hole, a deep hunger not only in the body but in the soul. Its divine nature becomes twisted and the soul 'food' leaves a grotesque ache. The hunger cannot be satisfied; *out of control* becomes a craving where entrances into the body, whether by injection or sniffing, are all *mouths*. A lack of satisfying nourishment has taken on monstrous proportions, wherein madness and violence become the answer if it not appeased.

The dance-movement therapist does not give milk, but, in an imaginary way, seeks to create an atmosphere of a lost world, where they can begin to re-choreograph dances they never danced. Sitting still, lying down, sleeping, standing, moving, jumping, running ... what is a movement of satisfaction? How can they begin to perceive a *satisfied* self without the aid of a drug? First and foremost comes recognizing sensations, then feeling. Reawakening their capacity to feel brings with it pain and confusion.

With difficulty, P. gets up to move. Like a tall, lanky adolescent who hasn't settled into her skin, she attempts to move her 27-year-old body to the group's pulse and rhythm. Music and dance essential for the worship of Dionysus become part of our group ritual, a way into a body/mind that has cut off its ability to feel. But there is torment and suffering here; her eyes flit from one to another in the group. Awkward and embarrassed, she knows that as part of the group's contract she can sit down and not participate at any time. Freedom and autonomy of movement is the *rule*. Bringing consciousness to what she chooses to do is the following step. P. stops, crosses her arms, closes her body inward and looks at the group with disdain.

Uncomfortable and mistrustful of her body, she precipitates the group's task by falling and fracturing her right wrist in the sixth session. (The group was comprised of ten women seen for two hours, once a week, for twenty-seven weeks.) The task was to begin to heal a 'split.' Dionysus, dismembered and torn apart physically and psychically, a true savior god, brings P., the author, and the group closer to the renewal, the rebirth for which the myth constantly asks.[4] Bringing any one of the senses into focus reawakens the self and can bring with it pain. This pain may aid them in confronting the past and in dealing with the present. The light touch of a hand on P.'s leg brings pain and tears, revealing a confused and unknown territory. Touch meant for comfort was perceived as such but could not be tolerated. The use of bodily contact — the sense of touch — is a dance-movement therapist's powerful instrument, and is used with extreme care. P. both wanted and feared this *light hand*. It will be a risk for her to feel. It will be *death* for her not to.

Embodying this ambivalence, in one of the last group sessions, P. stood up to reveal her paralysis. After almost seven months of work, she was now able to feel and allow her body to *speak* consciously — although she began many sessions with the declaration, "I don't want to feel."

Standing sideways to the group, she planted her right leg forward and left leg behind with the right arm reaching forward, leading the body towards *where she was going*. Her left hand touched her chest, the left elbow leading backwards towards her leg. With pain in her heart she was going forward, out of the group, out of the community, to the next phase of recovery — reentry — still caught in the ambivalence of her feelings.

Stillness as much as movement, silence as much as music — the dance therapist approaches the duality of Dionysus in the same spirit, working with him in every session. She is able to sit still and hold the passivity, as well as limit and define the over-zealous activity and action when it comes. Her body takes on the feeling of numbness, fear, joy, or sadness, and carefully feeds these feelings back to members of the group in order for them to claim these as their own.

Dance, music, play, and movement are para-doxically Dionysian tools which the dance-movement therapist uses to restore consciousness and feeling to the recovering substance abuser. Called to give homage to this god as part of human nature. Dionysus will be felt and heard.

The dance-movement therapist honors his presence by restoring a form of ecstasy in life to the recovering substance abuser, who now can have more respect for his powerful force.

REFERENCES

1. Hamilton E: Mythology, 49. Mentor Books, 1940.
2. Otto W: Dionysus. Myth and Cult, 86-91, 106-110, 143. Spring Books, 1965.
3. Kestenberg J: The Role of Movement Patterns in Development, 14-22. Dance Notation Bureau Press, 1977.
4. Fierz-David L: Woman's Dionysian Initiation, The Villa of Mysteries in Pompeii, 19. Spring Publications, 1966.

CHAPTER 75

Culture, Self and Body-Self:
Dance/Movement Therapy Across Cultures

Patrizia Pallaro

CULTURE AS SIGNIFICANT VARIABLE

Culture may be seen as behavioral constellations or patterns, replete with symbolic meanings which are characteristic of all humankind. Different expressions of such patterns cluster around particular sets of symbols, values, and ideas — which are transformed and selected throughout history — resulting in the configurations of different cultures.[1]

Linton, describing culture as "the configuration of learned behavior and results of behavior whose components and elements are shared and transmitted by the members of a particular society,"[2] suggests that behaviors may consistently change and vary within different cultural systems. During the last twenty years, a substantial body of writings has been developed on the implications of counseling and psychotherapy with culturally different populations, as well as on the delivery of mental-health services across cultural barriers. Culture is a persistent and inevitable yet sometimes overlooked variable in the enterprise of psychotherapy.[3-5]

Substantial evidence supports a consistent relationship between achieved levels of psychological development, forms of pathology, and cultural context, while "dominant forms of pathology are uniquely characteristic of the culture in which they emerge."[6] Cultural characteristics must also be considered within the therapeutic relationship, since some of the functions of psychotherapy and counseling are "to reintegrate the client into the culture, and to enable him or her to respond to cultural roles and to meet cultural expectations."[7] The role of psychotherapy becomes more complex when the therapeutic intervention addresses specific issues of a definite cultural minority in its interactions with a dominant, *host* culture. The problems brought to light may be the result of a clash between the different cultures' values. Mental-health professionals are encouraged, therefore, to take cultural variables into consideration, especially in countries which have been shaped by a variety of different ethnic groups.

The latest trends in cross-cultural psychology, which reflect the current mainstream in the social sciences, tend to reevaluate the subjective experience of the individual as pivotal to comprehension of human behavior.[8] Human behavior cannot be explained totally in terms of physiological processes, personality structures, cognition and affect patterns, environment adaptations, and so forth. The self may be considered as an entity unto itself, distinct from social role, and that behavior is therefore the product of the relationship, at times conflictual and always subject to change, between experiences of self and one's social role expectations.[8] Since behavior changes considerably within cultures, it has been postulated that cultural traditions shape one's sense of self and that the self will have particular ways, inherent to that particular culture, of engaging itself with external experiences.[9, 10]

SELF AND DEVELOPMENT OF OBJECT RELATIONS

Object-relations theory describes the experience of being a person as a process of synthesis and adaptation between inner life and outer reality. The sense of *self* is attained through the ongoing process of differentiation of internalized images of one's own self and those of external objects.[11-19]

Many authors agree that as the child internalizes the integrated image of the mother (or other primary caretaker) as *good* and *bad*, he/she develops a more complete and realistic sense of the mother as a person, and different from the child.[11-15, 20-29] At the same time, the child gradually acquires the sense of him/herself as both *good* and *bad*, and also as a unique person, distinct from others. Failure to integrate the all-good and all-bad images of the mother (and therefore of one's self) will lead to impairment of the sense of self and its function throughout adult life, subject to a variety of splits in its overall organization.

Object-relations theory has an intrinsic validity beyond cultural differences because of its *relational* structure and interpersonal focus.[30-33] Stages of psychosexual development are different in different cultures, varying in time span, meaning, and tasks to master, whereas the constructs of early development such as images of self and object are dynamically linked to each other in every culture. Each simultaneously shapes and is shaped by the other. This interlocking pattern, further colored by culturally determined socialization and developmental experiences, profoundly affects the ways in which individuals view and interact with each other.

Subjective experience as it is lived through the body is the crucial and principal organizer of object representations in infancy. The core of the mother-infant relationship is the same across cultures, as described by several authors,[10, 11, 29, 31-34] and punctuated by bodily-felt experiences which are the infant's first sources of learning.

MOVEMENT THERAPY

As defined by the American Dance Therapy Association,[35] movement therapy is "the psycho-therapeutic use of movement as a process which furthers the emotional and physical integration of the individual." Since its first appearance in the U.S. mental-health system (during the 1940s), movement therapy has continually refined its theoretical foundations through the contributions of many fine clinicians, whose work has solidly connected the pioneers' intuitive assumptions with the larger body of psychological theory and practice. All movement therapists share a belief that "body movement is the most primary means of communication,"[34] and utilize a variety of bodily techniques aimed at fostering self-awareness and connecting inner psychic processes with feelings and experiences in the outer world. Individual styles reflect each practitioner's preference for one or more of the major psychological frames of reference, providing a variety of different approaches, such as Adlerian, Jungian, Gestalt, systemic, psychoanalytic, experiential, transpersonal, and so forth.[36, 37] Movement therapists have also exhibited a growing interest in self-psychology, and discovered a "direct relation-

ship between the fundamental premises and work within the field of dance/movement therapy and object-relations theory."[34]

Within this frame, movement therapy carries forward its process of integration utilizing the notions of body-self and spatial self as configured by Wyman,[38] who proposes a model for individual growth and therapeutic process in movement therapy based on concepts of "merging" and "differentiating." The process of merging and differentiating is present throughout one's life, but determined by one's earliest experiences in infancy. Merging and bonding of the infant with the mother consequently allow the child to experience separateness and identification, resulting in differentiation.[11, 14, 21, 28, 29, 39, 40] Without merging and bonding, there is no possibility for the infant to acquire a distinct sense of self. In this relational model, merging with and consequently differentiating from the mother allows the infant to merge with his/her own body and thus differentiate his physical identity from those of others. When personal identity is thus established, the individual will again merge, this time in groups, first in the family and then in the socioculturally determined group, identifying him/herself with the values of that group, and eventually differentiating him/herself by choosing only those values that the individual feels befit his/her own needs and convictions.

BODY-SELF AND INNER SENSE OF SELF

The fact that Freud stated that the ego "is first and foremost a bodily ego"[41] was somehow subsequently overlooked by both Freud and his followers.[42] Thanks to developmental and object-relations theorists, the primary experience of the body as conveyer of the individual's sense of self has regained attention and significance in psychoanalysis. Stern asserted that "some senses of the self exist prior to self-awareness and language."[26] Over time, the whole of our subjective experience is built upon these senses, transformed, decoded, recoded, and further integrated. This *core self* includes the sense of agency, the sense of physical cohesion, the sense of continuity, the sense of affectivity, the sense of a subjective self, the sense of creating organization, the sense of transmitting meaning, all based on the body as agent, container, vessel, mirror, probe, and vehicle of exchange. As Mahler says, "the core of ego development, the first orientation toward external reality, is the differentiation of body image, which is the psychic representation of the bodily self."[43]

It is through the baby's repeated experiences of contact with the mother's body, her warmth, texture, rhythms, and constant ministrations, as well as the subsequent emergence of and contact with the feeling of his/her own body, that the infant develops a sense of his/her own body boundaries, as delimiting and containing his/her own sense of self. Mahler further states that "the beginning of the sense of individual identity and separation from the object is mediated by bodily sensation."[40] Thus, in the psychotherapeutic process, in order to strengthen, modify, or integrate the representations and the experiences of one's own inner self, it is absolutely necessary to start from the body and its experiences. The movement therapist, therefore, will facilitate clients' awareness of bodily sensations through explorations of various parts of their bodies, finding different (opposite and/or complementary) ways of moving those parts, exaggerating and intensifying movements, releasing inner tensions, and exploring one's own bodily rhythms.

The following examples are illustrative, and by no means inclusive. The therapist may ask clients to slap and pat themselves all over in order to clarify body boundaries and increase awareness of body parts. Or clients may be asked to move across space while imagining one part of his/her body (i.e. head, chin, hand, elbow, chest, etc.), leading the person forward, backward, or sideways. A person may be gently pushed by another and led through space, thus simultaneously experiencing external action and control and his/her own body's resistance or acceptance. *Centering* will allow the client to experience being balanced or off balance, possibly creating a metaphor for an inner emotional state. Eyes may be closed while breathing exercises are performed. Imagery can be used to facilitate the free flow of breath, enabling the client to visualize a stream of energy (or light) pouring through the whole body.

Exploration of one's own bodily rhythms in relation to stimuli from within and from without will enable the person to get in touch again with the body, promoting integration and cohesiveness of the sense of self. The therapist may suggest that clients tune in to their inner bodily rhythms as a way of *centering* themselves, or to explore rhythms created by hand-clapping, foot-stamping, torso fluctuations, etc., in order to discover many different rhythmic variations and broaden their experiential range. Thus, awareness of the body-self allows and enhances awareness of one's own sense of self.

SPACIAL-INTERACTIONAL SELF AND INTERPERSONAL SELF

When the body image is established and body boundaries developed, "this demarcation between inside and outside of the body makes it possible for the infant to direct affective impulses beyond the body-self boundary and to recognize on a motor-kinesthetic level an outside-of-the-body world."[44]

Similarly, in the psychotherapeutic process, "once an individual is able to relate to his/her own body, he/she can then begin to merge and differentiate from others on the spatial-interactional level."[38] Deep and meaningful relationships are determined by the individual's capacity for merging with others and at the same time retaining (differentiating) his/her sense of self. Johnson states that the interpersonal self finds its configuration in "states of mind associated with interpersonal experiences featuring explicit communication in dyadic and small groups involving direct, reciprocal interaction."[45] Thus, the object of a therapeutic process directed at fostering one's sense of self in relation to others will be awareness of feelings and states of mind associated with interactional movements. Movement experiences such as mirroring, leading, and following will provide the frame for the body-self to experience reflection, empathy, and engagement in relation to others. The movement therapist will enable clients to become aware of the different ways in which they interact with the therapist, either in a one-to-one relationship or with other partners if the setting features a group situation.

The therapist will facilitate merging by asking the client to follow another partner, for example, mirroring his/her walk stance, his/her walk rhythm, the movements of his/her arms, hands, etc., and then to resume (differentiating) one's particular way of walking, standing, moving, etc. The experience of merging and then differentiating, in this case, will enable clients to realize their own personal modes of being and to draw attention to differences and similarities between their personal experiences and the embodied experiences of others. The therapist may also encourage clients to relate their postures and movements to feeling states, helping them to "clarify the relationship between the affective experience and the kinesthetic one."[38] Movements, in fact, are used as metaphors for inner emotional states,[38, 46, 47] allowing clients to experience their own particular feelings, emotions, or personal qualities, as well as others', in order to promote integration at the emotional level.

Clients can be asked to find ways of embodying and moving sets of polarities, easily conceivable and translatable into movement, such as large/small, open/closed, warm/cold, heavy/light, strong/weak, fast/slow, etc., and then to associate the kinesthetic sensation experienced with the feeling or emotion arising. For example, clients may be encouraged to first center themselves, then to shrink and then grow, passing through the centered position again. While experiencing this polarity, different clients may get in touch with different feelings. Feelings such as helplessness, fear, and desire for protection may arise while shrinking, whereas feelings of power, strength, or happiness may surface while growing. Verbally sharing these feelings will enable the clients to realize the variety of subjective experience. Asking them to re-embody those feelings in a way that is particular and familiar to them and/or alien, will allow them to expand the range of their experience, and eventually promote integration of unknown or previously disavowed aspects of their own personalities.

Movement experiences lead to a greater capacity for acceptance of body-self and coping strategies of the social self. Kupka says, "... the body-self can be thought of as inner experiencing while the social self is the experience of the self interacting with the environment. The movement process focuses first on a quieting, tuning inward to the body-self experience and then, from this bodily-felt knowledge, [focalizes on] an expanding of the social self's interactions and experiencing with the environment ... It is through the body-self experience that we come to know what we need; it is through the social self interactions that we are able to get what we need."[48]

By facilitating the process of merging and differentiating, first within one's own body, and then in relation to others, exploring the everyday social interactions in terms of embodied conflicts and polarized body movements, awareness of one's own social self is attained and integration of appropriate coping strategies with culturally determined social experiences is achieved.

REFERENCES

1. Kroeber AL, Kluckhohn C: Culture: A Critical Review of Concepts and Definitions. New York: Vintage Books, 1952.

2. Linton R: The Cultural Background of Personality. Englewood Cliffs, NJ: PrenticeHall, 1945.

3. Draguns JC: Resocialization into culture: The complexities of taking a worldwide view of psychotherapy. In Brislin RW, Bochner S, Lonner WJ (eds), Cross-cultural Perspectives on Learning. New York: Sage, 1975.

4. Price-Williams D: Modes of thought in cross-cultural psychology: An historical overview. In Marsella AJ, Tharp R, Ciborowski T (eds): Perspectives on Cross-cultural Psychology. New York: Academic Press, 1979.

5. White G, Kirkpatrick J (eds): Person, Self, and Experience. Berkeley, University of California Press, 1985.

6. Phillips L: Human Adaptation and its Failures. New York: Academic Press, 1968.

7. Draguns JC: Cross-cultural counseling and psychotherapy: History, issues, current status. In Marsella AJ, Pedersen PB (eds), Cross-cultural Counseling and Psychotherapy. New York: Pergamon Press, 1981.

8. Marsella AJ, De Vos G, Hsu F (eds): Culture and Self: Asian and Western Perspectives. New York: Tavistock Publications, 1985.

9. Lock A: Universals in human conception. In Heelas P, Lock A (eds), Indigenous Psychologies: The Anthropology of the Self. New York: Academic Press, 1981.

10. Roland A: Psychoanalysis in civilizational perspective: The self in India, Japan and America. Psychoanalytic Review 71(4):569-590, 1984.

11. Mahler M, Pine F, Bergman A: The Psychological Birth of the Human Infant. New York: Basic Books, 1975.

12. Kernberg O: Internal World and External Reality. New York: Jason Aronson, 1980.

13. Kohut H: The Psychoanalysis of the Self. New York: International Universities Press, 1971.

14. Kohut H: The Restoration of the Self. New York: International Universities Press, 1977.

15. Winnicott DW: Collected Papers: Through Pediatrics to Psychoanalysis. New York: Basic Books, 1958.

16. Winnicott DW: The theory of the parent-infant relationship. International Journal of Psychoanalysis 41:585-595, 1960.

17. Stolorow R, Lachmann F: Psychoanalysis and Developmental Arrests. New York: International Universities Press, 1980.

18. Engler JH: Vicissitudes of the self according to psychoanalysis and Buddhism: A spectrum model of object relations development. Psychoanalysis and Contemporary Thought 6(1):29-72, 1983.

19. Jacobson E: The Self and the Object World. New York: International Universities Press, 1964.

20. Bowlby J: Attachment and Loss (2 Vols). New York: Basic Books, 1969-1973.

21. Fairbairn WR: Psychoanalytic Studies of the Personality: The Object Relation Theory of Personality. London: Routledge & Kegan, 1976.

22. Guntrip H: Psychoanalytic Theory, Therapy and the Self. New York: Basic Books, 1971.

23. Kestenberg JS: Children and Parents: Psychoanalytic Studies in Development. New York: Jason Aronson, 1975.

24. Kohut H: The Search for the Self (2 Vols). New York: International Universities Press, 1978.

25. Piaget J: The Child's Conception of the World. Peterson, NJ: Littlefield & Adams, 1965.

26. Stern DN: The Interpersonal World of the Infant. New York: Basic Books, 1985.

27. Winnicott DW: The Child, the Family, and the Outside World. London: Penguin Books, 1964.

28. Winnicott DW: The Maturational Process and the Facilitating Environment. London: Hogarth Press, 1965.

29. Winnicott DW: Playing and Reality. London: Tavistock, 1971.

30. Foulks EF, Schwartz F: Self and object: Psychoanalytical perspectives in cross-cultural fieldwork and interpretation. Ethos 10(3):254-278, 1982.

31. Roland A: The self in India and America: Toward a psychoanalysis of social and cultural contexts. *In* Kavolis V (ed), Designs of Selfhood. Cranbury, NJ: Associated University Presses, 1984.

32. Kakar S: Psychoanalysis and non-Western cultures. International Review of Psychoanalysis, 12:441-448, 1985.

33. Ng ML: Psychoanalysis for the Chinese: Applicable or not applicable? International Review of Psychoanalysis 12:449-460, 1985.

34. Bernstein PL: Object Relations, Self Psychology and Dance/Movement Therapy. *In* Bernstein PL, Singer DL (eds), The Choreography of Object Relations. Keene, NH: Antioch University, 1982.

35. American Dance Therapy Association: Proceedings of the Ninth Annual American Dance Therapy Association Conference, 1974.

36. Bernstein PL (ed): Eight Theoretical Approaches in Dance/Movement Therapy. Dubuque, IA: Kendall/Hunt, 1979.

37. Bernstein PL (ed.): Theoretical Approaches in Dance/Movement Therapy, Vol II. Dubuque, IA: Kendall/Hunt, 1984.

38. Wyman W: Merging and Differentiating. Unpublished Master's Thesis, University of California, Los Angeles, 1978.

39. Winnicott DW: Mother and Child. New York: Basic Books, 1957.

40. Mahler M: On Human Symbiosis and the Vicissitudes of Individuation. New York: International Universities Press, 1968.

41. Freud S.: The Ego and the Id. London: Hogarth Press, 1923.

42. Fliess R: Ego and Body Ego. New York: Schulte, 1961.

43. Mahler M: On child psychosis and schizophrenia: Autistic and symbiotic infantile psychosis. Psychanalytic Study of the Child 7: 286-305, 1952.

44. Naess J: A developmental approach to the interactive process in dance/movement therapy. American Journal of Dance Therapy 3:44-55, 1982.

45. Johnson FA: The Western concept of self. *In* Marsella A, De Vos G, Hsu F (eds), Culture and Self: Asian and Western Perspectives. New York: Tavistock Publications, 1985.

46. Dosamantes Alperson E.: The intrapsychic and the interpersonal in experiential movement psychotherapy. American Journal of Dance Therapy 3:20-31, 1979.

47. Dosamantes Alperson E.: Contacting bodily-felt experiencing in psychotherapy. *In* Shorr JE, Sobel GE, Robin P, Connella JA (eds), Imagery: Its Many Dimensions and Applications. New York: Plenum, 1980.

48. Kupka N: The Effects of Movement Therapy on Body-self and Social-self Acceptance. Unpublished Master's Thesis, University of California, Los Angeles, 1979.

CHAPTER 76

Dance Therapy/Group Therapy — Theory and Practice: The 'Here and Now'

Linda Marie DiNoto

Within the field of psychotherapy, many conduct groups with a *here and now* focus. This refers to a type of group process guided by the therapist toward calling attention to and exploring the experience of being in a group. Participants are encouraged to examine the types of exchanges and feelings they are having as a result of being group members.

Here and now is an orientation that comes out of existentialist therapy, which is more of an attitude in therapy than a technique.[1] This therapeutic adaptation is based upon the theories of Victor Frankl, a World War II concentration camp survivor and psychotherapist, who postulated that if one can give meaning to one's experience, one is more likely to transcend life's trials and sufferings. The ideas and attitudes contained in this approach are the psychotherapeutic counterpart to the European existentialist philosophical movement, which emphasizes the ability of the individual to fashion from his/her activities and circumstances an heroic journey that gives existence purpose and value. The existentialist perspective in therapy recognizes the uniqueness of the individual process in a search for meaning which is considered the project of every person's life. Dance therapy operating within a group-therapy format — dance therapy/group therapy — can be seen as essentially an existentialist method because it is a form that establishes one's personal interpretation and awareness of one's body and movement as the source of insight and change in therapy.

The idea that modern humans are "cut off" or "out of touch" with themselves and their reality as physical, sensate organisms may well be central to treatment within a *here and now* framework. Keleman elaborated on this theme in his examination of how one can organize one's musculature around biological, psychological, and sociological constructs that exist as patterns both within and of the body:

The loss of somatic reality is a current existentialist dilemma. We are exhorted to 'be ourself,' 'develop ourself,' 'be true to ourself.' Many of us, however, have no felt experience of what is meant by these phrases. Either we live through images, trying to transfer mental experience to the rest of ourselves, or we try to enliven or intensify experience through chemical substances, social involvement, meditative withdrawal, or physical fitness. Self-knowing may increase, but not necessarily somatic understanding.[2]

Here and now, within body-centered modalities such as dance therapy, can be given to mean a somatic understanding of oneself through the body and the senses. This way of experiencing one's reality implicitly starts with the reference point of the body as it exists in time and space; physical existence expands into time and space.

Modern physics, which is increasingly being incorporated into the field of psychology and psychological thought, has proposed that nothing exists apart from the subjective experience of the physical laws of time and space; from this viewpoint, these factors constitute *here and now* reality.[3]

Dance therapy, in working with body movement, addresses the factors of time and space as they relate to human perception and experience. Dance therapy in theory and practice encompasses aspects of space and time within its use and implementation of the *effort/shape* system as developed by Rudolph van Laban and Warren Lamb for describing and notating qualitative changes in movement. Dance therapy applies itself in use of the *space effort*, considered the attentional factor in movement; and the *time effort*, thought to be the decision factor presented through movement. Body action also involves space awareness, the awareness of oneself as an object moving through space, and engages the duration element of time, i.e. tempo.

Dance therapy further explores somatic reality by focusing on the kinesthetic (bodily sensation) aspect of experience.   As a result of being encouraged to connect with body awareness through movement, the dance therapy/group therapy member is brought into the realm of impulse and perception, thoughts, feelings, and sensations. A sense of integration in this context may begin to arise as one becomes conscious of oneself as a physical, sentient being existing in time and space.

A *here and now* approach within a modality stressing the development of somatic awareness sees the individual as being in a continuous process of dynamic interaction with his/her environment. In keeping with the tenets of existentialist therapy, the dance-therapy group form, by validating the body and movement as a reliable and viable reservoir of information, fosters the individual's capacity to impart meaning to his/her life. The issues of *self* and *other* that arise within a group are seen as emanating from personal experience and perspective.   In the dance therapy/group therapy format, individual realizations are brought to the attention and scrutiny of the group both verbally and in movement. The dance-therapy form, by utilizing the elements of space, time and kinesthetic awareness, as well as qualitative movement factors, graphically illustrates habits, reactions and posturings that group members adopt as personal and interpersonal styles of relating to self, others and the environment.   The dance therapist develops and guides the emerging group process and dynamics by providing a format that engages and contains a creative process. This is done via use of structures derived from the art form of dance improvisation, and by putting into action the elements of dance and movement.

Much has been written about what is often referred to as the *creative process* from the standpoint of many disciplines — art, science, philosophy, psychology and education. This is frequently used to describe a procedure of initiating a project without necessarily knowing what the outcome will be. Creativity, as so defined, begins as the desire to create, an urge which is not clearly defined or organized, but which moves toward completion. The creator is sparked by an original idea or impulse which, through discipline, s/he brings to fruition as a tangible form. This type of creative process is often spoken of in terms of a surrendering to a process rather than the imposition of a concept into form.[4]

The dance-therapy group form, with its traditional sequence of beginning, middle and closure, provides the structure within which to develop and guide group- and individual creative processes, and furnishes the tools and building blocks with which to inform this process by introducing and applying the elements of movement and dance.

Dance therapy/group therapy embodying can be seen as a means of embodying one's reality through physical properties of body movement. Movement has qualitative features which can be associated and correlated to psychological themes, issues and values. The observation and identification of these qualitative features of movement (effort), along with the use of the elements of movement and dance — space, time and shape — are employed by the dance therapist in order to highlight themes within a dance therapy/group therapy session, and then develop them through a creative process which uses movement as its main medium.

REFERENCES

1. Yalom I: The theory and practice of group psychotherapy, 2nd ed, 87. New York: Basic Books, 1975.
2. Keleman S: *In* Hendrix G (ed), Embodying Experience, Forming a Personal Life, 1. Center Press, 1987.
3. Dossey L: Space, Time and Medicine, 42-43. Boulder, CO: Shambhala, 1982.
4. Maslow A: The Further Reaches of Human Nature, 59. New York: Viking, 1971.

CHAPTER 77

Dance for Hope

Joan McConnell • *Donald E. McGill* • *Teena McConnell*

The history of Western culture has been characterized by the dichotomy between science and art — science, with its support of reason and precision, as opposed to art, with its praise of emotivity and imagination. The objective values of science have stimulated analysis of the external world, while the subjective ones of art have encouraged introspection. The victory of science and reason has eliminated the cathartic and communicative functions of art at the societal level. Because of scientific advances, art has been pushed into the peripheral sphere of spectacle and entertainment.

Throughout history, art has not always been considered an ancillary activity. For many intellectuals, dance was the most exalted of all the arts. Carlo Blasis, the famous Italian dancer/choreographer who codified ballet technique and theory in the early nineteenth century,[1] maintained that dance was born as a natural response to song. The twentieth-century historian Curt Sachs[2] defined dance as the mother of all the arts.

In oral cultures, dance has always had a synchronic and a diachronic function. As a socializing activity, it reinforces the individual's identity as a member of the community at a particular point in time. As a religious or magical function, it transmits common cultural traditions from generation to generation. Since the movements and gestures of body language externalize inner feelings, dance could be defined as visual verbalization whereby words become meaningful gestures in space.[3] The dancers *speak* to their audience through this body language, while the viewers *read* the messages in the dancers' movements.

The development of literacy has stripped dance of the ritualistic power it once wielded in oral cultures. As the written word displaced the spoken one, the language of dance no longer communicated the traditions of the past and the community experiences of the present.[4, 5]

Dance today is moving closer to the world of medicine, and thereby regaining, in a modern setting, some of its former prestige in healing the body and the soul. The true story of the author (TM), a former soloist with the New York City Ballet, illustrates how dance played a significant role in restoring her inner equilibrium, reducing her anger, and helping her establish contacts — old and new — with the outside world.

At twelve minutes past five on a cold Christmas day, the wooden safety match that TM had just lit broke. The wooden stick fell on the rug, but the burning tip landed on her chenille robe. In a few seconds, the flames spread wildly over the fluffy fabric, and imprisoned the young woman in a torch of fire. At 5:13, her charred, scorched body lay agonizing on the kitchen floor. She was alive only because her father, hearing her hysterical screams of pain, raced to the kitchen and threw himself on top of his burning daughter to smother the flames. One minute of fire had changed Teena's life. She lost her career as a ballerina, her professional security, and, for more than two years, her physical and emotional independence.

After extensive skin grafts, TM began a program of physical therapy to strengthen her leg muscles, which had deteriorated from the forced inactivity. Her mood was one of angry, aggressive despair. She hated the dull, repetitive exercises on the machines, as much as she hated her badly scarred body, which no longer functioned as a perfectly trained instrument. Anyone watching her work out could read the anger and frustration in her movements.

One day, she rebelled against the rehabilitation program. She told her doctor that she wanted to rebuild her muscle tone through ballet exercises, because this was the only language that her body understood. Although she was still angry as she practiced her frappés, jetés and battements, these familiar ballet movements slowly brought her back to her own world. As the days passed, her movements and her posture lost their rigid, angular lines. A six-year-old girl, who had lost both her parents and all her fingers and toes in a tragic fire, was the first to notice this transformation. "Please teach me to do those beautiful movements," she pleaded. The next day, this unlikely pair — a burned ex-ballerina and a disabled child — moved their arms, legs, and heads as they worked to rebuild their bodies and their souls. They had began their *dance for hope*.

The value of dance therapy for injuries, post-operative rehabilitation, and even general fitness, is hardly new to medicine. Dance therapy is generally considered a physical means to improve or restore specific physical and/or emotional conditions.[6] The client is encouraged to externalize inner feeling and translate this message into movements and gestures. This approach does not maximize the therapeutic potential of dance. People who lack a keenly developed body perception have a limited range of expressive movements, because they feel uncomfortable with their bodies. Although the modern or free-style dance permits greater freedom in individual interpretation, it does not teach them how to move the body. One of the shortcomings of dance therapy is the lack of disciplined movement instruction.

The story of the author's struggle demonstrates the therapeutic efforts of her ability to transform the artistic body language of her ballet career into the practical instrument for her physical and emotional recovery. The success of her body-mind integration encouraged her to apply the ballet approach in helping other young women who had suffered the physical and psychological trauma of burns.* The rigid physical discipline presupposed a corresponding intellectual control so that the body and mind would function as a harmonious and complementary unit. The beauty of dance has always reflected this magical collaboration.

Classical ballet can also reduce the ambivalent feelings that some women, especially those with physical scars from injuries or accidents, have towards their bodies. Ballet strips woman of her earthly sensuality and idealizes her an ethereal sylph who, through dance, transcends the limitations of this earth. In ballet, movement comes from the extremities.[4] The

*Note: *TM did not work with men, primarily because many American men still equate ballet with women. This prejudice would have intensified the psychological stress she experienced in working with burn patients.*

legs perform aggressive, dynamic movements, while the arms and hands add grace, harmony, and symmetry. Some women feel comfortable with the asexual body language of ballet, because this dreamy ideal enables them to escape their 'flesh and blood' identity.

Modern dance, with its emphasis on the torso and hips,[7] thereby accentuates woman's sexuality. The trauma of physical disfiguration is often heightened by modern dance, because the dancers move their bodies as real, earthbound women, not as airy, immaterial sylphs.

Physical and emotional recovery after a serious injury is a long, painful experience which scars the body and the mind. There is no one sure remedy to relieve this suffering. Ballet uses fantasy, while modern dance is grounded more in reality, but both can help restore inner equilibrium. You can dance for art, you can dance for joy, but in the author's words, sometimes you must *dance for hope*.

REFERENCES

1. Blasis C: An Elementary Treatise Upon the Theory and Practice of the Art of Dancing (Mary Stewart Evans, trans). New York: Dover, 1968.
2. Sachs C: World History of Dance (Bessie Schonberg, trans). New York: WW Norton, 1963.
3. Pei M: The Story of Language, 11. New American Library, 1949.
4. Bentivoglia L: La Danza Moderna, 15, 30-36. Milano: Longanesi, 1977.
5. H'Doubler M: Dance: A Creative Art Experience. Madison: University of Wisconsin, 1957.
6. Lego S (ed): The American Handbook of Psychiatric Nursing. Philadelphia: JB Lippincott, 1984.
7. McDonagh D: The Rise and Fall of Modern Dance, 20. New York: New American Library, 1970.

SUGGESTED READING

1. Comucci N (ed): L'Allenamento muscolare ed organico. Firenze: FIGC, 1971.
2. Dolan A: Pas de Deux: The Art of Partnering. New York: Dover, 1969.
3. Grant G: Technical Manual and Dictionary of Classical Ballet. New York: Dover, 1967.
4. Guillot G, Prudhommeau G: The Book of Ballet (Katherine Carson, trans) Englewood, NJ: Prentice-Hall, 1976.

5. McConnell J: Language and Culture. Tokyo: Seibido, 1981.
6. McConnell J, McConnell T: Ballet as Body Language. New York: Harper & Row, 1977.
7. Ong WJ: Orality and Literacy: The Technologizing of the Word. New York: Methuen, 1982.
8. Sachs C: La Storia della Danza. Milano: Longanesi, 1966.
9. Sapir E: Language. New York: Harcourt, Brace & World, 1921.
10. Wilson HS, Kneisl CR: Psychiatric Nursing. Menlo Park: Addison-Wesley, 1988.

PART VI

MUSIC EDUCATION

CHAPTER 78

The Art of Practicing®:
Movement, Sensory and Relaxation Techniques
for Pianists and Other Musicians

Madeline Bruser

In practicing music, we experience an alternation between pleasure and frustration, insight and confusion, freedom and struggle. The Art of Practicing® is a discipline of recognizing and cutting through habitual strain and confusion, thereby releasing innate musical ability. This discipline combines physiological principles, sensory awareness, and relaxation of heart and mind to cultivate a natural ease, clarity, and joy in making music.

Strain is frequently caused by faulty movement patterns. Strain also occurs when we focus more on conceptual ideas of musical phrases than on actual perception of sounds. Although basic ease can be established by applying kinesiological principles, techniques for fully listening and deeply experiencing the vibrations of music in the body bring an entirely new level of physical fluidity and precision, which may be called natural command, or mastery. Kinesiological and sensory capacities of the body become integrated, enabling each other to function more fully.

PREPARATION FOR PRACTICING

The Art of Practicing begins with establishing a state of physical and mental ease before practicing. Preparatory exercises include stretching and mindfulness of breathing, which energize the body and clear the mind, allowing more vibrancy and intelligence in practicing. Reflection on the motivation to practice opens the heart, creating further relaxation and energy.

USING THE BODY WITH EASE

The body has a natural way of working. When we move in a loose and comfortable way, our energy is free to create both power and subtlety.

Upright posture allows easy support of the upper body, uplifting and expanding the torso so that the heart and lungs can function well. The heart area becomes open and expressive, and blood and oxygen can flow freely, supplying the brain and entire body with nourishment. This posture also enables the arms to move freely. Further, uprightness creates a comfortable balance of the vertebrae, with a lack of pressure on the nerves extending from the spine, allowing maximum sensitivity in movement and in sensory perception.

Looseness of the fingers, including the ability to move one finger without others reacting more than necessary, allows speed and expressive subtlety. Flexibility of the wrist allows energy to flow freely between the hand and arm.

Independence of the arms from the back enables the torso to remain upright, which allows full visceral receptiveness to the music. The arms are free to produce a warm, penetrating sound with minimum effort of because they can move freely instead contracting and grasping.

SYNCHRONIZING THE MIND
WITH THE SENSE PERCEPTIONS

In the effort to produce sound, musicians frequently lose their awareness of actual sounds — the original joyful experience of being a listener. Similarly, in the effort to move, we often lose our awareness of the actual sensations of moving and touching our instruments.

Our sense perceptions are innately acute. By putting our attention on the details of our sensory experience, we can relax into a full and natural receptiveness to the music. This process is called synchronizing our mind with our sense perceptions.

Techniques for putting our attention on each individual sound allow us to relax our impatience for results and to fully engage with the music. Such mindfulness of pure sound ensures complete hearing and suspends expectations and preconceptions about the sound. With this clarity and sensitivity to *space* (duration), the *articulation* of that space (by means of impulses from struck notes) into phrases and textures can occur in a spontaneous way — which is the sense of *playing* the music. In this way, a large part of what is called *music theory* becomes living experience of sound and pulsation, and the intellect is free to operate with a natural brilliance.

Putting our attention on our sensations of touch and movement awakens our joy and sensitivity in using our body. By cultivating an awareness of pure sensation, we discover the full vibrant potential of our sense of touch and the full expansiveness and freedom of our movements. This vibrancy and freedom allow our personal energy to come through in the sound, which becomes rich and full. Because our movements are harmonious and unencumbered, we experience a natural precision and security.

Mental synchronization with our sense perceptions forms of balance between the effort of producing the sound and the receptive pleasure of hearing, moving and touching our instrument. In a state of full receptiveness, struggle and excessive movement fall away.

RELAXING THE HEART AND MIND

The heart has a basic warmth and the mind a basic openness. By practicing with gentleness towards ourselves, we can let go of mental speed and continually rediscover our natural vulnerability and inquisitiveness.

Having created a state of physical ease and mental clarity, we can easily notice interruptions in this state which arise in the form of habitual types of struggle. Various emotional styles of struggle, such as dramatic overstatement and aggressive forcing of the music, are recognizable through their accompanying physical patterns of grasping, contracting, and stiffening.

Mindfulness of these types of struggle and a gentle attitude towards ourselves allow us to return to a relaxed and genuine way of playing. Following our natural curiosity as we practice develops our intelligence and makes practicing more enjoyable and productive.

In sum, by practicing being receptive to both ourselves and the music, we replace habitual struggle with ease, clarity, and joy. In discovering the full range of our movements and the full richness of sounds, we release our artistic power, and we become a vehicle for the music.

CHAPTER 79

Freeing the Caged Bird:
Developing A Common Language
for Teaching Injury-Free Piano Playing

Barbara Lister-Sink

Why is the field of performing still so tragically plagued with injury? Is there a connection between injury and the relatively small ratio of success proportionate to the number of talented students? Why, for most performers and teachers today, is an understanding of how to play the piano freely and without injury still enshrouded in mist and obscurity?

It is historically accurate and only fair to acknowledge that art and science — music and medicine — have joined forces for more than a century to attempt to unravel the mysteries of injury-free piano playing. For the greater part of the twentieth century, pianists have had access to a 250-year-old legacy of written information, albeit not always scientifically validated, on how to master the keyboard technically. Included in this legacy are C.P.E. Bach's *Essay on the True Art of Playing Keyboard Instruments*, as well as various writings on or by great pianists and teachers of the nineteenth and twentieth centuries. These include technical masters such as Hofmann[1] and Gieseking.[2]

Over the last century, pianists have drawn extensively on medical and scientific knowledge for explanations of injury-free playing. As early as 1903, Tobias Matthay, in his essay *Act of Touch*, summarized the causes of unnecessary strain and injury and gave detailed explanation of how to develop natural and injury-free piano technique.[3] In 1929, the great teacher/performer Abby Whiteside began publishing clear, succinct explanations of the characteristics of effortless, injury-preventive technique in *The Pianist's Mechanism*.[4] The scientifically exhaustive *Physiological Mechanics of Piano Technique* by Otto Ortmann appeared concurrently.[5] Other exhaustive analyses followed in the second half of this century, including George Kochevitsky's *The Art of Piano Playing, A Scientific Approach*[6] and *On Piano Playing*

by Gyorgy Sandor.[7] Although many of the hundreds of books and articles on piano technique written in the twentieth century have been scientifically invalid and specious, numerous writings have been both valid and eloquent.

The authors worthy of respect from the scientific community have agreed on three critical points:

1. Injury from playing the piano is unnecessary; it almost always results from faulty, inefficient use of the body — primarily misuse, compounded by overuse — and a lack of understanding of the biomechanics of playing.

2. Maximum achievement in the art of playing is impossible without an understanding and mastery of the science of playing. Although understanding and mastering the biomechanics of playing will not in itself produce great art, it is a necessary component in developing artistic potential. Without this mastery, expressing the breadth, depth, and height of human emotions and experiences is compromised.

3. Command of the science of playing is possible for all pianists. Technical ease, freedom, and mastery are teachable skills, not merely products of talent. They result from an understanding and step-by-step application of the principles of efficient body use, from the simplest to the most complex gestures. The pianist is an athlete as well as an artist. The physical activity of playing the piano is a complex, kinetic one, on a level with the most complex athletic activities. As such, the pianist needs to develop an awareness of all aspects of the science of playing, the biomechanics-muscle tension and release, alignment, balance, and good coordination. *Effortless* playing is within the grasp of any pianist.

One of the most effective and eloquent teachers of our century, Abby Whiteside, stated it thus, "When the student is balanced in muscular adjustment the playing of the artist is no longer a miracle — the gift of the gods. It becomes a thing that can be clearly analyzed..."[8]

The success of the great teachers was and is proven in the ability of their own students to play freely, effortlessly and without injury. Added to this list of teachers and their students are the great pianists of this century and last who played with remarkable freedom and ease. Arthur Rubinstein was one of the finest examples of the perfect marriage of technical mastery and artistry. Even the giants of the piano, however, did not always hold the key to communicating the science of playing.

Added to our scientific and medical knowledge are the contributions from related areas, including dance, yoga and other eastern disciplines, chiropractic, the Alexander Technique, and athletics. *The Thinking Body* by Mabel Elsworth Todd,[9] *Zen in the Art of Archery* by Eugen Herrigel,[10] and *The Warrior Athlete, Body, Mind & Spirit* by Dan Millman,[11] are invaluable sources of knowledge on any movement activity, including piano playing.

Modern, 'state-of-the-art' piano technique is very old. Although not widespread, the knowledge of how to prevent injury and to play effortlessly has nevertheless been available for a long time. Why, then, with the available knowledge of the last two-and one-half centuries, are pianists still grappling with discomfort, pain, injury and disease? Will the addition of yet more intricate scientific explanations and analyses move us closer to our goal? Will the dazzling tools and stunning knowledge of modern-day science and medicine rid us once and for all of the unnecessary injury and tragic waste of talent? Or, like some elusive constellation, will this knowledge appear only to fade or disappear for yet another era of haphazard learning and senseless waste?

We now have an unprecedented opportunity, thanks to advances in communications and technology, to spread globally this knowledge of how to cure and prevent injury — of how to teach piano playing, and playing of all instruments, as a joyful, healing experience.

The critical question is: Will we be able to communicate this vital knowledge? All of our assembled knowledge is like a beautiful bird which sings only if freed from the prison of its cage. Finding a key to unlock the cage becomes the critical factor.

The ability to use our knowledge to cure and prevent injury — to heal ourselves — will free artists and scientists, musicians and physicians, to devote our attention to the use of both music and medicine to heal a wounded world.

The key is the development of a *common language*. This language will be a means of communicating effectively, from the medical/scientific world to the musical/artistic world, all available knowledge. It must be a universal, non-controversial language that all musicians will be able to understand and use. It must be a language which precludes ambiguity and equivocation, which sweeps away the mists of obscurity.

What is the nature of this common language? It is the language most appropriate to the world of healing and music. It is the language of *physical sensation — kinesthetic, visual, and aural.*

The great stumbling block in communicating existing knowledge — and therefore eradicating the plague of injury once and for all — has been the reliance on the written or spoken word as the primary language in teaching. For the musician — child or adult — the word, at best, underscores what has already been sensed. At worst, it confuses and obfuscates. Even if valuable as a means of confirmation, the word alone can never teach a physical feeling or sensation. And it is precisely this physical sensation of ease, good coordination, and balance that is the foundation for injury-free technique.

How do we develop this common language? The first stage will require scientists and artists to share their knowledge. Scientists can share with performers and teachers their knowledge of biomechanics, biochemistry, and efficient body use. Performers and teachers who have shown, through their playing and effective teaching, that they understand this same knowledge can share how they came to this knowledge and how they communicate it to others.

The second stage will be the distillation of this knowledge into a system of common values, of sensations essential to achieving technical mastery and freedom. This system of values will be stated in a practical, jargon-free language understandable by all.

The critical third stage will be the imparting of these values, these sensations, to all musicians, from beginners to advanced players by means of a holistic, multifaceted language of the senses — aural, visual, and kinesthetic. The word will be used only to reinforce these sensations. This will be the critical stage wherein the possibility of confusion and distortion of knowledge is finally eliminated.

The development of this common language is an enormous yet exhilarating challenge for both artists and scientists. It is a pioneer attempt to build a bridge between two radically different worlds of learning, thinking, and doing. The creation of this bridge, however — this common language — will serve to clarify and affirm the value of both worlds. In building this bridge, we may rediscover that these are not two worlds, but one world dedicated to healing and making whole. Once this common language, this key, is used, then the songbird can sing forever outside the bars of its cage.

REFERENCES

1. Hofmann J: Piano Playing and Piano Questions Answered. New York: Dover Publications, 1976

2. Gieseking W, Leimer K: Piano Technique. New York: Dover Publications, 1972.

3. Matthay T: The Visible and Invisible in Piano Technique. London: Oxford University Press, 1979.

4. Whiteside A: The Pianist's Mechanism. New York: Schirmer Books, 1929.

5. Ortmann O: The Physiological Mechanics of Piano Technique. New York: EP Dutton & Co, 1929.

6. Kochevitsky G: The Art of Piano Playing, A Scientific Approach. Evanston, IL Summy-Birchard Company, 1967.

7. Sandor G: On Piano Playing. New York: Schirmer Books, 1981.

8. Whiteside A: Indispensable of Piano Playing. New York: Coleman-Ross Co, 1955.

9. Todd ME: The Thinking Body. Brooklyn, NY: Dance Horizons, 1937.

10. Herrigel E: Zen in the Art of Archery. New York: Pantheon Books, 1953.

11. Millman D: The Warrior Athlete, Body, Mind & Spirit. Walpole, NH: Stillpoint Publishing, 1979.

SUGGESTED READING

1. Anderson B: Stretching. Bolinas, CA: Shelter Publications, 1980.

2. Barrett W: The Illusion of Technique. Garden City, NY: Anchor Press/Doubleday, 1979.

3. Camp M: Developing Piano Performance: A Teaching Philosophy. Chapel Hill, NC: Hinshaw Music, 1981.

4. Hahn TN: The Miracle of Mindfulness. Boston: Beacon Press, 1987.

5. Last J: The Young Pianist. London: Oxford University Press, 1960.

6. Lederman R: An overview of performing arts medicine. American Music Teacher, 12-15, 70-71, February-March 1991

7. Leibowitz J, Connington B: The Alexander Technique. New York: Harper & Row, 1990.

8. Penneys R: Motion and Emotion in Piano Playing. Unpublished. © Penneys R, Eastman School of Music.

9. Plato: The Republic. Part II, Bk X. 85-92. (Translation by FM Cornford) New York: Oxford University Press, 1945.

10. Stark F: Gray's Anatomy, A Fact-Filled Coloring Book. Philadelphia: Running Press, 1980.

11. Sternberg R: The Triarchic Mind, A New Theory of Human Intelligence. New York: Viking Penguin, 1988.

12. Taylor H: The Pianist's Talent. New York: Taplinger Publishing, 1979.

CHAPTER 80

Introduction to The McClintock Piano Course: A New Experience in Learning

Lorene McClintock

I have always had the conviction that everyone should be able to read music and play the piano and to experience the benefits of a music education. That is why I have spent more than thirty years of research and experimentation preparing *The McClintock Piano Course* — testing it with teenage and adult beginners of all backgrounds and capabilities. Among the most gratifying and rewarding — and, at times, almost overwhelming — experiences I have had during the evolution of the course have been the responses of patients in hospitals, the physically handicapped, mentally and emotionally distressed, and drug-dependent individuals.

During the years of my work with students who were learning to read music and play the piano, I observed one difficulty after another, and then looked for the particular principle that would resolve it. The recognition of a principle introduced new ideas that enabled me to see everything in a new way.

I made many discoveries concerning the principles and learning processes involved not only in developing the skills of reading music and playing the piano, but also in developing an awareness of the deeper and more subtle aspects of playing the piano musically.

As the text of the course was written, each new idea and procedure was analyzed, tested, and refined until it could be easily understood and practiced by all of my students. The result was *The McClintock Piano Course: A New Experience in Learning*, a series of 201 lessons (music and corresponding text) arranged in progressive order for self-study or for use by teachers and students.

In the course, students are given all the principles I have discovered, and they are led in a simple and direct way through the application of those principles as each experience of their study unfolds.

The purposes in writing *The McClintock Piano Course* were: 1) to enable those with no previous knowledge of music or the keyboard to learn to read music and play the piano and to receive a complete music education — with or without a teacher; 2) to provide a simple and direct approach that would dispel the fears of those who have always wanted to play the piano but felt it was too complicated and difficult to learn; 3) to provide a complete course, embodying both the theory and the practice of music, in order to lift the general level of music education; 4) to provide a model not only for teaching, studying, and learning music, but also for teaching, studying, and learning in all areas of education; 5) to enable everyone not only to become musically literate, but also to develop a musical consciousness, thereby becoming a more active and appreciative listener; and 6) to provide a discipline that is both enjoyable and stimulating in order to help awaken the individual to a broader interest and awareness intellectually, culturally, and spiritually.

The instructions in the course provide the student with an immediate, in-depth experience, rather than rules and information which must later be translated into an experience. Underlying each experience is a principle to which the student innately responds.

The text is a guide that captivates and inspires the student and leads him through a structured series of procedures, which result in the ability to analyze, understand, and play both classical and popular music. The course includes compositions from folk music through the classics, with examples from such composers as Bach, Handel and Chopin, as well as original compositions which I wrote especially for the purpose of explaining and teaching various aspects of music.

In the early lessons, simple cardboard devices — the McClintock Keyboard Concealer and McClintock

Interval Keyblocks — are employed to aid students in establishing eye-hand coordination as they are learning to read music and play the piano.

From the beginning, the course teaches students theory as they are learning to read music, thereby immediately establishing confidence and understanding. The lessons provide students with a thorough comprehension of the principles of rhythm, melody, and harmony as they are applied not only to the study of piano and composition, but also to the study of other musical instruments and the voice. The course proceeds through advanced work in theory and composition, which students (including graduate-level) have found invaluable in their study. The instructions guide students through all aspects of piano playing that contribute toward producing a musical performance as well as an all-around musical consciousness. Students are prepared for advanced study in any field of music they may choose.

The course is designed to give the student the unique experience of actually being the student and teacher simultaneously. The sense of observation is developed to such an extent that students are able to catch themselves in the act of violating a principle; therefore, they can easily recognize and correct their own mistakes, if any should occur. The philosophy and approach have wide application to all areas of learning.

Some advantages of *The McClintock Piano Course* are: 1) No previous knowledge of music or the keyboard is required; 2) Individuals may use the course as a unique and invaluable guide for teaching themselves to read music and play the piano and receive a complete music education as they study at home, at their own pace; 3) Teachers may use the course as a format for individual and group instruction; 4) The course provides excellent preparation for college entrance exams and for teacher certification; 5) Retired persons may use the course as a vital and rewarding new interest and experience — learning to read music and play the piano, without a teacher; 6) Working with the course is remarkably effective as a method of relaxation and stress release; 7) The course may be used as "learning therapy" for the physically handicapped, to develop coordination and confidence, and for mentally and emotionally distressed and drug-dependent individuals, to enable them to focus their attention, learn a new skill, and gain self-esteem.

Students who have worked with the course have gained insights into every area of their daily activities. The experience of studying the course not only has made the students aware of their own capabilities and potentialities in relation to music, but has given them courage to develop and pursue other interests as well. An adult student wrote, "Your unique method of teaching piano has done more than one thing for me. I have gained self-discipline, self-confidence, concentration ability, and most of all, appreciation of the detailed mechanics of music composition and piano technique. I see that it is possible to learn the correct way of playing the piano at any age, and I was amazed at the ingenuity and logic incorporated in the structure of *The McClintock Piano Course*."

CHAPTER 81

Therapeutic and Educational Aspects of Shinichi Suzuki's Mother-Tongue Method

Ewa Klimas-Kuchtowa

The source of Suzuki Mother-Tongue Method was his observation of infants during the 1920s and '30s. He then drew conclusions about the analogy between speech and music-learning. Suzuki found that every normally developed child can learn to speak and can develop his language ability if repeated stimulation is provided. Suzuki supposed that the same could be with true musical talent, which is the synonymous with musical ability. Every normally developed child can learn to play in the same way he learns to speak. Honda writes: "The fundamental ideology is based on the assumption that originally all humans are born with considerably high potential for developing themselves...This wonderful ability to learn is developed by the environment."[1] One cannot help noticing how optimistic and deeply humanistic this opinion is.

Starr submitted the following: "Imagine, if you will, a Mozart or a Beethoven brought up from birth to cacophony, to every variety of unmusical sound. My own observations tell me that we would not have had a Ninth or a Jupiter Symphony."[2]

The primary instructors and guides of an infant through the mysterious world of first experiences are his parents. A mother and father speak to him and play with him, and a baby begins to imitate their movements and voices. If they sing, play an instrument, or play recordings of music regularly from the first days of a child's life, he will listen, learn, and probably try to imitate some of these sounds. The music should be an integral part of the child's environment. This way, music can begin to be synonymous with household warmth and feelings of security, laying a foundation for good relationships with others. Parents can create not only a positive attitude toward music, but also an opportunity for the child to begin learning to play at a very young age.

The learning should be always positively motivated. The first impulse for it is a positive experience, and the next steps should be the same. A teacher never should tell a pupil he is playing badly; rather, he should say, "You can do better." The atmosphere of lessons is playful, full of games and humor — especially with small children — relaxing but activating at the same time. It is far from the stressful, tense atmosphere at some music schools.

The child is not alone with the teacher during his lesson. A parent is present, in addition to the pupil whose lesson preceded and the pupil whose lesson is to follow, along with their parents and sometimes a sister or brother. All of them can participate in games, and they represent an audience for the child's performance. He senses their attention and positive feelings toward him. They are not his competitors, they are his friends, and they wish for his best performance. He learns to perform for an audience, and that it can be stress-free. The connection between playing, performing, a playful atmosphere, positive feelings, and people's warmheartedness is created.

A similar situation is experienced during music marathons, which are usually held monthly. All children of Suzuki's school play together during this ceremony. It is truly a ceremony, sometimes in a concert hall. Children are dressed up, as is the audience, which includes parents, relatives, neighbors, and friends. There is applause after each performance, but the atmosphere is still playful and relaxed. Children learn to play with a group (of course, string instruments only), and learn to compare their own performing with those of other members of the group. Very young pupils play only a few pieces, but they listen to the whole program or play games with an instructor in another room. First and foremost, they learn to play in a concert hall with a real audience — an audience that is friendly and full of positive feelings toward the performers.

The day after the marathons, solo recitals are held. It is a more stressful day, but the audience is the same.

A special place in the Suzuki method is given to home lessons and home concerts. A parent, usually a mother, is a second teacher. She participates in school lessons and helps her child practice at home. Practice should take place every day, of course, and its atmosphere should be playful. The home lesson offers an opportunity for close contact between parent and child, as well as for playing together with instruments or with musical games. Suzuki points out that when a child does not like to practice at home, the reason is usually that his parents are not correctly working with him. Home lessons should help the child to play better and strengthen the relationship between parents and child. The same is true with home concerts which are held from time to time and involve the participation of friends, relatives, or neighbors. The ceremony is similar to official solo recitals, but with a smaller audience. Each home concert should provide positive reinforcement for the child. Even if progress is not substantial, listeners' approval reinforces the child's efforts. It should consolidate the will of playing and feelings of safety on stage, and, most importantly, intensify friendship and love between a child and his family and close friends.

Another important aspect of Suzuki's theory is the assumption that every child has his own rate of progress, which involves many factors and subjective characteristics. A Suzuki teacher must be patient, because this is the one and only way to success. Suzuki does not use the word *patience*, however. This idea means, in his opinion, controlled frustration, but there is no place for frustration in his method. School teacher and home teacher should be helpful, understanding, and friendly. Patience is a result of those features.

Supporting a child's own rate of musical development is connected to the encouragement of individuality. Honda said: "The children are encouraged to hear the records of famous artists. They must absorb the feeling, expression, and musical sensitivity of these artists. But it is difficult to acquire all these, and each child receives different feelings and develops his own sensitivity. We cannot lose our individuality even if we are taught from the same books, the same religion, the same living."[1] Landers continues this idea: "At lessons and group recitals teachers often hear students play in various ways in order to test their flexibility and true knowledge of the repertoire; for example, tempo and dynamic changes and different interpretations are sometimes requested. Thus, the child actually learns many ways to perform; he learns a flexibility that helps him to find his own creative flow and style".[3]

These are, of course, only some of the many principles of the Suzuki method. They particularly support the psychic health of the music student and teach him positive relations with environment. Ultimately, a good Suzuki student should be not only a good musician, but also a good, psychically healthy man of worth, with good feelings toward others. Suzuki noted: "Our understanding of the phrase 'Talent Education' does not only apply to knowledge or technical skill, but also morality, building character, and appreciating beauty ... Thus, our movement does not mean to raise prodigies. We must express it in other words as a 'total human education' or enriched environment."[4] That is why Landers, in a dedication in his book about the Suzuki method, wrote: "To Shinichi Suzuki, who taught me to expect much of all people."[3]

REFERENCES

1. Honda M: A Program for Early Development Tokyo: Early Development Association Press, 1972.
2. Starr W: The Suzuki Violinist. A Guide for Teachers and Parents. Knoxville: 1976.
3. Landers R: The Talent Education School of Shinichi Suzuki: An Analysis. Chicago: 1980.
4. Suzuki S: Nurtured by Love.   New York: Exposition Press, 1968.

PART VII

MUSIC MEDICINE

CHAPTER 82

Hand and Upper Extremity Injuries in Instrumentalists: Epidemiology and Outcome

William J. Dawson

INTRODUCTION

Many conditions can interfere with the ability to play a musical instrument; overuse syndromes, nerve entrapment, arthritis and trauma are but a few. The literature on this subject describes primarily music-related overuse problems, with publications in both American[1-3] and international[4] journals. Less has been written about trauma to the musician's hand[5, 6] yet the sequelae of injury may be as devastating as those from any overuse condition. Few studies in the arts-medicine literature have described the long-term follow up or end results of any of these problems.[6-9]

The author has treated and followed many instrumentalists for various traumatic conditions affecting the upper extremity. This chapter presents that experience, with follow-up to an end result in a majority of cases. Various epidemiologic and etiologic factors affecting this group are discussed, especially those that may affect the performer's return to playing. It is the author's intent to alert those caring for such instrumentalists to the significant frequency of hand injury in this important group, and to the potential consequences of such trauma.

MATERIALS AND METHODS

All instrumentalists with hand- and upper-extremity problems cared for by the author and his orthopaedic colleagues from 1981 through 1990 were surveyed. Patients were divided into six categories, depending on degree of musical activity (Table 1). The 468 patients seen during this interval included 262 (56%) in classes *A*, *B*, *C* and *D* — the performing and teaching professionals, university-level music majors and dedicated amateurs. Trauma to the upper extremity was the cause of symptoms in 239 (51.1%) of the 468. There were 113 instrumentalists in classes *A-D* with traumatic problems, constituting the author's basic series. This group formed 43.1% of all 262

patients in classes *A-D*, and 47.3% of all 239 with traumatic problems.

Table I: *Musician Classification*

Class *A*:	professional performing musicians
Class *B*:	music teachers (who also perform to some degree)
Class *C*:	conservatory or university music students
Class *D*:	active, dedicated amateurs who play at least weekly with an organized group
Class *E*:	elementary- or high-school musicians
Class *F*:	recreational amateurs who play mainly for personal enjoyment or social functions

Long-term evaluation was performed on 100 patients followed to an end result; those not able to appear in person for examination were contacted by phone, using a standardized questionnaire to determine current status. The other 13 included 11 lost to follow-up and 2 in whom a final result had not yet been obtained.

Of the 113 subjects, 74 (65.5%) were male. There were 19 in the second decade of life (ages 10-19), 33 in the third, 21 in the fourth, 18 in the fifth, 14 in the sixth, and 6 were above age 60 (oldest was 83). The primary instrument played by the 113 patients is noted in Table 2. As in other series,[1, 3] string- (40.7%) and keyboard players (38.9%) formed the majority of this group. Among the strings, guitarists comprised 54.3%, two-thirds of whom were in class A; two-thirds of the pianists, by contrast, were in class *D*.

Table II: *Series by Class and Instrument*

Instrument Class	A	B	C	D	Total
Strings	30	1	3	12	46
Keyboards	16	4	4	20	44
Woodwinds	2	0	1	3	6
Brasses	2	0	2	2	6
Percussion	3	0	3	4	10
Miscellaneous	0	1	0	0	1
TOTAL	53	6	13	41	113

RESULTS

The etiology of trauma was sports participation in 36 (31.9%), with almost two-thirds of these due to ball sports; this prevalence has been reported previously[10,11] as a significant cause of disability. Household accidents occurred in 28 (24.8%); this included 16 lacerations from knives or broken glass. Another 24.8% were sustained by falls or direct blows outside the home or automobile. Motor-vehicle accidents accounted for 13 (11.5%), while non-musical work-place accidents produced 8 (7.1 %) injuries.

Diagnoses are listed in Table 3. A majority of the fingertip injuries were occupationally related. Neck- and shoulder strains usually followed motor vehicle collisions and often were accompanied by additional diagnoses. Late sequelae of injury included joint stiffness or contracture, tendon rupture, nerve palsy or dystrophy, epicondylitis and joint instability. Instrumentalists with these complaints had obtained their initial care elsewhere and presented to our office long after their primary injury.

Table III: *Diagnoses (118)*

Type	Number	Percent
Contusion/crush	8	6.8
Sprain/strain	25	21.2
Fracture/dislocation	42	35.6
Laceration	21	17.8
Late effect/sequel	21	17.8
Burn	1	0.8
TOTAL	118	100.0

Details of treatment of these injuries is beyond the scope of this paper, which emphasizes epidemiology and end results. Standard orthopaedic/hand care principles were followed in all

cases, however; surgical treatment was required for 35 of the 118 diagnoses made.

Criteria for inclusion in the end-result group included healing of the acute injury with return to the highest possible level of musical function and activities of daily living. Maximal possible rehabilitation must have been achieved and secondary or reconstructive procedures accomplished, if decided upon by patient and surgeon.

The 100 patients in this group described a range of symptoms related to their original diagnosis (Table 4). The author found 86% to be asymptomatic or with minimal symptoms, but 14% mentioned significant long-term difficulties. Table 5 shows the comparison of return to playing as related to the original diagnosis. As in the previous table, most patients (73%) described a complete recovery; however, 24% indicated a significant change in their ways of playing, and 3 others were forced to give up playing altogether.

Twenty-six of the 100 patients reported some residual deformity or loss of motion in the injured area. This subset included 2 of 8 patients with contusion/crush injury, 3 of 25 with sprains or strains, 8 of 42 with fracture or dislocation, 5 of 21 with lacerations, and 8 of 21 exhibiting late sequelae of injury. Although the numbers are small, musicians suffering lacerations or having late effects of injury seem to be the most likely to experience persistent stiffness or deformity.

This special group was categorized according to their answers to the questionnaire (Tables 6 and 7). Six of the 26 had no symptoms, and only 11 returned to full, unrestricted musical performance. Although the number of musicians in this group is small, the functional significance of residual deformity and/or stiffness can again be implied.

Table IV: *End Results: Symptoms*

Answer	Contusion/ Crush	Sprain/ Strain	Fracture/ Dislocation	Laceration	Late Sequelae	Total
Cured	7	11	29	13	5	65
Cure/recurred	0	1	0	0	0	1
Mild/infrequent	0	7	6	4	3	20
Fewer/persistent	1	4	1	1	5	12
Not improved w/R	0	0	0	0	2	2
TOTAL	8	23	36	18	15	100

Table V: End Results: Return to Playing

Answer	Contusion/ Crush	Sprain/ Strain	Fracture/ Dislocation	Laceration	Late Sequelae	Total
Full return	7	16	32	13	5	73
Minimal problem	0	5	0	4	3	12
Change style, technique, frequency	0	1	4	1	5	11
Some instruments	0	0	0	0	1	1
Changed instrument	0	0	0	0	0	0
No, due to symptoms	1	1	0	0	1	3
TOTAL	8	23	36	18	15	100

Table VI: Deformity/Motion-Loss Group: End Results—Symptoms

Answer	Number
Cured	6
Cured/recurred	0
Mild/infrequent	11
Fewer/persistent	7
Not improved with treatment	2

DISCUSSION

Non-music-related trauma has not been discussed widely in the arts-medicine literature. The current series is the largest known, and only the second to describe outcomes. Since termination of the follow-up period, several patients whose treatment was incomplete have achieved a final result; another 12 have been added to the group under active treatment. Thus, the study is an ongoing one, with further data to be compiled and considered for future reports.

The large number of guitarists as well as pianists in class *D* reflects the author's practice mix, which is more characteristic of a general hand-care practice than an arts-medicine one.[5] Additionally, class *D* amateur musicians constituted 36.3% of the 113 patients in this study.

The high frequency of sports-related trauma is disturbing; almost two-thirds involved some kind of ball, especially American baseball and softball.[12] I believe those musicians who engage in sports or physical fitness activities should use appropriate protective equipment, warm up correctly and recognize that infrequent or casual participation may be more likely to result in injury.

Each specific injury will produce a certain period of time in which the patient will be away from his or her instrument, and a second period during which performance skills are regained. The former period is determined by the relative healing time for a specific injury; many factors, such as handedness, type of instrument played, and side of injury, will be more pertinent to the latter period. Additionally, the timeliness of seeking medical care, the precision of treatment, and the effects of both physical and artistic rehabilitation will have a profound effect on both periods.

The determinants of an end result in this study have been presented. Each diagnosis has a different duration of disability until a final result can be determined — a period lasting from a few days to a few years. In general, these times are shorter for contusions and strains, longer for fractures and dislocations. Rehabilitation times from tendon- and nerve injuries may indicate that patients with these conditions might take longer than all others to achieve a final result; indeed, one woman with a complete ulnar nerve laceration at the wrist was still showing improvement in piano technique 3.5 years after repair. Patients with late sequelae such as joint stiffness or contracture may never regain the motions needed for "normal" or pre-injury performance levels. The data presented herein would seem to confirm this, although the numbers are too small to be statistically significant.

CONCLUSIONS

This study has shown that non-music-related trauma to the musician's hand and upper extremity can be a significant cause of disability and time away from one's instrument. The spectrum of etiologies and diagnoses is characteristic of a general hand practice, with sports trauma and household accidents predominating in the former, and sprains/strains and fractures representing the majority of the latter. Hand- and wrist lacerations from knives or broken glass are most likely to cause major functional losses, irreparable or with incomplete return of function. Significant interference with performance can result from many types of injury, with technical losses and (often) financial consequences to the patient. Very few instrumentalists, however, had to give up playing because of such trauma.

REFERENCES

1. Lederman RJ, Catabrese LH: Overuse syndromes in instrumentalists. Med Probs Perf Artists 1(1):7-11,1986.
2. Fishbein M, Middlestadt SE: Medical problems among ICSOM musicians: Overview of a national survey. Med Probs Perf Artists 3(1):1-8, 1988.
3. Hochberg FH, Leffert RD, Helter MD, Merriman L: Hand difficulties among musicians. J Amer Med Assn 249:1869-1872, 1983.
4. Fry HJH: Overuse syndrome of the upper limb in musicians. Med J Australia 144:182-185, 1986.
5. Dawson WJ: Hand and upper extremity problems in musicians: Epidemiology and diagnosis. Med Probs Perf Artists 3(1):19-22, 1988.
6. Crabb DJM: Hand injuries in professional musicians: A report of six cases. Hand 12:200-208, 1980.
7. Knishkowy B, Lederman RJ: Instrumental musicians with upper extremity disorders: A followup study. Med Probs Perf Artists 1(3):85-89, 1986.
8. Fry HJH: The treatment of overuse syndrome in musicians: Results in 175 patients. J Royal Soc Medicine 81:572-575, 1988.
9. Manchester RA, Lustilc S: The short-term outcome of hand problems in music students. Med Probs Perf Artists 4(2):95-96, 1989.
10. Dawson WJ: Sports and the instrumentalist: The hand at risk. Presented at Sixth Annual Conference on Medical Problems of Musicians and Dancers, Aspen, CO, July 1988.
11. Dawson WJ: Upper extremity injuries in high-level instrumentalists: An end-result study. Med Probs Perf Artists 5(3):109-112, 1990.
12. Dawson WJ, Pultos N: Baseball injuries to the hand. Ann Emergency Med 10(6):302-306, 1981.

CHAPTER 83

The Impaired Upper Limb in Musicians: Diagnosis and Treatment Considerations

Richard G. Eaton

The elbow and forearm, linking proximal shoulder support with the rapidly adaptive hand and wrist, are often the site of overuse and entrapment syndromes. Many of the muscle groups which empower the wrist and fingers have a portion of their proximal attachments at or around the elbow. These musculoskeletal insertions may become inflamed with excessive stress creating pain localizing to the elbow region. Furthermore, all the major nerves in the arm must pass through or between these muscle groups and are thus vulnerable to entrapment sufficient to produce hand and wrist pain, weakness, and sensory abnormalities.

LATERAL EPICONDYLITIS (TENNIS ELBOW)

The powerful wrist extensor muscles, key forces in wrist and hand function, arise from the lateral epicondyle of the elbow joint. With rapidly repetitious or powerful gripping activities, the fibromuscular attachments of these muscles may develop micro-tears which produce inflammation and pain proportional to the extent of these tears. Contraction of these muscles, particularly with both the elbow and wrist extended, puts tension on these areas of inflammation, increasing pain at the lateral epicondyle and/or along the course of the muscles.

In the normal healing process, the tissue involved softens as it remodels. Traction applied at such time in the healing cycle may cause further micro-tears in the already inflamed areas, thereby perpetuating the pathologic process. This accounts for the aggravating chronicity so characteristic of lateral epicondylitis.

Treatment is most successful when the cyclic nature of the process is thoroughly understood. Unless pain is disabling, complete immobilization of the elbow is not indicated nor practical. Effective rest can be accomplished with a wrist extension splint which immobilizes and relaxes the distal segment of these two-joint spanning wrist extensor muscles. Another device often effective for activity-induced pain is the tennis elbow strap, which partially stabilizes the proximal muscles and reduces the tension on their epicondylar origins during contraction. Anti-inflammatory medications are an important supplement in treatment, the most effective being a short course of systemic prednisone. The author personally avoids steroid injections in this region because of the collagen-altering nature of highly concentrated corticosteroids and the potential for further micro-ruptures.

Severe intractable lateral epicondylitis can be corrected surgically by one of several simple procedures. The need for surgical correction, however, is the exception rather than the rule.

CUBITAL TUNNEL SYNDROME

Compression of the ulnar nerve as it passes through the cubital tunnel, behind the medial epicondyle of the elbow, is a relatively frequent occurrence in musicians. Clinical manifestations of such compression takes the form of weakness of pinch or intrinsic muscle power, or wasting when motor fibers are involved, and pain, tingling, and numbness of the fourth and fifth fingers when the sensory fibers are involved. Anatomically, the ulnar nerve passes through a fibro-osseous tunnel behind the epicondyle, which funnels the nerve into a hiatus between the common muscular origins of the wrist and finger flexor and pronator muscles. Because of this distal fixation, the nerve must undergo a 1-3 cm stretch as the elbow moves from full extension to full flexion.[1] Many instrumentalists — particularly violinists and flutists — when playing, require a marked degree of elbow flexion, which may be repetitious and/or constant. This causes the nerve trunk to be stretched, which, in turn, produces varying degrees of compromise of the nerve's circulation. Transient tingling or intrinsic muscle clumsiness would suggest such an occurrence. Engorgement of the flexor-pronator muscles through rapid repetitious wrist or finger movement may further compress the circulation of the oxygen dependent nerve.[2] The resulting perineural swelling may progress gradually to fibrous thickening around the nerve and the surrounding structures, producing a chronic ulnar nerve compression condition known as the cubital tunnel syndrome.

The diagnosis is confirmed by hypersensitivity to manpulation of the nerve at the medial epicondyle, alteration of sensibility of the fourth and fifth fingers, and measurable pinch strength weakness. Nerve dysfunction can be confirmed by electrodiagnostic testing; however, a negative examination does not rule out cubital tunnel syndrome.

Conservative treatment includes modification in arm posture while playing, reducing elbow flexion as much as possible, avoiding acute elbow flexion and direct compression of the ulnar nerve during sleep, and systemic steroids as discussed under lateral epicondylitis. These may be quite effective when instituted early. Intractable sensory symptoms, documented weakness, or muscle wasting are indications for surgical decompression.

The best surgical results in treating cubital tunnel syndrome involve anterior transposition of the ulnar nerve from its posterior cubital tunnel location.[3] This reduces the entrapment and creates longitudinal relaxation of the nerve trunk. Several techniques of anterior transposition have been advocated. The author prefers a simple, minimally invasive technique which creates a subcutaneous sling to maintain the decompressed ulnar nerve anteriorly and emphasizes immediate postoperative motion.[4] Patients are able to return to low-key playing of their instruments within 48 hours of this procedure. Barring irreversible fibrosis within the nerve trunk or additional proximal compression, such as with cervical radiculitis, the results of this technique are quite satisfactory.[5]

MUSCULOTENDONOUS OVERUSE

The majority of the muscles which produce finger and wrist movement arise around the elbow and in the proximal forearm. They are connected distally to the wrist and fingers by tough cord-like tendons. Both these muscles and tendon structures are vulnerable to stress-induced inflammation. Musicians, particularly those who, in preparation for a special performance, tend to dramatically increase their practice activity, both in duration and intensity, are uniquely vulnerable to such inflammation. The condition is generally known as *overuse syndrome* and may effect one or several muscle groups. Pain develops in either the muscles themselves, their proximal origins, particularly at the medial epicondyle, or in their distal tendinous extensions. A characteristic pain pattern then develops.[6] The well-coordinated musician is readily able to reduce the stress to the inflamed and painful area simultaneously with an unconscious transfer of stress to another set of muscles capable of achieving essentially the same sounds. However, the overuse of these secondary musculotendinous units rapidly creates new inflammation and pain. This compensatory process repeats itself and pain migrates to other muscle groups or tendon insertions. Such migratory musculotendinous pain is pathognomonic of overuse syndrome. The wrist flexor and extensor muscles are the most frequent primary participants in this syndrome.

In treatment, recognition of the pathomechanics of overuse syndrome is the first step in successful management. The syndrome is most frequent in the student and young professional. Once the overuse cycle is understood, the problem rarely recurs. Complete cessation of playing is never indicated unless pain is constant and completely disabling.[2] In such situations, immobilization of the wrist and systemic steroids are indicated. Pain occurring only with playing can be managed by reducing the duration and intensity of practicing sufficiently to limit pain to a level of 4-5 on a pain scale having a maximum of 10. *To completely stop practicinq initiates a disuse-pain cycle by which long-established tissue conditioning is lost and progressive weakness develops until even minimal activity induces pain.* Preventing this advancing disuse-fragility state is a major goal in treatment.

DEQUERVAIN'S STENOSING TENDINITIS

Overuse of wrist and forearm musculotendinous systems effects two specific mechanical configurations. The first and most common involves tendons which have no specific retinacular restraints en route to their distal insertions. The second configuration includes a limited number of tendons which pass through a retinacular pulley system or sheath, designed to increase their mechanical efficiency. These pulley systems, with increased stress and repetitive to-and-fro tendon excursion, often develop inflammation of their gliding membranes, and characteristic pain patterns ensue. In the hand, such tendon entrapment is known as a trigger finger or thumb. In the wrist, the stenosing tendinitis of the abductor pollicis longus and extensor pollicis brevis is called DeQuervain's disease. It typically produces pain at the radial styloid, an area approximately 2 cm proximal to the base of the thumb, and is aggravated by flexion and extension of the thumb and ulnar deviation of the wrist.

Since DeQuervain's disease is a mechanical entrapment of the abductor pollicis longus and extensor pollicis brevis, the most effective treatment is complete immobilization of the wrist and proximal thumb for up to three weeks. Because of the obvious "friction" within this retinacular pulley system, even decreased practicing is unlikely to reverse any but the most minimally inflamed tendons. In addition to the full-time splinting regimen, a brief course of systemic steroids is a valuable adjunct to the treatment. Failure to dramatically reverse these symptoms in 3-4 weeks indicates an intractable inflammatory state which can be dramatically relieved by a mechanical (surgical) decompression of the stenotic sheath, a 15-minute surgical procedure performed under local anesthesia.

CERVICAL RADICULITIS

A significant amount of arm and hand pain is due to intermittent compression of the proximal nerve roots by arthritic spurs in the cervical spine. All the nerves to the upper limb arise within the spinal cord and must pass through bony foramina, or channels, through the surrounding cervical vertebral column. Previous trauma, chronic poor posture, or prolonged asymmetric positioning of the head and neck while playing a musical instrument may create osteoarthritic spurs which encroach on these neural foramina and are capable of pinching these nerve roots with rotation or bending of the neck. Such compression can occur while awake or even during sleep.

The radiation of pain or tingling to the upper limb caused by irritation of the cervical nerve roots is known as cervical radiculitis. Electricity-like shooting pains or tingling caused by this compression may radiate to any site in the limb. Depending on the nerve roots involved, the radicular symptoms can even simulate common compression neuropathies such as cubital or carpal tunnel syndrome. Since cervical arthritis is so common, some element of radiculitis may coexist with any limb pathology, involving both motor as well as sensory nerves. Unrecognized, it is often the cause of persisting neurologic symptoms after surgical decompression of tendon or nerve entrapment syndromes or, for that matter, after any

surgical procedure performed to correct a painful upper limb condition.

Diagnostic evaluation includes cervical spine radiographs to rule out obvious cervical disc disease or congenital anomalies. The presence of radiographic arthritic changes has minimal diagnostic value, since there is very little correlation between the magnitude of radicular symptoms and the degree of arthritic involvement. Neck range of motion is often limited and, occasionally, reproduction of symptoms occurs with testing the mobility of the cervical spine. Reproductions of symptoms or radiation of electricity-like responses (Tinel's sign) by rolling the nerve trunks against the underlying bone is also strongly suggestive of prior episodes of proximal nerve compression with ongoing regeneration to the level where the Tinel sign is elicited. When this sign is elicited proximal to the classic site of nerve compression, it suggest that some element of cervical radiculitis is present. Electrodiagnostic studies, unfortunately, are rarely dependable unless muscle degenerative changes are picked up in the paraspinal or shoulder muscle groups. A negative test, however, does not rule out cervical radiculitis.

In most cases, effective treatment is quite simple. Once radiculitis is suspected, a simple exercise program which produces improved spine alignment will bring about definite improvement within 2-3 weeks and eventually completely reverse the radicular symptoms.[2] Simple upper trapezius strengthening exercises which simultaneously improve paraspinal muscle tone are all that are necessary. These are done with the arms abducted and extended from the side and elevated 20° above the horizontal plane of the shoulder. Clockwise and counterclockwise rotation of the arms is done until trapezius fatigue is maximum and the arms cannot be maintained above the horizontal plane. These are best done before a mirror, to be certain the arms remain symmetrically above the horizontal plane, thereby emphasizing upper trapezius activity. Neck rotation or head tilting exercises should be avoided because of the high risk of additional nerve root compression in the neural foramina.

INDICATIONS FOR SURGERY

In all the acquired conditions discussed above, the initial treatment should be conservative, using some combination of reduced activity, anti-inflammatory medication, and/or immobilization. In *non-entrapment* conditions, improvement is usually gradual with a finite though somewhat flexible endpoint. Such an endpoint means that, essentially, normal activity is possible without pain. In *entrapment* conditions, however, where mechanical compression is the pathology, a more definite time limit for resolution should be established. Failure to respond to a well-disciplined, conservative program within 4-5 weeks indicates a non-reversible entrapment of the tendon or nerve, and surgical decompression should be strongly considered.

Conservative treatment should not be viewed as open ended or of infinite duration. Disuse and tissue fragility develop rapidly when normal activity and stress to a limb or musculotendinous system is withheld. At some point between 6 weeks and 3 months of the onset, a disuse-tissue fragility cycle develops if normal activity is curtailed, a phenomenon which compounds the musician's problem. With the inevitable reversal of the inflammatory condition, whether through conservative or surgical means, the underused tissue, i.e. muscle, tendon, ligament, and joint capsule, is sensitive even to previously normal level activity or stress. A gradually progressive exercise program, including return to one's instrument, must be instituted as early as possible. Periodic monitoring of pinch and grip strength will provide a reliable index to both the loss as well as restoration of strength in the involved muscles. Practicing is permitted up to a pain level of 4-5 on a maximum scale of 10, after which a period of rest is indicated.

REFERENCES

1. Apfelberg DB, Lanson SE: Dynamic anatomy of the ulnar nerve at the elbow. Pl & Reconstr Surg 51:76-81, 1973.
2. Eaton RG: Entrapment syndromes in musicians. J Hand Therapy (publication pending).
3. Dellon AL: Review of treatment results for ulnar nerve entrapment at the elbow. J Hand Surg 14-A:688-700, 1989.
4. Eaton RG: Anterior subcutaneous transposition. *In* Gelberman RH (ed), Operative Nerve Repair & Reconstruction, Vol 2, 1077-1085. Philadelphia: JB Lippincott Company, 1991.
5. Townsend PF, Eaton RG: Stabilized anterior transposition of the ulnar nerve: Long-term follow-up. Presented at Annual Meeting, American Academy of Orthopedic Surgery, Washington, DC, Feb 21, 1992.
6. Eaton RG, Nolan WB: Diagnosis and surgical treatment of the hand. *In* Sataloff RT, Brandfonbrener AG, Lederman RJ, Textbook of Performing Arts Medicine, 205-227. New York: Raven Press Ltd, 1991.

CHAPTER 84

Surgical Treatment of Acquired Hand Problems

William B. Nolan

GENERAL PRINCIPLES OF MANAGEMENT

The performing artist is frequently required to execute movements which are subtle or rapidly repetitious. These demands may far exceed normal manual activity. Afflictions of extended mechanical stress such as tendinitis, synovitis, and arthritis often ensue.

When these syndromes have become intractable, serious consideration should be given to surgical correction. Surgical release of the mechanical entrapment syndromes and degenerative processes provides an excellent prognosis and should return the performer to rapidly increasing function within three to six weeks. Despite the natural reluctance to undergo surgery, repeated courses of unsuccessful conservative treatment serve only to prolong the disability and in time create serious career anxieties. Most surgical procedures are brief, simple, and can be done under local or regional anesthesia on an outpatient basis. In the appropriate instance, surgery offers a high likelihood of completely resolving the problem with a great reduction in the musician's period of disability.

Early recognition of the primary site of pathology and overuse patterns is vital in order to prevent major distortions in motor patterns. Performance disabilities in artists and musicians have the best prognosis when corrected early, before compensatory patterns, muscle and ligamentous weakness, and discouragement set in. Most of the symptomatic ligament strains and tendinitis states will begin to respond within three to four weeks with a carefully managed rest- and anti-inflammatory regimen. However, certain specific painful tendon and nerve entrapment syndromes such as trigger fingers, De Quervain's disease, and carpal tunnel syndromes, may not completely reverse or may recur soon after medical treatment has been discontinued. In these cases, surgery may greatly benefit the patient.

ACUTE INFLAMMATORY PROBLEMS

Treatment is frequently divided into non-operative and operative approaches. Non-operative treatment includes splints, oral anti-inflammatory medications, and injectable steroids. When non-operative treatment does not produce prompt clinical improvement, surgical decompression of the nerve is in the best interest of the patient. Of particular importance is the presence of motor paralysis. When this occurs, operative decompression should not be delayed beyond three months. Prolonged compression of a peripheral nerve may result in permanent neural damage with atrophy and fibrosis of the denervated muscle. Most compression neuropathies that do not respond to conservative treatment within three months rarely will improve without surgical decompression.

Carpal Tunnel Syndrome

Carpal tunnel syndrome is the most common nerve entrapment syndrome in the upper extremity. The arrangement of the median nerve and nine tendons in the carpal tunnel permits compression of the nerve between the flexor tendons and the transverse carpal ligament. In addition, any structure which occupies space in this enclosure can compress the median nerve. This can be synovium, a bony tumor, carpal bone dislocation, an anomalous blood vessel, a ganglion, a lipoma, or fat.

Carpal tunnel syndrome is usually the result of synovial swelling. The repetitive motion of wrist flexors, commonly part of playing an instrument, may result in hypertrophy of the synovium. An increase in synovial volume inside of this limiting space results in median nerve compression.

In the absence of muscle atrophy, a trial of conservative therapy is appropriate with splinting and oral anti-inflammatory medication. Anti-inflammatory medication can also be injected into the carpal tunnel. Injection of a corticosteroid into the carpal tunnel must be done with great care. The needle can damage the nerve and skin depigmentation or atrophy may occur due to the steroid. While injection of the carpal tunnel has advocates, it has been estimated that in the absence of a reversible systemic etiology such as pregnancy, 65-90% of patients will have some recurrence of symptoms. The use of nonsteroidal anti-inflammatory medication is of limited benefit in the treatment of this problem. In the case of pregnancy, treatment should be conservative, as the majority of patients will stop having symptoms when peri- and postpartum hormonal changes resolve.

The indication for surgical release of the nerve is failure of conservative measures. If symptoms persist beyond three months, or if there is evidence of motor loss, there should be prompt surgical decompression to avoid a permanent disability. Decompression of the carpal tunnel is accomplished by division of the transverse carpal ligament. This can be done with local or regional anesthesia on an outpatient basis. The length of time necessary for recovery of the median nerve depends on the severity of the nerve compression. Frequently, patients report almost immediate relief from the symptoms of night pain and painful tingling. If the nerve has sustained internal injury secondary to severe or prolonged compression, recovery takes months rather than hours and depends on the regenerative capacity of the individual and the condition of the nerve. Recovery time is approximately six weeks for the artist to return to a performance level.

Tendon Entrapment

The extensor- and flexor tendons pass through a fibrous pulley system as they enter the digits. At the site where the tendons enter the pulley system, there is considerable friction. With overuse, varying degrees of inflammation, the tendon synovium may hypertrophy and become swollen.

Trigger Thumb and Fingers

Tenosynovitis in the thumb or fingers is a common cause of hand problems in the professional musician. It is occasionally associated with systemic diseases such as diabetes, rheumatoid arthritis, and gout. In the musician, however, repetitive flexion and extension of the digit probably contribute to frequent occurrence.

Triggering or snapping occurs as the patient tries to flex and extend the digit. If the swelling around the tendon becomes great enough, it is impossible for the tendons to glide past the point of constriction. The digit is then locked in either flexion or extension. This is referred to as a *locked trigger*.

Non-operative treatment consists of oral steroids or a local injection of a steroid into the fibro-osseous tunnel at the level of the MP joint. Failure to achieve complete relief in three to four weeks is an indication for surgical release of the tendon sheath, a simple and reliable surgical procedure that permanently relieves the symptoms.

Surgical treatment involves a small incision over the appropriate MP joint and division of the proximal pulley under direct vision. The surgery is done with local anesthesia, and the patient is then asked to flex and extend the digit. A full range of motion confirms that the problem has been corrected. The hand is placed in a soft dressing and the sutures are removed at approximately ten days. Full active motion is usually achieved within one month.

De Quervain's Disease

Stenosing tenosynovitis of the first dorsal compartment of the wrist is another common cause of wrist- and hand pain in the performing artist. The patient reports pain associated with thumb motion, localized on the radial side of the wrist. There is frequent swelling over the first dorsal compartment, at the level of the radial styloid process. When these symptoms are reported, it is important to examine the basal (carpometacarpal) joint of the thumb, which can produce similar complaints. These problems are differentiated by x-rays and physical examination of the basal joint. It is also important to examine the patient for evidence of tenosynovitis of the second dorsal compartment, intersection syndrome.

Non-operative treatment consists of oral steroids or local steroid injection, or systemic anti-inflammatory medication in combination with a splint that immobilizes the wrist and thumb. This treatment usually results in relief of pain. However, in the absence of a medically correctable condition that is responsible for De Quervain's, such as pregnancy or an endocrinopathy, the symptoms frequently recur with the resumption of activity.

Surgical decompression of the first dorsal compartment is done with local or regional anesthesia on a outpatient basis. The wound is allowed to heal for two weeks with the wrist held in a plaster shell. The prognosis following surgery is excellent.

CHRONIC-DEGENERATIVE PROBLEMS

The second general category of performance-related hand problems includes the chronic-degenerative disorders. Osteoarthritis is the most common problem in this category. It is frequently seen in the general population. The incidence of hand involvement in the general population increases with age. In the age group of 18-24 years, less than 3% of people have radiographic evidence of an arthritic hand condition. By age 75, however, 80% of men and 90% of women have arthritic changes. In the vast majority of the population, the radiographic changes seldom have clinical significance. However, the performing artist frequently subjects the hands to forces that can exacerbate an arthritic condition and become a source of disability.

Basal Joint Arthritis

The highly mobile basal joint of the thumb owes its great range to its metacarpal trapezium "saddle" articulation. Such mobility, however, has its price as this joint develops earlier and significantly more disabling degenerative changes than other joints of the hand. In a random radiographic sampling of women past 50 years of age, one in six demonstrated moderate to advanced osteoarthritic changes in the thumb metacarpal-trapezium joint.

Prolonged and repetitious compression in time may cause loss of cartilage or aggravate existing arthritic changes, leading to the pain and stiffness of osteoarthritis. The patient complains of pain and weakness that is worse with activity and relieved by rest. The pain is diffuse, and is frequently localized to the radial side of the wrist. The point of maximum tenderness can be identified by pressing directly over the trapezium-thumb metacarpal joint. Decreased pinch strength and lateral subluxation (attempted dislocation) of the metacarpal on the trapezium are also frequently present. A radiograph with attempted lateral subluxation is called a stress view. These radiographs which induce lateral subluxation of the metacarpal on the trapezium are useful in demonstrating the degree of joint capsule laxity.

Radiographs are utilized to determine the degree (stage) of degeneration. Radiographic staging of degenerative arthritis is important because it helps to establish the extent of damage, which, in turn, helps determine the type of reconstructive surgery necessary, should symptoms become intractable.

In Stage I, the joint is hypermobile and inflamed. Radiographs show less than one-third subluxation of the joint and normal articular contours. With acute inflammation, molded splints and anti-inflammatory medications frequently resolve the symptoms. If symptoms persist, reconstruction of the volar ligament restores stability, resolves the pain, and reduces further degeneration.

In Stage II, early cartilage damage is present. Radiographs show more than one-third subluxation, joint space narrowing and calcific fragments along the joint margins less than 2 mm in size. Clinically, Stage II is similar to Stage I and its treatment is the same.

Stage III has significant joint-space narrowing and articular degeneration. Larger debris with fragments greater than 2 mm in size is seen. All involvement noted on the x-ray is confined to the metacarpal-trapezium joints. The scaphotrapezial joint has no visible degenerative changes. In this stage, stiffness and deformity have developed. Crepitus may be noted with twisting of the basal joint. Thenar muscular atrophy and decreased key pinch strength may be present. Conservative treatment is similar to Stages I and II.

If conservative treatment of Stage III fails to relieve the symptoms, relief can be obtained by reconstructive surgery. Arthroplasty which reconstructs the ligaments and interposes soft tissue between the irregular joint surfaces has been highly successful. Four weeks of immobilization in a cast and two to three months of therapy are required for optimal results.

Stage IV is a diffuse arthrosis with involvement of both the thumb metacarpal-trapezium and scapho-trapezial joints. There is severe joint-space destruction associated with cystic and sclerotic subchondral bone changes of all the trapezial joint facets. Clinically, these patients have signs and symptoms similar to Stage III patients. Treatment for this advanced stage includes trapezial resection, implant arthroplasty, and ligament reconstruction.

Ligamentous Laxity of the MP Joint of the Thumb

The thumb of the bow hand of large-upright string-instrument players (i.e. cello, bass) is particularly prone to chronic ligament stress. Long hours of continuous longitudinal pressure while 'pinching' the bow create varying degrees of stretching of the ligaments of the metacarpophalangeal joint. A very tight gripping technique is particularly stressful for the ligaments. Biomechanical studies have shown that for each kilogram of force transmitted to the tip of the thumb, twelve times that force crosses the basal joint and six times the terminal force crosses the metacarpophalangeal joint.

Short-term splinting and a modification of playing technique will often relieve such symptoms. Once a ligament has become significantly stretched, however, it is unlikely to shorten or contract to a more physiologic tension. Surgical management of intractable pain due to ligament laxity involves reconstruction of the ulnar collateral ligament of the MP joint, usually utilizing the palmaris longus tendon as a graft. There is absolutely no residual functional deficit from taking away this 'spare' palmaris tendon.

CONSIDERING SURGERY

The thought that one has been 'sentenced' to surgery is always a shock, particularly when it involves the hands of a musician or artist. Fortunately, the pathologic conditions discussed herein, if not responsive to conservative management, are quite predictably corrected by surgery, with an excellent long-term prognosis. The recurring tragedy among musicians are the inordinately long periods of disability so often associated with easily correctable conditions. Months may stretch to years of non- or under-performance, either because of the dread of surgery or lack of information as to the prognosis for this type of surgery. The procedures described are simple, minimally painful and highly predictable. The patient should be healed and rehabilitated sufficiently to be utilizing maximum force without pain in a relatively short period of time.

CHAPTER 85

Acupuncture-Moxibustion and Related Techniques for Artists

Kerong Dai • *Xiaokui Hou* • *Xueyong Shen*

Acupuncture-moxibustion is the science of prevention and treatment of diseases by stimulating the meridian-collaterals and acupuncture points with needles, moxa, or other means. According to the theory of traditional Chinese medicine, the meridian-collaterals are the pathways in which the *qi* (essential substances to maintain vital functions and activities) and blood of the human body are circulated. They pertain to the viscera interiorly and extend to extremites and joints exteriorly, integrating the tissues and organs into an organic whole to keep the functions and activities of all parts of the body in harmony and balance relatively. Acupuncture points are the specific sites through which the *qi* and blood of viscera and meridians are transported to the body surface. Acupoints are not only the loci of response to diseases, but also the stimulating sites to prevent and treat diseases.

The science of acupuncture-moxibustion is ancient, with a long history of steady development, and yet it is young in terms of modern scientific knowledge. It has been shown to produce full vitality and has won great popularity and attraction in the world today. Artists and athletes, in general, dislike the use of chemicals because of their potential toxicity and side effects. In fact, acupuncture-moxibustion is without toxicity and side effects, thus a more suitable and effective therapy for their occupation-related diseases.

The authors believe that, as a nonpharmaceutical treatment, acupuncture-moxibustion will be accepted by more and more artists and athletes all over the world, and will play an important role in the field of arts medicine.

ACUPUNCTURE TECHNIQUES

The needle should be inserted, in general, coordinately with the help of both hands. Generally, the needle should be held with the right hand, known as "the puncturing hand." The left hand, known as "the pressing hand." presses the area or supports the needle body.

The function of the puncturing hand is to hold the needle and to perform manipulations. The function of the pressing hand is to fix the location of a point and to grip the needle body to help the puncturing hand insert the needle.

In the process of insertion, angle and depth are especially important in acupuncture. Correct angle and depth help induce the needling sensation, bring about the desired therapeutic results, and guarantee safety. There are three possible angles of insertion:

(1) *Perpendicular*: The needle is inserted perpendicularly, forming a 90° angle with the skin surface. Most points on the body can be punctured in this fashion.

(2) *Oblique*: The needle is inserted obliquely to form an angle of approximately 45° with the skin surface. It is used for the points in which deep insertion is not advisable.

(3) *Horizontal* (also known as subcutaneons or transverse insertion): The needle is inserted transversely to form an angle of 15°-25° with the skin. It is suitable for the points on thin skin or muscle.

The fundamental manipulation techniques, in general, can be divided into two types:

(1) *Lifting and thrusting*: This is a method by which the needle body is perpendicularly lifled and thrust in the point when the needle is inserted to a certain depth.

(2) *Twirling or rotating*: This refers to the manipulation by which the needle body is twirled or rotated forward and backward continuously after the needle has reached its desired depth. The manipulation is done by the thumb, middle and index fingers of the right hand, which holds the needle body.

During the needling sensation, the patient has soreness, numbness, a distended feeling, or heaviness around the point. At the same time, the operator may feel tenseness and a pressing sensation around the needle.

Retaining means to keep the needle in place after it is inserted into a point. The purpose of retaining is to strengthen the needling sensation and to facilitate the manipulation of the needle. In general, the needle is retained for 10-20 minutes.

Upon withdrawal of the needle, press the skin around the point with the thumb and index finger of the left hand, rotate the needle gently, and lift it slowly to the subcutaneous level; then, withdraw it quickly and press the punctured point with an alcohol cotton ball for a while to prevent bleeding.

WARM MOXIBUSTION

Moxibustion is an external method of preventing and treating diseases by ignition of moxa to stimulate the points. There are many types of moxibustion:

(1) *Mild warm moxibustion*: This method utilizes moxa sticks. Put the lighted end of a moxa stick over the selected point to warm it up, at about 3 cm from the point. It is good for the patient to feel warm, comfortable, and pain-free. Every session may last 10-20 minutes, until the skin around the point becomes flushed.

(2) *Moxibustion with warming needle*: This method combines acupuncture with moxibustion. It is used for conditions in which both the retaining of the needle and moxibustion are needed. Manipulation is as follows: After the arrival of *qi* and with the needle retained in the point at proper depth, ignite the moxa wool, wrapping the handle of the needle until the moxa wool is burnt out completely; or, put the needle handle into a moxa stick, 1-2 cm long, and ignite the stick in order to conduct heat into the body through the needle.

EAR ACUPUNCTURE THERAPY

The auricle is just like a fetus with the head downwards and the buttocks upwards. The auricular points are distributed as follows: The points located on the lobule are related to the head and facial region; those on the scapha, to the upper limbs; those on the antihelix and its two crura, to the trunk and lower limbs.

After routine asepsis, put a seed of *vaccaria vegetalis* or a radish seed on a piece of adhesive plaster of 0.5 x 0.5 cm, and tape it to a corresponding sensitive spot or auricular point. The practitioner presses the seed by various manipulations to produce local sensations of soreness, distension, pain, heat, and others. The patient is asked to press the seed 3-5 times a day by himself; each pressing lasting 2-3 minutes. Generally, retain the seed on the sensitive spot or the acupuncture point for 3-5 days. A series of 5-10 treatments constitutes a course.

TECHNICAL ERRORS AND SIDE EFFECTS

Fainting: This is due to improper position, nervous tension, delicate constitution, or, in some patients, too forceful a manipulation. Some of the manifestations are sudden dizziness, nausea and vomiting, and pallor. In case of fainting, stop needling immediately and withdraw all needles. The symptoms will disappear after a brief rest.

Stuck needle: This is an abnormal condition in which the needle, after insertion and retaining in place, is difficult or impossible to manipulate, such as to twirl, lift and thrust. In this condition, you will ask the patient to relax, leave the needle in place for a while and, after the local muscle is released, withdraw the needle.

Bent or broken needle: Needles can be bent or broken by improper operating manipulation. When this happens, the practitioner must remain calm, ask the patient not to move, and manage each case accordingly.

ACUPUNCTURE PRESCRIPTIONS

Lumbago:

Shenshu (BL 23), Weizhong (BL40), and Ashi points (pressure pain points) in the lumbar region. Supplementary points:

(1) Acute lumbar sprain: Shuigou (DU 26) should be added, and the Weizhong (BL 40) should be pricked to cause bleeding.

(2) Chronic lumbar muscle strain: Qihai (RN 6), Fuliu (KI 7).

Sprain and Contusion:

Ashi points. Supplementary points:

(1) Ankle joint: Xuanzhong (GB 39), Sanyinjiao (SP 6).

(2) Knee joint: Xiyan (EX), Neiting (ST 44).

(3) Wrist joint: Yangchi (SJ 4), Waiguan (SJ 5).

(4) Neck: Tianzhu (BL 10), Shuigou (DU 26), Houxi (SI 3).

Tennis Elbow:

Ashi points, Quchi (LI 11), Shousanli (LI 10), Hegu (LI 4).

Plantalgia and Painful Heels:

Ashi point. Supplementary points:

(1) Painful heels: Taixi (KI 3), Shenshu (BL 23).

(2) Hot or cold sensation in the center of the sole: Yongquan (KI 1).

Tenosynovitis and Tonovaginitis of Flexor Digitorum:

Ashi point.

Periarthritis of the Shoulder:

Jianyu (LI 15), Jianqian (EX), Jianzhen (SI 9), Binao (LI 14), Xuehai (SP 10), Tiaokou (ST 38) through Chengshan (BL 57). Supplementary points:

(1) Pain in the lateral aspect of the shoulder and over the scapula: Houxi (SI 3), Tianzong (SI 11), Yanglingquan (GB 34).

(2) Pain in the anterior aspect of the shoulder: Hegu (LI 4), Quchi (LI 11), Zusanli (ST 36).

(3) Pain in the medial aspect of the shoulder: Chize (LU 5), Yinlinquan (SP 9).

Hoarseness:

Tianding (LI 17), Lieque (LU 7), Hegu (LI 4), Taixi (KI 3).

Simple Obesity:

Jianyu (LI 15), Quchi (LI 11), Liangqiu (ST 34), Biguan (ST 31), Lianmen (ST 21), Guilai (ST 29), Zusanli (ST 36), Fenglong (ST 40).

Cigarette Addiction:

Hegu (LI 4), Tim-Mee, Neiguan (PC 6).

Wrinkles of Facial Skin:

(1) Wrinkles on the forehead: Yangbai (GB 14), Yuyao (EX), Toulinqi (GB 15).

(2) Wrinkles on the sides of the outer canthus: Tongzilao (GB 1), Sizhukong (SJ 23), Taiyang (EX).

(3) Wrinkles between the eyebrows: Yintang (EX), Cuanzhu (BL 2).

(4) Wrinkles on the cheek: Sibai (ST 2), Juliao (ST 3), Quanliao (SI 18), Jiache (ST 6), Xiaguan (ST 7), Yingxiang (LI 20).

CHAPTER 86

Posture and Movement in Making Music

Ans Samama

As in sports, in making music, posture, movement, and coordination are of vital importance. The cause of many complaints, such as pain and numerous in-juries, lies in not using the musculoskeletal system optimally, or even using it incorrectly. Physicians and other prac-titioners, in general, are not fully acquainted with the demands made on the body when music is performed at a high level. In this chapter, a number of general principles are outlined, as well as a number of specific aspects of posture- and move-ment problems. The author's observations are based on years of experience in treating performing musicians for pain.

Any form of making music necessarily involves muscle tension. It is a prerequisite condition for athletes and musicians alike that they make correct use of, and train, both the muscles that determine posture (*static* or *tonic* musculature) and the muscles that primarily execute movements (*dynamic* or *phasic* musculature). Daily training is necessary in order to be able to make music without excessive strain. Insufficient training leads to insufficiently relaxed music making, which, in turn, leads to pain symptoms and sometimes also to stress syndrome.

The music profession is a complex one, requiring a versatility of talents. Musicians, however, often do not realize that physical training is necessary to them, as it is to athletes. In fact, the music itself is the focus, while not enough attention is paid to the physio-technical aspects of music making. This is not solely a musician's problem; a physical training program also plays a minor role in education. Learning good posture and correct movement patterns from early childhood could, in many instances, prevent deformities and complaints related to the muscular system at a later age. Unfortunately, this aspect receives relatively little attention from family- and school doctors.

It is very difficult, of course, to motivate young children to work hard on their physical condition; preventing problems that may occur at a later age

does not mean much to them. Nevertheless, efforts in this regard should be made. This applies *a fortiori* to children of extraordinary musical talent, who begin studying music at age five or even younger.

Physical complaints are common among musicians. These complaints are often caused by incorrect muscle use. This insight is not always sufficiently apparent to doctors and music teachers. Musicians themselves often hold the misconception that pain is a natural side effect of music making, and that one must spare one's muscles as much as possible in order to make music in a relaxed way. This is both curious and incorrect; no athlete would dream of entering a league game untrained. Musicians, on the other hand, come to a concert well prepared as far as the musical technique is concerned, but often with a muscular system that has not been trained. This is even more striking because performing a (major) concert demands great physical exertion, as can clearly be seen, for instance, in television shots. It would seem logical that in learning to play an instrument, one should learn and train the correct posture and movements at the very outset. Training muscles, *not* sparing them, is what is requisite.

All activities of the body involve two kinds of muscle activity. One group of muscles works pri-marily at keeping the body in balance. We may call these *posture* muscles; in reference works, we also find the terms *static* or *tonic* muscles. They will be referred to herein as *balance* muscles. Other muscles are used mainly for the carrying out of movements. This group of muscles, also sometimes referred to as *dynamic* or *phasic* musculature, will be referred to as *playing* muscles, considering the present concern with music making.

The balance muscles are the cervical muscles, those of the back, the abdomen, and the lower extremities. The playing muscles, depending on the nature of the music making, are located in the face, the throat and neck area, and in the upper extremities.

Obviously, this division into two muscle groups is not absolute and may vary for different activities. Compare, for instance, a tennis player and a cyclist.

When an instrument is being played, and in almost any other activity, all muscles are more or less tensed. It is of great importance that all muscles are tensed correctly — in other words, that the balance muscles are used mainly for posture and the playing muscles for movements. This is not a spontaneous way of using muscles, but one that must be consciously acquired, initially under the supervision of an expert. Ideally, every (professional) musician should work out a daily training program and learn how to make the acquired movements an integral part of his/her daily life. The importance of this training is demonstrated by the large number of deformities among musicians.

String Players

Violinists often develop thoracic scoliosis due to incorrect bending of the spinal column, either towards the violin or away from it. When playing the violin, the spinal column should be kept straight. Back complaints may be prevented by keeping the pelvis tilted backwards a little, in standing as well as in sitting posture. Neck- and shoulder complaints may arise due to incorrect position of the head in relation to the shoulder support.

Controversy exists concerning the shoulder support for violinists. The violin should rest upon the triangle that is formed by the left clavicle, the upper side of the left shoulder, and the lateral part of the neck. This is often well-aided by the shoulder support. Violinists with short necks can hold the violin between chin and shoulder without shoulder support. If, for holding the violin, the left shoulder is continually raised or the head is forcibly kept in a particular position, severe pain may ensue. When up-bowing, the right shoulder is often raised in order to achieve an enhanced tone. Another acquired bowing mistake is excessive pronation of the forearm. Tennis elbow is a frequent injury among violinists. Thus, learning to use one's bow to perfection may also prevent complaints.

The problems outlined above also apply, to varying degrees, to players of other string instruments. Cellists and bass players must pay particular attention to the way they sit. 'Embracing' the instrument, perhaps combined with a torsion of the spinal column, may lead to problems in the nape of the neck, the shoulder, and the back.

Patient A. is a 23-year-old female concert violinist, established in her career. She complained of pain in the upper region of the back, right paravertebral. Examination revealed an S-shaped scoliosis with slight thoracic gibus. Until recently, this deformity had caused little trouble. Experience, however, shows that in such a case, without specific training, the severity of the complaints may well increase, rendering it impossible to make music at a top level. Even after a short period of intensive training, significant improvement appeared to have come about, largely owing to the patient's own dedication, effort, and concentration. She must, however, continue this training.

Wind Instrument Players

The highest incidence of complaints of wind-instrument players is found among flutists; in particular, neck problems due to incorrectly turning the head, back problems due to incorrect standing posture (torsion of the spinal column), and pain in the upper extremities caused by holding the instrument in the wrong way. The flute should be held rather loosely in the hands, resting lightly on the thumb to the right and on the metacarpal articulation on the side of the index finger to the left. The elbows should hang loosely down and not be raised.

Patient B. is a 22-year-old female flutist, in her first year of music college. She was suffering from tendinitis in both thumbs and from breathing problems. After observation of her playing, it became apparent that this patient's posture was very poor and that the held her flute incorrectly. She held it much too tightly with the thumbs and, moreover, raised her elbows too much. Specific exercise alleviated the tendinitis. Improvement of posture and breathing technique increased the width of her thorax considerably. Gradually, all her complaints disappeared.

Keyboard Players

Of major importance in playing keyboard instruments is sitting properly. Where possible, the feet should be placed on the floor, in a straight line down from the knees, and the back should be sufficiently stretched. It is not surprising that back problems are common among pianists. Pain in the articulations of the upper extremity are often caused by incorrect distribution of work between balance muscles and playing muscles. Playing forte, for example, is often done with too much tension in the arm muscles and with wrist joints kept stationary. If one keeps the wrist flexible and plays forte with the fingers, while the back muscles are tensed as counterforce, the arm muscles can bear the right tension without being overtaxed. The hand- and finger movements of pianists are often too brisk. Just as when in walking the foot is flexed down, so must wrist and fingers be flexed down. The fingers should not be placed down tight and then released. Placing the fingers down carefully is of the greatest importance, much more so than lifting them.

Patient C. is a female fourth-year piano student at a college of music, 23 years old. She suffered from fierce pain in the upper arms and forearms, and paraesthesia of the fingers. According to her general practitioner, there was tendinitis in both forearms and possible neuritis in both upper arms. Observation of her playing revealed extremely narrow spreading ability of the hands, and a postural anomaly in the shoulders, i.e. protraction combined with hypertonicity and shortening of the Mm pectorales. These two anatomic factors, which can barely be influenced, simply make many pieces of music for this patient technically impossible to play. As she was not aware of her handicap, she had nonetheless tried, in the course of her education, to overcome her technical difficulties, overtaxing her muscles and articulations. This is a striking example of someone who should have been informed at an early age that the piano was not a suitable instrument for her. Her physical limitations had not been recognized by former or present teachers, so she was nevertheless assigned difficult passages. Although the patient's handicap cannot be eliminated, relaxation exercises and technical advice have resulted in alleviation of pain. She now knows her limits, however, and can adjust the selection of her repertoire accordingly.

Organ players additionally use their feet during play, so the support of the feet cannot be counted on for the sitting posture in this case, due to which the back muscles are overtaxed. This makes training of the back muscles all the more important.

Patient D. is a male graduate organ player, 28 years old, who complained of pain in the left shoulder, the nape of the neck and back, as well as perpetually cold hands. It was noticed during observation of his playing that his left shoulder was higher than his right, and that this was a case of cervicothoracic torsion scoliosis. It was obvious that unbalanced taxing of neck- and back muscles during an activity that completely relied on these muscles could be a major causal factor, which is why the patient had to specifically train his back

muscles before and during play. After several months, all complaints were gone, including that of cold hands.

As indicated previously, physical complaints of musicians are often caused by insufficient training and inadequate correction of technical mistakes. In many instances, such specific training can reduce or eliminate the complaints. It is more important, however, that these problems are prevented. Both musicians and music teachers have, on the whole, insufficient insight into the physical demands involved in making music.

In very young children, coordination of the musculoskeletal system has not yet been fully developed. This does not come about before the age of eight or nine. Consequently, when training extremely young performers of music, one should begin training the larger muscle groups. In music lessons, attention must be paid to correct posture and the large movements of the arms. The smaller muscles, which control the finer motorium, are dealt with at a later stage of training. The finer motorium, too, must be learned quite consciously and, in the beginning, even over-accurately, in order for the correct movements to be carried out automatically later.

A special group are the very talented children who begin playing an instrument when they are three or four years old. Curiously enough, these children often spontaneously carry out the large and small movements in proper coordination. Some of them, however, start wondering during puberty exactly how they are playing their instrument. When they start thinking about their motorium consciously, problems may arise and erroneous habits may be acquired after all. Thus, it is very important that children with natural talent are also consciously guided during their motor development.

Another factor in the generation of physical complaints is an incorrect way of studying; for example, practicing a very difficult passage too long at a stretch. This may naturally cause overtaxation of certain muscle groups. Sufficient variation during study prevents overuse and makes studying more enjoyable, as well.

The author is a practitioner whose daily concern is the treatment of musicians. In general however, the musician who has pain symptoms will initially go to his general practitioner. Physicians, too, lack specific training in this field. The G.P. will often treat the complaints symptomatically, or refer the patient to a physiotherapist. The average physiotherapist, however, does not have specific knowledge related to musicians. The number of doctors and therapists who do have the necessary knowledge of this field is small, but steadily increasing. If the musician does find someone who has expertise in this field, problems related to reimbursement by health insurers may arise. It would seem to be desirable to have special facilities available to assist and advise musicians, possibly coupled with a separate qualification. Indeed, it cannot be expected that every doctor and physiotherapist undertake extensive study in this area.

At the outset of music education, a specific medical examination is advisable, comparable to the examination for young athletes. Patient C. illustrates that timely medical advice may prevent the selection of a less suitable instrument. Such a medical examination should be made compulsory for first-year students at colleges of music. This points to the problem noted above, however; there are few practitioners with sufficient expertise in this field.

Not all complaints can be traced to a cause in the musician himself. Causal factors are often found in the job situation. Making music *freely*, with a sense of sufficient room to move, is impossible in most orchestras. Space in the orchestra pit is often limited for reasons of economy. This sometimes causes the musician to sit more or less hunched up while playing, without adequate room to move the arms or place the feet properly. Furthermore, lighting is often poor, especially in the orchestra pit, so the musician must bend over too much in order to be able to read the music properly. This means that the cervical musculature is unnecessarily and chronically taxed. Another complaint frequently encountered among orchestra musicians is that the conductor is not clearly visible, usually in connection with the aforementioned lack of space. The chair of an orchestra musician is a problem in itself, and one that is rarely given

attention. The seat of the chair must be horizontal; the height of the chair must be the same length as the lower leg for the feet to properly function as support. This means that chairs of various heights must be available — either by providing different types of chairs or making the chairs adjustable in height. One additional practical problem is the fact that the chairs must also be easy to stack. A challenge to industrial designers!

When a plea is made for better training and treatment of musicians, the question arises as to where the necessary knowledge is to be obtained. This question is not easily answered. The author would suggest the establishment of a working group for the study of medical aspects of music making. Based on a study of available reference material and original research, such a working group could formulate meaningful advice, both for the benefit of musicians themselves and those who are to guide and assist prospective musicians.

SUGGESTED READING

1. Holding DH: Human Skills. Chichester/New York/Brisbane/Toronto: J Wiley & Sons, 1980.
2. Journal of the International Society for the Study of Tension in Performance. London: Kahn & Averill, Nov 1985.
3. Ostrander S, Schroeder L: Super Studiel.. Baarn: De Kern, 1979.
4. Samama ALW: Stress bij musii. Haags Conservatorium, 1983.
5. Samama ALW: Epta (piano journal).
6. Samama ALW: Esta 6:1, 1981/82, en 9:4, 1985.
7. Samama ALW: Medici voor musici. Medisch Contact 40(45): 1409-1410, 1985.
8. Samama ALW: Muscle Control for Musicians. Amsterdam: Bohn Scheltema & Holkema, 1981.
9. Wolsh R: Towards and Ecology of Brain. MTP Press Ltd, 1981.

CHAPTER 87

Hearing Loss in Conservatory Students

J.M. Schmidt • *J. Verschuure* • *M.P. Brocaar*

INTRODUCTION

Workers exposed to noise may suffer from hearing loss. Criteria have been put forward for the maximum amount of noise to which a worker may be exposed without risking hearing loss. The criteria differ from country to country, but it has generally been accepted that no measurable hearing loss occurs as long as the noise level is below 80 dB(A). Above this level, measurable damage occurs, depending on the duration of the exposure.

With regard to music, we tend not to think of noise, but of pleasant sound. Yet, played loud enough, music can become a possible threat to the human ear. The question arises as to whether professional musicians suffer from hearing loss caused by their music-playing. It is of particular interest because musicians depend on their hearing for carrying out their profession.

Apart from the loudness, the spectrum is also important in the damaging effect of sound. The spectrum is not the same for music and for factory noise. In music, the lower frequencies dominate. Lower frequencies are less damaging to the ear partly because the stapedius muscle attenuates the low frequencies more effectively,[1,2] and partly because the ear is less sensitive at lower frequencies. A third important aspect is the temporal pattern of music. A worker in a factory will be exposed to a constant level of noise for almost an entire working day. A musician usually plays during a period of a couple of hours, usually with only short peaks of excessive sound. Between these periods, there usually are quieter intervals during which the ear gets a chance to recover. These aspects make it hazardous to apply industry norms to musicians, prior to further research.

Basically, there are two ways to investigate noise damage among professional musicians: (1) measuring the intensity of the sound to which a musician is exposed and see whether it exceeds the 80 dB(A) threshold; and (2) assessing musicians' hearing.

REVIEW OF THE LITERATURE

Intensity measurements were carried out by several authors under different circumstances: Lebo, et al.[3] measured the intensity level of the music played by a symphony orchestra. The measurements were made in the center of the orchestra section of a symphony hall. They found levels varying between 76 and 100 dB(A), with an average of 90 dB(A). They also measured the intensity level of the music produced by a rock-and-roll group. This time, the measurements were in the central part of the hall. They found levels varying between 107 and 116 dB(A), with an average of 111 dB(A). In both cases, the highest intensity was found in the frequencies below 2 kHz. An extensive review of this subject is given by Irion.[2]

A review of the existing literature on hearing loss in musicians was published by Sataloff.[4] He described the differences in approach in the various studies and stated that neither the results nor the quality of the studies were consistent. One of the preliminary conclusions, however, was that there was evidence indicating that noise-induced hearing loss occurred in both pop- and classical musicians, and was related to exposure to loud music.

Strongly supporting this conclusion is the finding of asymmetrical hearing losses among musicians; worse hearing in the left ear was found in violinists,[2,5-7] and the opposite was found in flutists,[5,8] French horn players,[8] and piccolo players.[5] The differences were explained by the fact that the sound source is closest to the left ear in violin players and to the right ear in the other instruments.

Very little is known about the hearing of musicians at the beginning of their careers, i.e. conservatory students and the damage caused to their hearing. The aim of the present study is to assess the incidence of hearing loss in these students and to examine the relationships between type of music played and hearing loss.

MATERIALS AND METHODS

All students of the graduating class of the Rotterdam Conservatory were asked to participate in the study. Seventy-nine agreed, and 14 refused. Nine teachers participated, forming a total of 88 musicians (59 male, 29 female). The median age was 25 years, with a range of 21-62 years. Subjects were distributed in the following way, among the four sections of the school: classical music (42), light music (31), pop music (5), ethnic music (2), and un-known (8).

All musicians were seen at the ENT department of the Rotterdam University Hospital, and the following tests were performed:

- standard pure-tone audiometry, consisting of air-conduction thresholds at the octave frequencies between 250 and 8000 Hz, and 3 and 6 kHz; and bone-conduction thresholds at the octave frequencies between 500 and 2000 Hz.

- extended high-frequency audiometry, consisting of air-conduction thresholds at 8-20 kHz, in steps of 2 kHz.

- speech-reception thresholds in quiet.

The musicians were asked to complete a questionnaire regarding the type of musical instruments they played, how long they have been playing, how often they played, and possible other causes of hearing loss.

RESULTS

Number of hearing losses (Table):

A low-frequency perceptive hearing loss was defined as a hearing loss = > 20 dB for the frequencies 250 or 500 Hz in one or both ears. A high-frequency perceptive hearing loss was defined as a

hearing loss = > 20 dB for the frequencies 3, 4, 6, or 8 kHz in one or both ears. A noise dip was defined as a hearing loss greater = > 20 dB for the frequencies 3, 4, or 6 kHz, with the two nearest frequencies at either side of this dip at least 10 dB better. This definition of a dip matched exactly our intuitive interpretation of audiograms. An extended high-frequency perceptive hearing loss was defined as a hearing loss = > 20 dB for the frequencies 10, 12, or 14 kHz in one or both ears. The reference curves described by Dreschler, et al.[9] were used. The frequencies 16-20 kHz were not included, because the SPL levels used in determining these thresholds are often so high that a broadband noise is detected in the low frequencies.

The incidence of hearing loss was then submitted to age correction. As reference curve for age, the ISO 7029 was used for frequencies up to 8 kHz, and the data published by Dreschler, et al.[9] for extended high frequencies. The same criteria were applied to obtain age-corrected values.

Results show that age correction reduces the incidence of hearing loss in the high-frequency region and in the extended high-frequency region.

Subsequently, possible other causes of hearing loss were excluded: musicians with a history of noisy hobbies, military service, recurrent otitis media, meningitis, head concussion, ototoxic medication, and Menière's disease (n = 16). This resulted in a reduced incidence of hearing loss in the high-frequency region. The incidence of noise dips was not reduced.

Conductive hearing loss:

It was defined as an air-bone gap = > 10 dB at any of the frequencies 500, 1000, or 2000 Hz. It was not found in any of the examined persons.

Speech perception:

Most musicians had excellent speech perception in quiet. In only eight persons, the speech perception threshold was shifted 10-15 dB in one or both ears.

Magnitude of hearing loss:

After age correction, and excluding other causes of hearing loss, the magnitude of the hearing loss was as follows (Fig. 1):

Table: *Number of conservatory students with earing loss in different frequency regions with and without correction.*

	low-frequency perceptive hearing loss	high-frequency perceptive hearing loss	noise dip	extended high-frequency perceptive hearing loss	no hearing loss
no correction (n = 88)	11 (12.5%)	24 (27%)	11 (12.5%)	66 (75%)	14 (16%)
after age correction (n = 88)	11 (12.5%)	19 (22%)	11 (12.5%)	45 (51%)	27 (31%)
after age correction and excluding causes of hearing loss other than music	8 (11%)	12 (17%)	10 (14%)	32 (44%)	24 (33%)

- low-frequency hearing loss between 20 dB and 25 dB.

- median high-frequency hearing loss of 25 dB, with a range of 20-40 dB.

- median noise dip of 25 dB, with a range of 20-45 dB

- median extended high-frequency hearing loss of 25 dB, with a range of 20-80 dB.

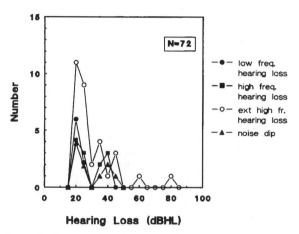

Figure 1: Number of musicians with hearing loss by amount of loss, correcting for age and other causes.

Hearing loss per conservatory section:

The Mann-Whitney U test was used for comparing the different hearing losses for students of the various sections of the conservatory. Noise dips were much more frequent among pop musicians than among classical musicians (p<0.01). No other significant differences were found.

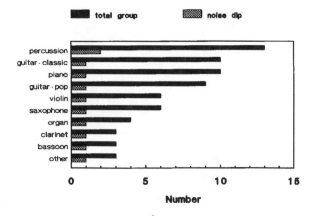

Figure 2: Number of musicians with a noise dip, by instrument group, excluding 21 who played another instrument.

Noise dips per instrument:

Percussionists represent the largest group (11), and also have the largest number of noise dips (2). Because of the small size of the individual instrument groups, and the small overall number of noise dips, it was difficult to establish statistical significance (Fig. 2).

Relationship between noise dip and extended high-frequency loss:

Among the 11 musicians (12 ears) with a noise dip, 7 ears also had an extended high-frequency loss, thus implying that noise dip and extended high-frequency loss are not correlated.

Asymmetrical hearing losses (comparing both ears):

The Wilcoxon test was used to assess hearing-loss asymmetry at all frequencies, by instrument group. The same procedure was used for cases with hearing loss. No significant differences were found. This might be due to the small number of cases per group, and the usually small amount of loss.

Average exposure of a conservatory student:

The exposure to music of a conservatory student was assessed by the length of his/her musical career. Most students started to play music between the ages of 6 and 9. Before they began their studies at the con-servatory, the median number of hours they practiced was 7 per week. During their school period, this increased to 18 hours per week (3 inside and 15 outside the school).

They usually started to perform publicly at the age of 16, but not for more than 1.5 hours per month. This increased to 5.5 hours per month during their school period. They usually attend concerts 1-2 times per month. They listen to music on CD, LP, or cassette, for an average of 10 hours per week. Most claim they listen at a moderate volume. One-third use headphones when listening to music.

DISCUSSION

A high number of noise dips (11/88) and high-frequency losses (24/88) were found among conservatory students. The median hearing loss was still rather small (25 dB for noise dips and 25 dB for high-frequency losses). After age correction, and after excluding other possible causes of hearing loss, the number of noise dips is not reduced. They were much more frequent among pop musicians than among classical musicians.

This seems to confirm the hypothesis that music is hazardous to musicians' hearing. Because most musicians studied were at the beginning of their careers, the diagnosed hearing losses pose an even greater threat to their professional lives.

The authors are currently investigating a reference group of medical students, with the same age and sex distribution, to see whether similar hearing losses are present in this group of non-musicians.

The high incidence of extended high-frequency loss (66/88) raises the question of Dreschler, et al.'s[9] reference curves being applicable to this group. Consequently, the authors will be creating their own reference curves, using in-house equipment.

This study shows a high incidence of hearing loss in conservatory students, emphasizing the need to teach music students the risks of high-level sounds and ways of protecting themselves from hearing loss.

REFERENCES

1. Axelsson A, Lindgren F: Hearing in pop musicians. Acta Otolaryngol 85:225-231, 1978.
2. Irion H: Musik als berufliche Lärmbelastung? Bundesanstalt für Arbeitsschutz und Unfallforschung Dortmund (Forschungsbericht Nr. 174).
3. Lebo CP, Oliphand KP: Music as a source of acoustic trauma. Laryngosc 78:1211-1218, 1968.
4. Sataloff RT: Hearing loss in musicians. Am J Otology 12(2):122-127, 1991.
5. Flach M, Aschoff E: Zur Frage berufsbedingter Schwerhörigkeit beim Musiker. Z Laryngol 45: 595-605, 1966.
6. Frei J: Gehörschäden durch laute Musik. Das Orchester 29:630-641, 1981.
7. Ostri B, Eller N, et al: Hearing impairment in orchestra musicians. Scand Audiol 18:243-249, 1979.
8. Axelsson A, Lindgren F: Hearing in classical musicians. Acta Otolaryngol (Suppl 377):3-74, 1981.
9. Dreschler WA, vd Hulst RJAM, et al: The role of high frequency audiometry in early detection of ototoxicity. Audiology 24:387-395, 1985.

CHAPTER 88

A Cryotherapeutic Approach to Relieving Upper Body Pain and Restriction Experienced by Performing Artists

Elizabeth T. Morris

When the general public thinks of physical therapy, accident victims or injured athletes are usually envisioned. Performing artists with restricted muscles, however, need physical therapy intervention every bit as much as football players with dislocated shoulders. Restricted muscles cause more than pain in performing artists; they inhibit coordinated movement and make artistic achievement even more difficult. An artist's joy in his performance, and his ability to express himself freely, depend upon the comfort and flexibility of his body. Artistic overuse or accidental trauma frequently cause restriction of the cervical, thoracic, scapular, and brachial musculature, along with elevation of the shoulder girdle, and shifting of its burden from the rib cage to the skull and cervical spine. Our professional challenge is to free this restricted musculature and restore normal posture and full flexibility to the upper body.

There is an interesting mechanical relationship between the musculature of the upper arm, the thorax, and the cervical area. The key to this relationship is the structure of the sternoclavicular joint. Except for this bony connection of the upper extremity with the axial skeleton, the shoulder girdle floats freely in musculature.[1] The sternoclavicular joint is responsible for the motions of elevation, depression, protraction, retraction, and circumduction of the shoulder. When movement at this joint becomes restricted, the shoulders assume a raised and hunched position. The use of cryotherapy permits the realignment of these structures at the sternoclavicular joint within a few treatment sessions without extensive corrective exercise. *Scapular drop* is the name given to the mechanical repositioning of the shoulder girdle downward and backward at the sternoclavicular joint.

To achieve scapular drop, it is necessary to work with all of the musculature of the upper body, not just that of the painful area. Scapular drop cannot be achieved without the use of ice. Treatment is given while the patient is lying on his side, presenting both the anterior and posterior portions of his body in a plane neutral to gravity. Mobilization of the sternoclavicular joint and all of the involved musculature of the trunk and shoulders can easily be achieved in this position. When the patient is then turned onto his back and the cervical musculature is iced and massaged, the shoulder girdle will drop downward and backward at the sternoclavicular joint, allowing restoration of normal, youthful posture.

Muscular restrictions in artists occur gradually unless an individual experiences trauma. Often, muscular restrictions are so complex that practically all of the musculature of the upper body is involved. Restrictions may be subtle and difficult to detect. The subscapularis muscles of violists, for example, often become restricted, preventing the scapulae from sliding freely on the rib cage. This condition is accompanied anteriorly by intercostal and pectoral muscular restriction and shortening of the elbow flexors within the brachial portion of the arm. The cervical muscles also become restricted after hours of practicing. Slowly, and almost imperceptibly, the artist becomes trapped in a painful body. A musician may have accompanying restrictions of the forearm musculature which may result in nerve entrapment syndromes. The pattern of muscular restriction differs between bowing and fingering arms. These problems may be effectively treated with moist heat, ultrasound, cryotherapy, massage, and gentle stretching techniques.

Although all of the modalities are important to the treatment regimen, ice is the key modality for achieving scapular drop. Ice applications over the full length of the muscle groups slow the biochemical activity of the muscle tissue, causing it to relax. Ice is not harmful to muscle tissue if applied loosely.[2]

The ice is wrapped in a medium-weight, wet, terry-cloth towel and then laid along the full length of the muscle group to be treated.   Maximum muscle relaxation is achieved within seven to ten minutes, depending upon the depth of the muscle tissue. During the icing process, the artist's core temperature is maintained by the application of a large abdominal hot pack and by wrapping him with flannel blankets. This prevents shivering which can cause muscle spasm and reduce the effectiveness of the treatment.

This treatment intervention also utilizes gentle stretching exercises to restore and maintain muscular flexibility.   Stretching, used alone, can relieve mild muscle spasm. It becomes a more powerful treatment tool, however, when it is combined with ice. Stretching can also be combined with Fluoromethane spray, a cold anesthetic spray, to release soft tissue restrictions.[3]

Massage, used in conjunction with ice, is an essential aspect of the treatment. Gentle, transverse fiber friction massage is incorporated into the treatment regimen to restore flexibility to areas of soft tissue which have adhered to themselves. Contractile tissue is inherently irritable and this may be increased if massage is used too vigorously. Massage is best applied when the muscle belly is in a relaxed position or in a plane neutral to gravity.

Although there may be slight variations for individual artists, the treatment protocol follows a standard pattern. Following application of full-body hot packs, ultrasound is applied to all of the involved musculature. The patient is then placed on his side with one pillow under his head and two pillows between his knees. The most painful side is treated first. With an abdominal hot pack in place, an ice wrap is applied to the anterior chest extending from the clavicle downward along the rib cage to intersect posteriorly with the paraspinal musculature. After ten minutes, the ice is removed and the artist is assisted in deep intercostal breathing to restore chest mobility. Four or five deep breaths will usually relieve inter-costal muscle restriction. If no intercostal motion occurs, the lower ribs may have to be iced. For this area, place an ice pack transversely across the body, wrapping the lower ribs. Repeat the assisted deep breathing exercises. Pectoral flexibility can now be restored by gently pulling the bent elbow posteriorly. By passively drawing the elbow backward, one can stretch the pectoral musculature and the anterior deltoid.   This motion occurs at the glenohumeral joint. Next, place the ice wrap on the paraspinal musculature of the posterior thorax for ten minutes. Remove the ice and manually assist all scapular motions. Check for restrictions of the subscapularis and middle trapezius, and fully mobilize the scapula on the rib cage. Muscular restrictions can be relieved by alternately stretching the shoulder at the gleno-humeral joint and applying gentle transverse fiber friction massage.   Icing and stretching must be repeated frequently. When all the muscles on the first side have been released, turn the patient to the opposite side and repeat the entire procedure. This treatment sequence is important because opposing muscle groups must be released to achieve scapular drop. Treating the front and back of the chest at the same time restores balance to the musculature of the entire thorax.   Freeing the scapula posteriorly enhances movement at the sternoclavicular joint anteriorly.

Because there is an intimate relationship between restrictions of the upper arm, thorax, and cervical area, it is also necessary to relieve any restrictions of the axillary and brachial musculature. This can be accomplished by encircling the axillary area with an ice wrap for ten minutes. Remove the ice and passively stretch the shoulder through all motions at the glenohumeral joint.   If brachial muscular restrictions are present, encircle the musculature of the upper arm with an ice wrap. After ten minutes, remove the ice and passively stretch the shoulder backward at the glenohumeral joint, keeping the elbow straight. This motion stretches the biceps at both the elbow and shoulder joints. Gently rotate the entire arm internally as the posterior movement is made.   Rotational movement frees the restricted muscle fibers of the upper arm. Gently twist and untwist the arm while moving it passively through the entire arc of motion from behind the body to overhead. Use massage to free any residual muscular restrictions.

Finally, the cervical musculature is treated. The patient is supine, an abdominal hot pack is in position, and there is no pillow under the head. Wrap the neck with ice for ten minutes. Remove the ice and gently stretch the cervical musculature in all directions. Tenderness, swelling and tightness can easily be palpated in the anterior and posterior cervical musculature. While applying straight manual traction to the skull, gently tilt the head from side to side, noting any differences in the restrictions of the muscles in the right and left sides of the neck. Depress the shoulders, together and singly. Notice restrictions of movement and work with massage and gentle stretching to mobilize the soft tissue. Stabilize one shoulder against the rib cage and rotate the head to the opposite side. Repeat with the other shoulder.

Always work to achieve a balance of movement between the two sides of the neck, interspersing massage and stretching. Fluoromethane spray can also be used to increase the flexibility of the neck musculature. Fluoromethane spray works effectively on the head and facial musculature to relieve TMJ and headache pain. When indicated, cervical manipulative techniques may be used. Two or three strong manual traction pulls, in the method of Cyriax, will generally relieve the headaches that sometimes accompany restricted cervical musculature.[4] A final icing of the neck will remove any residual tissue irritation caused by massage. Each treatment lasts approximately 2½ hours, and treatments are given two or three times a week. This allows time for the patient's body to reorganize following therapy. Repositioning of the shoulder girdle generally occurs within two to four treatment sessions.

A home-therapy program is an important adjunct to the clinical program. The cervical area and all of the involved shoulder and chest musculature are iced three times daily. Relaxed stretching of the upper body and deep intercostal breathing is done for 15 seconds of every waking hour to maintain flexibility of the soft tissue. Repetitive activities that involve the upper extremities are kept to a minimum. This speeds recovery and helps prevent recurrence.

In order for the overall treatment to be effective, the therapist must help the artist to understand the mechanics of his problem and teach him how to modify his performance activities to allow his body to change. Dancers should avoid carrying heavy dance bags over their shoulders, and musicians should carefully move heavy instruments if they want to keep the muscles of the upper body from becoming irritated. Artists should stand up, breath deeply, and stretch for 15 seconds of every hour during practice. They must become aware of where their muscles are tight and what makes them tight. Then, they must change their position, correct their posture, or modify the activities that keep their shoulders elevated.

Stress-reduction techniques should be addressed. Artists must realize that whatever is happening in their emotional lives is reflected in their muscles. Before auditions and performances, artists are especially vulnerable to the effects of added stress. The lives of performing artists are both satisfying and grueling. Their days are long, the competition is keen, and their stress levels may be high. The upper-body muscular restrictions that so many artists develop, however, do not have to be debilitating, and they certainly need not signal the end of performing careers. Cryotherapeutic techniques make it possible to eliminate artists' muscular restrictions, allowing them the full range of motion and freedom from pain that they need in order to achieve full artistic expression.

REFERENCES

1. Brunnstrom S: Clinical Kinesiology, 143. New York: Harper & Row, 1970.
2. Grant AE: Massage with ice (cryokinetics) in the treatment of painful conditions of the musculoskeletal system. Arch Phys Med Rehabil 45:233-8, 1964.
3. Travell JG, Simons DG: Myofascial Pain and Dysfunction: The Trigger Point Manual, 65. Baltimore: Williams & Wilkins, 1983.
4. Cyriax J: Orthopaedic Medicine Volume Two — Treatment by Manipulation and Injection, 90. Baltimore: Williams & Wilkins, 1971.

CHAPTER 89

Postural Disorders in Music and Medical Students:
A Comparative Study

M.D.F. van Eijsden-Besseling • B. Kap • M. Kuijers • H. Stam

INTRODUCTION

Complaints and lesions of the locomotor apparatus often occur in musicians, interfere with their musical performance, and obstruct their practice.[3,4] Analysis of the basic posture of musicians and its influence on making music hereupon can support the knowledge about the pathogenesis of complaints and lesions.[5]

The purpose of this study was to assess the nature and extent of misalignment of the locomotor apparatus in music students.

MATERIALS and METHODS

Physical examination of freshmen of the Rotterdam Conservatory in 1989 was performed as part of the acceptance procedure. This examination was voluntary and accessible to every freshman. At least 73 students participated (85%). They were compared to a control group of 59 1989 freshmen medical students of the Rotterdam Medical Faculty, who participated voluntarily as well. Both groups were age- and sex-matched.

Thirty-nine male and 34 female musicians and 19 male and 40 female medical students were involved. Figure 1 shows the distribution by instrument.

The first part of the examination was carried out by a physiatrist of the Department of Rehabilitation of the Rotterdam Academic Hospital. The examiner knew who studied at the Conservatory and who was a medical student and also the instrument played.

The Royal Conservatory of The Hague examination check-list was used to assess postural disorders, such as abnormal thoracic kyphosis or lumbar lordosis and scoliosis, as well as asymmetry of shoulders and pelvis (Table 1).

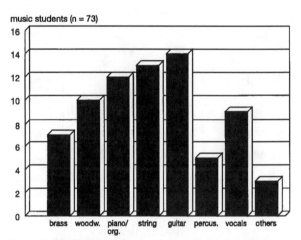

music students (n = 73)

Figure 1: *Distribution of the music students by instrument.*

Table 1: *Distribution of postural disorders within instrument groups: kyphosis, lordosis, scoliosis, shoulder, pelvis asym.*

	KYPH.	LORD.	SCOL.	SH.	P.
	6	0	9	14	9
WOODWIND	17	15	6	14	14
KEYB0ARD	22	31	31	21	20
STRINGS	11	8	3	10	9
GUITAR	28	23	28	17	29
PERCUSSION	6	8	13	10	9
VOCALS	6	15	9	10	11
OTHER	6	0	0	3	0

Thereafter, the group of music students was examined with their instrument by the first examiner and musician consultants. The influence of playing the instrument on the basic posture was assessed. Playing instruments by medical students was left aside. At the end of the examination a medical and occupational advice was given.

RESULTS

The postural disorders encountered in both groups, standing or sitting, with or without their instrument, are displayed in Figure 2. The distribution of disorders within instrument groups is shown in Table 2.

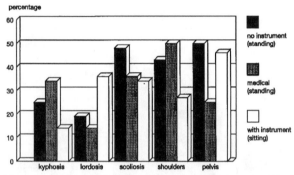

Figure 2: Incidence of postural disorders in music and medical students.

DISCUSSION

It is possible that, because of the selection process, students with many or just a few complaints did not participate. However, the large voluntary turnout for the examination and the fact that the results bore no consequences on their being allowed to continue their education, suggest any such bias to be minimal.

The postural disorders clinically. This method makes it impossible to give further differentiation of the results and statistical significance. Blanken et al.[2] showed that, with this method, the intra-observer reliability was acceptable.

There were no large differences in basic posture between medical and music students. Abnormal thoracic kyphosis was found more often in music students and abnormal lumbar lordosis more often in medical students. Abnormal scoliosis, asymmetric shoulder position and pelvis position appeared more often in music students. Albeit statistical significance

Table 2: The Royal Conservatory of The Hague postural examination check-list.

SHOULDERS posterior view	☐ neutral position
	☐ left depressed ☐ right depressed
PELVIS posterior view	☐ level
	☐ lateral tilt; high on left
	☐ lateral tilt; high on right
LEG LENGTH	☐ equal
	☐ left leg longer ☐ right longer
THORACIC SPINE side view	☐ normal curve; slight post. convexity
	☐ accentuation of thoracic kyphosis
	☐ diminuation of thoracic kyphosis
	☐ structural ☐ non-structural
LUMBAR SPINE side view	☐ normal curve; slight ant. convexity
	☐ accentuation of lumbar lordosis
	☐ diminuation of lumbar lordosis
	☐ structural ☐ non-structural
THORACIC SPINE posterior view	☐ normal; straight in drawing
	☐ C-curve; convex toward left
	☐ C-curve; convex toward right
	☐ structural curve ☐ non-structural
	☐ deviation to plumb-line
	☐ non-deviation to plumb-line
LUMBAR SPINE posterior view	☐ normal; straight in drawing
	☐ C-curve; convex toward left
	☐ C-curve; convex toward right
	☐ structural curve ☐ non-structural
	☐ deviation to plumb-line
	☐ non-deviation to plumb-line

could not be estimated in this study, Bejjani et al.[1] did prove that similar musculoskeletal differences were the result of playing an instrument in professional musicians who sarted at an early age. One could imagine that, if playing an instrument has an influence on the locomotor apparatus, this will become more evident later on in their career. Abnormal thoracic kyphosis and shoulder misalignment more often appeared with the instrument in place than without. This did not affect scoliosis, abnormal lumbar lordosis or pelvis misalignment.

This may be explained by the fact that the students were examined with the instrument in a sitting position (except vocalists) and without instrument in a standing position. In a sitting position abnormalities of the pelvis and low back region are less clear and the influence of leg-length is minimal.

Compensatory scolioses can also disappear in the sitting position. There seems to be a prominence of postural disorders in the piano/organ and guitar subgroups. This remains unexplained.

REFERENCES

1. Bejjani, F.J, Nilsson, B., Kella, J.J. Effect of the instrument on the musician's musculoskeletal system. *In:* D.A. Atwood, & D. McCann (eds.), Proceedings of the 1984 International Conference on Occupational Ergonomics, vol. I. Toronto, Ontario, Canada: Human Factors Conference, Inc, 1984, pp.247-251.

2. Blanken, W.C.G., et al. Inter-observer and intra-observer reliability of postural examination Med Probl Perf Arts; 6(3):93-97, 1991.

3. Brandfonbrenner, A.G. An overview of the medical problems of musicians J. Am Coll Health; 34(4):165-69, 1986.

4. Lederman, R.J. Medical Problems of violinists and violinmakers. Journal of the Violin Society of America; X(3):21-45, 1989.

5. Samama-Polak, A. Muscle control for musicians. Netherlands: Bohn, Scheltema, Holkema, 1981.

CHAPTER 90

What Can Happen to Musicians?

Marjon D. F. van Eijsden-Besseling • *E. Terpstra-Lindeman*

INTRODUCTION

In the eighties, it became more and more clear, that many musicians suffer from mis-/overuse syndromes and from that point of view can be compared to athletes.[1,2] Especially professional musicians who practice "top sport." Therefore they have - like top athletes - the right to (para)medical support, both curatively and preventively. The (para)medical coaching of musicians requires specific knowledge about the function and endurance of the locomotor apparatus and playing techniques in relation to the instrument.[2] Particularly in blowers and vocalists, knowledge about respiration and breathing techniques are of great importance. As a specialty, Physical Medicine and Rehabilitation is engaged in impairments of the locomotor apparatus and the resulting disabilities and handicaps,[3] thus making it an ideal medical specialty for the diagnosis and treatment of musicians' musculoskeletal disorders.

MATERIAL

During the period 1987-1990, thirty-five musicians visited the "Polyclinic for musicians" in the outpatient Department of Physical Medicine and Rehabilitation of the Dijkzigt Hospital Rotterdam. In 1990, an inventory on these musicians was started. Nineteen male and 16 female musicians, age 17 to 64 years (mode 21-25), were involved. Twenty-nine were professionals and 6 were amateurs[1] (Figure 1). Fifty percent of all musicians were conservatory students. The amateurs were found especially in the older musicians. Among these were also some with an acute trauma (Figure 2). Thirty-two musicians were right-handed. The main instruments they played were: piano (9), guitar (8), violin/viola (7).

COMPLAINTS and SYMPTOMS

Most of the complaints were physical, of which

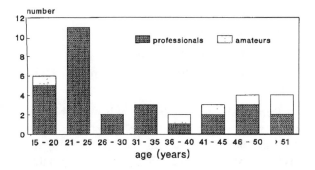

Figure 1: Age Distribution of the Professional and Amateur Musicians (n = 35) Examined.

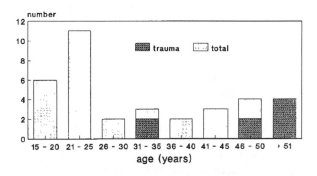

Figure 2: Distribution of Traumatic vs. non-Traumatic Ailments in Musicians (n = 35), by Age Groups.

pain was the most frequent (25).[1] Psychological problems were also present (8). With regard to complaints/symptoms/diagnoses no difference between males and females could be found. Pain in violinists and violists especially concerned the neck, shoulder girdle, and upper arm. In pianists and guitarists, pain was especially the distal part of the arm and hand. Neither side nor handedness seem to have any effect on the complaints and symptoms. Duration of the latter varied from 1 to 2 months up to 20 years with a peak at 2 years and appeared to be an important prognostic sign.

DIAGNOSES

- Musculoskeletal disorder (22):
    - muscle-tendon overuse arm/hand (7)
    - cervico-scapular muscle pain (9)
    - shoulder impingement or instability (6)
    - elbow tendinitis (2)[1]

- Postural disorder (17):
    - aggravated by playing the instrument (11)
    - functional (13)
    - structural (4)

- Psychological disorder (8)

- Vegetative disorder (4)

- Peripheral nerve disorder (3)

- Others (13): trauma, cerebral palsy, ganglion, premorbid disease.[2]

Remarkable was the finding of hypermobility in 7 musicians, giving rise to their symptoms. In 5, a blocked lumbar column (Lumbar Schober 10/≤12) was found with a hypermobile thoracolumbar column and hips. This was not related to lumbar pain. Multiple diagnoses were common. Occupational cramp, often mentioned in the literature, was not seen in this group. Additional tests were performed in 14 cases, and were positive in 10 (EMG, shoulder ultrasound, Doppler, X-rays).

Also noteworthy was that 6 out of 8 guitarists displayed functional postural disorders, aggravated by playing the guitar.

TREATMENTS

1. Rest, i.e. not playing the instrument (10); followed as soon as possible by slowly restarting to play, according to a building-up regimen.

2. Continue playing the instrument, but following a gradually increasing regimen (9)

3. Mensendieck therapy by therapists specialized in musicians (10)[4]

4. Sports, mainly swimming (10)

5. Haptotherapy (7)

6. Adaptations to the instrument (7)[5]

7. Posture and technique adjustments (6)[4]

8. Physiotherapy (5)

9. Psychotherapy (3)

10. Others (10): injections, medicaments, and surgery (2)

11. Advice regarding footware (6)

Several times more than one treatment was prescribed per musician. Always instructions were given regarding prevention (e.g. warming-up, cooling-down etc.).

RESULTS

Twelve musicians were very satisfied with the result of the treatment; and 17 had less complaints/symptoms; while 3 did not have any reduction thereof. In three musicians the results are yet unknown (Figure 3). The best results were seen in those musicians whose complaints had less than two years duration at the time of consultation. The three musicians with bad results, who were forced to put a stop to their career, had complaints for 5 to 20 years.

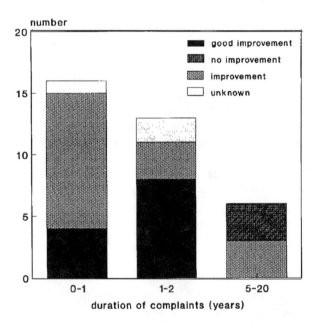

Figure 3: Musicians Treatment Results as a Function of Duration of their Complaints.

CONCLUSIONS and RECOMMENDATIONS

This inventory shows that musicians, mainly professionals, like top athletes, are predisposed to mis-/overuse syndromes. Many factors are responsible, especially wrong playing- and training techniques (lack of warming-up, cooling-down), postural disorders aggravated by playing the instrument, and discrepancy between instrument and anthropometric measures (Table 1).[1,2,6] Psychosocial factors can also play a role, such as health insurance uncertainties - mainly in free-lance musicians - or risk of loosing one's place in the orchestra.[7] The older the musicians, the more serious their symptoms. The

Table 1: Predisposing Factors for Misuse and Overuse in Musicians.

INTRINSIC FACTORS	EXTRINSIC FACTORS
Body Size and Shape	Changing Instrument(s)
Joints Mobility	Bad Playing Technique
Range of Movements	Repertoire too Demanding
General Conditioning	Bad Training Habits (no warm-up, excessive playing)
Local Conditioning	Technique Changes
Degenerative Changes of Musculoskeletal System	Traumatic Injury
Scoliosis	Bad Posture
Mood and Personality Profile	Psychosocial Stress

resemblance with top athletes is obvious and implies that, musicians also, need preventive directed (para)medical support from the very beginning of their career.

In the Netherlands, the newly founded MedArt Nederland needs to coordinate the national health service for musicians. This would certainly help keep costs down, while providing this section of the population with much needed help and support.

In 1988, a research program was started at the Rotterdam conservatory to investigate the locomotor apparatus of about 70 first-year conservatory students, in relation to their instrument. In 1989, this research program was enlarged by comparing 73 first-year conservatory students with 59 first-year medical students, serving as controls.

REFERENCES

1. Lederman, R.J. Medical Problems of violinists and violin makers. Journal of the Violin Society of America, X(3): 21-45, 1989.
2. Wallace, H. Performance-related injuries-a dark continent? The Strad, 102(1213): 396-404, 1991.
3. Lankhorst, G.L. et al. The international classification of impairments, disabilities and handicaps for the WHO. Dutch Journal of Medicine, 134: 212-213, 1990.
4. Samama-Polak, A. Muscle control for musicians Netherlands: Bohn, Scheltema & Holkema, 1981.
5. Benham, B. Emus and Owls. The Strad, 102(1213): 406-408, 1991.
6. Hartsell, H.D., Tata, G.E. A retrospective survey of music - related musculoskeletal problems occurring in undergraduate music students. Physiotherapy Canada, 43(1): 13-18, 1990.
7. Inglis, A. Going for Broke. The Strad,102(1213): 410, 1991.

CHAPTER 91

Classical Notes: Beethoven's Medical History

T.G. Palferman

INTRODUCTION

Ludwig van Beethoven was baptized in Bonn on December 17, 1770, and died in Vienna on March 26, 1827, after a 30-year struggle against progressively poor health, including the infamous insidious deafness.

The medical literature and original sources have been reviewed and reinterpreted, resulting in new conclusions. Particular emphasis is placed on the likely rheumatic diseases, in view of the suggestion that Beethoven's many disorders were compatible with a connective-tissue disease. In addition, a new, single diagnosis is proposed for the multisystem disorders.

HISTORY

Beethoven's medical history is summarized in Table I. From 1813 to his death in 1827, he was increasingly tortured by pain and debility from his many, relapsing, and progressive illnesses. The results of the post-mortem examination held the day following his death are shown in Table II. Table III presents the main rheumatic symptoms, and a differential diagnosis is attempted by considering these in light of his general medical history and in conjuction with the autopsy findings.

The picture is incompatible with systemic lupus erythematosus (SLE) or polyarteritis nodosa, as have been suggested.[1] One of the main objections relates to Beethoven's liver disease. It seems likely that macronodular cirrhosis was present from longstanding hepatitis. Lupoid hepatitis is chronic active hepatitis (CAH) unrelated to SLE,[2] and can result in a macronodular cirrhosis with associated joint, chest, eye, and bowel disease. Although a background of irritable bowel seems likely, the evidence weighs heavily against the presence of ulcerative colitis or Crohn's disease. Alcoholic cirrhosis has been a popular notion,[3] but this is highly unlikely, since a micronodular picture results and it also fails to explain the extra-hepatic complications and overlooks the

Table I: *Summary of Beethoven's Medical History*

- Probable smallpox in childhood.
- Contact with tuberculosis, from which mother (1787) and at least one brother (1815) died.
- Deafness:
  - ☐ Onset circa 1797, to total hearing loss — 1817.
  - ☐ Heiligenstadt Testamaent — 1802.
- Recurrent bouts of depression — from 1787.
- Chest symptoms and 'asthma' — from 1787.
- Repeated episodes of 'kolik,' i.e. diarrhea and abdominal pain, sometimes debilitating — from before 1800.
- Recurrent infections.
- Attacks of rheumatism — from 1826.
- Jaundice — first appearing 1821.
- Eye pain — April 1823-January 1824.
- Hemoptysis and spontaneous epistaxis — 1825 while in Baden.
- Dropsy, peripheral edema, and ascites — December 5, 1826.
- Probable septicemia — December 12, 1826.
- Abdominal paracentesis, large volumes drained — December 20, 1826-February 27, 1827.
- Death — March 26, 1827

Table II: *Autopsy Findings*

- Body 5 feet 6 inches. Wasted. Covered in petechiae.
- No significant abnormalities in the bony parts of his ears.
- Auditory nerves: Shrivelled and marrowless.
- Auditory arteries: Dilated to 'more than a crow's quill' and cartilaginous.
- Facial nerves: Considerably thickened.
- Skull vault: Uniformly dense, ½-inch thick.
- Liver: Shrunk to half volume. Leathery, greyish-blue, tuberculated surface. Cut surface — bean-sized nodules.
- Spleen: Twice normal size, black and tough.
- Pancreas: Large and indurated with a dilated duct.
- Kidneys: Pale and chalky calyceal concretions size of split peas: the whole enclosed in cellular membrane, one inch thick and dripping turbid fluid.
- Bowel: Distended with gas.

weight of evidence against Beethoven being alcoholic. Syphilis is another myth for which a case has not been made in more than 30 years;[4] the medical literature since has contradicted it.[5-8]

A combination of peripheral joint symptoms, back pain, and painful eyes suggests HLA B27-associated spondylarthropathy, with postdysenteric reactive arthritis a possible prodrome, as Beethoven drank the murky waters of many spas and resided in Vienna during its siege by Napoleon when the water supply would have been vulnerable and a decline in public health inevitable.

Table III: Beethoven's Main Rheumatic Symptoms

1816	December: 'Rheumatic feverish cold."
1817	Autumn: 'Fearful attack of rheumatism.'
1820	Bad year for health, culminating in rheumatic fever: 6 weeks in bed.
1822	'Gout on my chest' (thoracic gout).
1823	April-January 1824: Sore eye(s); eyes bandaged at night. Violent diarrhea; 'Abdomen and eyes wretched.'
	September 5: Baden, taking waters and drinking mineral waters.
1826	February: 'Plagued long with rheumatism or gout.' 'Pain in my back not severe but still there.'

Any attempt to apply Occam's Razor excludes all the conditions mentioned heretofore. Tuberculosis has been proposed as a unifying diagnosis;[9] it is unlikely, however, that miliary tuberculosis could be held responsible for 35 years of poor health, particularly as the deafness would result from eighth-nerve involvement from basal pachymeningitis, with its high mortality. Sarcoidosis, however, is a chronic, granulomatous, progressive, multisystem disorder, not mentioned in any of Beethoven's medical biographies. Sarcoidosis can present with skin involvement,[10] eighth-nerve involvement,[11] hepatitis,[12] portal hypertension,[13] splenic involvement,[14] arthropathy/arthralgia,[15] uveitis,[16] chest symptoms,[17] hypercalcemia and ureteric colic,[18] and, to complete the picture, deafness — found in association with widespread disease including uveitis and hepatomegaly.[19] Many components of Beethoven's medical history lure one to the possibility of sarcoidosis. The macronodular cirrhosis with the description at autopsy of bean-shaped nodules would fit with granulomatous hepatic change. The renal calculi, largely ignored in medical writings on Beethoven, relates to the hypercalcemia and hypercalciuria of sarcoidosis and would explain the bouts of prostrating abdominal pain. Eighth-nerve involvement can present so early that the diagnosis of sarcoidosis cannot be made until other features of the disease evolve. A recent suggestion that Paget's disease was responsible for the deafness[20] lacks foundation.

SUMMARY

A differential diagnosis is as follows:

(1) Sarcoidosis, as the possible single diagnosis encompassing all aspects.

(2) CAH with resultant cirrhosis and multisystem aspects.

(3) Cryptogenic/idiopathic cirrhosis; (2) and (3) leading to portal hypertension.

(4) Seronegative arthropathy

    (a) Postdysenteric 'reactive' arthritis.

    (b) Sacroiliitis/ankylosing spondylitis from (a).

    (c) Associated with inflammatory bowel disease.

(5) Irritable bowel syndrome.

(6) Paget's disease.

(7) Deafness of undetermined type. See specialized literature.

CONCLUSION

Today's diagnostic and treatment methods would have allowed an accurate diagnosis to be made, with analgesics now in routine use, together with corticosteroids and immunosuppressants, modifying or curing his diseases and their many symptoms. Perhaps his life would have been prolonged, yet all this begs the question of whether a more comfortable, peaceful Beethoven with hearing intact would have been driven and inspired to produce the Ninth Symphony and late string quartets. Could it be that Beethoven's increasing wretchedness, misery, and despair have ultimately been a blessing on the curse of mankind?

REFERENCES

1. Larkin E: Beethoven's medical history. *In* Cooper M (ed), Beethoven: The Last Decade, 488-489. Oxford: Oxford University Press, 1985.

2. Bresniham B, Jenkins W, Chadwick VS, Hughes GRV: Chronic active hepatitis in a patient presenting with SLE. J Rheum 6:38, 1979.

3. London SJ: Beethoven: Case report. Arch Intern Med 113:442-4488, 1964.

4. McCabe BF: Beethoven's deafness. Ann Otol Rhinol Laryngol 67:129-206, 1958.

5. Sorsby M: Beethoven's deafness. J Laryngol Otol 45:529-544, 1930.

6. Tremble E: The deafness of Beethoven. Can Med Ass J 27:456-459, 1932.

7. Asherson N: The deafness of Beethoven and the saga of the Stapes. Trans Hunterian Soc 6:24:7-24, 1965.

8. Baker D: The deafness of Beethoven. History Med 5:10-13, 1973.

9. Forbes E: Thayer's Life of Beethoven, 2nd revised ed. Princeton, 1967.

10. Scadding JG: Skin infiltrations in 500 cases of sarcoidosis. Praxis 61:133-136, 1972.

11. Delaney P: Neurological manifestations of sarcoidosis. Ann Intern Med 87:336-345, 1977.

12. Maddrey WC, John CJ, Boitnott JK, Iber FL: Sarcoidosis and chronic hepatic disease. Medicine Baltimore 49:375-395, 1970.

13. Rosenberg JC: Portal hypertension complicating hepatic sarcoidosis. Surgery 69:294-299, 1971.

14. Kataria YP, Whitcombe ME: Splenomegaly in sarcoidosis. Arch Intern Med 140:35-37, 1980.

15. Spilberg I, Siltzbach LE, McEwen C: The arthritis of sarcoidosis. Arthritis Rheum 12:126-127, 1969.

16. Karma A: Ophthalmic changes in sarcoidosis. Acta Ophthalmol Suppl 141:1-94, 1979.

17. Siltzbach LE, James DG, Neville E, et al: Course and prognosis of sarcoidosis around the world. Ann J Med 57:847-852, 1974.

18. Romer FK: Renal manifestations and abnormal calcium metabolism in sarcoidosis. Q J Med 49:233-247, 1980.

19. Scadding JG, Mitchell DN: Sarcoidosis, 307-308, 397. London: Chapman & Hall, 1985.

20. Naiken VS: Did Beethoven have Paget's disease of bone? Ann Intern Med 74:995-999, 1971.

CHAPTER 92

Relationship Between Painful Hands of Pianists and Piano Techniques

Naotaka Sakai

INTRODUCTION

Recurrent medical problems of performers are often related to specific playing techniques. Thus, it may be possible to some of these problems by improving education. Japanese pianists with medical problems were evaluated and treated during the period 1982-1990, and a propensity of some special piano techniques (especially octave) to bring about painful hands was found.[1] This paper studied the relationship between painful hands from overuse and piano techniques.

SAMPLE

The sample included 40 Japanese profes-sional pianists or students with painful hands because of overuse during playing piano, not due to trauma or diseases such as rheumatoid arthritis or tumor. They were 4 men and 36 women with 13 right, 13 left, and 10 bilateral painful hands. Their ages ranged from 16 to 53 years, averaging 23.5.

RESULTS

Diagnoses are shown in Table I. The enthesopathy, such as lateral or medial epicondylitis, distal pain of flexor carpi radialis or ulnaris, was most frequent, then tenosynovitis such as de Quervain's disease. First MP joint pain was seen in two cases, one at the radial collateral ligament and the other at ulnar collateral ligament; whereas 5th PIP joint pain was seen at the radial collateral ligament.

Thirty pianists attributed their physical ailments to some special piano technique (Table II). Octave, chord and six degrees were responsible for 77% of the cases.

DISCUSSION

Many studies have attempted a scientific approach to piano technique and education since the beginning of this century.[2-6] Medical problems of

Table I: *Diagnoses of Pianists in Study*

Diagnosis	*Number of Cases*
Lateral epicondylitis	10
Medial epicondylitis	2
Pain at olecranon	3
Forearm extensor pain	3
Forearm flexor pain	1
Pain at distal end of FCR*	3
Pain at distal end of FCU**	2
Dorsal wrist pain around scaphoid	1
Pain at 4th extensor retinaculum	2
Pain at 5th extensor retinaculum	1
De Quervain's disease	7
3rd flexor tenosynovitis	1
5th flexor tenosynovitis	1
Pain of thenar muscle	2
Pain of abductor digiti minimi	2
1st MP joint pain	2
5th PIP joint pain	3
4th PIP joint pain	2
3rd PIP joint pain	1
2nd PIP joint pain	1
Neck pain	4
Scapular pain	1
Finger cramp	4

* FCR = Flexor carpi radialis
**FCU = Flexor carpi ulnaris

musicians have recently been differentiated from writer's or telegrapher's cramp."[7-9] Musicians were often told by their medical doctors that only rest could cure their conditions, but this means an end to their performing. Even if rest helped, they still worried that problems might recur when they went back to playing. This led many Japanese musicians to stop consulting medical doctors, and seek instead Oriental treatment such as acupuncture. Some musicians were cured, but many were not, forcing them to abandon their professional careers.

Table II:: *Techniques Responsible for Painful Symptoms*

Technique	Number of Cases
Octave	15
Chord	6
Six degrees	2
Fortissimo	2
Quick passage	2
Arpeggio	1
Wide-extent passage	1
Staccato	1

If the medical problems are caused by trauma or diseases such as arthritis, the first treatment will be effective. But when problems are caused by overuse or instrument-playing techniques, it is necessary to study the kind of technique that caused them. With this study, the means of treatment or prevention of musicians' medical problems could be established. Here, the value of *music medicine* was demonstrated.

Piano techniques such as octave, chord and six degrees were responsible for 77% of all cases. These techniques have in common the abduction of thumb and small finger and the stabilization of the wrist joint. Thus, it is foreseeable that they could cause lateral epicondylitis, forearm extensor pain, pain at distal end of FCR or FCU, pain at 5th extensor retinaculum, de Quervain's disease, pain of thenar muscles or abductor digiti minimi, 1st MP joint pain and 5th PIP joint pain. In Table I, these diagnoses represented 58% of all cases. This helps establish a relationship between wide-extent techniques and painful hands. Thus, it may be possible that painful hands can be prevented by education.

The size of the hand may also play a role in these ailments, because pianists with small hands have difficulty playing wide-extent techniques such as octave and chord. In this sense, Japanese pianists are at a disadvantage compared to their European and American colleagues. It has also been suggested that not only octave but trills and arpeggios can cause to extensor forearm or dorsal hand pain,[10] perhaps suggesting some difference in anatomic predisposition between Japanese and American musicians.

REFERENCES

1. Sakai N: Painful hands of pianists. Musicanova, Supplement:123-126, 1988 (in Japanese).
2. Matthay T: The Act of Touch.   London: Longmans Green & Co, 1903.
3. Matthay T: The Visible and Invisible in Piano Forte Technique. London: Hollen Street Press Ltd, 1932.
4. Marek C: Lehre des Klavierspiels.   Zurich: Atlantis Verlag, 1939.
5. Ortmann 0: The Physiological Mechanics of Piano Technique. London: Routledge & Kegan Paul Ltd, 1929.
6. Schultz A: The Riddle of the Pianist's Finger. New York: Carl Fischer, 1949.
7. Dawson WJ: Hand and upper extremity problems in musicians: Epidemiology and diagnosis. MPPA 3:19-22, 1988.
8. Fry HJH: Overuse syndrome of the upper limb in musicians. Med J Aust 144:182-185, 1986.
9. Manchester RA: The incidence of hand problems in music students. MPPA 3:15-18, 1988.
10. Hochberg FH, Leffert RD, Heller MD, et al: Hand difficulties among musicians. JAMA 249:279-282, 1983.

CHAPTER 93

Preventive Home Conditioning for Musicians

Dwight M. Tamanaha, and Julie A. Plezbert

NOMENCLATURE

Pelvic Tilt[4,15]:While supine with knees flexed and hip flexed at about 45°, using the abdominal muscles to slowly push the lower back firmly to the floor simultaneously tilts the pelvis posteriorly. Pelvic tilt can be achieved in different positions (i.e., against the wall, bending, reaching, sitting, etc.).

Plastic Pipe exercises: Using a horizontally-oriented (across the torso), approximately 1-1.5 inch diameter plastic pipe, lay on adjacent levels starting from the upper back (as far up the vertebra as you can reach) moving down to the gluteal folds. Lay on each horizontal level for ten seconds. With the pipe vertically-oriented, continue from the vertical middle of the body between the gluteals, moving as far lateral to the side of one gluteal/trochanter.

Steady Thoracic Lock[1]: With relaxed neck muscles and a neutral head position (looking straight ahead), tightening of the anterior chest and upper thoracic muscles.

INTRODUCTION

Both athletes and musicians must practice gross and fine motor patterns, between a hundred to thousands of repetitions, in order to perform complex athletic movements and difficult arpeggios as well.[1] These motor patterns require highly-focussed mental imagery, strength/dynamic control, speed, coordination and timing/tempo (Table 1). Musicians must sit and position themselves through long practice and performance sessions. Both athletes and musicians must contract relevant muscles which, if not kept at a functional length and strength, will inevitably lead to a vicious cycle of secondary compensatory mechanisms, setting them up for chronic overuse syndromes.

Overuse syndrome involves frequent, repetitive, long duration motions; and movement patterns on a gross and fine level that result in eventual demonstrable pathology or disability. Restoration of proper joint biomechanics implies that all surrounding tissues, such as tendons, ligaments, muscles and fasciae are in proper dynamic functional balance.

The limbic system is a functional area of the brain in the older part of the cerebral cortex and is

Table 1: Comparison Chart Between Athlete and Musician.

Characteristic	ATHLETE	MUSICIAN
GENETICS	X	X
PRACTICE	X	X
STRENGTH	X	DYNAMIC CONTROL
SPEED	X	X
TIMING	X	TEMPO
COORDIN.	X	X
MENTAL IMAGERY	X	X
MOTOR PATTERNS	GROSS	FINE

generally considered to be the central neural mechanism governing behavior and emotion. A positive attitude and imagery obviates the negative activation of the limbic system sympathetic response. The limbic system bridges somatic and psychic functions which influence muscle tone.[2] Emotional stress typically increases tone in the shoulder, low back and pelvic floor area,[3] which can lead to chronic overuse syndromes.

BREATHING

Coordinated breathing can be a beneficial avenue in dealing with stress emotionally and physiologically. Paradoxical or chest breathing is a common cause of abuse and overload of the scalene muscles. To coordinate breathing, one should initially exhale, then inhale with only the diaphragm, and then exhale. Ideally, with practice, one should breathe in a more natural rhythm, moving the chest and abdomen synchronously in and out together.[4]

NUTRITION

Optimal nutrition is also a valuable adjunct to good health, though it is often neglected. Minimal toxicity coupled with optimal absorption of necessary nutrients will significantly enhance a musician's health. Maintaining an optimal lean body mass (regardless of bodyweight) is also healthy. Sitosterols (phytosterols), a plant sterol and soluble fiber, can be a valuable aid for large serum cholesterol reduction.[5] The largest amounts of phytosterol occur in oils of wheat germ, common bean, rye, corn germ, corn gluten, dry hull of hempseed, and kale and broccoli leaves.[6]

If necessary, and for only a brief period of time (two weeks), musicians can follow a no less than a 1200-1500 calorie, nutritionally-balanced with a diverse food variety (mostly complex carbohydrates, no more than 30% fat and 20% protein) diet. Consuming high-calorie meals in the earlier part of the day until the mid-afternoon is recommended, because increased metabolic rate occurs during/after/between exercise and morning hours, including breakfast. Focus should be on complex carbohydrates (grains, veggies, fruits), limited lean meat/fowl (one to two times weekly), fish (four times weekly), and drinking a lot of water. Sodium, fat and sugar intake should be reduced. Using a seven-day diary, it is recommended to plan and prepare balanced-calorie meals with the afore-mentioned recommended proportion of protein, carbohydrates and fat.

CONDITIONING

The reasons for conditioning are[14,15]:

- it decreases tension and rigidity in the back, shoulder and arm;
- it improves posture for fine, repetitive movements, and gross, static positions, especially in musicians;
- it elevates the mood through endorphin release;
- it prevents and reduces the severity of musculoskeletal pain episodes;
- it keeps myofascial tissue at an optimal functioning length.

It is essential to carry out the activities of daily living (ADL) ergonomically, along with a conditioning exercise program. Artful positioning of the head, trunk, upper and lower extremities and sitting, lifting, reaching, carrying, wearing cloths, sleeping and other

ADL must be conceptualized for simplified applications.[4,7,9] Special attention should be given to practice, in musicians:

- frequent breaks;
- total playing time not to exceed 30-40 hours per week;
- precede practice or performance with light aerobics, such as walking;
- play as relaxed as possible;
- vary tempo and dynamics, duration and intensity, to gradually prepare for difficult passages;
- mentally focus on extremity lock (aikido): imagine a "wave of strength" traveling from the upper thoracic spine (strongest) down to the wrist (weakest), and coordinate breathing.

Functional stabilization (Figure 1) is a trained, symmetrical unloading response,[10] which offers the musicians protection in both their professional and dailing living activities. The *steady thoracic lock, pelvic tilt*, and abdominal exercises,[4] along with the subsequent, properly balanced, stretching of the trunk and proximal upper and lower extremity muscles is critical in unloading spinal discs and extremity joints.[11,12] Lumbar lordosis correction with abdominal muscle strengthening seems to be more effective than lower back flexion or extension exercises.[13]

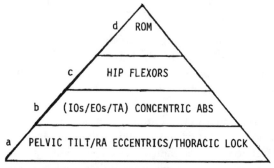

***Figure 1**: Functional Stabilization/Symmetrical Unloading, from Longer to Shorter Cycles. a to d, conditioning; d, stretching.*

Basic conditioning exercises include tennis or racketball, *plastic pipe* and chairs. Daily conditioning and stretching exercises have been extensively covered in the literature.[1,15,16] It is recommended not to stretch until mastering the *steady thoracic lock* and the *pelvic tilt*, and to conclude the conditioning and stretching sessions with the *plastic pipe exercises*. These exercises can be done in less than 20-30 minutes, preferably first thing in the morning when one is stiffer, rather than just before retiring for the evening; a small time to invest in professional lifestyles. The general rules of stretching are:

- a mild to mederate stretch should last 30 sec. minimum;
- avoid bouncing;
- in case of discomfort (sharp excessive pain), stop or slowly reduce the stretch until the pain lessens, then hold it for up to 30 sec.;
- heavy passive stretch destroys beneficial reflexes[15];
- a transient, mild to maderate, stiffness period for up to three days, can be expected at the early stages of the conditioning/stretching program.

POSTURAL STRESS

Some of the most common overuse syndromes incidental to performing artists include back pain,[7,18] and various upper[20,21] and lower extremity[22-31] conditions. Instrumentalists often incur hand, wrist, proximal forearm myofascial pain (Table 2), and nerve (median, ulnar, radial/posterior interosseous branch) entrapments.[32] Trigger points in lower spinal torso muscle, causing low back pain, occur most commonly in the quadratus lumborum (QL), lower rectus abdominis, iliopsoas and serratus posterior inferior muscles.[4] The most common posture obviously is sitting and would entail all the stress associated with this posture. Depending on the instrument played, different areas will be stressed.

Table 2: *Pathophysiology of the Myofascial Syndrome.*

- Shortened unstretched muscles
- Strenuous use
- Prolonged, shortened position
- Sustained, repeated muscle contractions
- Cold, damp weather
- Fatigued muscle exposure to cold draft
- Sustained upward gaze with head extension

The force of gravity must constantly be balanced by muscular energy for postural control. Various practice positions will change where the center of gravity is and even by minute amounts can significantly alter where most of the loading on joints/muscles will occur. Postural control is a complex process of interrelating inputs/outputs of various sensory-motor responses to information.

Musculoskeletal functional measures of postural control are restrictive joint range-of-motion and muscle length-strength-endurance. In any particular joint, alterations or suboptimal conditions of any part of the musculoskeletal system can have far-reaching effects on other parts of the musculoskeletal system (i.e. foot-ankle dorsiflexion limitations can cause compensatory aberrant musculoskeletal patterns at the hip, pelvis, then lower back).

The British Medical Research Council's ten-year multicenter independent experiment, comparing chiropractic manipulation to conventional hospital treatment of acute and chronic mechanical low back pain, concluded that the former was more effective.[33] According to the New Zealand Government Commission of Inquiry into Chiropractic,[34] the chiropractic physician usually enjoys a greater, more varied, and more systematic exposure to spinal techniques.

REFERENCES

1. David Q, Plezbert JA: Stretching for olympic weightlifting. Part 1. International Olympic Lifter 10(10):14, 1991.
2. Guyton AC: Textbook of Medical Physiology (7th Ed.). Philaderphia, PA: Lea and Febiger, 1989.
3. Murphy DR: The neglected muscular system; it's role in the pathogenesis of the subluxation complex. Journal of Chiropractic, 27(12):38, 1990.
4. Travell J, Simons DG: Myofascial Pain and Dysfunction. The Trigger Point Manual. Baltimore. MD: Williams and Wilkins, 1983.
5. Pollack OJ: Reduction of blood cholesterol in man. Circulation 7:702-5, 1953.
6. Lange W: Cholesterol, phytosterol and tocopherol content of food products and animal tissues. J. of Americal Oil Chemical Society 27:414, 1950.
7. Sataloff RT, Brandfonbrenner AG, Lederman RJ editors: Textbook of Performing Arts Medicine. New York, Raven, 1991.
8. Hildebrandt RW: Chiropractic Spinography. A Manual of Technology and Interpretation (2nd Ed.). Baltimore, MD: Williams and Wilkins, 1985.
9. Cailliet R: Low Back Pain Syndrome, Pain Series, (4th Ed.). Philadelphia, PA: FA Davis, 1988.
10. David Q: Lower back conditioning for sports. Triton Junior College lecture, Illinois, 1991.
11. Thorstensson A, Arvidson A: Trunk muscle strength and low back pain. Scandinavian Journal of Rehabilitation Medicine 14:69, 1982.
12. Morris JM, Lucas DB, Bresler B: Role of the trunk in stability of the spine. Journal of Bone Joint Surgery 43-A(1):334, 1961.

13. Kendall PH, Jenkins JM: Exercises for backache: a double-blind controlled trial. Physiotherapy 54:154-7, 1968.

14. Klafs CE, Arnheim DD: Physical Conditioning for the Prevention of Sports Injuries. Modern Principles of Athletic Training, 5th Edition. Missouri, Mosby, 1981

15. Schafer RC: Chiropractic Management of Sports and Recreational Injuries, 2nd Edition. Maryland, Williams and Wilkins, 1986.

16. Beaulieu JE: Stretching for All Sports. California, Athletic Press, 1980.

17. Cailliet R: Low Back Pain Syndrome, 3rd Edition. Pennsylvania, FA Davis, 1981.

18. Fry HJH: Incidence of overuse syndrome in the symphony orchestra. M.P.P.A., 1:51-5, 1986.

19. Cibulka MT, Rose SJ, Delitto A, Sinacore DR: Hamstring muscle strain treated by mobilizing the sacroiliac joint. Physical Therapy 66(8):1221, 1986.

20. Andrews JR, Angelo RL: Arthroscopy in the diagnosis and treatment of rotator cuff injuries. Orthopedic Society of Sports Medicine presentation, Louisiana, 1986.

21. Upton A, McComas AJ: The double crush in nerve entrapment syndromes. Lancet 2:359, 1973.

22. Sola AE, Kuitert JH: QL myofascitis. Northwest Medicine 53:1003-5, 1954.

23. Corwin JM: Piriformis syndrome in the athlete. Am. Journal of Chiropractic Association 24:21-3, 1987.

24. Wing T: The piriformis syndrome: differential diagnosis in sciatic pain how full-time metering aids therapy. Dig. Chiro. Econo., 3:132-140, 1988.

25. Sammarco GJ: Diagnosis and treatment in dancers. Clinical Orthopedics 187:176-87, 1984.

26. Backrach RM: The relationship of low back/pelvic dysfunction. Orthopedic Review 17:1037-43, 1988.

27. Bachrach RM: Injuries to the dancers spine. Chapter 13. In: Ryan AJ, Stephens RE, editors. Dance Medicine. Illinois, Pluribus, 1987.

28. Marymount JV: Exercise-related reaction of the sacroiliac joint. Americal Journal of Sports Medicine 14:320-3, 1986.

29. Baratta R: Muscular coactivation. Americal Journal of Sports Medicine 16:113-22, 1988.

30. Hardakee WT: The pathogenesis of dance injury. Chapter 2. In: Shell CG, editor: The dancer as athlete. The 1984 Olympic Scientific Congress Proceeding:11-30, Illinois, Human Kinetics, 1986.

31. Micheli LJ, Solomon R: Training the young dancer. Chapter 3: In: Ryan A, Stephens RE, editors: Dance Medicine. Illinois, Pluribus, 1987.

32. Lederman RJ, Calabrese LH: Overuse syndromes in instrumentalists. Medical Problems of Performing Artists 1(1), 1986.

33. Meade TW, Dyer S et al: Low back pain of mechanical origin: randomized comparison of chiropractic and hospital outpatient treatment. British Medical Journal 300:1431-7, 1990.

34. Hasselberg PD: Chiropractic in New Zealand. Wellington, Government Printer, 1979.

CHAPTER 94

Trunk and Upper-Limb Pathology in Professional Musicians

Rubén Jaén • *Guillermo Bajares* • *César Restrepo*
Salvador Rivas • *Federico Fernandez-Palazzi*

Trunk and upper-limb disorders are common in musicians, the most frequent being overuse. They range from vaguely defined pain syndromes to classic presentations of the signs and symptoms of such conditions as tendinitis or tenosynovitis. Many of these result from repetitive stress or cumulative trauma. The location depends on the maneuvers or postures necessary to perform on a particular instrument. Also, as in any occupation where there is recurrent friction of tendon sheaths over joint surfaces, ganglions are frequently seen in the wrists of musicians.

A variety of nerve-compression syndromes occur in musicians. Most are related to postures assumed during playing. Carpal tunnel syndrome is extremely common in keyboard and string players who habitually posture the wrist in marked flexion. Many violinists hold the bow firmly pinched between the thumb and fingertips with the wrist flexed; this position can predispose to the same pathology. Cubital tunnel syndrome can occur in the left arm of violinists who habitually posture the wrist in marked flexion. Static loading can also result in digital nerve compression or compression of Guyon's canal in flutists.

All of these problems are amenable to postural modification if detected early. Chronic problems may require, in addition to postural change, surgical decompression.

Musical instruments have associated risks such as the posture taken by the musician, the frequency of repetitive actions required, or the size and shape of the instrument. Guitar players tend to hold the instrument so that both wrists are strongly flexed, frequently with some added radial deviation of the left wrist and ulnar deviation of the right wrist. The positions of the left arm, wrist and hand when playing violin and viola are comparable; the basic hazard for the left hand is caused by the hyperflexion of the left wrist accompanied by increasing degrees of ulnar deviation. Trumpet and flute players encounter many types of shoulder, neck, and arm problems, most of which are a direct consequence of the individual's own stance, arm position, and grasp of the instrument. Many of the medical problems of musicians, including those of trunk and upper limb, can be avoided entirely or reduced in severity.

An important key to prevention lies in proper conditioning of the musculoskeletal system. Good muscular tone, flexibility, and endurance depend on appropriate exercise, warming up before playing, cooling down and stretching after playing, and attention to maintaining a mechanically sound posture.

MATERIALS

During an eight-year period, 1982 to 1990, we examined 41 professional musicians, of whom 18 were violinists, 7 violists, 6 cellists, 8 bassists, and 2 trumpeters.

The most frequent clinical findings were cervical pain accompanied by contracture of the trapezius muscle in 14 musicians (8 violinists, 2 violists, 2 cellists, 2 bassists), followed by: synovial cysts at the dorsum of the wrist in 8 (4 violinists, 2 cellists, 2 bassists); postural dorso-lumbar scoliosis of less than 25° in 7 (3 violinists, 2 violists, 1 bassist, 1 trumpeter); shoulder bursitis in 6 (2 violinists, 2 violists, 1 bassist, 1 trumpeter) bicipital tendinitis in 2 violists; and elbow epicondylitis in 2 cellists. None of these patients required surgical treatment; their symptoms improved with conservative medical treatment, sometimes infiltrations with corticosteroids, and all of them went through a period of rehabilitation which included postural exercises, changes in technique and physical conditioning. At the end of treatment, all were able to resume their previous levels of performance.

CONCLUSIONS

Musicians demand high levels of skilled performance from their upper extremities to execute the greatly coordinated and complex movements required to attain excellence. Injuries most often occur from performance or practice, and most musicians experience overuse symptoms at some point. Prevention of these medical problems involves developing healthy habits of positioning the instrument, proper posture, good technique and adequate conditioning. The right mental attitude is also important. Once established, it can be very difficult for musicians to undo poor postures and relearn positions that are mechanically safer. Musical instruments are not custom-sized or shaped to fit the player. Of necessity, postures will vary among individuals as they adapt to their instruments. Postural fatigue is a common complaint of musicians, and poor posture may be associated with a mild functional scoliosis, which usually is a long thoracolumbar curve with no compensatory curves. The scoliosis is very flexible, disappearing on recumbency or when the patient is asked to stand straight; it does not progress or become structural. Corrective measures must be taken to increase back strength, namely passive and active postural exercises.

A good position should require a minimum of muscular exertion, especially of the back, and the musician should develop a relaxed posture and proper balance during performance, as well as playing movements that avoid extreme positions.

Most of the patients examined in our work had neck and shoulder pain accompanied by contracture of the trapezius muscles due to incorrect body positions while playing. Tendinitis or tenosynovitis often respond to a combination of activity modification, NSAIDs and, at times, steroid injections, a period of rest until pain and inflammation subside, followed by a progressive rehabilitation program until return to performance.

We compare musicians with high-level competitive athletes, and in order to avoid injuries they need to maintain a good physical condition to withstand long hours of study and practice and to cope with the stress that surrounds their performance.

SUGGESTED READING

1. Amadio PC, Russotti GM: Evaluation and treatment of hand and wrist disorders in musicians. Hand Clinics 6(3), 1990.

2. Blair S, Bear-Lehman J: Prevention of upper extremity occupational disabilities (editorial comment). J Hand Surg 12A:821-822, 1987.

3. Brandfonbrener AG: The epidemiology and prevention of hand and wrist injuries in performing artists. Hand Clinics 6(3), 1990.

4. Caldron P, Calabrese LH, Clough JD, et al: A survey of musculoskeletal problems encountered in high level musicians. Arthritis Rheum 28 (suppl 4):597, 1985.

5. Carragee EJ, Hantz VR: Repetition trauma and nerve compression. Orthop Clin North Am 19:157-164, 1988.

6. Fry HJH: Overuse syndrome in musicians: Prevention and management. Lancet 2:728, 1986.

7. Hochberg F, et al: Hand difficulties among musicians. JAMA 249:1869-1872, 1983.

8. Lederman RJ: Performing arts medicine. N Engl J Med 320:346, 1989.

9. Lockwood AH: Medical problems of musicians. N Engl J Med 320:221, 1989.

CHAPTER 95

Restoration of Performing Capacity in Wind Players Following Surgery for Sleep Apnea

David Sternbach

The author, a psychotherapist and professional french-horn player for twenty-five years, underwent surgery to relieve obstructive sleep apnea with consequent loss of ability to perform on this instrument. The specific cause was removal of the uvula, defeating maintenance of an air seal adequate to resist wind delivered under compression.

This chapter describes the discovery of an alternative solution that restores playing ability. As far as the etiology and treatment modalities of this disorder, suffice it for the purposes of this discussion to mention that it is a relatively newly diagnosed illness. It appears to be one of a number of disturbances of sleep in older persons, and is increasingly viewed as contributing to or directly causing daytime sleepiness, narcolepsy, fatigue, lack of energy, and even premature mortality.[1]

The author presented to several ENT specialists with complaints of blockages in the nasal system stemming from a long history of allergies, polypoid growths, and a deviated septum that had twice been operated upon with only partially successful results. Symptoms included inhibition of respiration waking and in sleep, daytime sleepiness, fatigue, and frustration at the limitations to maintaining a full schedule of work and exercise. There were recurrent sinus infections, and spousal reports of vigorous snoring. Dr Jeffrey Hausfeld, ENT surgeon and a specialist in treating sleep disorders, has indicated that in his experience, the spouse is frequently the first line of referral.[2]

Examination by one of several ENT specialists consulted resulted in exploration of a factor overlooked by others who perhaps were concentrating too exclusively on the presentation of pathology in the nasal system. This specialist noted an enlarged uvula and pursued possible sleep disturbance as a cause of the symptoms presented. A referral made to a sleep clinic and the results of an overnight stay on a variety of monitoring devices revealed a highly significant number of episodes of breathing cessation, i.e. 108 episodes in that one evening, averaging 23 seconds in duration, with one event having a duration of 48 seconds.

Discussion of these clinical findings, together with imaging evidence and the clinical impressions developed by examination, confirmed a diagnosis of severe obstructive sleep apnea. Non-surgical treatment for enlarged polyp formation and control of allergic symptoms with routine medication were indicated and succeeded in controlling the symptoms they were designed to address, but had no significant effect on the daytime sleepiness, general fatigue, lack of reserves of energy, and the snoring in sleep. The first line of treatment, CPAP, was rejected as unsatisfactory in this case. Surgery was advanced as the most likely route that could result in remediation of the problem, together with an extensive schedule of surgery on the nose and sinuses.

In the pre-surgery interview, potential benefits and risks were discussed. The most significant risk presented was probable loss of playing ability based on information that oboists and bassoonists were unable to play their instruments following similar surgery. The author, in subsequent consultations with physicians interested in music medicine, learned of brass players who also experienced loss of playing ability.

Nevertheless, weighing risks versus benefits, the author elected to follow the option for surgery, the physical and affective disturbances being sufficiently aggravated to demand attention. The author privately reserved the hope that the french horn might perhaps require sufficiently lower amounts of air compression compared to oboe or bassoon to leave open the prospect for a return to some level of performance ability.

Surgery took place in May 1990, followed by a recovery period during which the author set aside concerns about a return to the instrument. The surgery relieved the sleep apnea, restored normal employment of the nasal passages in respiration, and relieved the physical and affective symptoms. Surgery as the option of choice appears to have been validated on the basis of relief of symptoms and a return to full functioning in everyday life. This, however, left open the prospect of a return to playing ability.

After several months, exploration confirmed the limitations created by the surgery. While tones could be produced, nothing above C concert one octave below middle C (128 cycles per second) was useable. At that pitch and above, air compression required to vibrate the lips at these pitches is also sufficient to break the fragile air in the throat.

The net effects of the loss of an adequate air seal are, first, an audible rush of air through the nasal passages interfering with clear tone production. This is not only aesthetically distracting, it also limits the player's ability to hear and evaluate notes produced due to this noise of air rushing upwards through the throat and nose.

Secondly, no volume above piano is possible, and this exposes more obviously the sound of air escaping through the nose. Third, ascent into the lyric or high registers where virtually all of the literature for horn lies is virtually impossible. Finally, the ability to sustain a melodic line without unacceptably frequent interruptions for breaths is greatly restricted. In sum, this confirmed the prediction of loss of playing ability.

The author consulted Dr. Richard Norris, an expert in rehabilitation medicine and the field of arts medicine, who suggested two courses for possible remediation. First, further rest to assure completed healing of the musculature involved. Second, progressive challenge to the musculature beginning at very conservative levels until a return to full strength might be achieved. This prescriptive advice was followed, but it became evident that no further improvement would occur.

Further confirmation of this was supplied by Kendall Betts, principal Horn of the Minnesota Orchestra. Betts et al.[3] have conducted experiments testing compression rates generated by playing different wind instruments. Their studies indicate that french horn requires higher compression rates than other wind instruments, and substantially more than either oboe or bassoon. Given this information, the author turned to an exploration of alternatives to enable a return to playing.

Eventually, adapting an approach[4] to his specific concern, the author self-induced a trance state and processed a series of inductions in which he visualized performing on the instrument using a device that provided an air seal in the throat. What then appeared was essentially an image of the design the author now uses. There were, however, further steps to be traversed.

At that point, uncertain whether there existed any technology to construct such a device following the model the author envisioned, be consulted with his surgeon, Dr. Hausfeld, who suggested consulting a dentist specializing in prosthodontics. Dr. Hausfeld's pivotal contribution was the insight connecting the author's concept with his knowledge of devices made for cleft palate and cancer patients.

The author conferred with Dr. Conrad Schwalm, a prosthodontist in private practice, and after a description of the author's imagined device and requirements, Dr. Schwalm agreed to undertake the construction of a prosthodontic device, modified to fulfill the requirement for a tight air seal with air delivered under powerful compression.

The design arrived at through experimentation, custom-made to fit the author's physiology, has resulted in complete remediation of the loss experienced due to the surgical procedure. Wearing this removable prothodontic device, the author can play throughout the entire four-octave-plus range of the french horn, at all volumes and with breath control adequate for long phrases.

Several disadvantages associated with this design should be noted. The device requires accommodation to avoid a gagging reflex, with attention required to control abrupt movements of the head to either side or downward, which brings the device into contact with the back of the throat and can exacerbate the gag reflex. The device somewhat interferes with clear articulation of speech and initially provokes a plentiful salivary reaction. This reaction does appear to diminish over time.

With the current model of this device, a minute amount of leakage occurs when playing in the highest range at a high volume, but the author considers this to fall within an acceptable range of air loss since it does not noticeably affect playing efficiency. On balance, the author considers the disadvantages to be acceptable compared to the benefits derived.

In view of the fact that other players have suffered and may in the future suffer a loss of their playing ability following this type of surgery, it is recommended that physicians be aware of this alternative and offer it to patients where appropriate.

REFERENCES

1. Williams T, Ferguson J, et al: NIH Consensus Development Conference on the Treatment of Sleep Disorders of Older People. Washington: National Institutes of Health 8(3), 1990.
2. Hausfeld J: Preoperative discussion, 1989.
3. Betts K, et al: Private discussion, 1990.
4. O'Hanlon W, Davis M: In Search of Solutions; A New Direction in Psychotherapy. New York: WW Norton, 1989.

CHAPTER 96

Evaluation of the Injured Musician: Role of the Instrument

Caryl Johnson

Performers fall into one of four groups: student, amateur, professional/free lance, or soloist. Each of these groups has unique needs and expectations. A performing history which includes previous training, technique, current and previous repertoire, and performance schedule is important to treatment planning.

When evaluating an injured musician, the history and physical examination must include yhe musician playing his instrument. To carry this out the health care professional needs a knowledge of traditional instruments, how they are played, what physical demands they place on the player, and how different styles of music affect these demands. During the evaluation he observes the patient's body working with the instrument, his skill, musicality, and technical proficiency. Video tapes of this evaluation provide a valuable baseline by recording motions and sound.

A look at the workplace may provide clues about causes of injury. An otherwise efficient body-instrument interaction can be destroyed by working in uncomfortable space, with limited lighting, or under extremes of stress, injured one because of space, vision, or other workplace limitations.

The performer's attitude toward music and toward his injury are factored into the evaluation and treatment plans. His description of his problem or injury provides insight into his emotional potential for recovery.

The primary goal of treatment of the injured performer is a return to playing. This begins with a plan for general body conditioning to return a balance of strength and control away from and with the instrument. The patient moves through a graded progression of muscle strengthening, increased speed of response and motion, control, and coordination exercises, and exercises to increase endurance.

Graded exercises are composed for use at the instrument to guide the performer safely through critical technical areas. Repertoire is chosen from material specifically related to the cause of injury and its resolution.

Splints are sometimes constructed to use as an assistive and training device. These splints, worn while playing, may substitute for weakness or protect injured tissues.

Returning a patient to his instrument and his work is the goal and the reward of treating injured musicians.

SUGGESTED READING

1. Polnauer FF, Marks M: Occupational hazards of playing string instruments. Strad 1987.
2. Dawson WJ: Hand and Upper Extremity Problems in Musicians: Epidemiology and Diagnosis. Med Prob Perform Art 3, 1988.
3. Hoppman RA, Patrone NA: Musculoskeletal problems in instrumental musicians. *In*: Sataloff, R. (ed.) Textbook of Performing Arts Medicine, New York: Raven Press. 1963.
4. Schonberg, HC: The Great Pianists from Mozart to the present (ed. Fireside). New York: Simon and Schuster, 1963.
5. Hochberg FH, Harris SU, Blattert TR: Occupational hand cramps: Professional disorders of motor control. In: Amadio PC (ed) Hand Injuries in Sports and Performing Arts, Hand Clinics, 1990.
6. Poore GV: Clinical lecture on certain conditions of the hand and arm which interfere with the performance of professional acts, especially piano playing. 1887.
7. Lippman HI: A fresh look at the overuse syndrome in musical performers: Is "Overuse" Overused? Med Prof Perform Art. 1991.

8. de Quervain F: Ueber eine form von chronischer tendovaginitis. C-Blatt Schweizer Aerzte, 1895.

9. Finkelstein H: Stenosing tenovaginitis of the radial styloid process. J Bone Joint Surg. 1930.

10. Grundberg AB, Reagan DS: Pathologic anatomy of the foremarm: Intersection syndrome. J Hand Surg. 1985.

11. Lockwood AH: Medical problems of musicians. N Engl J Med. 1989.

12. Volz RG: Biomechanics update No. 2. Basic biomechanics: Lever arm, instant centers of motion, moment force, joint reactive force. Orthop Rev. 1986.

13. Koller W, Vetere-Overfield B: Usefulness of a writing aid in writer's camp. Letter. Neurol. 1989.

14. Marsden CD, Obeso JA, Traub MM, et al: Muscle spasms associated with Sudeck's atrophy after injury. British Medical Journal, 1984.

15. Newmark J, Hochberg F: Isolated painless manual incoordination in 57 musicians. J Neurol Neurosurg Psychiatry 1987.

16. Panizza M, Hallett M, Nilsson J: Reciprocal inhibition in patients with hand cramps. Neurology 1989.

17. Schott GD: Induction of involuntary movements by peripheral trauma: And analogy with causalgia. Lancet 1986.

18. Witt T, Jaeger M: Congenital subluxation of the metacarpophalangeal joint of the thumb as the cause of writer's syndrome. Z Orth, 1984.

CHAPTER 97

Misuse Syndrome in Musicians: Combined Medical and Musical Approach

Samuel Lehrer, Janet Weiss, and Pieter Kark

INTRODUCTION

A team of therapists has treated musicians with illnesses of the hands or arms acquired from playing their instrument. The core members of the team are a piano teacher who specializes in dealing with hand and arm problems, a flute teacher with similar expertise, and a neurologist who is an amateur flutist. When needed, the team has included physical and occupational therapists, a chiropractor who uses massage to decrease physical tension in muscles, and a psychiatrist with special expertise in hypnosis.

The musicians we have treated have had problems of pain, clumsiness, or focal dystonia. Six did not have a major surgical problem as the basis of their difficulties and have improved to being able to resume performing after learning to release unnecessary tension in muscles other than the prime mover as part of the warm up each time they practice or perform, and to keep the muscles relaxed while playing. The team approach may be useful in other cases.

CASE REPORTS

Case 1: JO is a 60 year-old flutist who began to make errors with the second finger on the left onto the "A" key. Over two years, he became unable to play the bulk of the orchestral and chamber repertoire.

Examination by JW revealed this dystonia, problems in the angle between the flute and the embouchure, problems where thumbs and fingers held the instrument, and movements off the embouchure while playing. All this decreased the quality of the tone and the ease of playing. He played a conventional, open-hole flute with all keys in line. The left wrist was markedly hyperextended and the angle of the right hand tended to push the left hand out of line.

Neurological examination (PK) revealed minimal decrease in sensation in the distribution of the medial nerve. In nerve conduction studies, motor distal latencies were mildly prolonged across both the carpal tunnel and Guyon's tunnel on the left when the wrist was hyperextended.

Wrist splints helped transiently. Chiropractic massage of arm muscles just before sessions allowed the flutist to work with JW or SL but the tension in antagonist muscles persisted when playing at home or in the orchestra. A flute crutch and changing the position of the keys on the flute 90 as to be more physically convenient for his hands (JW) helped transiently but over time the modifications had to be varied. Inderal helped little. Fast and difficult passages continued to be hard to play, and there were unexpected errors in concerts. Exercises designed to decrease or "release" unnecessary tension in muscles (SL) led to a marked improvement in the ability to play virtuoso passages and in tone.

The flutist had difficulty changing his habits. Performance deteriorated although lessons improved. There began to be a definite delay of nerve conduction across the left carpal tunnel. Surgical release was considered. he decided to pursue work with SL and JW more rigorously.

JW taught him to change registers by changes in embouchure rather than in the position of the flute's head-joint against the chin, and to maintain good postures when with the orchestra. Muscles were being contracted that were not necessary for the note he was playing. Some muscles were antagonists of those needed for the note. To demonstrate this to him, surface electrodes were placed over the extraneous muscles and surface EMG was displayed while he played.

Over two months, recordings were made over each of the unneeded muscles several times a week while he played, did "releasing" exercises, and continued to play. He had fortnightly or weekly sessions with SL and JW. In addition, he was now scrupulous about doing "releasing" exercises for all warm-ups and in intermissions. By the fourth month, there was a marked improvement in performances and nerve conduction studies became normal.

A fine tremor appered but responded to Sinemet. For the past year, the flutist has able to play 90 to 95% of the orchestral repertoire.

Case 2: GK is a 77 year-old amateur guitarist who took up formal weekly lessons and developed pain in the left forearm, hand and fingers while playing, 18 monr to our evaluation. The pain began near the elbow and radiated distally, in muscle bellies. Sometimes the third finger would lock in flexion. Symptoms ceased soon after each practice.

On examination, there was atrophy of a muscle in the hand, mildly decreased grip and mildly impaired sensation in the left C6 and C7 dermatomes.

He was shown how to release unnecessary muscle tension in the arm and hand before playing and whenever the pain developed. In a single 90-minute session, SL taught him to keep the accessory and antagonist muscles relaxed when playing. There have been no further problems in 5 months.

Case 3: LK is a 22 year-old master's student who had numbness of the ulnar aspect of the right hand and aching of the ulnar aspect of the forearm within 20 minutes of beginning to play any of several instruments.

When she played difficult passages on the flute, the right arm and hand were held rigid. Within a few minutes, sensation for light touch became impaired in the ulnar distribution of the right hand. There was mild slowing of sensory conduction in the right ulnar nerve across the elbow.

Within a few weeks of learning to release tension, sensory conduction across the right elbow was now normal. Her ability to play became normal.

Case 4: NH is a 29 year-old professional pianist had burning pain in the ulnar aspect of the right hand and a cramping ache in the right forearm for 6 months, exacerbated by 4 months of a heavy schedule, 90 that it was almost impossible to practice or to play chords and arpeggios. Writing and carrying grocery bags became difficult.

The intrinsic muscles of the right hand and grip were weak. Sensation was impaired in the median distribution. Nerve conduction studies were normal. After learning "releasing" exercises, she could perform and teach normally.

Case 5: AB is a 16-year-old cellist who had transient pain in the palm and fingers of the left hand while playing throughout the day at a music camp, pain which recurred after playing two days in a row with a youth orchestra.

There was tenderness in the left index flexor tendon at the distal palm crease, mild weakness of the left intrinsics, and impaired sensation in either the median distribution or cervical roots C6 and C7's. Motor latencies for the left median were dispersed, but both motor and sensory velocities were normal.

She was taught to keep unneeded muscles relaxed. She was able to play well until she tried to prepare two difficult pieces for a piano recital in three days. Her symptoms recurred. Once she learned to do "releasing" exercises first in all warm-ups and to study difficult passages slowly at first, she was able to play both instruments without difficulty.

DISCUSSION

A. Onset of problem:

In each instance, the problem began when the musician was preparing a virtuoso piece for a major audition or a major concert and was exacerbated by practicing difficult passages at tempo. Musicians should probably learn virtuoso passages very slowly until they have been mastered.

While persisting in playing, and trying harder despite the problem, both reflect well on attitude, harm appears to come from such persistence if the underlying problem is not addressed. We have only seen the problem corrected when the misuse of muscles was addressed, or when an underlying medical difficulty was treated.

B. Misuse vs overuse:

The term "overuse" has been applied to this syndrome. The term correctly alludes to the excessive physical, mental, and emotional work that takes place when the syndrome develops. "Overuse" has a good connotation: an illness due to working too hard.

However, the authors believe that "misuse" is the more correct term. In each case, the problem could only be solved by getting the musician to relax accessory muscles that were being used forcefully, but which were not needed to play the notes or phrases. Often, muscles were being used that were antagonistic to the movement needed to play.

C. Releasing Technique:

SL draws on a variety of techniques, including

Feldenkreis, Tai-Chi, Alexander, and combinations and modifications of these methods. He examines the individual musician's playing. In the light of this, and observations by other members of the team, he draws on a repertoire of exercises and adapts those that seem likely to help. Two sets of feedback are used to reenforce or modify the approach. First, one can hear whether there is improvement or worsening of playing within a few minutes in each session. Second, the other members of the team report changes in the musician's playing and its quality after several sessions.

Some exercises refine coordinated movements between large and small muscles during playing. At the same time, points of excessive or unnecessary tension are sought. Some exercises release or decrease unnecessary tension, make the musician aware of the unnecessary tension and help integrate the awareness into daily playing. The validity of each exercise is judged by whether it helps decrease symptoms and by whether the exercise seems to improve facility of playing, accuracy of pitch and quality of tone.

D. Modification of instruments:

JW has found how woodwind instruments can be held to the best physical advantage for the individual player. She has found ways in which individual differences in physical characteristics can influence techniques of blowing the instrument and of fingering the instrument, and has begun to understand how these problems contribute to the breakdown of playing in cases like those above. A number of flutists cannot manage the conventional flute. JW has designed changes that are physically convenient for these players but do not impair tone or pitch and intonation.

E. Pathophysiology

The authors speculate that the symptoms in our cases came from misuse: contracting agonist and antagonist muscles at the same time. As a result, various tissues may be compressed or stretched. The nature of the damage may depend on anatomical differences between individuals and these differences determine susceptibility. If an excessive compression or stretch happens each time a difficult passage is played, pain or an erroneous movement can result. This may lead to clumsy phrasing or perhaps even focal dystonia.

F. Release of unnecessary tension:

The authors also speculate that the common factor that improved the playing in each of these cases was the decrease or release of unnecessary tension in specific muscles while playing specific notes or passages. To some extent, there was relaxation of the whole body, indeed of the entire playing attitude.

CHAPTER 98

Use of Vibration to Enhance Finger Mobility in Musicians

A.S. Skuratovich

INTRODUCTION

Mechanical oscillations can be applied to the muscles of the fingers, via a device which operates by transforming the electric engine rotations into return-forward movements of pins exerting influence upon the fingers (Figure 1).

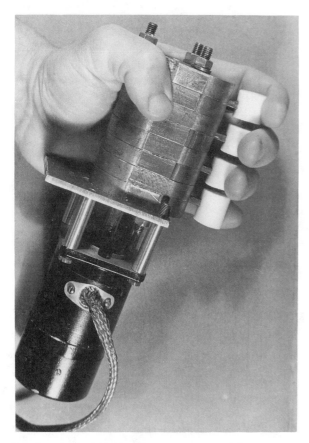

Figure 1: *Mechanical Oscillator Device. Model for Enhancement of Finger Mobility.*

MATERIALS and METHODS

This device was tested on three pianists, age 11 to 14 years. The period of study lasted for two weeks, comprising 6 training sessions of 20 minutes each.[1] To control the effectiveness of the device, the number of successive blows by the five fingers of both hands in 30 sec was registered, along with hand dynamometry.

RESULTS

The study showed that, after two weeks of training, the number of successive blows had increased by 10-17%. As for hand dynamometry, it remained largely unchanged with a tendency to slight increase. The subjects pointed out that application of the device helped decreasing fatigue. This vibration effect is achieved via a better blood circulation and a stronger influence on the muscles mechanoreceptors.[2]

INDICATIONS

The device can be used by musicians of various instruments, whose activities demand fingers mobility, for:

a. warming up;
b. rehabilitation after injuries;
c. increasing fingers strengths;
d. raising speed-strength endurance; etc.

It can also be used for the following diseases:

1. Nervous system diseases: neuritis, plexitis, neuromyositis, and posttraumatic affections of peripheral nerves;
2. Joint diseases: non-specific and degenerative dystrophic;
3. Post-injury: fracture, strain or sprain;
4. Restoration of mobility;
5. Prevention of or occupational injuries.

CONTRAINDICATIONS

Same as physical therapy in general:

1. Acute fever;

2. Any local acute process;
3. Acute stage of chronic diseases;
4. Susceptibility to blood-fluxes;
5. Varicose veins;
6. Thrombophleitis;
7. Vessel aneurysms;
8. Lymphadenopathy;
9. Non-malignant and malignant tumors.

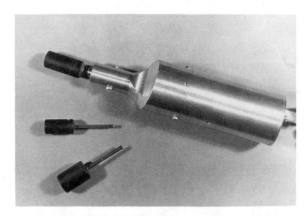

Figure 2: *Mechanical Oscillator Device. Model for Face Muscles.*

SPECIAL APPLICATION

Using the same principle, a modified device was designed for cosmetic application to face muscles (Figure 2).[2]

Due to its peculiar effect upon face muscles this new device can also rehabilitate vision at the initial stage of myopia.

This device can be successfully used for other aims and other muscle groups, both small and large, i.e., muscles of hand, fingers, back, shin, etc.

Changeable nozzles of various materials make it possible to locally affect muscles of different sizes.

Preliminary trials showed this device to be effective in the treatment of face injuries and bruises in boxers. It can also be used to relax vision tension and fatigue in microscheme fitters, who usually work all day long over a microscope, and video display terminal workers.

REFERENCES

1. Шейдин, А. И: Аппаратнъій Массаж Минск. Полъі мя, 38-42, 1988.
2. Назаров, В. Т.: Виомеханическая Стимуляция: Явъ и Надеж-дьі. Минск. Полъі мя, 5-26, 1986.

CHAPTER 99

Rehabilitation of the Brain-Injured Artist

Tedd Judd

INTRODUCTION

A patient, T., presented with loss of his musical abilities. He was a 32-year-old college-educated jazz guitarist and pianist who had had a mild head injury. T. reported that since his injury, he had difficulty concentrating and remembering, had lost his guitar technique and was quite anxious about this. He was assessed and treated for these problems, and a few months later, he returned to his usual work in jazz clubs.

The effects of brain damage on musical and other artistic abilities have been well-studied for over a century, and hundreds of case studies are available in the literature. Yet in all that time, very little has been written about how to help brain-injured musicians or artists recover their abilities. We know a great deal about creative arts therapies, that is, how to use the arts to aid in rehabilitation in general, and also about general rehabilitation of brain injuries. Knowledge in arts medicine is also growing. Until quite recently, however, these themes have not been integrated to deal with the rehabilitation of artistic impairments of artists with brain injuries.

The restoration of artistic ability in brain-injured artists is obviously only one part of a fully integrated rehabilitation program involving the conventional rehabilitation team presented: physiatrist, nurse, neuropsychologist, physical therapist, occupational therapist, speech pathologist, recreational therapist, creative arts therapist, social worker, vocational counselor, and art- or music teacher as needed. Ideally, rehabilitation of the brain-injured artist is a creative collaboration between the therapist and the artist. The therapist brings knowledge of brain injury and its rehabilitation, and the artist brings knowledge of his or her own art and the creativity to adapt that art.

ASSESSMENT

The assessment of artistic abilities consists of history, interview, and examination.

Artistic History

The artistic history can be organized by three questions: What? How? and Why?

What? What is it that the artist does and did artistically? It is important to determine not only the artist's strongest or most characteristic artistic activities, but also the breadth of the artist's work in order to find the most appropriate channels for rehabilitation efforts. The history is best obtained from a directed interview beginning with "What do you do (as an artist, musician, etc.)?" For musicians, this interview should include the instruments played and whether there is skill at music reading, playing by ear, improvising, composing, arranging, conducting, critiquing and/or teaching. For the graphic artist, this should include the media worked in, the subjects treated, teaching, critiquing, and so on.

How? This question includes styles of work, skill levels, settings and habits. Artists will usually readily explain their styles, but it is often necessary to consult others or examples of previous work to determine previous level of skill. The work setting can be important to rehabilitation, and a rehearsal or studio visit can sometimes be important. Habits such as playing music from the page vs. by ear or improvised, or drawing from models, photographs or imagination also give clues to rehabilitation strategies.

Why? To understand the artist's motivations in his/her work is to understand better what is to be rehabilitated. At a minimum, it is useful to know how the artist's art functions as a personal or emotional expression, as a personal identity, as recreation, as a career, and as a social activity. This taking stock of art's personal meanings is also a taking stock of life's meanings and is a therapeutic process in itself. It can also lead to reassessing priorities and choosing appropriate adaptations.

Interview

After the history, we try to determine what problems the artist is experiencing. The artist's description of these problems provides some of the initial hypotheses about what neuropsychological impairments might be producing them. The neuro-psychological test results and knowledge of the type of injury provide other hypotheses. These are then explored through examination.

Examination

It is critical to observe the artist in action. We need to ask the artist to do what (s)he typically does, as well as the things which are producing problems. A formal examination with standardized and normed tests is rarely possible. Instead, we must collaborate with the artist to explore the problem, trying creative variations of the problematic activities to discover what component skills are disrupted, what strengths remain to be built upon, what skills can be relearned and what adaptations can be made. An outline of a musical screening examination is shown in Table I.

Table I: Music Screening Tests

---

1.   Performance of Choice
2.   Preparing a New Piece
3.   Vocal Expression
     ☐   Sing familiar songs alone and with examiner
     ☐   Sing short, unfamiliar melodies by imitation
4.   Rhythmic Expression
     ☐   Reproduce tapped rhythmic patterns
     ☐   Repeat tapped rhythmic patterns in time with examiner
5.   Reading and Writing (when appropriate)
     ☐   Copy a musical text
     ☐   Transcribe a dictated melody
     ☐   Sight-read musical texts singing and on instrument
6.   Perception
     ☐   Listen to and comment on an unfamiliar piece in a familiar style, identifying instruments, structures, quality, etc.

When conducting an artistic examination, it is important to remember that the skills may be out of practice due to lengthy illness or disability. It may take months of directed practice to discover what the ultimate rehabilitation strategy will be.

TREATMENT PLAN

Table II illustrates T.'s treatment plan. He had complained that he lost his technique. Assessment shows that this was due to impaired attention, lack of practice, and anxiety. Through directed practice, he gradually recovered his technique at home, passing rapidly through the sequence of study he had originally learned with — scale exercises, chord progressions, etc. He then complained that he could not jam, or improvise with other musicians. This was due to distractibility, which is a form of attention impairment, and anxiety. He was directed to play with records, starting with easy chording along, gradually filling in more moving lines as he was able to do with security. He then complained that he could not play in clubs because he would be too distracted and awkward. Besides distractibility and anxiety, he had subtle impairments in his executive functions, especially planning, organizing, and social judgment. About this time, he got a job playing "space music" in a restaurant at lunch. This was a low-key job with limited distractions and a very forgiving musical format. It allowed him to work his way back to public performance. Further work on jamming at home with friends allowed him to return to his old jobs.

Counseling

A number of themes are common with the impaired artist and often need to be dealt with before other artistic rehabilitation can begin.

Despair: Dr. Samuel Johnson, the seventeenth-century British man of letters, awoke one night to discover he had suffered a stroke and could not speak, so he composed a prayer in Latin verse to test his intellectual skills. This was an example of a successful self-test of artistic abilities after brain injury. Many artists who suffer brain injury are similarly tempted to test themselves with their most difficult endeavor, such as a concerto as soon after their illness or injury as they can manage. Most are not as lucky as Dr. Johnson. When they fail, they often despair and may abandon their art.

Artists often have a very strong personal identification with their art and not uncommonly feel that any loss at all is a devastating blow to the self. This is particularly true for those who come from a highly competitive environment where technical virtuosity is prized.

The intervention needed to avoid or modulate this despair pattern involves educating the artist about the

Table II: *Treatment Plan*

ARTISTIC PROBLEM-ORIENTED TREATMENT PLAN

Artistic Problem	Components	Plan
Impaired technique	Impaired attention	Practice (slow)
	Lack of practice	Practice
	Anxiety	Relaxation training
Unable to improvise with others	Distractibility	Play with records
	Anxiety	Recognize tension, stop, relax
Unable to play jobs at clubs	Distractibility	Avoid noisy clubs, pressure
	Anxiety	Relaxation training
	Executive-function and social-skill impairment	Play with friends at home; check social perceptions with friends, therapist

NEUROPSYCHOLOGICAL PROBLEM-ORIENTED TREATMENT PLAN

Neuropsychological Problem	Artistic Consequences	Plan
Impaired attention	Difficulty practicing Difficulty playing Difficulty playing at clubs	Progressive attention training: (1) simple material at home; (2) complex material; (3) with records; (4) with friends; (5) quiet clubs; (6) noisy clubs
Anxiety	Fear of practicing and performing; fear of loss of art and work; fear of going crazy	Head-injury education; supportive counseling; relaxation training; gradual return to feared activities
Executive-function and social-skill impairments	Gullibility in business Alienating band and clientele, fear of failure	Practice with friends at home; check perceptions and judgments with friends and counselor

pattern, preferably before the self-test. This education should include information about the effects of lack of practice, the long time frame of recovery, possibilities for rehabilitation, and realistically optimistic stories about the recovery and adaptations of other artists.

Fixed Approaches

Many artists develop fixed and even obsessional or ritualistic approaches to their art. For example, consider the case of a painter with lupus, an auto-immune disease, which produced chronic fatigue. She had painted expressive landscapes, always working standing in the field, completing her large canvases in a single session. With lupus, she lacked the stamina to do this. She thought she could not be an artist, and stopped painting for months. This type of problem can be overcome by stripping away the nonessential parts of the fixed pattern. She was sent back to the studio to sketch small still lifes while sitting, interrupting and resuming work as her stamina dictated. She rediscovered her talent and ways to adapt her work.

Shift in Style

A brain injury can result in a shift of style either due to emotional reactions to the trauma or as a direct consequence of the brain damage itself. An example is the case of a mildly brain-injured painter who had changes in visual perception so that she was able to see scenes not according to the laws of perspective, but as if they were blotches of color on a sheet of glass. She was able to paint those blotches directly as she saw them, giving her works a new and intriguing ambiguity. She switched from insightful portraits to impressionistic landscapes, which turned out to sell better. The artist should be encouraged to explore new areas of self-expression, rather than trying to recapture and relive the old.

Recovery Time

People with brain injuries usually need to be told that recovery can continue for a year or two or even longer. Artists should avoid attempting too much too soon, and should avoid commitments to deadlines and performances until they have clearly reestablished and demonstrated their abilities. Recovery is an active process and requires exercise and practice.

Using Art to Recover

Art can be used to express the emotions resulting from the illness or disability. It can also be used to explore the disability itself and to communicate the experience to others. The artist can regard his or her new self as a new instrument or palette or medium to be explored. In this way the artist may not only achieve a new adjustment, but help others with their challenges and disabilities in ways that we clinicians can perhaps only dream of. Examples include May Sarton's journal, *After the Stroke*, and *Don't Worry, He Won't Get Far on Foot*, autobiography of the quadriplegic cartoonist, John Callahan.

Relearning

Where there is a realistic possibility of recuperation, relearning can be attempted, often through a condensed version of the original learning process, as with T. This process often parallels rehabilitation in other areas. It may be helpful to work on this process collaboratively with a teacher in the artist's field. The process also resembles cognitive rehabilitation, a set of techniques developed in the last decade to help people with brain injuries recover their thinking abilities. T.'s recuperation process was guided by the cognitive rehabilitation techniques of attention-process training. He progressed from sustained attention in his technical practicing, to selective attention when learning to play with records, to divided attention when relearning how to play with others and in clubs. For the graphic artist or crafts person, it may be necessary and possible to break artistic tasks down into their components and retrain the component skills as needed, following the principles of executive-function work used in cognitive rehabilitation.

Adaptations

When a skill or ability cannot be relearned or recovered, adaptation is sometimes possible. Rasaan Roland Kirk, the jazz saxophonist, adapted his saxes for one-handed playing after a stroke paralyzed his left side. A guitarist with an injured left hand switched to bottleneck or dobro style which uses open tunings and only one finger on the strings. Others use electronics to fill in what they cannot play. Oral musicians with memory impairments may resort to "Fake Books" with the lyrics to thousands of popular songs, or to reading music. A composer with visual impairments seen by the author functioned better with wide-lined staff paper. Count Geza Zeichy in the nineteenth century, and Paul Wittgenstein in the twentieth, commissioned compositions for piano left hand when they lost their right arms, and Cyril Smith arranged piano duets for three hands after his stroke.

Compensations

Sometimes the artist needs to curtail or abandon some artistic activities and compensate by emphasizing others more. Beethoven cut back conducting and performing in favor of composing when he became deaf. Sometimes this has unexpected benefits. Smetana wrote, "I have completed in these three years of deafness more than I had otherwise done in ten." A fabric-construction artist found new projects were difficult to organize in the months following a mild head injury, so she used the time to finish a backlog of routine projects. A composer with a right-hemisphere stroke was no longer able to compose or perform, so he emphasized his conducting, writing, and teaching.

CONCLUSION

Rehabilitation of the brain-injured artist is a creative challenge to both the artist and the therapist. The collaboration of these two can produce recuperation, inspiration and a better understanding of disabilities, art, and the human spirit.

PART VIII

MUSIC THERAPY

CHAPTER 100

Music and Medicine

Fred J. Schwartz

Music has been used therapeutically throughout history. Primitive tribes around the world used drum rhythms and chanting to treat the sick. The ancient shaman used these rhythms to reach altered states of consciousness, in the belief that this gave him the power to heal. Some of these ancient medicine men used this to reduce the pain and stress of childbirth. Shamanism is still a primary source of healing in parts of the world today. The ancient Egyptians used music to heal the sick, as well as for treating infertility. The Greeks also used music for healing, as evidenced by Apollo, the god of medicine, music, and poetry. Later, in Italy, during the fifteenth and sixteenth centuries, the tarantella, a type of spirited dance music, was designed to combat the frenzied agitation seen in patients who suffered tarantula bites. It was thought that this convulsive condition, which was impossible to control, could be suppressed and cured only by music with a fast rhythmical beat. The music was tailored to the particular temperament of the victim, who would call to the performers with desperate cries while dancing for hours or even days on end until he was completely exhausted. During these enforced pauses, he was covered with blankets and given a strong broth and wine to drink, causing him to perspire. A cure was achieved eventually, but only after having sweated out all the venom of the spider. In the 1800s, Franz Mesmer, the father of hypnotism, believed music could potentiate his hypnosis treatments. These were often carried out with a piano or glass armonica providing background music.

There are early twentieth-century written accounts of string quartets being brought into the delivery suite during childbirth. It was only after methods for playing recorded music were available that the medical use of music became more widespread. Dentists in America were actually the pioneers in using recorded music to decrease pain and anxiety in their patients, who could be subjected to some extremely uncomfortable procedures. In this situation, audio-analgesia was used to decrease pain through

intense auditory stimulation with music and white noise, and the sound volume would be turned up to mask the drilling sounds.

There is no doubt that the time before surgery is anxiety-provoking for patients. Many preoperative patients experience intense fear relating to such issues as loss of control, negative outcome, and anticipated pain. Table I lists many of the emotional changes noticed when preoperative patients listen to music.

Table I: *Emotional Condition Rating Scale*

Before Music	After Music
Depression, sadness, despair	Sense of well-being, confidence, acceptance
Psychological isolation, withdrawal from warmth and depth in relating to others, defensiveness, shallowness	Psychological openness, warmth, and depth in relating to others, honesty, genuineness
Anxiety, apprehension, tension	Sense of serenity, security, peace of mind
Difficulty in medical management, complaints, refusal of services, ill temper	Ease in medical management, amenability, openness to medical care and treatment
Preoccupation with pain and physical suffering	Tolerance to pain and physical suffering

Many of the harmful physiologic effects of the stress of the perioperative period (Table II) are mediated by the sympathetic nervous system (SNS). The hormonal mediators here are the catecholamines dopamine, epinephrine, and norepinephrine. Blood pressure, heart rate, and other body functions mediated by the SNS are usually in a state of balance. The system evolved to respond so that in stressful situations blood flow increases to the brain and certain brain functions are stimulated, and other body functions are stimulated or depressed. This system worked well when we were cave men either hunting our next meal or running from predators. The problem is that we have become so cerebral that

375

many of us are constantly sending messages that inappropriately activate the SNS. For patients, there are many deleterious effects. Blood pressure and heart rate increase, causing the heart to work harder. This increased heart rate can cause less blood to be delivered to the heart by the coronary arteries. For the patient with significant coronary disease, this can cause coronary ischemia or even myocardial infarction. While some of these patients will be on medication to blunt these effects, activation of the SNS can often override this, so music is very much of value here.

Table II: *Physiological Consequences of Preoperative Anxiety*

---

1. Hypertension
2. Tachycardia
3. Peripheral vasoconstriction/low blood flow
4. Increased anesthesia induction drug doses
5. Decreased immune function
6. Increased metabolism and oxygen consumption

It has been shown that music causes mild decreases in systolic and diastolic blood pressure and lower respiratory rates in patients having surgery under regional or local anesthesia. Music has been shown to decrease the drug dose needed to initiate general anesthesia. It is the author's experience that under regional anesthesia, many patients drift off to sleep themselves when music is added, as compared to patients who have had equal amounts of sedation but do not fall asleep without music.

The stress level of the surgical patient is very much affected by the operating-room environment, especially what is heard. When you talk to patients in a calm, reassuring manner as they go to sleep, they drift off more easily. Patients also hear and process information while they are under general anesthesia. Comments about losing sports teams can be misinterpreted, and the patient could think that the surgeon meant the operation was going poorly.

Music creates a warmer, more pleasant environment for the patient and staff. It provides a diversion, distracting the patient from monitors and the surgical setup. Music can prevent the patient from hearing inappropriate conversation. For the patient under regional anesthesia, the music muffles extraneous noises such as drilling, hammering, and sawing. When well-chosen music is played, members of the surgical team work in closer harmony because of decreased levels of frustration and fatigue. Appropriate rhythms may stimulate rapid, coordinated movements. The author has seen the length of time for facelift surgery

reduced by ten percent with music. For the patient who is somewhat awake during surgery, there is no doubt that music makes the time seem to pass more quickly.

There is increasing evidence that hearing and learning occur under general anesthesia. Recent studies have shown that when a recorded tape of positive suggestions is played to patients under anesthesia, they have a faster recovery. Typical positive suggestions used are: *The operation seems to be going well. You feel warm and comfortable; calm and relaxed. You will not feel sick at all. Your bladder and bowels will work normally. You will feel no pain at the site of your operation. You will recover quickly and completely.*

A study of hysterectomy patients given positive suggestions under general anesthesia showed significant benefits: less fever, fewer bowel difficulties and gastrointestinal problems, a smoother recovery, and an average of 1.3 days less time in the hospital recovering. Another study showed that these patients used 23% less self-dosed morphine via PCA pump during the first 24 hours after surgery. The author believes that music may potentiate the effects of positive suggestions during surgery. It has been shown, however, that when music is coupled with positive suggestions postoperatively, this is less effective for reducing pain than music or positive suggestions alone. This may be because patients experiencing pain cannot focus easily on music and positive suggestions at the same time.

At Piedmont Hospital, patients listen to music with headphones with an open air construction. This type of headphone enables patients to hear people talking to them, as long as they have not adjusted their volume too high. Many of the patients with premedication close their eyes and drift off.

In designing this system, the types of music channels used were dictated by patient requests. Many children and adolescents want to hear rock & roll, and although this is probably not what most of us would choose before surgery, it does work for them. Choice of music is very personal, and patients can alter their environment best when they listen to familiar music that connects with good feelings and emotions from past experiences. There is some evidence that slow, quiet non-vocal music lowers the physiologic stress response most effectively, so if a patient is undecided as to choice of music, New Age music is often suggested. Music preference for surgery is very much a cultural matter, and many of our patients request country music. In Germany, many patients choose nationalistic music to listen to preoperatively.

The music system consists of five carousel-type CD players with ten amplifiers which are wired to the main preop area, outpatient preop area, recovery room, and coronary care unit. The system is left on 24 hours a day, since many of the patients in the CCU with chest pain may need this during the night. The system is expandable and can be extended to several hundred patient locations. The next expansion will soon be to labor and delivery. It is also possible to use the hospital's existing TV cable system to have the music go into every patient room.

In regard to the coronary care unit, most patients are admitted there with the presumptive diagnosis of acute myocardial infarction. Anxiety is very common in these patients, and this can produce an increase in sympathetic-nervous-system activity, leading to an increase in cardiac workload and increased myocardial ischemia. Anxiety here is associated with increases in heart rate and blood pressure, palpitations, tightness in the chest, and peripheral vasoconstriction. A recent study has shown that when music was played to these patients, a significant decrease was seen in the following complications: persistent chest pain, cardiac arrest, severe congestive heart failure, and pericarditis. Many of our CCU patients elect to listen to the music. In one such patient with an acute MI and second-degree heart block, the ischemia lessened and the heart block disappeared. It is hoped that music will eventually be available to our open-heart-surgery patients and other patients in the intensive care units.

Music is also used effectively during labor and delivery. Couples coming to a delivery suite frequently perceive it as a foreign and unfamiliar environment over which they have little control. The act of choosing a musical program for labor and delivery allows a couple to exert some control. Since pain and enjoyment emerge as two distinct though related dimensions of the birthing process, music can express both the struggle and the joy of the occasion. The beauty of this technique is that it can be utilized for natural childbirth, with epidural anesthesia, and, if need be, during cesarean section.

The author has used music as part of the anesthetic approach in hundreds of C-sections over the past 15 years. There is often some discomfort, even with epidural anesthesia, as traction is put on the uterus before the baby is delivered. You don't want to give any sedation until after the baby is born, since you don't want to affect the baby. Music is an effective way to decrease the discomfort here. It is best to determine the type of music the couple and their baby find soothing. If they don't have an idea of what they want to hear, classical music or New Age music is usually suggested. These types of music seem to fit beautifully with C-sections. Overall, music for labor and delivery is best played through speakers rather than headphones, because the music is also beneficial for the husband and hospital personnel. It also may help the newborn know that a special event is occurring, and when the newborn comes into this world, the music, along with the familiar sounds of voices, is indeed special.

The negative effects of a hyperactive sympathetic nervous system in surgical and cardiac patients were previously described. In the laboring patient, elevated levels of catecholamines cause decreased effectiveness of uterine contractions, sometimes resulting in the need for a cesarean section. High levels of catecholamines also cause constriction of the uterine blood vessels. Intense anxiety as a cause of fetal death in the third trimester is well-documented. More commonly, the extremely anxious patient who is having trouble dealing with her labor will have high catecholamine levels, decreasing placental blood flow and causing fetal distress. This is further compounded if the laboring patient hyperventilates; the resulting alkalosis constricts the uterine blood vessels further. Music has been shown to lower stress hormone levels during labor and, in this situation, can be therapeutic.

Music has been shown to speed up the laboring process. Even if the labor is not accelerated, when music is played, the perceived length of labor decreases. Other studies have shown that when music is played, there is less need for pain medication during labor.

Music therapy is not widely available in obstetrical units. In this day and age of fierce competition for patients, perhaps we will see hospitals using this as a marketing ploy to attract patients. Ideally, music should be integrated as a basic part of hospital care for *all* patients.

SUGGESTED READING

1. Evans C, Richardson R: (1988) Improved recovery and reduced postoperative stay after therapeutic suggestions during general anaesthesia. Lancet 2:491-493, 1988.

2. Guzetta C: (1989) Effects of relaxation and music therapy on patients in a coronary care unit with presumptive acute myocardial infarction. Heart and Lung 18:609-616, 1989.

3. Kaempf G, Amodei M: The effect of music on anxiety. American Operating Room Nurses Journal 50:112-118, 1989.

4. McKinney C: Music therapy in obstetrics: A review. Music Therapy Perspectives 8:57-60, 1990.

5. McLintock T, Aitken H, Downie C, Kenny G: Postoperative analgesic requirements in patients exposed to positive intraoperative suggestions. British Medical Journal 301:788-790, 1990.

6. Moss A: Music and the surgical patient: The effect of music on anxiety. Association of Operating Room Nurses Journal 48(1):64-69, 1988.

7. Myers R, Williams M: Preventing fetal asphyxia. Clinics in Obstetrics and Gynaecology 9(2):369-414, 1982.

8. Oyama T, Sato Y, Kudo T, Spintge R, Droh R: Effect of anxiolytic music on endocrine function in surgical patients. In Droh R, Spintge R (eds), Music in Medicine, 169-178. Springer-Verlag, 1987.

9. Steelman V: Intraoperative music therapy. American Operating Room Nurses Journal 48: 64-69, 1990.

10. Tanioka F, Takazawa T, Kamata S, Kudo M, Matsuki A, Omaya T: Hormonal effect of anxiolytic music in patients during surgical operations under epidural anaesthesia. In Droh R, Spintge R (eds), Music in Medicine, 199-204. Springer-Verlag, 1987.

11. Thompson G, McMahon D: Music and analgesia. Problems in Anesthesia 2(3):376-385, 1988.

12. Updike PA, Charles DM: (1987) Music RX: Physiological and emotional responses to taped music programs of preoperative patients awaiting plastic surgery. Annals of Plastic Surgery 19: 29-33, 1987.

CHAPTER 101

Music-Based Models for Altering Physiological Responses

Bruce M. Saperston

This chapter provides an overview of two music-based models developed by the author for the purpose of altering various physiological parameters (e.g. heart rate, muscle tension, respiration) in patients. First, *physiologically interactive music* (PIM) will be discussed with regard to its theoretical basis, definition, research support, and practical applications in medical settings.[1] Secondly, *music-based individualized relaxation training* (MBIRT) will be described, and the various roles of music in this behavioral-medicine approach will be identified.[2]

PHYSIOLOGICAL INTERACTIVE MUSIC

The PIM model is based on entrainment (Huygens phenomenon) from the field of physics.[3] Entrainment refers to "the locking into phase of previously out-of-step oscillators." An oscillator is "anything that vibrates in a regular periodic manner."[4] Leonard claims that this phenomenon is universal:

Whenever two or more oscillators in the same field are pulsing at nearly the same time, they tend to lock in so that they are pulsing at exactly the same time. The reason, simply stated, is that nature seeks the most efficient energy state, and it takes less energy to pulse in cooperation than in opposition.[5]

Entrainment mechanisms have been identified and researched in the fields of physiology,[6] psychology,[7] and music therapy.[8] These studies, however, have largely dealt with circadian rhythms. As musical stimuli and physiological responses consist of oscillations, the PIM model is based on the premise that music could be systematically presented as a synchronizer *zeitgeber* to influence ongoing physiological parameters through entrainment. While a few studies were found which suggest that auditory stimuli or prerecorded music may be useful in entraining respiration[9, 10] and heart rate,[11] no studies

were found in which musical stimuli were systematically manipulated in relation to ongoing physiological responses in order to entrain such responses. The PIM concept was initially defined by the author in order to provide a basis for such research.

PIM is an hypothesized approach in which one or more elements of music (or combinations of the same element of music) are continuously presented in a systematic relationship to an organismic rhythm within the periodicity limits necessary for entraining the organismic rhythm. As the organismic rhythm changes, either in the desired direction (i.e. towards the musical synchronizer) or away from the synchronizer, the musical synchronizer is again presented within the new periodicity limits necessary for entrainment. The process is repeated in a continuous manner. The process is 'interactive' because of the hypothesized interdependent relationship which is set up between the musical stimuli and the physiological response.[1]

Method

The usefulness of the PIM concept was investigated by the author using a physiologically interactive tempi (PIT) condition to influence heart rate (HR).[1] Subjects' electromyographic (EMG) responses (frontalis muscle) were also recorded. Sixty-four university students were randomly assigned to one of four experimental groups (n = 16): Tempo 1, Tempo 2, PIT, and a no-music control. Excluding the control group, all subjects were presented with the same baroque music selections via a synthesizer. Tempo 1 subjects listened to music at a slower tempo ($\flat$ = M.M. 48) than Tempo 2 subjects ($\flat$ = M.M. 86). The PIT subjects were presented with music at tempi approximately one beat below their ongoing heart rates in an attempt to entrain their heart rates. Physiological data were recorded during four three-minute periods for each subject, one baseline and three treatment.

Students' t-tests were performed, comparing baseline means with means from each of the treatment periods.

Results

Data demonstrated that music presented at a slow tempo and at a moderately fast tempo resulted in minimal nonsignificant HR decreases and increases respectively, while the PIT music was the only music to significantly influence HR decreases ($p < .001$). Control group HR's decreased significantly ($p < .05$), but not as immediately or to the extent exhibited by PIT subjects. Fisher's LSD tests demonstrated significant treatment effects for the PIT and control group conditions ($p < .05$) over both of the other music groups during period 2 and over the Tempo 2 group during period 3.

Although no significant differences in EMG response occurred for any of the groups, the control group's EMG actually increased slightly across the treatment phase while the PIT group's EMG decreases were about twice the decreases exhibited by the other music groups.

Conclusions

These findings appear to indicate that music presented according to the PIT model can predictably influence heart-rate responses. A critical range within which oscillations must occur for entrainment to take place has been described in the fields of physics[3] and physiology.[12] The PIT music in this study ranged from 1 beat to 1.9 beats beneath HR. It is probable that entrainment occurred only periodically. As the PIT music followed a subject's HR responses, it may have occasionally entered some critical range necessary for entrainment.

The author is currently developing a computer-automated PIT system capable of presenting synthesized music at tempi within 1/100 of a beat per minute in relation to the subject's HR. Research will be directed towards determining whether a universal critical range exists for all subjects or whether each individual has his/her own critical range for entrainment.

Practical applications of this technique could include the control and stabilization of heart rate during various medical/surgical and recovery procedures, which might result in a decreased need for the use of drugs for these purposes. This technique may also be useful in the treatment of hypertension.

MUSIC-BASED INDIVIDUALIZED RELAXATION TRAINING

While behavioral medicine techniques (e.g. biofeedback, relaxation, imagery) have been successfully utilized in the treatment of anxiety, psychologically-related somatic disorders, and disorders of a purely somatic origin,[13, 14] the need exists for approaches that would benefit populations with cognitive and/or behavioral deficits (e.g. elders with cognitive deficits, developmentally disabled, severely disturbed) who have been unable to use traditional approaches and who are most commonly treated with medication.[15-17] The MBIRT approach was developed to meet the needs of such individuals.[2] Due to the comprehensive nature of this model, however, it may be employed with a wide variety of populations. The author has defined MBIRT as follows:

Music-Based Individualized Relaxation Training is a behavior-therapy approach in which one or more elements of music are incorporated in individualized task-specific training strategies designed to elicit and/or shape one or more behaviors identified as necessary in the eventual achievement of a generalized state of relaxation. The approach is 'music-based' because music serves a variety of functions during all phases of training. Training strategies are individualized and task-specific in order to meet the needs of each client at his particular level of functioning.[2] Music is applied in MBIRT as a means of circumventing learning- and behavioral problems. The various functions of music in MBIRT can be categorized within three general areas of the behavioral paradigm: music as a reinforcing stimulus, music as a structural prompt, and music as an eliciting stimulus. As patients with cognitive impairments may not understand the rationale for maintaining behaviors that are requisites for participation in relaxation training (i.e. lying still with eyes closed), music-listening is useful in initially engaging these individuals in relaxation training because: (a) considering the requisite behaviors, music is one of the few experiences that can be presented; (b) music provides meaning to the activity (i.e. the client participates by listening to music); and (c) music-listening is a reinforcing experience.[2] Other factors which make music a particularly powerful and efficient reinforcing stimulus include the fact that musical inputs are mediated at the thalamic level and arouse sensations, emotions, and feelings in lower functioning individuals who may not be accessible at a verbal (cortical) level,[18] and that the temporal aspect of music allows for its precise administration in conjunction with brief inappropriate motor responses and physiological fluctuations. "If music is structured in time concurrent with the behavior, it is generally being used as a structural prompt."[19] Applications of music as a structural prompt during MBIRT include the use of concept songs to improve comprehension and retention of relaxation induction skills, and the use of the patient's chanting of short phrases to develop breath control, slow respiration, and focus attention on the relaxation task. In addition, language cues to "breathe in" and "breathe out" are accompanied by rhythmic chord changes to teach diaphragmatic control skills.

A major factor in the presentation of music as an eliciting stimulus is the use of the *iso principle*.[20] The iso principle refers to matching musical stimuli to an individual's existing mood and then changing the musical stimuli in the direction in which the individual's mood is to be influenced[20]. The iso principle is employed throughout all phases of MBIRT in conjunction with several basic MBIRT assumptions related to the use of music preferences and the identification of music that elicits more relaxed physiological responding in specific patients.

MBIRT intervention strategies are designed. in general, to move the patient from respondent to operant procedures so that relaxation skills can be performed independently. MBIRT are sequenced according to four levels of intervention:

☐ Level I: Development of Enabling Behaviors;

☐ Level II: Development of Therapist-Directed Relaxation Responses.

☐ Level III: Development of Independent Relaxation Responses; and

☐ Level IV: Development of Transfer and Generalization Skills.

Case studies have demonstrated that these strategies have been successful in decreasing EMG activity, training psychophysiological control skills, reducing undesirable behaviors, and eliminating the need for medication for behavioral control.[2]

REFERENCES

1. Saperston BM: The effects of consistent tempi and physiologically interactive tempi on heart rate and EMG responses. *In* Wigram T, Saperston BM, West R (eds), Music and the Healing Process: A Handbook Of Music Therapy. Chichester, UK: Carden Publications, in press.

2. Saperston BM: Music-based individualized relaxation training: A stress-reduction approach for the behaviorally disturbed mentally retarded. Music Therapy Perspectives 6:26-33, 1989.

3. Pippard AB: The Physics of Vibration (Vol 1). Cambridge University Press, 1978.

4. Halpern S: Tuning The Human Instrument: An Owner's Manual. Belmont, CA: Spectrum Research Institute, 1978.

5. Leonard G: The Silent Pulse. New York: Elsevier-Dutton Publishing Co, 1978.

6. Minors DS, Waterhouse JM: Circadian Rhythms and the Human. Bristol, Wright: PSG, 1981.

7. Brown FM, Graeber RC: Rhythmic Aspects of Behavior. Hillsdale, NJ: Lawrence Erlbaum Associates, 1982.

8. Rider MS, Floyd JW, Kirkpatrick J: The effect of music, imagery, and relaxation on adrenal corticosteroids and the re-entrainment of circadian rhythms. Journal of Music Therapy 22:46-58, 1985.

9. Haas F, Distenfeld S, Axen K: Effects of perceived musical rhythm on respiratory pattern. Journal of Applied Physiology 62(3):1185-1191, 1986.

10. Lovell G, Morgan J: Physiological and motor responses to a regularly recurring sound: A study in monotony. Journal of Experimental Psychology 30:435-451, 1942.

11. Bason PT, Celler BG: Control of the heart rate by external stimuli. Nature 238(5362):279-280, 1972.

12. Wever RA: The Circadian System of Man: Results of Experiments Under Temporal Isolation. New York: Springer-Verlag, 1979.

13. Basmajian JV: Biofeedback: Principles and Practice for Clinicians. Baltimore: Williams & Wilkins, 1983.

14. Stroebel C, Sandweiss J: The Handbook of Physiological Feedback. San Francisco: Pacific Institute, 1979.

15. Ferrell BR, Ferrell BA: Easing the pain. Geriatric Nursing, 175-178, July/Aug 1990.

16. Harvey JR: The potential of relaxation training for the mentally retarded. Mental Retardation 17:71-76, 1979.

17. Menolascino FJ: Challenges in Mental Retardation: Progressive Ideology and Services. New York: Human Science Press, 1977.

18. Weigl V: Functional music: A therapeutic tool in working with the mentally retarded. American Journal of Mental Deficiency 63:672-678, 1959.

19. Jellison JA: Music instructional programs for the severely handicapped. *In* Sontag E, Smith J, Certo N (eds), Educational Programming for the Severely and Profoundly Handicapped. Reston, VA: Council for Exceptional Children, 1977.

20. Altshuler IM: A psychiatrist's experience with music as a therapeutic agent. *In* Schullian DM, Shoen M (eds), Music and Medicine. Freeport, NY: Book for Libraries Press, 1948.

CHAPTER 102

Use of Music and Paraverbal Techniques in Degenerative Diseases with Focus on Huntington's Disease

Helen M. Grob

Among the most commonly addressed degenerative diseases today are Alzheimers, Parkinson's, Huntington's and Acquired Immune Deficiency Syndrome. All are described as involving neurological deterioration reflected in motor and cognitive functioning associated with dementia. In most instances, dementia is associated with and includes, but is not limited to, memory and cognitive deficits, marked personality changes, aphasia, agnosia, anomia, apraxia, dysarthria, and other deficits.[1]

Among the aforementioned diseases, Huntington's disease has unique characteristics, one being that it is genetic. The mean age of onset has ranged from 35-42 years. Onset has also been reported prior to the age of 15 years and is characterized by intellectual decline, seizure disorder, and rigidity rather than chorea.[2-4]

In serving Huntington's disease victims who have reached the stage requiring residential skilled nursing care, the author has focused treatment on three other observed unique characteristics. Simply stated, while there are aberrant neuronal messages being transmitted from the brain, especially to muscles, manifested in choreiform and rigid movements, there does not appear to be a deficiency in peripheral nerve fibers effecting transmission of messages to muscles and back to the central nervous system.

Another characteristic observed is that while dementia is ascribed to all the diseases mentioned,[1] the Huntington's disease victims served, except for intermittent, fleeting loss of focus, are alert, oriented, aware, reveal adequate memory, have intact ego functioning, are social and, despite awareness of their disease, have keen, appropriate senses of humor.

Socially/affectively, all have histories of personality changes including depression, irritability, and poor frustration tolerance resulting in tantrums and combative and abusive behaviors. All the aforementioned do not represent a dementia but are justifiable, as these victims are accomplished people who are fully aware of their diagnosis and prognosis, experiencing continuous loss of faculties, progressive dependence on others for all functions, and are terminal. This is compounded by a gamut of other emotional factors, since a majority have spouses and children. The latter have the potential to have the disease or pass it on genetically. In some instances, some of the offspring have already manifested symptoms of the disease.

An example of their awareness was exhibited when the author informed the patients that she would not be present the following week due to attendance at an International Neuropsychological Society conference. One client inquired as to whether sessions on Huntington's disease would be included in the program. The author replied in the affirmative. Upon return, the same client wondered if any new information on the disease had been presented at the conference.

Communicatively, unlike the other degenerative diseases, the Huntington's disease victim's receptive ability and expressive speech content are intact and related. Expressive speech is characterized by a progressive dysarthria which eventually results in unintelligibility. Other characteristics are aprosody and aposiopesis, in that expressive speech lacks resonance, inflection, and rhythm of normal speech, and consists of abortive and explosive or inaudible phrases and sentences. None of these is related to cognitive functioning, but rather to muscular involvement, including the diaphragm.

Also unique to Huntington's disease is the type and variance of degeneration. Some have sudden extreme weight loss to the point of appearing emaciated, yet maintain the same level of external motor- and cognitive functioning. Others maintain cognitive functioning with sudden deterioration of motor functioning, manifested in inability to ambulate, and constant uncontrollable trunk-thrusting, flailing of extremities, grimacing, vocal emissions, and almost complete inability to communicate, the last resulting in extreme frustration and tantrum-like behavior. Deterioration is also evidenced in the digestive process.

The characteristic of intact peripheral nerve fibers for sensory input plays an important role in the treatment for inhibiting and decreasing these choreiform movements. Appropriate stimulation of these receptors which fire back to the central nervous system may modulate uncontrollable muscle contractions.

During treatment it has been revealed that peripheral, cyclic, sensory input of pulse and rhythm via tactile, auditory, visual, kinesthetic, and somesthetic approaches decrease/inhibit choreiform and rigid movements and increase more fluid movements.

The use of music with victims of degenerative diseases has been generally used. The unique characteristics associated with Huntington's disease, however, have been responsive to the use of music using paraverbal techniques, based on paraverbal therapy.

Paraverbal therapy was developed by Heimlich[5] in 1965 for the treatment of children with communication disorders, particularly those who were inaccessible to orthodox modes of psychotherapy. This aspect assumes importance, since children with Huntington's disease are sometimes misdiagnosed.

Paraverbal therapy uses the individual- and combined components of music along with rhythmic movement and the 'drama' associated with communication. In the nonverbal area, the drama consists of exaggerated facial expression, gesture, and body movement. In the verbal area, it consists of exaggerated changes in prosody-accent, dynamics, rhythm, pulse, and pitch. Responses may be verbal or nonverbal.

The success of the therapy is attributed to the approach's flexibility, in that the therapist responds to the client's behavioral cues. The approach has been modified and expanded to also include a neuro-psychological and developmental framework,[6] which plays an important role in the differential diagnosis of children[7] and in the assessment of status in the social/affective, cognitive, communicative, and motor areas in those with degenerative diseases.

This is revealed via the specific effects of the components of music, particularly to the right hemisphere, for spontaneous responses, as well as distinctive characteristics of music and specifically designed dual dependent rhythmic motor tasks.[6]

All music and tasks are designed by the therapist with focus on providing personal interaction. The piano and recorded music are not used, as the piano does not provide for personal interaction and recorded music intrudes only on one sense — auditory. For those who are sensory-impaired, it may serve as an additional stimulus which cannot be filtered or dampened. In addition, if this input is constant, it may foster unrelatedness compounded by the fleeting loss of focus associated with the disease. Recorded music does not allow for alteration of input in response to behavioral cues. Also, because of varied experiences and aberrant neurotransmitter functioning, the imagery created cannot be ascertained and may not be consistent with intended input.

Consequently, voice — the timbre to which most humans are responsive — is used, as well as designed materials and tasks that will provide personal interaction and appropriate sensory input specific for each client.[6]

The use of pulse and rhythm as organizing components, thought by some to be an innate response,[8] and changes in pitch, dynamics, tempo, melody, and harmony as attention securers, has been reported and documented similarly as the specific design of lyrics.[9]

Lyrics are personalized and reflective to conform with the psycholinguistic concept that verbalization stabilizes perception. The design of lyrics with these specifics attempts to secure and maintain focus and relatedness, as well as provide self/environmental awareness and ego functioning.

Repetitive, simple melodic line and harmonies are also used to facilitate auditory encoding,[10, 11] particularly for those who cannot tolerate complex auditory input, whether organically or emotionally based.

The specific intervals of the ascending perfect 4th and descending minor 3rd are the base of all music designed. Responses to these two intervals are well-documented, and it is conjectured that these responses may be due to 'physiological programming' in much the same manner as birds and specific animals respond to pitches.[6, 12, 13] These two intervals are also consistently utilized in *melodic intonation therapy* with unimpaired-right-hemisphere aphasic persons where prosody remains intact.[14]

The use of repetition of simple melodic line has been most effective in assisting in verbal apraxia, other forms of dysfluency, general motor planning, retention, recall, and various learning disabilities.[15] It also appears to be effective in eliciting spontaneous responses, in that it addresses the right hemisphere and does not require encoding.[7, 16] In effect, the right hemisphere assumes new material until routinized, at which time the left hemisphere assumes the role of conceptualization and integration.[17]

Most effective in providing the appropriate visual, auditory, tactile, kinesthetic, and somesthetic peripheral sensory input is the use of the afore-mentioned characteristics of music incorporated into dual dependent rhythmic motor tasks. The dual dependent rhythmic motor tasks designed for Huntington's disease clients require two or more people to perform a task in synchrony or in rhythmic turn-taking. The designed tasks involve tactile, kinesthetic, visual, and auditory senses, individually or concurrently, while offering physical support to assist in the performance of the task. The physical support and other tactile input are offered not only to assist in more fluid motor performance of the task, but to specific areas that require inhibition of choreic movements. The tasks are designed not only to provide more successful fluid motor experiences, but to encourage eye contact and social/communicative interaction.[6]

Huntington's disease clients are usually seen in groups to provide social and communicative interaction as well as cognitive stimulation. Since the Huntington's disease victim is acutely aware and oriented, when extreme degeneration in varied domains occurs in some clients, the composition of the group is changed for consistency of functioning in an attempt to curtail further depression.

Many people fail to realize the sudden absence of social, tactile interaction when one is admitted to a residential facility. Consequently, tasks are designed to provide appropriate tactile interaction. This interaction is one Huntington's disease victims seek and request. Many have become aware of the decrease in choreiform movements during this type of

interaction and input, and will seek the therapist's hands for input.

In some instances, the auditory and tactile input of the components of pulse and rhythm, and repetition of simple melodic line, appear to have an effect in modulating the contractions of the diaphragm and other muscles involved in respiration. This is manifested by vocalizations exhibiting more normal prosody, appropriate pitch, and sustained tones, with decrease in explosive vocal emissions.

Huntington's disease is a progressive, degenerative, terminal disease, of which its victims are aware. While remission or reversal of the symptoms is not possible at this time, the techniques and approach utilized attempt to offer some awareness of maintenance and successful performance in a variety of domains within a milieu of dignity.

REFERENCES

1. Bayles K: Linguistic communication disorders of dementing diseases. International Neuro-psychological Society Conference, San Antonio, TX, 1991.

2. Hayden M: Huntington's Chorea. New York: Springer-Verlag, 1981.

3. Brothers C: Huntington's chorea in Victoria and Tasmania. J Neural Sci 1:405-20, 1964.

4. Myers R, Martin J: Huntington's disease. Semin Neurol 2:365-72, 1982.

5. Heimlich E: Paraverbal techniques in the therapy of childhood communication disorders. Int J Child Psychother 1:65-82, 1971.

6. Grob H: The use of music and paraverbal techniques with children afflicted with AIDS. Proceedings of Canadian Music Therapy Association, 1990 (in press).

7. Grob H: The use of music in differential diagnosis. Twenty-fifth Annual National Conference, National Association for Music Therapy, Philadelphia, PA, October 22-26, 1974.

8. Mittleman B: Mobility in infants, children and adults. Psychoanal Study Child 9:142-177, 1954.

9. Grob H: Music therapy. *In* Valletutti PJ, Christopolos F (eds), Preventing Physical and Mental Disabilities: Interdisciplinary Programs, 197-210. University Park Press, 1979.

10. Kohut H: Observation on the psychological functions of music. J Am Psychoanal Assoc 5:389-407, 1957.

11. Mayer W: Live composers dead audiences. New York Times Mag 12:12-42.

12. Bjorkvold J: Child culture and music education. International Conference of Biology of Music Making: Music and child development, and personal contact.   University of Colorado, Denver, 1987.

13. Payne K: Elephant talk. National Geographic, August 1989.

14. Sparks R, Helm N, Albert M: Aphasia rehabilitation resulting from melodic intonation therapy. Cortex 10:303-316, 1974.

15. Grob H: The use of music and paraverbal techniques in the diagnoses and treatment of specific learning disabilities.   37th Annual Conference, National Association for Music Therapy, Chicago, IL, 1986.

16. Jackson H: Selected Writings of John Hughlings Jackson. London: Hoddler & Staughton, 1931.

17. Rourke B: Syndrome of nonverbal learning disabilities: manifestations in neurological disease, disorder and dysfunction. New York Neuropsychology Group, 1991.

CHAPTER 103

Mozart's Contribution to Music Therapy and Discussion of His Unknown Affliction: Tourette's Syndrome (?)

Benjamin Simkin

A fascinating relationship between young Wolfgang Mozart and the eminent Viennese physician, Doctor Franz Anton Mesmer, discoverer of animal magnetism and hypnotherapy, began in September 1767, when Leopold Mozart and his family paid their second visit to Vienna to participate in the wedding celebrations of the Archduchess Maria Josepha.[1] Scarcely a month after their arrival in Vienna, the Princess Josepha died of smallpox, and so Leopold wrote: "The Princess bride has become a bride of the Heavenly bridegroom."[1] As the smallpox epidemic raged, the court went into mourning, all musical activities ceased, and the Mozart children also contracted the disease. After their recovery, the Mozarts were graciously received at Court by Dowager Empress Maria Theresa and her Co-Regent son, Emperor Joseph II, who commissioned the 12-year-old Wolfgang to compose an opera buffa, *La finta semplice*.[1] Due to various intrigues and cabals, this work was never performed in Vienna; its first performance was in Salzburg on May 1, 1769.[1]

The Mozart stage work performed in Vienna during this visit was the German singspiel, *Bastien und Bastienne*, commissioned by Doctor Franz Anton Mesmer (1734-1815), a respected and fashionable Viennese physician, recently married and scarcely one year past graduation, who moved in the highest social and aristocratic circles. It was performed in the garden theater of Doctor Mesmer, who held musical open houses at his home in the Landstrasse district.[2] Mesmer's birthplace was Iznang, a village near Lake Constance on the Swiss-German border, in the Holy Roman Empire province of Swabia. His education for the priesthood was supervised by the Bishop of Constance at a monastic school, followed by doctoral degrees in philosophy and theology at the universities of Dillingen and Ingolstadt in Bavaria. Opting for a career in medicine, Mesmer, in 1760, began six years

of studies at the University of Vienna; an exciting time to be a medical student in the Capital.[3-5]

Empress Maria Theresa had assembled some of the best minds in Europe for the Faculty of Medicine, famous in medical annals as the Old Vienna School. These included Baron Gerhard van Swieten, President of the Medical Faculty, a pupil at Leidin of Hermann Boerhaave, the century's foremost physician; Anton de Haen, also a pupil of Boerhaave, who was Europe's best teacher of clinical medicine; and Anton von Stoerck, a young Swabian appointed to the new Chair in Pharmacology. Mesmer's graduation thesis was entitled, "The Influence of the Planets on the Human Body." His interest in the teachings of Paracelsus led him to believe that the stars and planets influenced the health and general condition of human beings by way of a subtle, all-permeating and invisible fluid called the *universal fluid*. This subject was in keeping with the dominant Newtonian physics of the new scientific Age of Reason, and sought to explain the effect of gravitation on human physiology. Although Newton described the laws of gravity, the cause of gravitation remained unknown. Mesmer hypothesized that universal fluid explained not only gravitation, but other intangible properties such as magnetism, electricity, light, and heat. The direct influence of the universal fluid and its indirect influence by way of heavenly bodies made us healthy or ill. This force was the cause of universal gravitation and the basis of all bodily properties, which he called *animal gravitation*. When Mesmer later changed the concept of animal gravitation to *animal magnetism*, he came into conflict with his medical and scientific peers.[6]

In 1768, at the age of 34, Mesmer's brilliant marriage to a socially prominent, vivacious, and good-humored widow ten years his senior brought him a number of material advantages: high social status, inherited wealth, a shared adoration of music and cultural refinement, and a large house on the Landstrasse with sufficient space for a clinic, a dispensary, a research laboratory, rooms for board-and-care inpatients, a music room, and a garden theater. Mesmer's musical parties soon rivalled those of Baron Gottfried van Swieten, son of the President of the Medical Faculty, and arbiter of musical taste throughout the Viennese Classical Period.

Reasons for Mesmer's patronage of the *wunderkind*, Mozart, included social prestige, a shared Swabian ancestry with Leopold Mozart,[7] and German nationalism. At a later time (1777), Mozart spoke of meeting a strong proponent of German national opera in Munich who "heard me play at young Herr von Mesmer's house."[1] As a staunch supporter of German national theater,[1] *Bastien und Bastienne* was the first of five singspiels composed by Mozart, leading to the flowering of German national opera.[8]

A fourth bond between Mesmer and Mozart concerned music therapy and was revealed in a series of letters written by Leopold Mozart to his wife in the summer of 1773 from Vienna, where he accompanied his now 17-year-old son on a two-month visit. Of the twelve 1773 letters dispatched from Vienna, the Mesmer name was mentioned in eight, with varying degrees of discussion of Doctor Mesmer, his family, his home, and his musical and professional activities.[1] The ambience was one of easy familiarity with the homes and inhabitants of the Landstrasse — Mesmer and his wife, his wife's son, Herr von Bosch, posted in the War Department, and Fraulein Franzl, a live-in, board-and-care patient who, after her cure, later married Mesmer's stepson.

Mesmer was an accomplished amateur musician who excelled in an exceedingly unusual musical instrument, the glass armonica, which Leopold Mozart certified in the following manner:[1] "Do you know that Herr von Mesmer plays Miss Davies' armonica unusually well? He is the only person in Vienna who has learnt it and he possesses a much finer glass instrument than Miss Davies does. It cost him about 50 ducats [$112.50] and it is very beautifully made. Wolfgang too has played upon it." The Mozarts were intrigued by the glass armonica, which they first encountered five years earlier in 1768, during the European tour of Marianne Davies, who performed on and introduced to Europe the new instrument improved by Benjamin Franklin. During the tour, she also met Doctor Mesmer.[1,9] Wolfgang

Mozart's last encounter with the glass armonica took place in May 1791, when he composed a work for another Marianne, Marianne Kirchgessner, a blind performer on the armonica who undertook numerous successful concert tours. This composition was an exquisite quintet for armonica, flute, oboe, viola, and cello, *Adagio and Rondo in C minor and major, K617*, which she first performed in Mozart's presence at the National Theater of Vienna on August 19, 1791.[1] Benjamin Franklin's 1761 invention, which he named *glass armonica*, consisted of musical glasses fitted concentrically (the largest on the left) on a horizontal rod activated by a crank attached to a pedal.[10] The performer could produce chords and runs with increased ease. The heyday of the armonica in Europe lasted until about 1830, and its distinctive timbre of vibrant, piercing sweetness caught the imagination of various French and German Romantic writers, including the great Goethe.

Doctor Mesmer had an additional professional interest in the glass armonica, as an ideal means of inducing a dream-like hypnotic state in his patients.[10] In the interval between the 1768 and 1773 Mozart Viennese visits, Mesmer had undertaken studies of the treatment and cure of nervous disorders by animal magnetism with controlled transfers of the universal fluid from inanimate to animate objects. He always began a therapeutic session by sitting at his armonica and playing slow, unearthly music, which served to induce a state of drowsiness and contentment, rendering his patients receptive to his magnetism treatments. He then rhythmically passed his hands over the patient's brow, temples, cheeks, throat, and arms down to the fingers, in gently stroking motions. Meanwhile, he would gently talk to the patients, tell them they were being magnetized through himself, and he would gently issue instructions to them, until he awakened them at the end of each session.[4]

What dream music could Mesmer and Mozart have played? One of Mozart's distinctive early symphonic contributions was replacement of the usual galant andante by his inimitable "dream" andantes.[11] First encountered in his *Old Lambach Symphony*, K45a, in 1766, in the ensuing period up to 1773, "dream" andantes were found in seven symphonies and serenades.[12] It is likely that Mesmer was familiar with them, since several were performed in Vienna. This was serenade-style music with a dreamy, far-off romantic ambience, the spirit of fancy and fairyland, and an instrumental texture of muted violins and reduced winds with the flute replacing the oboe over the pizzicati of the cellos and bass.[13] The progression of Mozart's early dream music, with its flute-like textures and muted sweetness of the upper strings to the peculiar glassy timbre of the armonica, is illustrated by symphonic excerpts from K45a, 43, 100, and 131, and the armonica quintet K617.

Mesmer was in the habit of conducting his therapeutic work in open public view. Leopold Mozart's letters of 1773 avidly followed the day-to-day progress of Fraulein Franzl, who was treated for excruciating pains in her ears and teeth, migraines, vomitings, fainting fits, and screaming attacks. That Wolfgang was somehow involved in her treatment was indicated in one of Leopold's letters:[1] "She is so much better now that she has knitted in bed a red silk purse for Wolfgang which she has given him as a remembrance." The happy denouement of her cure was documented in Wolfgang's first 1781 letter from Vienna:[1] "I hardly recognized her (Frau von Bosch), she has grown so plump and fat. She has three children . . . "

Stories of such remarkable cures by mesmerism brought 17-year-old blind piano virtuoso Maria Theresa von Paradis to seek Mesmer's professional help to restore her sight. Daughter of the imperial court secretary and godchild of Empress Maria Theresa, she was blind since age three and the recipient of a lifetime imperial pension. Musically talented, she studied with Kozeluch, Righini, Salieri, and Abbé Vogler. As a child prodigy she performed in private salons such as Mesmer's, along with Mozart. She was reputed to have committed 100 concertos to memory.[14] All attempts by Viennese and French oculists to restore her vision failed. Mesmer accepted her as a board-and-care patient in his own home, and painstakingly worked with her for six months.[4] As her vision slowly began to improve, her piano playing started to deteriorate. She lost her concentration while watching her fingers. She lost her facility, stumbled over difficult passages striking wrong notes, and her once fabulous memory was now betraying her. Rumors circulated that Mesmer was a seducer of young girls, and that Demoiselle Paradis' pension would be rescinded, prompting the frantic family to withdraw their daughter from Mesmer's care in June 1777. Mesmer's professional colleagues, previously supportive, turned on him, accused him of practicing magic, and in 1778 ordered him to leave Austria. Mesmer settled in Paris, taking with him only his papers and glass armonica.[3, 4] Once more completely blind, Maria Theresa von Paradis returned to her musical studies and became a first-rate piano virtuoso. In August 1783, she embarked upon an extensive three-year concert tour of Europe, at the beginning of which she stopped off at Salzburg to visit Mozart, and commissioned him to write a piano concerto (K456 in B flat) for her use on the tour.[15]

It is of interest that Mesmer and Mozart independently journeyed to Paris in 1778 to seek fame and fortune, unaware of each other's presence in the French capital. As is well known, mesmerism achieved fantastic success in Paris, where the French dubbed his fashionable salon *L'Enfer des Convulsions*,[4] whereas Mozart's venture ended in failure, marked by his mother's death and his contempt for the Parisians. In view of Mozart's immense genius, fully recognized by his contemporaries, it would appear that defects of personality prevented him from reaching the top rungs of material success. Fully cognizant of Mozart's fairy-tale childhood, Empress Maria Theresa,[16] in 1771, advised her son not to degrade his service with "useless people" such as the Mozarts, who went "about the world like beggars." In 1772, the new Archbishop Colloredo brought an unwanted oppressive and tyrannical atmosphere to the Salzburg court, in which Mozart was constantly intimidated and bullied, in part because of his short, unprepossessing stature and appearance. Repeatedly, both father and son, Leopold and Wolfgang Mozart, remarked on his unfavorable, small, undistinguished, and insignificant appearance.[1] In 1778, Baron Grimm wrote to Leopold from Paris:[1] "To make his fortune I wish he had but half of his talent and twice as much shrewdness . . ." In Vienna, salon hostess Caroline Pichler recalled Haydn's and Mozart's lack of education and intellect and their penchant for silly jokes — and, in Mozart's case, an irresponsible way of life. Mozart's coarseness and scatological humor were not beneficial to his cause.[18]

The absence of a satisfactory explanation for the surprising scatology found in Mozart's letters was the impetus for the author's tabulation of his scatology. Scatology was present in 39 of 371 letters by Mozart, an incidence of 10.5%, whereas his father, mother, and sister contributed one such letter each. Mozart's scatology focused primarily on anal vulgarities and defecation, with frequent use of such words as shit, arse and arse hole, muck and fart, words also used in Shapiro et al.'s 1978 series of New York patients with Tourette's syndrome.[19] The involuntary utterance of obscenities or socially unacceptable words is termed coprolalia. Several letters had additional bizarre features, such as word games and scrambling, repetition of words by another (echolalia), and repetitions of his own words (palilalia); there was a total of 23 such 'bizarre' letters, an incidence of 6.2%. The amalgam of coprolalia, echolalia, and palilalia found in a total of 63, or 17%, of Mozart's letters, along with cited biographical evidence of motor tics, oral scatology and obsessive hyperactive behavior, suggests Mozart's plausible affliction with Tourette's syndrome (TS), a syndrome of both vocal and motor tics.[19-24]

Facial and body motor tics were described by Mozart's sister-in-law, Sophie Haibel,[25] the Irish tenor Michael Kelly,[26] and in Stendahl's plagiarized 1814 biography of Mozart.[27] The evidence for Mozart's vocal tics was meager, consisting of three citations: (1) his brother-in-law Joseph Lange's description[18] of Mozart's confused, disconnected speech with "sudden outbursts of vulgar platitudes" while composing; (2) Mozart's own revelation to his father of public after-dinner recitations of scatologic rhymes on several occasions in Mannheim;[1] and (3) Caroline Pichler's anecdote[28] that Mozart "miaowed like a cat" after improvising on the fortepiano.

Although there is abundant evidence of written scatology (coprographia) in Mozart's letters, no other reference to coprographia could be found in the TS literature or in the clinical experience of a distinguished neurologic consultant.[29] A suggested mechanism for Mozart's written scatology is mental coprolalia[19] (the repetitive thought of an obscene word), which Shapiro's group found in 8% of their patients. In this connection, Shapiro et al. refer to the not infrequent occurrence of lavatory coprolalia in TS.

In an alternative opinion, Doctor Peter Davies attributes Mozart's scatology to a hypomanic manifestation of a cyclothymic personality disorder.[7] One of his principal arguments is a presumed relationship between Mozart's creative surges and upward hypomanic swings. Careful tabulation of Mozart's Work List fails to support such a relationship, including specific consideration of five such periods listed by him. It is the author's conclusion that Mozart was a remarkably consistent and productive composer whose output was largely unrelated to his emotional state, but could be further stimulated by external factors such as the demands of concert life and the need to earn money.

Finally, careful study of Mozart's bizarre letters, the *Baslebriefe*, revealed several common thought processes:[30] (1) scatology (coprolalia or "vulgar platitudes"); (2) repetition of word sounds and rhyming; (3) echolalia-palilalia principle; (4) mirror imaging or reversal of words and sentences; (5) expansive free word association; (6) word scrambling; and (7) make-believe names and word tomfoolery. In 1777, Mozart wrote to his father:[1] "Even by signs and gestures I cannot express my thoughts and feelings... But I can do so by means of sounds, for I am a musician." It is the author's belief that the thought processes of the letters have musical counterparts and can be found in Mozart's music.[30] Some examples are the following:

(1) *Scatology* ("vulgar platitudes") — The musical equivalents are sudden chromaticisms and held discordant dissonant notes peppered through his early symphonies and serenades,[31] starting at age nine.[32] These are later transfigured into the fabric of great music in the opening Allegro of K271[33] and the emotionally wrenching dissonances of the great Adagio of K563.[34]

(2) *Repetition of sounds and phrases* — heard in Mozart's canonic writing and famous echo effects.

(3) *Echolalia-palilalia principle* — The rondo is a prime musical example of this principle. Mozart had a lifelong preoccupation with the elaboration of sonata-rondo form.

(4) *Mirror imaging or sentence reversal* — Mozart's most famous musical equivalent is his use of invertible counterpoint in the coda of the contrapuntal finale of his *Jupiter Symphony*, K551.

(5) *Word scrambling* — This is the basis of the infinite variety of Mozart's music within well-defined musical forms, best heard in his sonata-form recapitulations, and in the development and recapitulation episodes of his sonata-rondos.

In conclusion, Mozart exhibited the principal features of TS, which is suggested to have been a major factor in his failure to secure a musical post commensurate with his immense genius. Had he been treated by current drugs (haloperidol, pimozide, clonidine), the effect on his creativity could have been disastrous because of the uniform cognitive impairment induced by these drugs, presenting the modern therapist with a cruel therapeutic dilemma.[19, 23, 24] As for Mozart, he invoked the memory of Mesmer in the Act I finale of his 1790 opera, *Cosi Fan Tutte*: "This is that piece of magnet, Mesmer's stone, that originated in Germany, then was so famous there in France."

REFERENCES

1. Anderson E (ed): The Letters of Mozart and His Family, 3rd ed, 71, 74, 79-83, 87-91, 93, 198, 233-246, 276, 289-291, 350, 363, 367, 373, 597, 698, 713, 890-891, 953. New York: WW Norton & Co, 1985.

2. Abert AA: The operas of Mozart. *In* The New Oxford History of Music, vol 7, 107. London: 1973.

3. Goldsmith M: Franz Anton Mesmer. Encyclopedia Britannica, vol 15, 202, 1968.

4. Wydenbruck N: Doctor Mesmer, An Historical Study, 13-15, 32-43, 44-69, 70-97, 117-126. London: John Westhouse, 1947.

5. Buranelli V: The Wizard from Vienna. New York, Coward, McCann and Geoghegan, 1975.

6. West LJ: Hypnosis in Medical Practice. *In* Lief HI, Lief VF, Lief NR (eds), The Psychological Basis of Medical Practice, 510-513. Hoeber, 1963.

7. Davies PJ: Mozart in Person, His Character and Health, 3. New York: Greenwood Press, 1989.

8. Einstein A: Mozart, His Character, His Work, 470. New York: Oxford University Press, 1962.

9. Baldwin O, Wilson T: Cecilia Davies. *In* Sadie S (ed), The New Grove Dictionary of Music and Musicians, vol 5, 273, 1980.

10. King AH: Musical Glasses. *In* Sadie S (ed), The New Grove Dictionary of Music and Musicians, vol 12, 823-825, 1980.

11. Girdlestone CM: Mozart's Piano Concertos, 39-40. London: Cassell & Co Limited, 1948.

12. Between 1766 and 1773 Mozart's "dream" andantes were found in three symphonies, K45a (1766), K43 (1767) and K45 (1768); the three 1769 orchestral serenades (K63, K99, K100); and the 1772 divertimento for winds and strings (K131).

13. Zaslaw N: Mozart's Symphonies, 143. Oxford: Clarendon Press, 1989.

14. Angermüller R: Maria Theresa von Paradis. *In* Sadie S (ed), The New Grove Dictionary of Music and Musicians, vol 14, 175, 1980.

15. Mozart WA: Concerto in B-flat major for Piano and Orchestra, K456 (1784).

16. Pestelli G: The Age of Mozart and Beethoven, 140. Cambridge University Press, 1984.

17. Sadie S: Wolfgang Amadeus Mozart. *In* The New Grove Dictionary of Music and Musicians, vol 12, 685, 1980.

18. Steptoe A: Mozart's Appearance and Character. *In* Landon HCR (ed), The Mozart Compendium, 104-108. New York: Schirmer Books, 1990.

19. Shapiro AK, Shapiro ES, Bruun RD, Sweet, RD: Gilles de la Tourette Syndrome, 143. New York: Raven Press, 1978.

20. Eldridge R, Sweet R, Lake CR, Ziegler M, Shapiro AK: Gilles de la Tourette's syndrome: Clinical, genetic, psychologic and biochemical aspects in 21 selected families. Neurology 27:115-124, 1977.

21. Erenberg G, Cruse RP, Rothner AD: Tourette syndrome: An analysis of 200 pediatric and adolescent cases. Cleveland Clin Q 53:127-131, 1986.

22. Walton J: Gilles de la Tourette syndrome. *In* Walton J (ed), Brain's Diseases of the Nervous System, ed 9, 350. Oxford Press, 1985.

23. Golden GS: Tourette's Syndrome. *In* Johnson RT (ed), Current Therapy in Neurologic Disease. Toronto, BC: Decker Inc, 1987.

24. Menkes JH: Textbook of Child Neurology, ed 4, 150- 152. Lea & Febiger, 1990.

25. Jahn O: Life of Mozart (Townsend PD, trans), vol 2, 419-420. London: Novello, Ewer & Co, 1891.

26. Kelly M: The Reminiscences of Michael Kelly, vol 1, 255. London: Henry Colburn, 1826.

27. Stendahl HB: Haydn, Mozart and Metastasio (1814). *In* Coe RN (ed, trans, intro), 163. New York: Grossman Publishers, 1972.

28. Landon HCR: Mozart's Last Year, 1791, 38. New York, Schirmer Books, 1988.

29. Benson F: Personal communication. Dr. Benson, Augustus Rose Professor of Neurology at UCLA School of Medicine, graciously reviewed some of the material concerning Mozart's scatology.

30. Simkin B: Common thought processes in Mozart's bizarre letters and his music. *Presented*: Society for the History of Medicine, Cedars-Sinai Medical Center, Feb. 28, 1991; BioMedicine and the Performing Arts Lecture Series, The Royce Two-Seventy, UCLA Center for the Performing Arts, May 16, 1991.

31. Zaslaw N, Cowdery W (eds): The Compleat Mozart, 165. New York: WW Norton, 1990.

32. Early quirky chromaticisms and "vulgar platitudes" are found in the opening allegros of symphony K19 (1765) and orchestral serenades K63 and K100 (1769); the jig rondo-finale of symphony K22 (1765); segments 6, 13 and 14 of Gallimathias Musicum, K32 (1766).

33. Mozart Piano Concerto No. 5 in E flat, K271 (*Jeunehomme*, 1777).

34. Mozart Divertimento in E flat for Violin, Viola and Cello, K563 (1788).

CHAPTER 104

Music and the Limbic System: Implications for Use of Music Therapy in Work with Patients with Dementia

Concetta M. Tomaino

Mr. A. was admitted to the skilled nursing facility after having suffered several strokes. He presented himself as silent, with an almost flat affect. Initial diagnosis included dementia. During the music-therapy group session on his unit, Mr. A. remained on the periphery, showing no initial response to the music presented other than eye contact. With each successive session, Mr. A. became more attentive and rocked his head slightly to the rhythm of the music. The author began to work with him, presenting traditional Yiddish songs and noting any response. At first, he just watched and rocked slowly, then he cried, silently. Next, he made humming sounds and, after several weeks, sang a word from the song — his first word in over two years. Eventually, more words followed during the singing. Then, speech — meaningful speech — occurred without music.

As a music therapist with over 12 years of experience in working with patients with dementia, the author has experienced many such 'breakthroughs' as with Mr. A. They pose the question of underlying mechanisms of preserved functioning in some areas of speech and memory which are otherwise clinically silent if not for the spontaneous responses to music which these patients present. Studies in the music-therapy literature indicate that there is a significant preference for the songs which were popular during the patient's second and third decades of life.[1] Long-term memory for songs exists with recall of lyrics enhanced with melodic cuing.[2]

REVIEW OF NEUROANATOMY

Auditory Pathway

To appreciate the importance of music as a stimulus for reaching patients with dementia, a review of the basic auditory and memory processes is necessary. In examining the ascending and descending pathways of the neural connections of the auditory nerve,[3] one notes immediately the bilateral representation of a sound stimulus. The auditory nerve divides as it enters the brain stem and sends fibers to both the dorsal and ventral cochlear nuclei. It branches further, making connections as shown in Fig. 1.

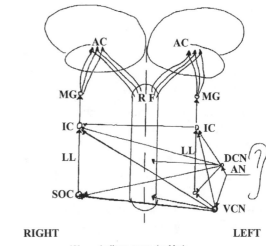

AN	Auditory nerve (cochlea)
VCN	Ventral cochlear nucleus (brain stem)
DCN	Dorsal cochlear nucleus (brain stem)
SOC	Superior olivary complex (midbrain)
IC	Inferior colliculus (midbrain)
LL	Lateral lemniscus (midbrain)
RF	Reticular formation (midbrain)
MG	Medial geniculate (thalamus)
AC	Auditory cortex (cerebral cortex)

Figure 1: Schematic drawing of the ascending auditory pathway.[2]

Descending pathways to the brain stem and spinal cord allow for reflex-type responses to sound, serve to inhibit lower auditory centers, and elevate the threshold of hearing. Ascending pathways serve to alert the cortex to the upcoming signal. Studies in which the classical auditory pathways have been cut show a return of the ability to respond to sounds using this alternate auditory pathway through the reticular formation. Kaufman states that the bilateral representation of sound has important clinical implications.[4] Though lesions of the acoustic nerve or damage to the ear itself may cause deafness in that ear, unilateral lesions of the brain stem or cerebral hemisphere will not cause any hearing impairment. Since central-nervous-system lesions do not impair hearing, patients with CVA, brain tumor, or Alzheimer's disease typically have normal hearing acuity.

Higher cortical areas responsible for cognitive functioning, memory storage, language, and visual processing are usually affected by Alzheimer's. Though a sound can evoke a simple reflex response, e.g. attention, music reflective of an individual's past, (songs of childhood, homeland, key life events) result in emotional reactions. It is the connections of the auditory nerve to key limbic structures that account for such emotionally charged responses to familiar music stimuli.

Limbic System

The limbic system is composed of the following parts:

Hippocampus — involved in the storage of events (long-term memory).

Amygdala — plays a role in feelings of aggression and fear; flight and defense. It is possibly involved in mnemonic information processing.[5] It is argued that the human amygdala is responsible for activating or reactivating those mnemonic events which are of emotional significance for one's life history and that this (re)activation is performed by charging sensory information with important emotional cues.

Hypothalamus — has many connections to other areas of the brain. It is connected to the pituitary gland and is involved in homeostasis.

Pituitary gland — major gland that controls release of hormones into the bloodstream.

Thalamus — major relay between sensory input and cortex. It is involved in arousal and activation of cortical association areas.

Another section of the limbic system is the *entorhinal* area. It has many connections from the frontal, temporal, and cingulate neocortex as well as the olfactory cortex, indicating that it is the final link between sensory systems of the neo- and transitional cortex on the one hand and the hippocampus and dentate gyrus on the other.[6]

Our deepest emotions are rooted in this area. Sensory input, such as a familiar song, sound, or smell, elicit an immediate sense of *déjà vu*. One recalls an event, picture, etc., by just hearing the song. Clynes suggests that music seems to be processed as integral, holistic auditory images.[7] Barbizet stated that *memories persist when they have some personal importance for the subject. A certain perception, a commonplace object, a musical phrase, a landscape, is retained because it has been experienced intensely in some affective context: love, joy, hope, surprise, fear... In due course, these events inevitably become tied to these sentiments and each occasion that they are experienced will be submitted to a fresh recall and evaluation...*[8] Research also suggests that the auditory cortex may not be necessary for hearing and that many auditory discriminations may be medicated at subcortical levels.[9]

Memory

There are three factors that influence storage of short-term memory: (1) emotionally strong information, (2) rehearsal, and (3) lack of interference.

Of long term memory, *recall* memory is said to involve the search and retrieval of information in storage.

Recognition memory is thought not to involve retrieval at all, but matching stored information with events in the environment. This type of memory remains better preserved in the elderly than does recall memory. Damage to the connection between the reticular formation in the brain stem and the limbic system could be the cause of retrograde amnesia as the patient is unable to retrieve information. Lesions in the limbic zones, especially the hippocampus, lead to disturbances of the selective imprinting of traces. Many neurons of the hippocampus serve to compare stimuli with traces of past events.[10]

Squire and Zola-Morgan[11] proposed that there are two distinct memory processes — procedural and declarative (Fig 2). Damage to diencephalic or hippocampal-temporal structures in humans results in marked deficits in the formation of declarative memory, but not procedural memory. They further propose that declarative memory may be a new development in evolution that corresponds with the elaboration of the hippocampus and other higher brain systems. Procedural memory, then, would include more classical conditioning tasks.

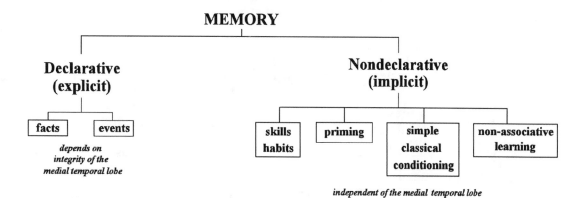

Figure 2: *The two memory processes.*[10]

Crystal et al.[12] found that an 82-year-old musician with Alzheimer's disease showed ability to play previously learned piano compositions from memory while being unable to identify the composer or titles of each work. A preserved ability to learn the new skills of mirror reading, while being unable to recall or recognize new information, was also shown. They concluded that both anterograde and retrograde procedural memory may be relatively spared in this disease.

Sensory systems do provide a convenient and advantageous entry into the complex neural events underlying learning.[13] Although practicing a performance skill such as piano playing is different from listening repeatedly to a favorite song, the retrieval mechanism may be similar in that both utilize processes involving procedural memory. Studies have shown that animals can store long-term information if the hippocampus has been removed, through rehearsing new patterns again and again. The components of the limbic system involved in the integration of affective inputs, whether from the immediate sense (visceral responses to autonomic activity) or from memory areas involved in the storage of the relationships between affect, action, and sensory input, may serve to control the level of repetition of recent information to the cortex by the hippocampus. If the cortex serves as an amplifier and analyzer and the limbic system retains associated states, it would explain why patients with even severe cortical damage can respond to certain stimuli — in particular, music.

It has been proposed that associative areas have fewer prior commitments than primary areas.[13] At all ages, their plasticity is much greater and their participation in the retention and recall of memory is probably determined, to a large extent, by the history of the organism.

Such procedural memory may be retained because of two neuroanatomically distinct loops — the hippocampo-reticular and the mammillo-reticular (Table).[12] These two loops have different limbic components — mammillary bodies versus hippocampi — but a shared midbrain component. Both limbic structures are connected with the same group of reticular nuclei. The mammillary system is more critical in learning situations that involve direct and effective reward, and the hippocampal system to more indifferent information such as word-learning. According to this model (Fig. 3), the fornix is an auxiliary component which serves to connect the two systems, and lesions to the fornix would be expected to have the least impact on memory.

Table: *Hierarchic Pairwise Comparison of the Components of Two Memory Circuits*

Level	Mammillary System	Hippocampal System
Mesencephalic	Ventral tegmental nucleus area	Ventral tegmental nucleus area
Posterior Limbic	Mammillary bodies	Hippocampi
Anterior Limbic	Hypothalamus	Amygdala
Thalamic	Anterior thalamic nucleus	Dorsomedial thalamic nucleus
Cortial	Cingular cortex	Neocortex

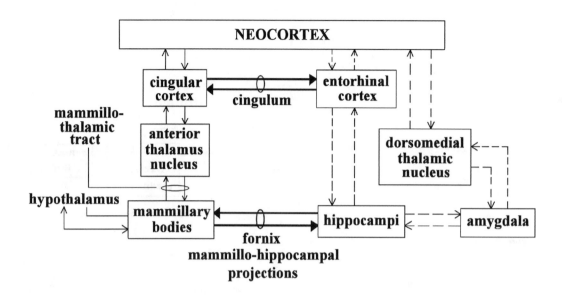

Figure 3: *Two circuits of reverberation related to memory: the mammillary system (thin solid line) and the hippocampal system (broken line). Interface between the two systems is indicated by thick solid line.*

Much has been written about cognitive deficits following hippocampal lesions, but the literature is not as extensive on damage to the mammillary bodies. In studies of subjects with profound retrograde amnesia, early-life memories tend to be less affected. These memories also tend to be affectively more significant than more recent memories.

As cortical dysfunction increases and the older person loses capacity for storing or making sense of new information, the old memories become more salient, since they are the most familiar.

Recent studies indicate that normal brain function depends on a continuing arousal reaction generated in the reticular formation, which, in turn, depends on constant sensory bombardment. Sensory stimuli have the general function of maintaining this arousal and they can rapidly lose their powers to do so if restricted to a monotonously repeated stimulation of an un-changing environment. Since a person with dementia already has a compromised cognitive system, an environment which is unfamiliar or non-stimulating can only add further to the decline.

IMPLICATIONS FOR MUSIC THERAPY

Studies have shown the many inter-connections of the auditory system with various brain systems, especially its connections to subcortical regions, i.e. the limbic system.

Music involves much more than one element of sound. Even with some neurological deficit, there is the probability that some aspect of the music will be received. Because of the redundancy effect that occurs in songs, there is an inherent *rehearsal effect* which may assist in musical material being stored much more easily in long-term memory.

Since recognition memory is preserved in persons with Alzheimer's disease and other dementias, there are many implications for use of music to *reach* these patients.

The more powerful the associations one has to the song presented, the more likely it is that a response will occur. One patient, diagnosed with leuko-encephalopathy, had limited verbal responses, walked and avoided obstacles, but could not dis-tinguish between a cup and what was in it (everything ended up in her mouth). During a music-therapy session, she walked up and spontaneously sang the songs played by the author, complete with lyrics. She was able to sing with feeling and yet could not speak or recognize familiar family members.

Familiar songs associated with key life events will evoke attention, emotional response, and recognition/sense of the familiar. By reviewing a patient's history, including song/music preferences, the therapist will have the resources needed to make initial contact with the patient. During the initial sessions, it is essential to use a variety of songs and rhythms, including songs which may have some personal associations for this individual, in order to evoke attention and response. The therapist must then make careful observations and change music accordingly to stimulate as well as support any reactions by the patient.

The repetition of such familiar songs during the music-therapy session and subsequent sessions will promote increased recognition, enhance memory recall, and increase eye contact, as well as attention and self-awareness. It reduces restlessness in some early-Alzheimer's patients by providing a sense of the familiar.

Rhythm serves to stimulate attention and promote spontaneous movement which would otherwise not occur, thus enhancing muscle flexibility, joint range of motion, and prevention of contractures. Often, the patient's automatic responses will be synchronous with the rhythm of the music.

Various instruments can be used by patients to further engage them in the music, to help focus their attention, and to reinforce their sense of their own activity.

CONCLUSION

Since music/sound stimulates the subcortical areas best preserved in persons with dementia, it serves as an important connecting device to stimulate higher cortical areas. With consistent use of appropriate music, the patient's attention, word finding, self-awareness and orientation to the immediate environment are improved.

REFERENCES

1. Gibbons AC: (1977). Popular music preferences of elderly people. Journal of Music Therapy 14(4):180-189, 1977.
2. Bartlett JC, Snelus P: Lifespan memory for popular songs. American Journal of Psychology 93(1):551-560, 1980.
3. Hodges DA (ed): Handbook of Music Psychology. Kentucky: National Association for Music Therapy, 1980.
4. Kaufman DM: Clinical Neurology for Psychiatrists. New York: Grune & Stratton, 1981.
5. Sarter M, Markowitsch HJ: The amygdala's role in human memory processing. Cortex 21(1):7-24, 1985.
6. Gregory RL (ed): The Oxford Companion to The Mind. London: Oxford University Press, 1987.
7. Clynes M (ed): Music, Mind and Brain. New York: Plenum Press, 1983.
8. Barbizet J: Human Memory and Its Pathology. San Francisco: WH Freeman & Company, 1970.
9. Martin FN: Introduction to Audiology. Englewood Cliffs, NJ: Prentice-Hall, 1975.
10. Luria AR: The Working Brain. New York: Basic Books, 1973.
11. Squire LR, Zola-Morgan S: The medial temporal lobe memory system. Science 253:1380-1382, 1991.
12. Crystal H, Grober E, Masur D: Preservation of musical memory in Alzheimer's disease. Journal of Neurology and Psychiatry 52:1415-1416, 1989.
13. Squire LR, Butters N (eds): Neuropsychology of Memory. New York: Guilford Press, 1984.

SUGGESTED READING

1. Aronson MK: Understanding Alzheimer's Disease. New York: Charles Scribner & Sons, 1989.
2. Ball MJ, et al: A new definition of Alzheimer's disease: A hippocampal dementia. Lancet 8419:14-16, 1985.
3. Bear DM: Temporal lobe epilepsy: A syndrome of sensory limbic hyperconnection. Cortex 15:357-384, 1979.
4. Botwinick J: Aging and Behavior. New York: Springer Publishing, 1978.
5. Bright R: Music Therapy and the Dementias. St. Louis, MO: MMB Music, 1988.
6. Brun A, Gustafson L: Distribution of cerebral degeneration in Alzheimer's disease. Archiv fur Psychiatrie und Nervenkrankheiten 223(1):15-33, 1976.
7. Campbell DG: Introduction to the Musical Brain. St. Louis, MO: MMB Music, 1986.
8. Casino GD, Adamo RD: Brainstem auditory hallucinosis. Neurology 36(8):1042, 1986.
9. Clynes M: On music and healing. Somatics: 20-27, 1987-88.
10. Critchley M, Henson RA: Music and the Brain. London: William Heinemara Medical Books Limited, 1977.
11. Diamond MC, Scheibel AB, Elson LM: The Human Brain Coloring Book. New York: Barnes & Noble Books, 1985.
12. Garelik G: Exorcising a damnable disease. Discover, 74-84, Dec 1986.

13 Harvard Medical School Health Letter. Alzheimer's Disease, 13(6), 1988.

14. Jarvik LF, Winograd CH (eds) Treatments for the Alzheimer's Patient. New York: Springer Publishing, 1988.

15. Kandel ER, Schwartz JH (eds): Principles of Neural Science. New York: Elsevier Science Publishing, 1983.

16. Loftus E: Memory. Reading, PA: Addison-Wesley Publishing, 1980.

17 MacLean, PD: Atriune Concept on the Brain and Behavior. Toronto: University of Toronto Press, 1973.

18. Maces AR: Learning and memory disorders and their assessment. Neuropsychologia 24(1):25-39, 1986.

19. Mazziotta JC: Tomography and auditory stimulation. Neurology 32:921-937, 1982.

20. Mazziotta JC: Tomography mapping of human cerebral metabolism: Sub-cortical responses to auditory and visual stimulation. Neurology. 34(6): 825, 1984.

21. McDuff T, Sumi SM: Subcortical Degeneration in Alzheimer's Disease. Neurology 35(1):123, 1985.

22. Pribram K: Holographic memory. Psychology Today, 71-76, Feb 1979.

23. Restak RM: The Brain The Last Frontier. New York: Warner Books, 1979.

24. Sacks O: Neuropsychiatry and Tourette's. *In* Mueller (ed), Neurology and Psychiatry: A meeting of the Minds, 156-174. Basal: Karger, 1989.

25. Sacks O, Tomaino CM: Music and neurological disorder. International Journal of Arts Medicine 1(1):10-12, 1991.

26. Scientific American, The Brain. San Francisco: WH Freeman & Co, 1979.

27. Terry RD, Gershon S (eds): Neurobiology of Aging. New York: Raven Press, 1976.

28. Terry RD, Katzman R: Senile dementia of the Alzheimer's type. Annals of Neurology 14(5):497-506, 1983.

29. Wenk G, et al: Neurotransmitters and memory. Behavioral Science 101(3):325-332, 1987.

CHAPTER 105

Multicultural Music Therapy: A World Music Perspective

Edith Hillman Boxill

"Music must serve a purpose; it must be a part of something larger than itself, a part of humanity . . ."

Pablo Casals

The vision and orientation of Music Therapists for Peace, Inc. is presented, with a focus on multicultural music therapy as the conscious use of music within the context of world peace. Emphasis is on the possibilities of assimilating the basics of a variety of world musics, thus pointing in the direction of the cross-cultural role of music therapists--in effect, music therapists as ambassadors of world peace through musical and interpersonal communication.

ABOUT THE ORGANIZATION

Music Therapists for Peace, Inc. is a worldwide network of music therapists dedicated to meeting the challenge of the most critical and urgent issue of the modern age world peace. Through innovative approaches to the use of music therapy methods within the context of peace, it is committed to making a vital contribution to the betterment and healing of Planet Earth on multicultural and multisocietal levels. Thus, in expanding the scope of the field of music therapy and extending the services of the field by reconceptualizing the role of the music therapist, it brings a world perspective to the profession that has not heretofore been explored or put into action.

The role that Music Therapists for Peace has assumed is that of establishing music therapists around the world as ambassadors of peace who are carrying the message through crosscultural/ multicultural musical and healing traditions. By expanding the scope of the field to the grand context of world peace, it is reaching beyond the treatment room out to humanity at large. Commonalities and differences in musical expression are acknowledged, cultural and societal barriers are broken down, creating bonds in ways that are felt through direct experience rather than understood intellectually.

Music Therapists for Peace is on the cutting edge of the action needed for an intensive and expansive developmental — evolutionary — shift in our field.

Carrying out the vision of this worldwide network, a critical mass of like-minded music therapists is in the process of doing the work of peacemaking through music making on many levels around the world. These music therapists are serving as guiding lights for an international exchange of innovative approaches, imaginative ideas, and creative methods for multicultural music therapy, holding a world music perspective that bespeaks a new wave of the future.

ABOUT THE FIELD

Broadly defined, the modern treatment modality of music therapy is the skilled, conscious use of music to bring about mind-body healing and positive attitudinal change. In humanistic terms, techniques and methods unique to this discipline are designed to improve the quality of intrapersonal and interpersonal relationships, to increase communication abilities on individual and collective bases, to enhance well-being holistically, to empower becoming "fully human."

It is interesting to note that the profession of music therapy evolved in the United States from a need to address the multifaceted problems -- psychological, physical, mental, and psychosocial -- that beset World War ll veterans who were pouring into hospitals at the end of the war. With the realization that more than offering musical performances and sing-alongs was necessary to deal with the conditions presented -- that service (therapia) through music on deeper levels was required, a group of musicians, music educators, and psychiatrists convened at the Menninger Clinic in Topeka, Kansas. This meeting resulted in the establishment of the first academic training program in music therapy at Michigan State University in 1944.

By 1950, the National Association for Music Therapy (NAMT) was formed, and in 1970 the American Association for Music Therapy (AAMT) came into being. Both national associations grant registration (RMT) or certification (CMT) in fulfillment of their respective requirements to graduates of an approved college/university music therapy training program or of an alternative route as specified by AAMT. Since 1983, The Certification Board for Music Therapists, Inc. has been granting Board Certification (BC) to candidates who fulfill its requirements. And, in 1989, AAMT instituted Advanced Certification (ACMT).

Currently, in addition to the United States, there are training programs and various certification designations in Canada, Europe (including the United Kingdom, France, Germany, Norway, Italy, Spain, and the Netherlands), Japan, Australia, Israel, and South America (Argentina and Brazil) as well as music therapy associations internationally (including Africa, India, Japan, South Korea, the Philippines). Qualified music therapists are practicing in countries throughout the world.

MULTICULTURAL MUSIC THERAPY

As we move toward the 21st century, our world is fast becoming the global village perceived by the cultural historian Marshall McLuhan. Planetary phenomena are in the foreground of people's minds as never before in the annals of mankind. We explore the mysteries of the universe. We share concerns about the survival of mother Earth. We fly to remote lands rapidly encircling the globe. We contact people instantaneously in the farthest reaches of the planet.

Indeed, we live in a global village--a multicultural world that calls out for more peaceful relations, more harmonious coexistence, more commonalities awareness, more appreciation of differences, more consciousness of the essences of humanness.

Such an essence is music, one of humanity's most ancient and most natural means of expression, communication, and healing. Its universality makes it a quintessential part of life itself: As quantum physicists so poetically and metaphorically put it: "We are not matter, we are music!"

In comparatively recent years, this universal form of expression has emerged as the therapeutic agent of the modern treatment modality, music therapy. As a profession, it can be said to be a continuation of a thirty-thousand-year-old tradition of music and healing, as practiced in biblical times and so-called primitive cultures.

In point of fact, rituals in various world cultures provide contemporary evidence of the continuity of music and healing traditions that have come down through the ages. Without being designated as music therapy per se, music as therapy is currently flourishing in countless tribal and other non technological societies in Asia, Australia, Europe, and North and South America. Documenting this in ethnomusicological literature, a survey of world music traditions reports on nineteen cultures. Among those represented are Indonesian, Australian aboriginal, African tribal, North American Indian, South American Indian, and Alaskan Eskimo (May, 1983).

Music therapy, like music itself, is a multicultural phenomenon (Moreno, 1988). In this article, the author points out that the issue of cross-cultural music communication is becoming increasingly important, to the degree that it is essential for music therapists to assimilate and incorporate non-Western as well as Western musical and cultural traditions. The primordial power of indigenous musics affects the human being on many organismic levels--emotional, auditory, visual, kinesthetic--serving to link peoples of diverse origins in ways that bridge differences and affirm similarities.

In speaking of indigenous musics, let us take a kaleidoscopic look at the simple yet complex attributes and human interconnectedness of the folk song. Through this genre of music, direct lines of communication can open up, much can be learned and transmitted: qualities of life-style, attitudes, feelings, customs, unique traditions, stories and tales that paint dynamic pictures. The galvanizing effect of such material has a highly significant yield for the music therapist. Among especially rich sources for a great variety of these kinds of songs are *Echoes of Africa in folk songs of the Americas* (Landeck, 1961), *Children's songs for a friendly planet* (Weiss, 1986), *A treasury of folk songs* (Kolb, 1951), *Folk songs of North America* (Lomax, 1960), *Worlds of music: An introduction to the music of the world's peoples* (Titon, 1984), and *A discography of folk, traditional, and ethnic music* (Boxill, 1985). Obviously, an organic tie with the folk idiom is the wealth of indigenous musical instruments as found in Musical instruments of the world (The Diagram Group, 1978).

A NEW PARADIGM FOR MUSIC THERAPY

By encompassing knowledge and experience of world music, the music therapist's heightened awareness strengthens the deeply-rooted, natural bonds that already exist in human life. The English scientist J.E. Lovelock (1989) holds the assumption that our symbiotic relationship with Gaia (Mother Earth) is such that we do not live on this earth but that we are an integral part of its life. As an analogue, our relationship with music is such that it is not only an expression of human beings, it is an integral part of our beingness.

When music therapy is the conscious use of music within the context of world peace, the boundaries between human beings that have existed begin to disappear, horizons are broadened and enriched, possibilities for interrelating and coexisting harmoniously are enlarged and enhanced. This context for music therapy is evolutionary--truly a context whose time has come!

Fundamental to our work is the establishing of human contact. One technique, *reflection*, is a music therapy strategy that is a first means of making contact with a person or persons of a different culture and language by reflecting/mirroring sounds, gestures, rhythmic patterns, melodic phrases.

Another strategy that is basic to this perspective is The *contact song*, a song that has personal or social meaning that can be shared, thus creating a bond through awareness of common interests, concerns, feelings, experience (Boxill, 1985, 1986).

Of great importance in building relationships and interpersonal connectedness is the phenomenon of rhythmic entrainment or *synchrony*[1]. Taking a cue from tribal healing rituals in which people who are drumming or singing or moving "slot" into common rhythmic patterns, toning, or movements (Blacking, 1983), the music therapist brings people into alignment and resonance with each other through this phenomenological occurrence.

Musical improvisation, vocally and instrumentally, on rhythm, and melodic percussion instruments, offers opportunities for self-expression without requiring musical training or skills. The use of the pentatonic scale--particularly on Orff xylophones and gamelan chimes--makes this kind of music production tonally synchronous. It is impossible to strike a wrong note!

REFERENCES

Bentov, L. (1980). Sound waves and vibration. *In* L. Bentov (Ed.), Stalkina the wild Pendulum: On the mechanics of consciousness. New York: Bantam Books.

Blacking, J. (1983). Trends in the black music of South Africa. *In* E. May (Ed.), Musics in many cultures: An introduction. Berkeley, CA: University of California Press.

Boxill, E.H. (1985). Music therapy for the developmentally disabled. Austin, TX.: Pro-Ed, Inc.

Boxill, E.H. (1986). Music therapy for living. St. Louis, MO: MMB Music, Inc.

Hart, M. (1991). Planet drum: A celebration of percussion and rhythm. New York: Harper Collins Publisher.

Kolb, S. & J. (Eds.) (1951). A treasury of folk songs. New York: Bantam Books.

Landeck, B. (compiler) (1961). Echoes of Africa in folk songs of the Americas. New York: David McKay Company.

Lindsay, J. (1979). Javenese gamelan. London: Oxford University Press.

Lomax, A. (1960). Folk songs of North America. New York: Doubleday.

Lovelock, J.E. (1989). Gaia: A new look at life on Earth. Oxford, England: Oxford University Press.

May, E. (Ed/) (1983). Musics of many cultures: An introduction. Berkeley: University of CA Press.

Moreno, J . (1988) . The music therapist: Creative as therapist and contemporary shaman. The Arts in Psychotherapy, Vol. 15, 271-280.

Moreno, J. (1 988). Multi-cultural music therapy: The world music connection. Journal of Music Therapy, XXC(1), 1 7-27.

Musical instruments of the world (1976). An illustrated encyclopedia by The Diaaram Group. New York: Bantam Books.

Olsen, D. (1983). Symbol and function in South American Indian music. *In* E. May (Ed.), Musics of manv cultures: An introduction. Berkeley, CA: University of California Press.

Titon, J. (Ed.) (1984). Worlds of music: An introduction to the music of the world's peoples. New York: Schirmer Books.

---

[1]Acoustically, sympathetic resonance occurs when a string of one violin is bowed and the same string on another violin is observed to humming--to be "locked into" the same vibrational energy, pulsing at the same frequency/wave pattern. Also, there is the example of fireflies, at first blinking on and off at random, who are seen to develop an order--the blinking is soon in unison. The phenomenon is called rythmic entrainment (Bentov, 1981). The law of entrainment, discovered by the Dutch scientist Christian Huygens in 1665, "holds that if two rhythms are nearly the same and their sources are in close proximity, they will always lock up, fall into synchrony, entrain. Why?...nature is efficient and it takes less energy to pulse together than in opposition. Because we are part of nature, it is likely that we are entrained with the larger planetary and universal rhythms that surround us" (Hart, 1991).

CHAPTER 106

Supportive Effects of Music on the Therapeutic Process: Energetic Release Techniques with Improvised Music

Ann C. Bowman • *John Snyder*

Developmental Phases of the Collaboration Between Energetic Therapy and Improvised Music

Phase I — Artists in Individual Therapy: In individual therapy with clients who are artists, it became clear that their artistic process was an asset to their therapy. Their art forms provided them with:

☐ a focus for discovery and exploration of their recurring patterns, which originated in childhood;

☐ a creative expressive force in their sessions, which freed them emotionally;

☐ a way to rewarding relationships, which was cleared in working to remove blocks to creative expression; and

☐ motivation for full participation in their creative fields, which contributed to fulfillment in their professional and personal lives. This was true for painters, sculptors, dancers, actors, singers, and musicians.

Phase II — Group Therapy/Art as an Extension of Therapy: Incorporating the arts in residential groups, 4-7 days in duration.

☐ Improvised theater and dance as workshops and warm-ups.

☐ Art, painting, and sculpture as workshops and lectures.

Phase III — Group Therapy/Music and Therapy: These groups joined energetic exercises and improvised music on specific instruments. This simultaneous collaboration added an interaction between the art form and the energetic exercises. The music and therapy are responsive to each other and, through mutual flow, they lead and follow the needs of the group.

Purpose of this Collaboration

☐ Emotional support and energetic guidance to facilitate:

■ the emergence of new material from the subconscious;

■ circumvention of their usual control, which allows freedom from inhibitions;

■ expression of their repressed feelings; and

■ acceptance and integration of their therapeutic experiences.

☐ To introduce experientially the concept of the creative process to:

■ introduce the creative approach into their professional and personal lives; and

■ build trust in their unique vision.

Substantiating Information

According to Dr. John Diamond[1]:

☐ All sounds have a definite and demonstrable effect on our life energy.

☐ There are two separate systems of hearing — the ear and the acupuncture system of the body. These effects are apparent only with low frequencies up to approximately 1,000 Hz and above 50 KHz.

☐ Each acupuncture meridian responds to specific frequencies:

■ Each meridian responds to a particular consonant.

■ Vowels relate to the thymus, a calibrator of the acupuncture meridian system.

■ Each meridian relates to a specific emotional state.

☐ Music is primarily a property of the right cerebral hemisphere.

It has been shown that vibrations create form and that complex combinations of vibrations create complex forms analogous to animal tissue.[2] Dancing, chants, drumming, and rattling have been used for thousand of years in shamanic healing practices among cultures throughout the world.[3]

Methods

This coaction requires a musician who is a skilled improviser, sensitive and alert to energetic movements and feelings. These are general outlines, subject to exceptions and extensions as in any creative process.

☐ As an opening exercise, the music is used as a soothing tool to create a contemplative mood; this is combined with guided imagery to:

▪ release surface tension to aid the discharge of mental 'chatter,' relaxation of their muscles, and deepening of the client's breathing; and

▪ bring internal focus to make a conscious assessment of the material they will focus on in their session, choice of their goals for the session, and commitment to these goals.

☐ As a closing exercise, the music and guided imagery utilize the energetic and bodily awareness which have been achieved through the workshop. The music is used to bring an internal focus, and the didjeridu is played close to the energy centers. This maximizes the effectiveness of the vibrational qualities of the music. The guided imagery becomes more specific in relation to the energetic movement through their bodies. This verbal and musical combination is used to:

▪ aid acceptance and integration of their experiences;

▪ help clarify their goals; and

▪ confirm their commitment to continue the pursuit of their goals daily.

Energetic Exercises and Improvised Music

The general progression for the use of the exercises would be:

☐ stretching exercises, using specific forms to generate and release energy.

☐ exercises to release anger and other aggressive feelings from regressed and present material.

☐ exercises for releasing feelings of longing and sadness, past and present.

☐ affirmation exercises which honor their sexuality.

☐ grounding exercises for claiming their empowerment.

Musical Instruments — Descriptions and Choices for Specific Uses

Factors Determining Choice of Instruments

☐ Available and familiar.

☐ Sounds which express/mirror a wide range of human experience.

☐ Portability to move around and among the participants, in order to play close to them.

☐ Sounds which affect deeply and evoke strong responses.

The choice of an instrument to use at a given moment and what to play are intuitive. They must be empathetic with the participant's work at the moment and in keeping with the desire to support that work with sounds which may complement, reinforce, contrast, soothe, or aggravate. Three instruments which are most versatile for this work are:

☐ the *frame drum* — a round wooden frame 2-3 inches thick and 1-2 feet in diameter, covered with an animal skin. A large diameter is preferable, allowing for rather deep sounds from the middle, as well as high sounds from the outer edges. Drums and synthesizers elicit and aid the release of aggressive expression. These instruments often reveal intense fears.

☐ the *didjeridu* (this name being most likely of European origin) — the aboriginal wind instrument traditionally from Arnhem Land in Northern Australia. This instrument comes from the oldest continuous culture in the world, having roots which go back at least 40,000 years. It is made from a branch or trunk of one of a variety of species of the eucalyptus tree. Termites nest in a naturally hollow space and enlarge the cavity. The aborigines cut the branch or trunk and clean out the debris left by the termites, sometimes slightly enlarging the bore by scraping. The piece is then stripped and painted, often with bark-painting techniques depicting animal totems, symbols of clan history, and geographical or botanical representations. The smaller end (mouthpiece) is often coated with beeswax or vegetable gum for more comfort and a better seal. Thus is fashioned a very simple wooden horn which is typically 3½-5 feet long. It accompanies singing and/or dancing in large celebrations or small clan gatherings. The larger instruments are sometimes used for special ceremonies. The didjeridu produces a powerful, penetrating sound which encourages the client to: (1) become centered; (2) enter his/her subconscious to discover new material; (3) increase cognitive ability to make choices beyond one's usual patterns; (4) experience support to release sadness; (5) receive a comforting effect during regressed states; and (6) sense an unrestricted flow of energy.

☐ the *waterphone* — a contemporary instrument made of steel and brass. Two stainless-steel mixing bowls are welded face to face with a hole in the top center, from which protrudes a foot-long metal tube. Around the lips of the bowls are welded brazing brass rods of varying lengths. Water is poured inside the bowl. The rods are struck or bowed, creating very unusual sounds of water and space, dreams and the imagination, terror and suspense. The waterphone has a wide range of sound effects and can be useful in either enlivening or giving soothing support.

Results

Support is the most important element contributed by the music. This support allows clients to:

☐ experience healthy equality in a nurturing interaction;

☐ expand their concept of mutual assistance and cooperation, which (1) dispels their beliefs that they are alone and alienated, (2) develops trust in the resources available to them, and (3) assists in giving themselves permission to experience beyond their previous boundaries; and

☐ promote trust and understanding of their energetic movements, to:

■ reveal and clarify their intuitive processes;

■ integrate their cognitive processes with their intuition; and

■ know their physical bodies in a way which provides them with (1) an integration of their mental and emotional processes with their physical bodies, (2) knowledge of how to use physical ailments as a vehicle for emotional growth, and (3) direction and methods for relieving ailments expressed through their bodies.

REFERENCES

1. Diamond J: The Life Energy in Music, Vol 1, 119-121. Archaeus Press 1981.
2. Jenny H: Cymatics. Basilius Press, 1972
3. Harner M: The Way of the Shaman, 65-69. Harper & Row, 1980.

SUGGESTED READING

1. Bealiea J: Music and Sound in the Healing Arts. Station Hill Press 1987
2. Diamond J: The Life Energy In Music, Vols II and III. Archaeas Press, 1981 and 1986.
3. Eliade M: Shamanism. Princeton University Press, Bollingen Series, 1964.
4. Garfield LM: Sound Medicine. Celestial Arts, 1987.
5 McClellan R: The Healing Forces of Music. Amity House, 1988.
6. Rouget G: Music and Trance. University of Chicago Press, 1985.

CHAPTER 107

Therapeutic Uses of Vocal Harmonics

Jonathan Goldman

INTRODUCTION

Since ancient times, the voice has been used as a healing instrument. In various spiritual and shamanic traditions, the ability to create distinct, audible harmonics has been utilized for transformational experiences. This paper focuses upon the creation of vocal harmonics — the sounding of two or more notes simultaneously.

THE SCIENCE OF HARMONICS

Harmonics, or overtones, are sounds within sounds that are created by the vibrations of any one note. While pure tones do exist and can be created through synthesizers, they do not exist in nature. The natural sounds that are created through acoustic instruments, nature sounds, or our voices are full of overtones. These overtones, in fact, are responsible for giving different instruments and our voices their *timbre*, or tone color. Specific overtones are more distinct and present in different instruments, which result in the sounds of these instruments.

The most prominent overtones which contribute to the recognition of the tone character and establishment of the tone color are called *formants*. They are the area of the sound spectrum where the sound energy is most largely concentrated.

Harmonics exists as simple mathematical ratios of any given fundamental. The first overtone which is created from a fundamental frequency will be vibrating twice as fast as the fundamental, at a ratio of two to one. If the fundamental is vibrating at 100 cycles per second, the first overtone created vibrates at 200 cycles per second. The next overtone vibrates three times as fast as the fundamental and, in our example, would be vibrating at 300 cycles per second. The next overtone vibrates four times as fast as the fundamental, at 400 cycles per second, and so on. Theoretically, these harmonics can continue to infinity, with each overtone following the same mathematical formula. Of course, since most of us cannot perceive vibrations above 15,000 Hz, even if these overtones were created, it would be impossible to hear them.

Scientists have found that the whole-number ratios of musical harmonics correspond to an underlying framework existing in physics, chemistry, architecture, crystallography, astronomy, spectro-analysis, botany, and the study of other natural sciences.[1] The relationship of the elements in the periodic table of elements, from which all matter is formed, resembles the overtone structure in music, as do the orbital distances between the planets.

Through the experiments of Jenny, a Swiss medical doctor who spent ten years examining the effects sound had upon shape and formation, there exists visual proof that sound has the ability of creating form.[2] Jenny photographed liquids, plastics, pastes, powders, and other substances as they were being vibrated by sound; they took on extraordinarily geometric and lifelike forms, looking like starfish, human cells and organs, underwater- and microscopic life. The shapes of these structures were reportedly due to the harmonically related frequencies utilized.

VOCAL HARMONICS

While vocal harmonics exist whenever we talk or sing, we have the ability to produce and amplify specific harmonics in our tonal spectrum. This ability to create vocal harmonics may be an extremely ancient technique. Until recently, however, these techniques and their uses as tools for transformation have been shrouded in many of the sacred and magical esoteric traditions of the world, including the *One Voice Chord* of Tibetan Buddhism and the *Hoomi* of Mongolian shamanism. Vocal harmonics have been used in these traditions as a tool to help induce altered states of consciousness and to communicate with various deities and spirits. They may also have been utilized as a tool for creating resonance of the body.

This ability to create specific vocal harmonics is due to the formants contained within the different vowel sounds. Each vowel sound stresses particular overtones. Through sounding the different vowels, one can to learn to create vocal harmonics and sing two notes at once.

THERAPEUTIC USES

Through learning to hear and then create vocal harmonics, we are altering and enlarging the sound spectrum of our hearing and our voices. According to Tomatis, our voices contain only those harmonics which the ear can hear.[3] Thus, by opening our listening to the world of harmonics, it is possible to actually alter the tonal spectrum of our voices. We may also be creating other physiological affects.

Through affecting the cranial nerves via the ear, it is believed that certain sounds stimulate and charge the cortex of the brain and give energy to the body.[3] In particular, these are sounds which are rich in overtones and quite high in the frequency spectrum.

Many people report feelings of extreme relaxation and calming while creating vocal harmonics. Others also report being quite energized after these sonic experiences. Initial investigation into the effects of toning, chanting, and other self-created sounds seems to indicate that these sounds affect and lower heartbeat, respiration, and brain waves. Resonance of the cranial bones has also been observed. Through sounding vocal harmonics, it is possible that we have rediscovered a technique which has many applications in therapeutic fields.

REFERENCES

1. Kayser H: Akroasis: The Theory of World Harmonics. Boston, MA: Plowshare, 1970.

2. Jenny H: Cymatics, Vols I and II. Switzerland: Basilus, 1974.

3. Gilmour TM, Madaule P, Thompson B: About the Tomatis Method. Phoenix, AZ: Listening Center, 1988.

SUGGESTED READING

1. Berendt JE: Nada Brahman: The World is Sound. Rochester, VT: Destiny, 1987.

2. Goldman J: Healing Sounds: The Power of Harmonics. Rockport, MA: Element Books, 1992.

3. Levarie S, Levy E: Tone. Kent State, OH, 1968.

CHAPTER 108

Using a Mercury Switch to Improve Posture During Music Practice and Leisure

Jean C. Abell • Mary R. Burch • Jon S. Bailey

The behavioral deficits of severely mentally and/or physically challenged individuals may be so great as to require thousands of repetitions of a simple training contingency to produce even the smallest change in adaptive behavior. Lesser handicapping conditions are dealt with through relatively well-known interventions such as one-on-one training sessions or small group instruction with repeated prompts and opportunities to engage in appropriate task-related behaviors.

Expecting staff to carry out programs requiring thousands of applications of a simple contingency with a person with severe handicaps can cause rapid burn-out, reduction in the effectiveness of training, and subsequent ineffectiveness of the program itself. What appears to be needed in such cases is an automated system to determine when a behavior has occurred, and an automatic means for a reinforcer to be delivered. Electronic switches/devices that can be adapted to a wide variety of physical responses appear to provide an additional therapeutic tool to be used in addition to personalized one-on-one training and activities. These devices can be used to define very particular physical responses and deliver reinforcers in a consistent manner with no errors or variability.

Thus far, electronic devices have been used with persons who are mentally challenged in the self-delivery of reinforcers,[1] to establish controlled motor movements using contingent stimulation,[2,3] and as classroom tools designed to teach specific functional skills.[4]

Electronic devices can also be used to improve physical problems. Several studies have investigated the effects of automated equipment in improving the posture of persons with physical and/or mental handicaps.[5-8]

The purpose of this study was to determine the effects of using a mercury switch to deliver contingent music and television in the music-practice and leisure activity settings of the participant.

METHOD

Setting and Participant

This study was conducted at a 64-bed Intermediate Care Facility for the Mentally Retarded. The participant in this study was a 31-year-old man who was blind and non-ambulatory as a result of a bicycle accident at the age of 6 years. He functioned in the moderate range of mental retardation intellectually and in the severe range of adaptive behavior due to physical impairments.

Prior to implementation of the study, the participant generally sat in a "slumped over" position as shown in Fig. 1, which resulted in the following problems: (1) The physical therapist reported that this posture was causing further permanent damage to the participant's spine. (2) The speech therapist reported that this sitting posture was affecting the participant's speech production (i.e. he was inaudible when he was not sitting correctly). (3) Staff reported that this sitting position resulted in drooling, which greatly reduced social acceptability.

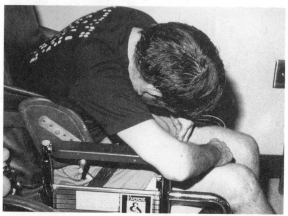

Figure 1: Subject prior to implementation of treatment.

Equipment

The equipment used included (1) a battery-operated Casio Keyboard, (2) a General Electric battery-operated AM/FM radio which had the capability to receive television channels, and (3) a mercury switch which was sewn into a base-ball cap. The mercury switch (Radio Shack #275-025) was attached to one end of a 30-inch (76.20 cm) piece of 22-gauge speaker wire. A ¼-inch square (.63 cm) of brass was soldered to the other end of the wire.

To activate the equipment, the hat containing the mercury switch was placed on the participant's head. A 10° tilt forward would activate the mercury switch. The brass square was inserted in the keyboard or the radio between a battery and the metal contact. When the participant's head was upright, the switch was in the 'on' position, and slumping over resulted in the switch turning the equipment off.

Procedures

Prior to the study, two activities which functioned as reinforcers were identified. These were: (1) practicing music on a Casio keyboard, and (2) listening to a TV game show. In baseline, at the beginning of each session, which lasted 10 minutes, the hat was put on the participant and he was given the verbal instructions: "During this session, try as hard as you can to sit up straight." The mercury switch was not connected to the keyboard during baseline.

In the treatment condition, the participant was given no verbal instructions. The mercury switch was connected so that the keyboard and radio were activated contingent on correct sitting posture.

Throughout the study, in the music-practice sessions, the participant practiced playing scales, chords, and portions of simple songs which he had learned several weeks earlier in music-therapy sessions.

Data was recorded in 15-second intervals for 10-minute periods in both the music-practice and leisure settings. In order for the participant to be scored as having "correct" posture, he had to be sitting upright for the entire 15 seconds of the interval. Two observers were present when the sessions were conducted. In baseline, the participant was scored as having "correct" posture if (1) his shoulders were against the back of his high-top wheelchair and (2) his head was upright. With this particular participant, pilot observations had indicated that putting his shoulders back automatically resulted in his head being held upright. During treatment, scoring procedures were the same as in baseline. In addition, observers could hear the equipment when the mercury switch was activated.

In each session in the leisure setting, the participant listened to the final 10 minutes of a 30-minute game show, the part that he had previously identified as his "favorite part."

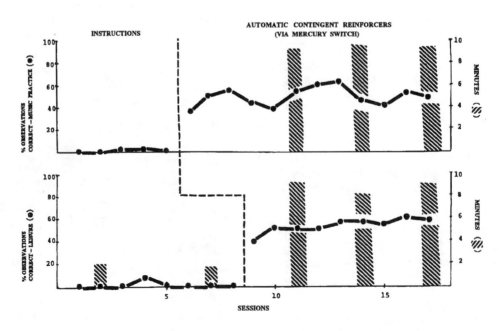

Figure 2: Correct posture in music-practice and leisure settings.

In order to demonstrate that effects seen were not due to one specific reinforcer but to the contingency relationship between "correct" posture and the delivery of the reinforcer, two different reinforcing activities were used.

RESULTS

Baseline data in both the music-practice and leisure settings show that instructions had no effect on getting the participant to sit up during music practice sessions, as shown in Fig. 2.

In the music-practice setting, when the mercury switch was activated during treatment, the participant sat up for as much as 63% of the intervals observed ($x = 49\%$). In the leisure setting (i.e. listening to a game show), the participant sat up an average of 52% of the observed intervals during the treatment condition.

Data from both settings indicate the participant sat in the correct posture for longer periods of time during treatment, suggesting that he was gaining physical strength and endurance over time. In treatment, the participant was sitting in the correct posture for as long as 9 minutes 27 seconds of a 10-minute session, whereas in baseline, the longest total time he sat in the correct posture during a 10- minute session was 2 minutes 28 seconds.

Reliability data was obtained for 35% of the observations. Reliability scores ranged from 98% to 100%, with an average of 99%. Reliability was calculated using the formula: Agreements/Agreements + Disagreements x 100.

DISCUSSION

This study demonstrates that electronic (e.g. mercury) switches can be used effectively as therapeutic tools to correct improper posture during functional daily activities. Previous work pertaining to the use of electronic equipment has generally not been data-based. Much of the data-based work that does exist has had limitations including (1) a failure to demonstrate with experimental control that electronic devices can be used to mediate consequences which provide therapeutic benefits automatically; (2) a failure to present reliability data; and (3) the presentation of data which shows no clear results.

The need for empirical studies pertaining to electro-mechanical technology has been identified in the literature.[9] This study is one of the first data-based investigations to demonstrate adequate experimental control and provide reliability data. Unlike much of the previous research in this area, it also demonstrates that the use of electro-mechanical equipment can be effectively incorporated into functional daily activities. The activities chosen in this study (music-

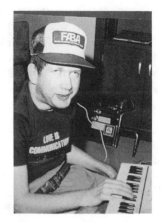

Figure 3: Subject during treatment.

practice and television-listening) were 'normalized' hobbies that were engaged in almost daily with no apparent satiation. The treatment in this study had socially significant results, in that it resulted in the participant being able to sit in the correct posture for a significant portion of an activity session, as shown in Fig. 3. It also enabled him to participate in a vocal choir, where his singing was now clearly audible, and resulted in a solo performance in a community-based program.

Due to physical weakness of the participant, it was possible to employ the procedures only in 10-minute periods of time. Thus, follow-up work is warranted to investigate methods for increasing physical strength and durability and for further generalizing the behavior gains seen in this study.

A subsequent application of the mercury switch is being used for treatment of a 7-year-old female, diagnosed with cerebral palsy with spastic quadriplegia, microcephaly, seizure disorder and cortical blindness. Her functioning level is in the 3-4-month range. Auditory function is normal. While sitting, her head is forward, chin resting on her upper chest. Physical therapy determined that while there was limited neck control, she could physically withstand an upright head position without assistance if so motivated.

When assessed by the music therapist and presented with recorded male-vocal music, significant facial changes were demonstrated — smiles, widening of eyes, cooing sounds. A 1-point mercury switch was sewn on a bonnet, positioned to activate a cassette tape of her preferred music if her head was lifted upright.

Training is being conducted 3 times per week. To allow for maximum opportunity for learning cause and effect, however, her bonnet is worn during all times she is in her stander or chair. Recent data taken during a 15-minute treatment period shows an increase in number of lifts, 0-7, as well as increased length of time correct position is maintained, 7 seconds-90 seconds per lift.

Cognitive levels differ between the child and the adult. Also, the time frame in which the behavior was demonstrated differs — 9 months and 3 months, respectively.   The treatment strategy, however, appears to promote a similar result — that of increased muscle tone.

The benefits of appropriate sitting and head postures are numerous. Vocal production can improve. Feeding can occur without restraint. Improved social acceptability can lessen the degree to which the individual is perceived as handicapped. And depending upon the client's cognitive level, training in the areas of self-help, daily-living and leisure-time activities may be addressed.

Further investigation into additional areas for switch placement is recommended.   Given the contingency of a meaningful reinforcer, this simple device could provide the individual with a pleasurable experience while independently working toward improved physical change.

REFERENCES

1. Bailey JA, Meyerson L: Effect of vibratory stimulation on a retardate's self-injurious behavior. Psychological Aspects of Disability 17: 133-137, 1970.

2. Fehr M, Wacker D, Tresize J, Lennon R, Meyerson L: Visual, auditory, and vibratory stimulation as reinforcers for profoundly retarded children. Rehabilitation Psychology 26:201-209, 1979.

3. Murphy R, Doughty N: Establishing controlled arm movements in PMR students using response contingent vibratory stimulation. American Journal of Mental Deficiency 82:212-216, 1977.

4. Burkhart L: More homemade battery devices for severely handicapped children. Millville, PA: L Burkhart, 1982.

5. Azrin N, Rubin H, O'Brian F, Ayllon T, Roll D: Behavioral engineering: Postural control by a portable operant apparatus. Journal of Applied Behavior Analysis 1:99-108, 1968.

6. Ball T, McCrady R, Hart A: Automated reinforcement of head posture in two cerebral palsied retarded children. Perceptual and Motor Skills 40:619-611, 1975.

7. Grove D, Dalke B, Fredericks HD, Crowly R: Establishing appropriate head positioning with mentally and physically handicapped children. Behavioral Engineering 3:53-59, 1975.

8. Wolfe DE: The effect of automated interrupted music on head posturing of cerebral palsied individual. Journal of Music Therapy 27:184-206, 1980.

9. Nietupski J, Hamre-Nietupski S, Ayres B: Review of task analytic leisure skill training efforts: Practitioner implications and further research needs. Journal of the Association for Persons with Severe Handicaps 9:88-97, 1984.

CHAPTER 109

Surgeons and Music:
A Psychophysiological Investigation

Karen Allen

Although it has become relatively common for music to be played during surgery, and many studies exist that have explored music's possible effects on *patients* in a variety of therapeutic settings, little is known about how the music being played affects the *surgical team*. Patients have been studied from a variety of interesting perspectives, with a wide range of findings regarding the therapeutic benefits of music during medical procedures.[1-7] While it is beneficial to know the effect of music on patients, it appears equally important to increase our understanding of the effects music may be having on the physiological reactions and performance ability of the individuals in whose hands we literally place our lives. Although to date the reactions of surgeons to music have not been studied from the perspective of psychophysiology, a considerable literature exists that has looked generally at the relationship between listening to music and physiological responses.[8-13] These investigations have employed a wide variety of methodological approaches, and findings have ranged from strong support for the effect of music on physiology, to no effect at all. In an attempt to increase understanding of the potential influence of music on physiology, the study described herein was developed as an initial exploration of what happens to the cardiovascular reactivity of surgeons when they listen to music. It focused on the autonomic responses of 50 surgeons while they performed a stressful task in a psychophysiology laboratory in which music was played.

HYPOTHESES

It was hypothesized that: (1) subjects would have lower measures of physiological reactivity in the condition in which their self-selected music was played as compared with other conditions, and (2) subjects would be more accurate at the task in the condition in which their own music was played as compared with other conditions.

SUBJECTS

Subjects were 50 male, Caucasian surgeons ranging in age from 31-68 years (mean age = 52 years). All subjects were self-reported music lovers or amateur musicians who regularly played music during surgery, and who volunteered for the study because they were interested in learning about their physiological responses to music. All said they played music often because they loved music and felt it had stress-reducing properties. To qualify for the study, subjects could not be on any medications that would affect heart rate or blood pressure (e.g. beta blockers or calcium antagonists), and could not have hypertension or cardiac complications.

METHOD

Subjects came to a psychophysiology laboratory and participated in an experiment consisting of performing a stressful task (mental arithmetic consisting of rapid serial subtraction) under *each* of the following three conditions: (1) self-selected music, often played in surgery, (2) a control piece of music chosen by the experimenter which was *not* chosen by any of the subjects — Pachelbel's *Canon in D Minor*, and (3) no music. Order of music conditions was randomized.

A standard laboratory paradigm was used, consisting of four 5-minute rest periods with three 2-minute task periods of mental arithmetic between the rest periods. Mental arithmetic, while certainly not a simulation of stress experienced in surgery, is an established laboratory stressor. In this study, mental arithmetic became increasingly difficult and started with counting backwards, aloud, by steps of 13, and ended with counting backwards by steps of 47. Task performance was continuously recorded on audio tape.

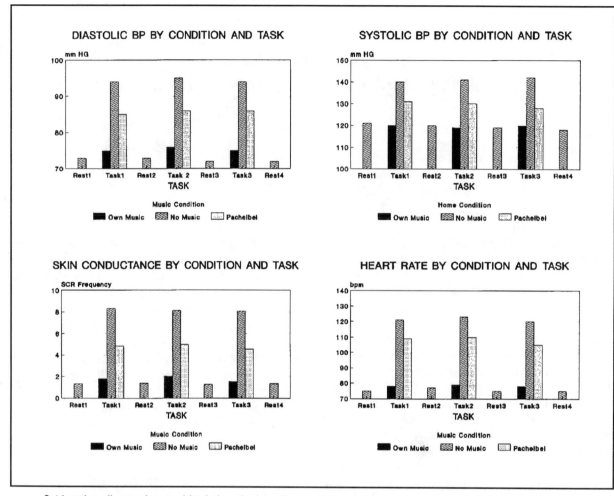

Subjects' cardiovascular reactivity during three music conditions: self-selected music, control piece, and no music.

PHYSIOLOGICAL MEASURES

Pulse rate (PR) was measured in beats per minute with a Panasonic photoplethysmographic pulse meter attached to the subject's right ear. Pulse rate was recorded every 20 seconds throughout the experiment. Skin conductance was recorded continuously using a Grass polygraph. Blood pressure was measured with a portable monitor (Health Check CX-1) from the index finger of the subject's left hand. Diastolic and systolic pressure were recorded once during the last minute of each rest period, and once during the second minute of the performance of each task.

RESULTS

A multivariate analysis of variance was performed with three within-subject factors (music condition, task, and period [baseline and performance]), using the four physiological measures (skin conductance response frequency [SCR], systolic blood pressure [SBP], diastolic blood pressure [DBP], and pulse rate [PR]) as dependent variables.

As hypothesized, subjects' cardiovascular reactivity was significantly lower (Wilks lambda = .063, $F_{(7, 67)}$ = 18.72, $p < .001$) when performing the task during the *self-selected* music condition than under the other two music conditions (Figure). In addition, the results support the hypothesis that *task performance* would be significantly better in the self-selected music condition than in the other music conditions. Data analysis also revealed no order effect for music condition, and no habituation effect for the task.

DISCUSSION

This study has extended previous research about the effects of music on physiology to a specific group of people (50 American surgeons) and has demonstrated compelling evidence that for some individuals, music can have a beneficial effect, in terms of both physiololgy and performance of a task while under stress. One might question the importance of knowing about cardiovascular reactivity when under stress. Considerable evidence exists that supports the idea that individuals who experience pronounced, frequent, or enduring autonomically mediated cardiovascular responses to stress may be at risk for the development of cardiovascular disease, and it appears that surgeons fall into this category. The fact that all of the surgeons in this study *believed* they were under frequent and enduring stress, and that music had a *calming* effect on them is an important factor to consider.

A significant aspect of this study is that it emphasizes the importance of familiarity, choice and control in the efficacy of music as a calming agent, extending the work of other researchers.[14] Although everyone in the experiment was affected by music, each individual was most favorably affected by the music he *chose*. Music selected by subjects included pieces representing a wide range of musical taste. For example, many subjects chose the vibrant, happy music of Vivaldi, but there were also jazz selections, several chamber pieces by Mozart, many instrumental opera arias (no one chose anything with lyrics being sung), a few Beethoven quartets, and even James Galway and the Chieftains playing traditional Irish music!

The idea of focusing on choice, familiarity, and control concerning music played during surgery is intriguing and should be extended to considering how the *lack* of such choice and control may be affecting *other* members of the surgical team, as well as the patient. Although all of the surgeons in this study said they regularly played music during surgery, not one had consulted other people in the operating room about *their* tastes and desires. They all said, in fact, that they chose what they played in surgery according to their *mood* at the time. That the Chieftains could exert a more calming influence than Pachelbel appears to lend especially credible support to the importance of choice.

Future investigations about the effects of music on human physiology would do well to consider control as a prominent factor, as well as the *type* of task being performed. Practical considerations precluded this experiment from being conducted during actual surgery, and the task performed required rapid response to a cognitive challenge. Since surgery is such a complex activity involving both cognitive and physical dexterity, future studies might employ a different type of task. Despite these methodological limitations, however, the results of this study demonstrate significant evidence supporting the position that there can be a powerful relationship between music and our minds and bodies.

REFERENCES

1. Locsin R: The effect of music on the pain of selected post-operative patients. Journal of Advanced Nursing 6: 1925, 1981.
2. Tanioka F, Takazawa T, Kamata S, Kudo M, Matsuki A, Oyama T: Hormonal effect of anxiolytic music in patients during surgical operations under epidural anaesthesia. *In* Spintge R, Droh R (eds), Musik in der Medizin/Music in Medicine, 199-204. Basel: SpringerVerlag, 1985.
3. Oyama T, Hatano K, Sato Y, Kudo M, Spintge R, Droh R: Endocrine effect of anxiolytic music in dental patients. *In* Spintge R, Droh R (eds), Musik in der Medizin/Music in Medicine, 223-226. Basel: SpringerVerlag, 1985.
4. Oyama T, Sato Y, Kudo T, Spintge R, Droh, R. Effect of anxiolytic music on endocrine function in surgical patients. *In* Spintge R, Droh R (eds), Musik in der Medizin/Music in Medicine, 169-174. Basel: SpringerVerlag, 1985.
5. Shapiro AG, Cohen H: Auxiliary pain relief during suction curettage. *In* Spintge R, Droh R (eds), Musik in der Medizin/Music in Medicine, 227-231. Basel: Springer-Verlag, 1985.
6. Davila JM, Menendez J: Relaxing effects of music in dentistry for mentally handicapped patients. Special Care in Dentistry 7:18-21, 1986.
7. Updike PA, Charles DM: Music Rx: Physiological and emotional responses to taped music programs of preoperative patients awaiting plastic surgery. Annals of Plastic Surgery 19:29-33, 1987.
8. Ries HA: GSR and breathing amplitude related to emotional reactions to music. Psychonomic Science 14: 62-64, 1969.
9. Landreth JE, Landreth HF: Effects of music on physiological responses. Journal of Research in Music Education 22:4-12, 1974.
10. Peretti PO: Changes in galvanic skin response as affected by musical selection, sex, and academic discipline. Journal of Psychology 89:183-187, 1975.

11. Kibler VE, Rider MS: Effects of progressive muscle relaxation and music on stress as measured by finger temperature response. Journal of Clinical Psychology, 39(2):213-215, 1983.

12. Perretti P, Zweifel J: Effect of musical preference on anxiety as determined by physiological skin responses. Acta Psychiatrica Belgique 83:437-442, 1983.

13. Thayer JF, Levensen RW: Effects of music on psychophysiological responses to a stressful fiom. Psycho-musicology 3:44-53, 1983.

14. De Jong MA, van Mourik KR, Schellekens HMC: A physiological approach to aesthetic preference. Psychotherapy and Psychosomatics 22:46-51, 1973.

SUGGESTED READING

Rohner SJ, Miller R: Degrees of familiar and affective music and their effects on state anxiety. Journal of Music Therapy 17:2-15, 1980.

CHAPTER 110

Composing a New Language

Barbara S. J. Balch • *Dennis Bathory-Kitsz*

The potency of musical memory, especially early musical memory, is undisputed. Fully orchestrated musical material is stored in the minds of people with little or no musical training; such music can be drawn complete and undisturbed from childhood.[1]

The authors propose the development of a new branch of diagnosis and therapy, offering music as a replacement for lost language, and using music to assess type and depth of loss, the progression of loss in disease, and as a prognostic indicator following injury.

Such a proposal is sweeping, and with serious obstacles at the very level of the definition of music. Stravinsky[2] called the song of a bird the promise of music, whereas Ohno[3] playfully suggests that both bird- and human tunes are governed by a "hierarchy of periodicities." Peretz[4] claims that autonomous brain systems process the melody and rhythm of music, but Laudon[5] speaks only of the magic of music and healing. Therapeutically, of course, via music per se there is participation, human contact, and a renewed or new language. Music is joy, capability, and power — these ideas exquisitely expressed in Dennison's novel.[6]

Largely because of these strengths (and these mysteries), many have attempted to use music as therapy — alas, too often by playing music *at* people — with almost no understanding of music, its therapeutic mechanisms, or, indeed, what it communicates emotionally or conceptually.

To understand music as a replacement for lost language, then, a deeper respect for music's communicative substance is essential. Music, while culturally dependent, is a singular model in universality of emotional expression. Kleinz[7] has demonstrated in a convincing manner the rudiments of a biological, cross-cultural melodic expression, far from Ohno's amusingly irreverent DNA-to-Bach transformations. Referring to emotionally communicative music, Kleinz states: "The more precisely you perform it, the more it conforms to a biologic form,

the more convincing, the more eloquent, the more contagious it is to convince others to change the state of feeling in the other person."

The authors suggest that it is possible to explore through music the relationship between expression and cognition, which, in turn, will provide some sense of what exists inside one who has lost the usual, measurable cognitive functions; in other words, "What's it like in there?" From a practical viewpoint, music is heard even in a comatose state.

Several researchers[4,8] have noted clear shifts in brain-hemisphere dominance and ear advantage among trained musicians. Secondly, then, the authors propose that learning music both as music and as language be explored through these questions: Can music retard the march of senility? Can music differentiate depression from organic disintegration? Can music touch those reaches of human experience remaining after horrifying injury, and invite recovery? Our premise is that music — and music alone — can.

The potential is both diagnostic and therapeutic. Research assumes that disorganization/disorientation of dementia occurs by stages, at a different rate and following a different path for each person (except when due to trauma, stroke, or other paroxysmal insult).

One possibility is that implementing this approach would retard the process of disintegration. If enough of a pattern[8] can be evolved from an individual in the early stages of loss, perhaps it can be retarded before the onset of advanced senility. If loss of function occurs little by little, then based on responses it might be possible to tell not only the degree of loss, but the areas in which this loss progresses. Further, it might be useful to differentiate physiologic disintegration from depression and other types of psychiatric disorders.

There is the possibility that the 'recentness' of the cognitive or memory loss would not be important, as musical memory is stored wholesale. Thus, the diagnosis and therapy may help with, for example, a 16-year-old accident victim. It is possible, however, that life experience and maturity may be required before certain musical material could be integrated.[4]

Studies have shown the integrity of an individual's musical memory despite severe physiologic assault. Gardner[9] has called music a "relative island of preservation in a sea of impairments," in speaking of retarded or autistic children. While many studies have sought to identify, usually via 'fractionalized' assays, the human brain's means for integrating music into experience, our purpose is to discover how to let music substitute wholesale as an individual language. "Music seems, sui generis, just like natural language."[9]

To implement the substitution of music or lost language, the following methodology is proposed:

Preparation: Progress in equipment used for virtual reality[10] will guide the somewhat simpler requirements of this proposal, i.e. the equipment used will be for the manipulation of real people (musicians) — manipulated, if you will, by people who have no other means to do it. Initially, the requirements will be for the most appropriate among hand sensors (gloves, balls), comfortable EEG equipment, galvanic skin sensors, eye switches, and cardiovascular sensors.

Following the development of this new hardware and the modification or adaptation of existing virtual-reality equipment, the research would proceed in three steps.

Stage One: A single-blind routine is established to test the validity of sensing- and feedback equipment, the viability of the premise where conditions are known, and the sensitivity of musicians and composers to the client. Among the musical techniques employed will be familiar music, voices, acoustic instruments, perfect-fifth resonances, and improvisation. Synthesizers (in the guise of 'virtual musicians') will form a part of Stage Two.

Stage Two: Personal history is researched on the client's contact with music, a menu of simple orchestrated musical material (together with bridges and modulations) is developed, a group of live performers is organized, and the feedback equipment and sensors (especially gloves) are provided. The playing is done in a comfortable, familiar environment. The musicians play through the menu, checking responses (as learned in Stage One). The menu is narrowed based on the responsive 'participation'; eventually, a composition is developed with the main themes and bridges that are specific to the client. This is the music of communication to the client, who is then provided with comfortable controllers (foam balls, eye switches) which may be used to control virtual-reality synthesizers (i.e., virtual musicians); the client can play along with this music. As it progresses, all play together. Musicians gradually yield 'solos' to the client, and a call-and-response pattern is evoked. Eventually, the client can improvise and compose as a method of communication, totally replacing the damaged verbal, visual or other motor responses.

Stage Three: As the individual communication is perfected from client to client, the 'noise' may be analyzed and dropped out, and common cultural/musical experiences remain from which to create communal music and communication. The group versus individual dichotomy is bridged as this form of language becomes more common.

This research must be done with care and be extremely personal or it will be both unsuccessful and inhumane. It is proposed so that those with language loss may be given back, in an alternative way, the power of communication and community. The musicians will have to understand the clients' lives and experiences, and through this new language, they will be as strangers suddenly becoming close friends. There must be no experiment-on, play-at mentality at work; the participants will share memory and a unique language. What each knows, all will know of each other. This is not just 'old people making music together' — it is new life.

REFERENCES

1. Sacks O: The Man Who Mistook His Wife for a Hat; and Other Clinical Tales. New York: Harper & Row, 1987.
2. Stravinsky I: Poetics of Music, in the form of six lessons. Cambridge MA: Harvard University Press, 1970.
3. Ohno S: Repetition as the essence of life on the earth: Music and genes. Haematology and Blood Transfusion 31:511-518, 1987.
4. Peretz I: Processing of local and global musical information by unilateral brain-damaged patients. Brain 113:185-1205, 1990.
5. Laudon RT: To lend a hand: The magic of music and medicine. Minnesota Medicine, 73:21-22, Nov 1990.
6. Dennison G: Luisa Domic, a Novel. New York: Harper & Row, 1985.

7. Kleinz M: Interview. *In* Angier J: What is Music? Nova broadcast, PBS, 1989.

8. LaBarba RC, et al: Cerebral lateralization of music perception in the dual task paradigm: Unfamiliar melody recognition in sinistrals. Neuropsychologia 27(2):247-259, 1989 .

9. Gardner H: Frames of Mind: The Theory of Multiple Intelligences, 99-127. New York: Basic, 1985.

10. Stedman N: Fields of dreams; Virtual reality systems launch video on a daring new quest for total immersion. Video, 30-33, May 1991.

CHAPTER 111

How Can the Use of Music in Medicine Be Promoted and Supported?

Olu-Birgit Jeppson

The use of music in medicine is not a new constellation. It has existed as long as mankind. In a review paper,[1] the author quotes the following Renaissance artists:

Conclusion Quotation

"Medicina Sanat Animam per Corpus, Musica Autem Corpus per Animam" ("Medicine heals the soul by the body but music heals the body by the soul"), states Giovanni Pico della Mirandola (1463-1494); and *"Musica itaque Medicinalis est..."* ("Thus music belongs to medicine"), states Johannes de Muris (1350).

Despite its nearly explosive development in recent decades, however, it is very likely that there are still many medical professionals who are not aware of this well-established phenomenon. A further step of development would be to include at least theoretical information regarding music in medicine in medical and nursing curricula. The physician should be responsible for the choice of therapy in collaboration with the nursing staff. Some hospitals use a printed referral form from the doctor to the music therapist for each patient. It is desirable that nurses also participate in this referral.

Another special group should also be included in this discipline. It is musicologists. They deal with all kinds of music, in theory, practice, and research, and their scientific contribution to the interdisciplinary medical team is necessary.

In the Scandinavian countries, there is to date only one doctoral dissertation in music therapy, which was prepared in the Department of Musicology of Oslo University, in Norway. To our knowledge, in Sweden, there is only one doctoral candidate in music therapy, in the Department of Musicology of Gothenburg University.

Ten years ago, a dissertation defense took place in the Department of Psychiatry of Lund University, Sweden, on the topic: *Music, Mind and Mental Illness.*

The discussant appointed by the university, a medical doctor from Gothenburg, was totally uninformed about music, so the advisor had to ask for a complementary discussant, an associate professor of music psychology at Uppsala University. Presently, Lund University enjoys a special Department of Music in Medicine-Music Therapy.

In Denmark, the founder of the Society for Music Therapy was a professor of musicology. In Italy, the *Minerva "Rivista di Musicoterapia"* is edited by a professor of psychiatry, and the Scientific Committee consists of about forty members, seven of whom are musicologists.

In France, Dr. Anne-Marie Ferrand-Vidal, founder of the International Association for Melody-Programmed Therapy of Speech (IAMPTS) states, in her book, *La Mélodie-Thérapie du Langage:* "Here we give only a 'model' of Corpus. This should be constructed by an interdisciplinary team comprising a neurologist, a psychologist (or psychoanalyst), a phoniatrician (or orthophonist), a linguist, and a musicologist. The latter is indispensable for the construction of the 'melodies' of the 'phrase-items,' in order to keep track of the pauses, pitches, and accents of the melodic scheme."[3]

It would also be of importance to find composers interested in writing music especially fitted for various medical purposes: "We need collaborative and cooperative investigations of the vibratory and frequency nature of musical tones and instruments, relate and correlate the results of these studies to the vibrations and frequencies of the human organism and compose music accordingly."[4]

There are numerous clinical and research applications to music in medicine. To name just a few: 1) the unborn child — delivery; 2) Alzheimer's disease — geriatrics; 3) oncology; 4) bone marrow transplants;

5) rheumatology — Bechterew's disease; 6) mental illness — psychiatry; 7) criminology — prison hospitals; 8) drug- and alcohol problems; 9) speech difficulties; 10) the incurable, dying patient; 11) anesthesia; 12) prophylaxis, etc.

CASE REPORTS

Case 1: An 11-year-old *worsting* (ill/bad) who had smashed the lips of one of his mates and crushed the spleen of another was expelled from school. After about two months with a music therapist and the aid of two simple recorders, he was discharged from the children's psychiatric clinic and could return to school like a normal boy.

Case 2: An elderly woman who, after a stroke, was considered a "hopeless case," without any medical treatment, regained her health by means of music therapy, such that she was able to participate in a handicapped tour from Copenhagen to the Greek island of Kos, and she also spontaneously conducted the nursing home audience in a refrain song.[5]

Case 3: A young schizophrenic patient, after three months of various conventional medical treatments to no avail, made significant strides with a psychiatrist/ music therapist and two drumsticks, from the very first session.[6]

In some countries, there is a great opposition to the conventional psychiatric medical treatment of mentally ill patients. Therefore, if the use of medicine should be reduced in this group, there will be a need for other forms of therapy to fill the gap. The above successful cases suggest that music therapy could very well fulfill this task.

REFERENCES

1. Jeppson OB: Musikterapin fran bibeln till dagens Sverige (Music therapy from the Bible to Sweden today). Läkartidningen 20:2045-2048, 1981.

2. Petiziol A: Rivista di Musicoterapia. Minerva Medica 3(6), Roma, 1988.

3. Ferrand-Vidal AI: La Mélodie-Thérapie du Langage, 35. Paris: Maloine SA, 1982.

4. Eagle CT: Music in Medicine, 406. New York: Springer, 1987.

5. Blichfeldt P: Kazooen er lige så dyrebar som Steinway flygelet (The ocarina is just as valuable as the Steinway grand piano). OPUS 3(1):12-14, 1983.

6. Strobel W: Miusiktherapie mit schizophrenen patienten. Musiktherapeutische Umschau 6(3): 177-298, 1985.

CHAPTER 112

Musical Concepts of Conservation in Mentally Handicapped Children

Joanna Kossewska

In handicapped children, revalidation music has cognitive, prophylactic, and therapeutic values. Listening to music helps develop musical intelligence, as well as understanding and use of musical language. Music also enables the listener to benefit from the culture of the past .

Music is the total complex of melody, rhythm, and meter, and, as each kind of human activity, makes use of a special collection of concepts. For the creative perception, understanding, and experience of the beauty included in musical compositions, it is necessary to use the concepts which are the basis of musical alphabet. These concepts evolve during the individual child's psychic development, following innate and social factors. These factors range from the emotional response, occurring when the listener has a pleasant auditory impression, to the ability of distinguishing between pitches, rhythm patterns, and meter.[1]

Differentiation between many auditory phenomena needs musical intelligence that permits the listener to move beyond the limits of his/her perceptual field, and to conserve the constancy of some musical dimension within the modification of others in temporal sequence. The listener is able to grasp tonal-rhythmic movement because s/he can separate tonal and rhythmic patterns from the total complex of sound.

Conservation is a necessary condition for all rational activity. These rational aspects consist of the intellectual controls of operational thought, according to research into the child's development of concepts of quantity, weight, and volume.[2] Differences between pre-operational and operational thinking result from the nature of the internal cognitive structures, perfected during the various stages of child development. They are not simply dependent on the results of learning.

This study concerns the rational aspects of handicapped children's musical development. Do their musical concepts of conservation develop in the same sequence as normals?[3]

Mentally handicapped children slowly develop according to the same developmental rules as others. They have difficulty passing from one level to another. A concrete operational stage is the highest level of mental development reached by a mildly handicapped child. Problems with understanding and perception of more complicated musical compositions follow the decrease of cognitive ability. In spite of these limitations, they can experience pleasure in listening to and making music.

MATERIALS AND METHODS

Two groups of 15 handicapped children with IQ>55 (by WISC) took part in the experiment:

· Group P: preoperational stage of mental development, without conservation of quantity, weight, and volume concepts; average chronological age 9.7 years; average mental age 6.9 years.

· Group O: concrete operational stage of mental development, concepts conserved; average chronological age 11.5 years; average mental age 8.3 years (as determined by Piaget's experiments with plasticine balls).

Six music tasks were divided to measure the ability to conserve meter, tone, and rhythm. They were analogous to the Piagetian tasks, and based on tasks described by Pflederer.[1] Each task was recorded on magnetic tape from the synthesizer, and had one musical element changed with the others conserved. Each child met individually with the investigator for a 10-minute session following the practice period.

The tasks were designed to study conservation of meter, tone, and rhythm: 1) conservation of rhythm pattern under deformation of tone (melody); 2) conservation of rhythm pattern under deformation of pitch; 3) conservation of melody under deformation of duration values; 4A) conservation of tone (pitch) under deformation of rhythm; 4B) conservation of melody under deformation of rhythm; 5) conservation of melody (tonal pattern) under deformation of pitch; and 6) conservation of meter — double (march), triple (dance).

RESULTS

Group O (operational level) obtained better results in tasks measuring musical conservation than group P (preoperational level). Group O had better average results and smaller individual differences in musical conservation in tasks 4A, 4B, and 6. The biggest differences among the two groups were in tasks 4A and B. Conserving melody under deformation of both rhythm and pitch was very difficult.

There were also large sex differences: Girls scored higher in tasks measuring rhythm conservation (1, 2) and conservation of meter (6), but lower in tasks measuring conservation of melody (5). Boys showed more variation in their level of musical conservation development than girls.

DISCUSSION

The above results were compared to Pflederer's,[1] serving as a control group. We were able to compare Polish and American children's results because, in spite of a large difference in chronological age, they had similar mental age and development (operational and preoperational) (Table 1).

The Polish children's results varied less between the two groups than Americans', except for tasks 4A, 4B, and 5. Polish children obtained higher scores in general than Americans, especially group P, except in tasks measuring conservation of melody under deformation of rhythm and pitch.

Pflederer found that the ability to conserve meter and rhythm followed the ability to conserve melody.[1] This study presents adverse conclusions. Indeed, handicapped children had no trouble with meter conservation, but considerable trouble with conserving melody and rhythm. The developmental rule stating the increase of melody conservation under

Table I: American and Polish Children's Music Conservation Results

Task	Group	P	Group	O
	Am.	Pol.	Am.	Pol.
2	78.3	71.7	72.0	86.7
3	50.0	78.3	99.4	98.3
4A,B	68.0	15.8	80.0	35.0
5	63.0	36.7	76.0	56.7
6	44.0	85.0	75.0	96.7

deformation of different elements (duration, pitch, rhythm) was confirmed.

It was easier to notice the conservation of melody under deformation of duration than under deformation of rhythm and pitch for both Polish and American children. The discrepancy between these results and Pflederer's might be due to the difference in preparing musical tasks or to the specific character of mentally handicapped children's thinking.

THERAPEUTIC APPLICATIONS

Musical tasks with conservation of melody can be used to develop logical thinking on the concrete operational level. The Botvin study showed that training in conservation of melody improved solution of the Piagetian conservation tasks in quantity, weight, and number.[4] Training was more successful when involving behavior (shaping). Learning effects transfer shows that both musical and non-musical types of conservation are dependent on the same cognitive structures.

It is very important that attention be given to the level of the children's cognitive development, taking into account their tendency to concrete activity. Activity connected with conservation of melody should be amplified to help develop other concepts.

During testing, the children used oral or nonverbal answers, so they could express their evoked emotions and experiences connected with music tasks and testing situations. Gratification of the need for pleasure and playing followed the use of metaphor (dance for little girl/boy and for grandmother/-father). This guessing was the basis of association between symbolic contents and melorythmic patterns.

It is a very important element of the global teaching in special schools for handicapped children. Nonverbal answers (movement, clapping, shaping) followed the spontaneous need for movement and reactivity of temperament. Movement is a basic source of practice and verbal intelligence development.[5]

Music improves the psychomotor functions in children with mental deficiency. It stimulates their intellectual and mnemonic activity and balances personality disharmonies and behavioral disturbances. Music can play an important role in revalidation and rehabilitation of children with brain damage, following perinatal and early childhood trauma.[6]

This experiment did not follow a common music-therapy model, because the main experience aim called for individual testing. The individual form of testing helped the children feel safe; using admission examples and encouraging them to realize that music tasks helped them to reduce fear of the unknown. Similar tasks in playing situations could help the children to come into contact with themselves, and to communicate and integrate in the group. It is very important to avoid using rivalry, considering that handicapped children have a decreased potential to reduce their state of stress and frustration. Competition could involve comparing.

REFERENCES

1. Pflederer M: The responses of children to musical tasks embodying Piaget's principle of conservation. J Res Mus Ed 12(4):251-268, 1964.
2. Fraisse P, Piaget J: Inteligencja. Warszawa: PWN, 1967.
3. Sterczynska J: Pojecia stalosci u dzieci uposledzonych umyslowo w stopniu lekkim. Unpublished master 's thesis, Krakow, UJ, 1988.
4. Serafin ML: Piagetian research in music. Bull C Res Mus Ed 62:1-21,1980.
5. Sekowska Z: Pedagogika Specjalna. Warszawa: PWN, 1981.
6. Schipkowensky N: Musical therapy in the fields of psychiatry and neurology. *In* Henson RA, Critchley McD (eds), Music and the Brain. London: Heinemann Medical Books Ltd, 1980.

CHAPTER 113

Effects of Music and Relaxation on Anxiety in Adolescent Pregnancy

Sammi S. Liebman, and Aileen Maclaren

REVIEW of LITERATURE

Pregnancy has been described as a difficult and turbulent period.[20] Early research addressing the effects of psychological tension in pregnancy has shown emotional factors, such as degree of anxiety and severe physical or emotional stress, to be involved in such pathology as habitual abortion and hyperemesis gravidarum.[11] McDonald[23] noted a relationship between increasing amounts of catecholamines and decreasing uterine efficiency, consequently inhibiting progress in labor. Other authors[21] also noted that increased levels of stress related hormones, such as norepinephrine, have been linked to incoordinate uterine activity.

Lederman, et al.[18] found that increased anxiety levels effected physiologic elevators of plasma epinephrine and were associated with decreased uterine contractility and prolonged labor. In subsequent research, the authors[19] found that specific psychological factors measured in the third trimester of pregnancy were predictive of progress in labor, thus confirming the relationship between increasing anxiety and obstetric complications.

Spielberger and Jacobs[30] have identified two different types of anxiety. They make a distinction between transitory emotional reactions to situational stress (state anxiety) and degree of anxiety-proneness inherent in personality (trait anxiety). The *State Trait Anxiety Inventory* (STAI) was developed to measure these two distinct concepts of anxiety. In these authors' review of studies using the STAI to examine anxiety levels during pregnancy, they found that consistently higher state anxiety levels during pregnancy were associated with the later development of obstetric complications.

The pregnant adolescent is often considered a high-risk patient because she is predisposed to (a) higher maternal and infant mortality rates, (b) pre-eclampsia, (c) anemia, (d) low-birth-weight babies, (e) size and date problems, and (f) multiple socioeconomic complications.[6]

The successful use of music therapy techniques with obstetric patients has been thoroughly documented.[5,13,25,33] Early approaches toward incorporating the application of music into the childbirth experience were for the purpose of distraction from pain,[4,24] promoting positive associations during labor and delivery, and to cue rhythmic breathing.[13] The effects of music during prenatal education classes have been found to be beneficial for the mother, albeit, statistically insignificant.[9,27] Recently, DiFranco[7] has outlined suggestions for using music as a wellness technique during childbirth education classes.

Given the fact that maternal psychological factors such as anxiety most definitely have an impact on pregnancy outcome, and that music therapy protocols have been successfully implemented to reduce anxiety, it was the sole intent of this study to investigate the effects of a music and relaxation intervention on third-trimester anxiety in adolescent pregnancy.

METHODOLOGY

Sample

Subjects for the study were drawn from the South Area Continuing Opportunities for Purposeful Education (COPE) Center School, Dade County, Florida. COPE Center South is designed to enable pregnant students (grades 6-12) to continue education.

The first 25 students to volunteer for the study were assigned to the experimental group and the following 20 students were assigned to the control group. Excluded from the data collection were the following students: those who were multiparous (n=2); those who delivered prematurely (n=2); and those who left school (one dropped out and one was hospitalized). Thus, a total of 39 students ranging in age from 13 to 18 years provided data for this study. Nineteen girls served as the experimental group and 20 girls served as the control group. Chi-square analyses indicated no significant difference between groups with respect to distribution of ages (χ^2 (2) = .53, p = .77) social class (χ^2 (2) = 1.5, p = .47), and race (χ^2 (1) = .21 p = .65). Therefore, age, social class, and race were not included as a factor in the final analysis.

Experimental Setting

Students in the experimental group received an individual music therapy session once a week. Each session took place in the clinic at the COPE Center and lasted approximately 15 - 20 minutes. With each subject sitting in a reclining chair, music was provided via headphones from a Panasonic dualcassette, auto-reverse deck/recorder (Model No. RXFW25). Subjects were included in the data analysis if they attended a minimum of 10 sessions.

Variables

The music therapy treatment served as the independent variable and consisted of progressive muscle relaxation training paired with music. Only those subjects in the experimental group received the music therapy treatment.

State- and trait- anxiety scores from the STAI served as the dependent variables. The trait anxiety inventory was administered to both groups at the beginning of the seventh, eighth, and ninth months of pregnancy (approximately at the twenty-eighth week, the thirty-second week, and the thirty-sixth week of pregnancy). The state anxiety inventory was administered weekly to both groups beginning at the seventh month of pregnancy for a total of ten weeks.

RESULTS

The statistical design employed in the study was a repeated-measures factorial design comparing the trait and state anxiety scores over time between the experimental group and the control group. The trait scores were analyzed with a 2 x 3 factorial design involving comparisons at weeks 28, 32, and 36 of pregnancy between the groups. The state scores used a 2 x 10 factorial design involving comparisons of the two groups from week 28 to 37 of pregnancy.

The repeated-measures ANOVA revealed a statistically significant main effect difference between the two groups on the trait anxiety scores (Table 1).

Table 1: *Repeated Measures Anova, Comparing Trait Anxiety Levels Over Time.*

Source	DF	SS	MS	F	P
Between	38	9058.31			
Groups	1	1415.13	1415.13	6.85	.012
Error	37	7643.18	206.57		
Within	78	2498.49			
Weeks	2	143.72	71.86	2.35	.1023
Weeks X Groups	2	93.15	46.58	1.52	.2246
Error	74	2261.62	30.56		
Total	116	11556.3			

Essentially, the experimental group showed significantly less trait anxiety than did the control group. No significant change over time was found in the anxiety level of the two groups. Also, no significant interaction between group and week was found.

As shown in Table 2, the repeated-measures ANOVA revealed a statistically significant main effect difference between the groups. Overall, the

Table 2: *Repeated Measures ANOVA Comparing Groups' State Anxiety Levels Over Time.*

Source	DF	SS	MS	F	P
Between	38	34274.1			
Groups	1	10137.8	10137.8	15.54	.0003
Errors	37	24136.4	652.3		
Within	351	28708.7			
Weeks	9	908.8	109.0	1.44	.1713
Weeks X Groups	9	2457.1	273.0	3.60	.0003
Error	333	25270.8	75.9		
Total	389	63045.3			

experimental subjects showed less state anxiety than did the control subjects. No statistically significant main effect differences were found across weeks. However, a statistically significant interaction between group and week was found.

Follow-up t-tests comparing the two groups at each week revealed that the state anxiety levels of the two groups differed significantly at weeks 30, 31, 34, 35, 36, and 37. It is apparent from Table 3 that the differences were greatest at weeks 35, 36, and 37.

Figure 1 portrays graphically the two groups' state anxiety means for weeks 28 through 37.

Table 3: *Follow-up Comparisons Between Groups on State Anxiety Group-Means for Weeks 38 thru 37.*

Week	Group	n	Means	Mean Diff.	t	p
28	E	19	35.63			
	C	20	41.65	-6.0	1.83	.076
29	E	19	32.0			
	C	20	40.30	-8.3	2.38	.022
30	E	19	31.73			
	C	20	41.30	-9.6	3.05	.004
31	E	19	33.84			
	C	20	45.70	-11.9	2.92	.006
32	E	19	34.84			
	C	20	43.00	-8.2	1.78	.083
33	E	19	35.58			
	C	20	37.60	-2.1	.48	.636
34	E	19	34.32			
	C	20	42.70	-8.4	2.20	.034
35	E	19	33.68			
	C	20	44.75	-11.1	3.29	.002
36	E	19	31.53			
	C	20	46.60	-15.1	4.38	.001
37	E	19	30.79			
	C	20	52.35	-21.6	6.44	.001

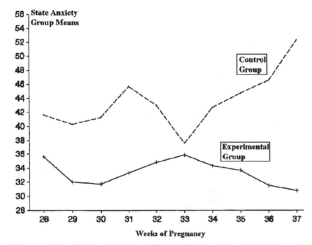

Figure 1: *State Anxiety Group-Means for Control and Experimental Groups for Weeks 28 thru 37.*

REFERENCES

1. Bacon, L. Early motherhood accelerated role transitions and social pathology. Social Forces, 52: 333-341, 1974.

2. Bernstein, D., & Borkovec, T. Progressive relaxation training: A manual for the helping professions. Champaign, IL: Research Press, 1973.

3. Biller, J., Olson, P., & Breen, T. The effect of "happy" versus "sad" music and participation on anxiety. Journal of Music Therapy 11: 68-73, 1974.

4. Burt, R., & Korn, G. Audioanalgesia in obstetrics. American Journal of Obstetrics and Gynecology, 88: 361-366, 1964.

5. Clark, M., McCorkle, R., & Williams, S. Music therapy-assisted labor and delivery. Journal of Music Therapy, 18: 88-100, 1981.

6. Corbett, M., & Meyer, J. The adolescent and pregnancy. Boston, Massachusetts: Blackwell Scientific Publications, 1987.

7. DiFranco, J. Relaxation: Music. *In* F. H. Nichols & S. S. Humerick (Eds.), Childbirth education: Practice, research, and theory. (pp. 201-215). Philadelphia, PA: Saunders, 1988a.

8. DiFranco, J. Music for childbirth, Childbirth Educator, Fall: 36-38, 1988b.

9. Durham, L., & Collins, M. The effect of music as a conditioned aid in prepared childbirth education. JOGN Nursing, May-June: 268-270, 1986.

10. Franklin, D. The impact of music on the level of anxiety of high and low music listeners as measured by Spielberger's State-Trait Anxiety Inventory. Dissertation Abstracts International 3419-B, 1981.

11. Grimm, E. Psychological tension in pregnancy. Psychosomatic Medicine, 23: 520-527, 1961.

12. Halpern, S. Sound health: The music and sounds that make us whole. San Francisco, CA: Harper & Row, 1985.

13. Hanser, S., Larson, S., & O'Connell, A. The effect of music on relaxation of expectant mothers during labor. Journal of Music Therapy, 20: 50-58, 1983.

14. Hanser, S. Music therapy and stress reduction research. Journal of Music Theapy, 22:193-206, 1985.

15. Isaac, S. & Michael, W. Handbook in research and evaluation. San Diego, CA: EDITS, 1985.

16. Konapaka, G. Life situational and psychodynamic factors in pregnancy experience of married adolescents. American Journal of Orthopsychiatry, 37: 265, 1967.

17. LaBarre, M. Pregnancy experiences among married adolescents. American Journal of Ortho-psychiatry 38: 47-55, 1968.

18. Lederman, R., Lederman, E., Work, B., & McCann, D. The relationship of maternal anxiety,

plasma catecholamines, and plasma cortisol to progress in labor. A.J.Ob.Gyn., 132:495-500, 1978.

19. Lederman, R., Lederman, E., Work, B., & McCann, D. Relationship of psychological factors in pregnancy to progress in labor. Nursing Research, 28: 94-97, 1979.

20. Leifer, M. Psychological effects of motherhood. New York: Praeger Publishers, 1980.

21. Levinson, G., & Shneider, S. Catecholamines: the effects of maternal fear and its treatment on uterine function and circulation. Birth and the Family Journal, 6: 167-174, 1979.

22. Lieberman, M. Does help help? The adaptive consequences of obtaining help from professionals and social networks. American Journal of Community Psychology, 6: 499-517, 1978.

23. McDonald, R. The role of emotional factors in obstetric complications. Psychosomatic Medicine 30: 222-237, 1968.

24. McDowell, C. Obstetrical applications of audio-analgesia. Hospital Topics, April: 102-104, 1966.

25. McKinney, C. Music therapy in obstetrics: a review. Music Ther. Perspectives, 8: 57-60, 1990.

26. Rohner, S., & Miller, R. Degree of familiar and affective music and their effects on state anxiety. Journal of Music Therapy, 17: 2-15, 1980.

27. Sammons, L. The use of music by women during childbirth. Journal of Nurse-Midwifery, 29: 266-270, 1984.

28. Shouse, J.. Psychological and emotional problems of pregnancy. In J. Zackler & W. Brandstadt (Eds.), Teenage pregnant girl. (pp. 161-186). Charles C. Thomas, 1975.

29. Smoke, J., & Grace, M. Effectiveness of prenatal care and education for pregnant adolescents: Nurse-midwifery intervention and team approach. Journal of Nurse-Midwifery, 33: 178-184, 1988.

30. Spielberger, C. Manual for the State-Trait Anxiety Inventory (Form Y). Palo Alto, CA: Consulting Psychologists Press, 1983.

31. Spielberger, C., & Jacobs, G. Maternal emotions, life stress and obstetric complications. In L. Zichella & P. Paneheri (Eds.), Psvchoneuro-endocrinology in reproduction (p. 540). Elsevier, North Holland: Biomedical Press, 1979.

32. Stoudenmire, J. A comparison of muscle relaxation training and music in the reduction of state and trait anxiety. Journal of Clinical Psychology, 31: 490-492, 1975.

33. Winslow, G. Music therapy in the treatment of anxiety in hospitalized high-risk mothers. Music Therapy Perspectives, 3: 29-33, 1986.

CHAPTER 114

Music Therapy in Treatment of Psychiatric Patients

Ingeborg Formann-Radl

It has been scientifically confirmed that even in the pre-Christian cultures, music was accorded a significant position within the framework of medical techniques. The beginnings of its utilization date back to the primitive — apostrophized by Herder in the eighteenth century as *Naturvölker* — when medicine men employed rhythmic chants in ritual ceremonies aimed at driving demons from a body considered immortal. Those ceremonial rites can be considered as forerunners of today's music therapy.

Among various cultures, music has retained its ceremonial rather than its entertainment value. Rhythmic song and dance are used to reach an ecstatic state facilitating the transition from reality into the spiritual realm.[1]

The primitive medicine man sang and danced together with members of his tribe in order to convince the pertinent patient of his ability to exorcise from his body the demon responsible for his sickness. His ritual was accompanied by instruments such as bells, metal rods, rattles, and clappers, which purportedly were imbued with magical properties. Psychic as well as somatic complaints were treated by the same methods. Healing was the responsibility of the entire tribe, and music played a significant part in its application.

During the seventh and sixth centuries B.C., it was the Pythagoreans who recommended the utilization of music as a psychohygienic and therapeutic medium. The actual effects of music therapy were not clearly defined, but through its harmonic patterns, music was expected to reestablish a balance of bodily and psychic function. In the eyes of the Pythagoreans, music served a cathartic, i.e. a psychohygienic, purpose. Even at that time, defined methods were employed in treatment of certain affective disturbances. Xenophiles and Jamblichon as well as many other authors of that period, described the manner in which music can be successfully employed in order to reestablish psychic well-being.

During the fourth century B.C., Plato asserted that "rhythm and harmony deeply affect the soul," and confirmed thereby the great significance he accorded the art of music as a therapeutic measure.

Aristotle had already classified emotion and reactive mood as affective segments of the individual personality structure. He also stressed the cathartic effect of music, an aspect shared by present-day advocates of music as a therapeutic agent, because this effect touches certain aspects of life style. It is important to mention that during the first century A.D., Aretaios of Capadocia observed the effect of music upon the disposition of the soul, on the formation of character, and on the ability to imitate certain characteristics.

During the first century A.D., Asklepiades employed music therapy in his treatment of split-personality cases. Later, it was Aristides Quintilianus who asserted that music has a specific effect upon the individual. As far as he was concerned, every obsession represented the symptom for an illness. Through the medium of music, he attempted to transport his patients into "the fitting psychic state." Depending upon the extent of the obsession, he suggested that the patient hear music or make music himself, thereby establishing the pilot-pattern for the passive-receptive or active music therapy of our time.

During the fifth century, it was primarily Boethius who attributed to music the regulative function which continued to be ascribed to it well into the time of the Renaissance. Later, a significantly in-depth psychological component was also ascribed to music.

At the beginning of the sixteenth century, the physician Cornelius Agrippa attributed to music a high therapeutic value — above all, to music produced by the human voice, which he considered best suited to swiftly alleviate psychic disturbances. Burton wrote: "Music is a powerful weapon against melancholia. It resuscitates and refreshes the languishing soul. It reaches not only the ears but every blood vessel, as well as the vital and animalistic spirits; it elevates the soul and sensitizes it."[2]

During the eighteenth and nineteenth centuries, the *sympaticotone* effect of music came under debate. Wackenroder asserted that of all the arts, only music promoted the most conflicting emotions in human beings; and Samuel C. Vogler described music — especially song — as the language of the soul. French psychiatry represented by Leuret, however, described several cases which had been negatively affected under the influence of music therapy.

Thus, history informs us that music therapy is not — as often assumed — an invention of our age. Throughout the twentieth century, it was influenced mainly by the experiences and conceptual definitions of American therapists. Arising from sociocultural differences, several independent teaching methods and areas of application developed, but today, all psychologic and psychotherapeutic concepts are united in the precept that the human being represents a homogeneous entity rather than a conglomerate of two separate ones, namely body and soul. In accordance with that precept, modern medicine again supports a homogenous therapy concept.

Only the human individual is capable of communicating on three separate levels[3] — verbally, emotionally, and actively. In those instances where communication on the verbal or active level is no longer possible, access to the individual should be sought via the emotional level. It is in this area that the value of music therapy becomes most apparent, although it must be stressed that it can never be more than an ancillary treatment method. As far as the therapist himself is concerned, however, it is important that two basic requirements are met: (1) due consideration must be given to the patient's entire social and cultural environment, and (2) acknowledgement of the fact that both patient *and* therapist are members of a sick society. The therapist is therefore expected to dispose of adequate insight into his/her own deep-seated psychological problems,[4] whereby special emphasis is placed upon the aspect of transference.

Basic research studies carried out at the Psychiatric University Clinic of Vienna, Austria, upon neurotic, psychotic, and psychosomatic case material, as well as on patients presenting diverse form of drug and alcohol abuse and behavioral aberrations, have shown that in many instances, music therapy provided an access to the psychotic patient which, in itself, effected an improvement in the patient's condition, or facilitated his acceptance and cooperation with regard to an appropriate medical treatment program.

We know that many psychiatric ailments are basically triggered by intrapsychic stress conditions connected with unresolved averse environmental influences, a combination which leads to the loss of psychosomatic balance. Patients lose their bearings and experience an ever increasing sense of inner loneliness; their social contacts deteriorate and they suffer from anxiety and panic attacks. At this point in the development of a psychic disturbance, i.e. when the patient's communicative abilities are negligible or no longer functional, music therapy provides a valuable substitute for verbal communication.[5]

Depending upon the severity of the psychic disturbance and following the establishment of a psychiatric diagnosis, it will be necessary to assign the patient to either individual- or group therapy. It has been affirmed that the criteria of diagnosis will not influence choice of the music-treatment program. This decision rests exclusively with the music therapist.

Guidelines specifying the type of music applicable in the treatment of individual types of psychic ailments are impossible to determine and do not in fact exist. Irrespective of the nature of the illness, this selection can be made only in consideration of the patient's own personality. The satisfactory relationship between physician and therapist represents an important prerequisite for a successful patient-therapist relationship, whereby the term *successful* has no bearing upon expectations for a positive reaction on the part of the patient. Even a negative reaction to music therapy may be of considerable significance. Our experience has shown that it does not serve to confront the patient with music in a manner resembling the offer of purchasable goods to a prospective buyer. For the individual patient, Bach does not equal Bach, Mozart not Mozart, and pop/rock not pop/rock. We should carefully avoid preconceptions. The therapist is called upon to carefully explore the preferences of each individual patient being treated, and this — if the therapy is to prove effective — demands of the therapist a very high educational and professional standard.

The relationship between music therapist and patient poses a greater demand on humane sensibilities than is required for the establishment of technical data determining, for example, the effect of music upon pulse rate and heartbeat rhythm; although the acquisition of such data is of great relevance, a fact which again illustrates the importance of a collaborative physician-therapist effort.

The studies at the University Clinic of Vienna have established certain similarities in the statements of the patients involved. A considerable majority of patients recounted experiences which could serve as a dominant part in effecting a psychic breakthrough. The effects of classical music by Bach or Beethoven, for example, must also be considered as beneficial. The research has shown that, with very few exceptions, patients undergoing music therapy experienced an improvement in their physical condition and a positive change in affectivity and reactive ability. Thus, music appears to be a powerful healing agent. It can also, however, elicit negative reactions if introduced indiscriminately or abusively utilized by destructive elements. The music therapist, therefore, must aim to counteract the diminishment of instinctively accepted or traditionally acquired positive values and, by reducing feelings of anxiety, reestablish a basis for communication in order to revitalize the general ethical concepts within the sociocultural framework. This aspect assumes even greater importance since, during the recent past, the world has experienced a downgrading of moral demands and social structures, and a general trend to emulate the undesirable — all developments which promote and support the establishment of a purely materialistic and performance-oriented society.[5]

All these considerations demand a reply to the question of how exactly the aims of a music-therapy program can be formulated. These aims are many and diverse, and their effectiveness depends largely on the highly individualistic reaction of the patient, irrespective of the psychiatric diagnosis. We can, however, summarize the aims as follows:

1. Emotional release.

2. Response to musical stimulation in form of primitive reactions.

3. Promotion of human contacts.

4. Integration into society.

5. Liberation from isolation.

6. Reduction of tension.

7. Attainment of a position within the sociocultural environment.

8. Relief from psychic pressure.

9. Promotion of will power.

10. Improved awareness of personal mood fluctuations.

11. Deflection from concentration on somatic ailments.

12. Promotion of self-disciplinary powers.

13. Reactivation of self-confidence.

14. Promotion of attainment experiences (learning through success).

15. Adjustment to life's problems.

16. Adequacy in dealing with daily requirements.

17. Improved ability to concentrate.

18. Recovery of learning ability and mnemonic capacity.

19. Stimulation of either collaborative or independently undertaken creative activities.

20. Suggestions for sensible hobbies.

21. Improved acceptance of demands imposed by duties or responsibilities.

22. Promotion of ability to face competitive situations.

23. Introduction to cultural activities.

24. Extension of the sphere of general interests.

In conclusion, the application of music as a healing agent appears as old as mankind itself and, in conjunction with magic rites, has accompanied and fortified attempts at medical treatment through the ages. Prominent musicians and composers — Mozart, Beethoven and, more recently, Kagel, to mention just a few — have stressed its suggestive powers.[6] Noted psychoanalysts such as Freud attribute to music the power to trace problems "which hide in the recesses of the soul in order to resolve them." Throughout the twentieth century, music therapy has won an established position within the medical profession. Recent developments indicate that mankind is becoming aware of the necessity to revitalize its social and cultural values.

Music undoubtedly will make an important contribution toward this process, and its significance as a therapeutic agent should find increasing recognition within a homogenous medical concept. The value accorded to music therapy in our time cannot, of course, be regarded as an indication for our society's cultural values, but within its scope, it can be effective in counteracting their deterioration. Seen from this perspective, music therapy appears to be an instrument capable of providing for some patients the humane and supportive environment so lacking in today's society. It should be our aim to assist those of our fellow men who find themselves unable to cope with the harsh realities of our society, and to prevent their apostrophization as "inferior." Music can make a considerable contribution toward such a goal.

REFERENCES

1. Revers WJ, Harrer G, Simon WC: Neue Wege der Musitherapie. Düsseldorf/Wien: Eccon, 1974.
2. Burton R (Cripps H, ed): Anatomy of Melancholy. Oxford, 1621.
3. Winter JA: Selbstüberwindung von Krankheit und Angst. Genf: Ramon Keller, 1972.
4. Radl I: Diplomarbeit, 1965.
5. Formann-Radl I, Kryspin-Exner R: Möglichkeiten der Musiktherapie bei Drogen abhängigen. Stuttgart, Thieme, Z Psychother med Psychol 26(3):85-92, 1976.
6. Geck M: Musiktherapie als Problem der Gesellschaft. Stuttgart: Klett, 1973.

SUGGESTED READING

1. Eggers C: Entwicklungspsychologische Apsekte der Anhedonie. *In* H. Heimann (Hrsg): Anhedonie — erlust der Lebens-freude. Ein zentrales Phänomen psychia-trischer Störungen. Stuttgart: Fischer, 1990.

CHAPTER 115

Music in Physical Rehabilitation in The Netherlands

Ineke Hansson-Bosma

Music therapy is considered to be of great value in the process of regaining complete psychological capability; this is why the act of making music tends to increase the patient's involvement in the process of rehabilitation.

Education as well as rehabilitation can be seen as a process of learning to cope with the demands of life. Music has been used throughout history in education. It has been looked upon in a numerous ways, throughout various culture. Action, communication and expression are value levels in on which music can have an impact. Therapists should be aware that rehabilitation is complete only if treatment has taken place on the three levels: activities; integration into communication with others; and integration into a person's view of his skills, values, and interests.

MATERIALS

The study described herein took place at the Revalidatie Centrum Hoensbroeck in 1990. The patients involved had been comatose for periods of six months to a year. They awakened with severe motor-, cognitive and social disabilities. Therapy had included group sensory-motor activities. The program included music, as well as visual and tactile elements.

As an occupational therapist, the author was convinced of the positive influence of auditory elements in rehabilitation of traumatically brain-injured adults.

METHOD

Auditory Elements

A group of patients sit in their wheelchairs around a table in the living room of the clinic. The author presents small musical instruments. One at a time, each participant plays his/her instrument in different ways (loud, low, fast, slow, etc.). Everyone listens to the player, who thus has the experience of being important in a positive way (emotional goal)

and experiences being listened to (preverbal communication, as a basic step in social behavior). The player is asked whether he has ever heard the sound before and is invited to describe his memories to the group (activating short-term and long-term auditory memory).

This design provides every member of the group with the opportunity of playing (*motor activity*), remembering (*cognitive activity*), listening (*social activity*), and associating memories hearing the stories of the other participants.

Socialization — First Stage

The participants are now asked to place their instruments in the middle of the table. The author invites them to request a different instrument. Again, one at a time, each plays the instrument and is asked to talk about the sound and its memories (training short-term memory). In addition, the participant is encouraged to exchange memories and associations with the former player of the instrument (social-skill training).

The period of listening and of recalling memories may require additional time because of the lack of memory in a post-coma patient. It is essential that he is supplied with enough time to learn to know himself, as he is now. That means how he feels, experiences and reacts.

As hemiplegia is frequent following coma, participants will have difficulties in using both hands. This is the reason for using small rhythmic instruments (Orff instruments) made of wood and metal. It is also possible to use other objects in the clinic, such as chairs, leaves of plants etc., or to use tapes with sounds of daily living; however, the chosen instruments should produce a quality sound. Adaptive equipment can be used to fixate the instruments.

In this phase, the joy of making music is of more importance than the motor- or technical aspect of making the sound.

Socialization — Second Stage

The next stage in therapy begins when a participant is ready to be invited to bring a tape with his favorite music. Most often, these will be popular songs, not classical music, especially if the age range of patients is 16-40 years.

While the participant presents this music, the group is asked to listen and react to the music (social goals). They are invited to play the rhythm of the music by hand on the table or, even better, on their own knee. It is also nice to accompany the taped music by playing the small instruments, and to form a small orchestra (guided motor- and cognitive activity).

The therapist has the important task of guiding the participants through their reactions, associations and memories about the music during this socialization process. Musical elements can be useful assessment and in helping the patient develop his tolerance, initiative, and activity level.

Consolidation of Cognitive Elements

As socialization develops, new cognitive elements are added: sounds (real instruments) and structures of sounds (tapes with classical music as well as popular and ethnic music). Repetition is necessary — in listening, playing instruments, and using sound elements as a part of games (e.g. musical goose-tray).

Thus, participants learn to identify auditory impressions and structures and they are encouraged to communicate them as well. Cognitive, social and motor ability are developed. *Problem-solving processes* can now be started, using musical elements to enhance re-education, analytical, and re-structuring skills.

Integrating New Skills into Social Behavior

Auditory elements and sound structures can be altered games such as passing a musical structure to another person, or playing and singing rondo.

It is of the utmost importance that the brain-injured adult develop a wide range of possible communicative reactions. Using music and musical structures, he is trained in a non-competitive way, and encouraged to react in a playful way.

As rehabilitation may take a year or even longer, there is sufficient time to practice ways of experimenting with music and social behavior. It may even be possible to continue music therapy in day-activity centers for brain-injured adults.

Expression

The brain-injured patient may experience a feeling of loss about his former abilities and social position. Listening to and making music can help him express anger or grief as a phase in the process of learning to accepting his present status. The music he himself is making is encouraged by the therapist, who, at that moment, acts as a creative arts therapist. This stage can take place at any point during the rehabilitation process.

Individual Treatment

Individual treatment with music in physical rehabilitation can be very successful for those with a special interest in music, if they can let go of the image of their former abilities.

A keyboard can be played even by a brain-injured adult with severe motor-, cognitive, emotional and social handicaps. Experience in this study with a severely brain-injured adult (following an overdose of contaminated heroin) resulted in his regaining emotional, cognitive and social and motor skills after a program of individual therapy with music using a JVC keyboard. A patient whose diabetes led to blindness and amputation of both legs below the knee was emotionally and physically rehabilitated by learning to play the piano as a form of recreation.

The Effect of Somatron and Music on Headache

Juanita McElwain

Studies which examine the effects of vibrotactile stimuli are fairly recent and therefore relatively few. Skille describes the field of vibroacoustic therapy (VAT) in Norway and its potential for music therapists, physiotherapists, psychologists, psychiatrists, physicians, chemotherapists, and chiropractors.[1] An overview is presented of the use of VAT in Britain, Finland, Germany, Denmark, and Estonia. Types of cases for which therapeutic benefits may result include Rett syndrome, autism, stress-induced depression, and general stress discomfort.

Darrow and Goll reported on a study of effects of vibrotactile stimuli on hearing impairment, in which the ability to identify rhythmic concepts was facilitated by supplementing auditory skills with vibrotactile stimuli.[2] Other studies include affective responses of musicians and non-musicians to a Somatron,[3,4] and an infant's crying and a Somatron.[5]

Specific research on the effects of vibrotactile stimuli and music with physiological dependent variables includes a study in which vibrotactile stimulation blunted perception of comfort and discomfort, with music preceding a dental drill reducing the drill's aversive effects, while the drill preceding music generally enhanced music's positive effects.[6] Neither music nor the dental drill, alone or in combination with vibrotactile stimulation, produced a consistent heart-rate response.

Stockton found no significant difference in respiration rates between subjects who listened to music with Somatron and those who listened to music alone.[7]

Studies of headache include migraine and tension headaches. Physiological measures assessed, including include heart rate, skin temperature, and skin resistance,[8] indicated no significant differences. Kroner found no differences in migraine response to conditions of stress, recovery, and relaxation when industrial noise and social discomfort stressors were followed by a recovery period. Relaxation was induced by verbal instructions accompanied by soft music. Lapp[9] found that music achieved superior results to biofeedback in decreasing severity, intensity, and duration of migraine headache, while both were superior to the control group. Interestingly, the music group was originally considered to be a second control group. Follow-up data at one year indicated that both biofeedback and music groups maintained change, but the subjects in the music group continued to show improvement in decreasing the frequency of headache.

Relaxation training combined with music reduced headaches in an 89-year-old, seriously ill nursing home patient with a 30-year history of tension headaches.[10] Epstein et al. presented music contingent on low electromyogram levels to determine effects of biofeedback on tension headache.[11] Results indicated that headache levels and medication requirements were low during biofeedback but increased when biofeedback was terminated.

Possible treatments for headache seem to include anti-depressants, muscle relaxants, relaxation, visual imagery, biofeedback training, and massage. The present study attempted to determine whether vibrotactile stimuli combined with music has an effect on headache.

METHOD

The purpose of the study was to determine whether or not music played through a Somatron has any effect on headache. The experiment was conducted in the Mr. & Mrs. Albert Sims Music Therapy Laboratory at Phillips University, Enid, Oklahoma.

Subjects

Subjects were volunteers who had any kind of headache at the time of treatment. No attempt was made to solicit subjects with a specific kind of headache. Kinds of headache included 20 tension, 2 migraine, 1 sinus, 1 allergy, and 1 other.

At the beginning of the session, subjects filled out a headache diary which indicated location of headache, what was happening and where subject was located at the onset of headache. Possible headache triggers including stress, alcohol use, tobacco use, and specific possible food triggers were listed. Additional information included on the consent form signed by each subject included kind of headache, if known, description of headache, and medication taken by subject.   At the close of the session, subjects completed the diary, indicating results of the session and approximate termination time of headache.

Aural Conditions

Subjects reclined on a Somatron Sound Lounge, an acoustic massage reclining chair, in a darkened room. Music, played on a Pioneer tape deck, was *Canyon Trilogy* by R. Carlos Nakai (Canyon Records Productions, Inc., CR-610). This is native American wooden flute music.

Design

Music was played through the Somatron for 30 minutes. Heart rate and skin-conductance level (SCL) were monitored through an Orion Model 8600 Biofeedback System. SCL is used in the Orion biofeedback system in place of galvanic skin response (GSR); this measurement is very similar in that it also measures skin perspiration and is a stress indicator.

Data collected included whether the session had successfully removed headache, based on subjects' reports, and continuous recordings of heart rate and SCL.

RESULTS

This study was designed to determine whether or not music played through a vibrotactile device (Somatron) would have any effect on headache. Analyses by Chi-Square of number of subjects who reported that headache had ceased at the end of treatment versus those who reported that headache had not ceased showed a significant difference at .001 level. All subjects with stress headache reported headache eliminated. The number of subjects with other headaches was too small to be significant. Results were: 20 stress headaches eliminated, 1 of 2 migraine headaches eliminated, 1 sinus headache eliminated, 1 allergy headache not eliminated, 1 other headache eliminated.

Changes in heart rate and SCL were not significant when analyzed by t-test. Heart-rate mean

for the first 3 minutes of sessions was 70.75 beats per minute and 75.14 beats per minute for the last 3 minutes. SCL mean for the first 3 minutes of sessions was 15.1, and 15.4 for the lats 3 minutes. The differences were not significant, but it was interesting to note a slight rise in both heart rate and SCL.

DISCUSSION

Most subjects were university students, who seem to be under a high stress level, possibly explaining the high percentage of subjects with stress headache.

Conjecture concerning the success of treatment includes a number of variables. Since the Somatron and music were an inseparable part of the treatment, the Somatron must be seriously considered as a contributing factor. This must address the direct application of vibration to eliminate or reduce pain. Further study comparing the three elements of Somatron vibration, music alone, and the combination of Somatron and music would seem to be indicated.

Relaxation, in all cases, did not seem to be a significant contributing factor, as indicated by the slight rise in heart rate and SCL. Some subjects reported an alertness after the headache ceased, which did not sound like verbal reports expected at the end of relaxation sessions.

Further study should determine whether the same results could be obtained using music without the Somatron. Another variable which should be studied is whether or not the same results would be obtained using other music. Some subjects reported effects of the wooden flute sound, which is a full round sound unlike that of the conventional flute. Reports included statements about the sound entering their heads and absorbing the pain. Other reports described the pain gradually moving to the neck before leaving.

REFERENCES

1. Skille O: VibroAcoustic therapy. Music Therapy 8(1):61-77, 1989.

2. Darrow A, Goll H: The effect of vibrotactile stimuli via the somatron on the identification of rhythmic concepts by hearing impaired children. Journal of Music Therapy 16(3):115-124, 1989.

3. Madsen C, et al: The effect of a vibrotactile device, "Somatron," on affective responses: Musicians versus non-musicians. Unpublished manuscript. Florida State University.

4. Madsen CK, Moore RS: Experimental Research in Music. Dubuque, IA: Kendall Hunt Publishing Co, 1974.

5. Geringer JM: The effects of Somatron and music on an infant's crying. Unpublished manuscript, 1989.

6. Standley JM: The effect of vibrotactile and auditory stimuli on perception of comfort, heart rate, and peripheral finger temperature. The Journal of Music Therapy 27(3):120-134, 1991.

7. Stockton J: The effect of music through speakers versus music through Somatron on respiration. Unpublished manuscript. Phillips University, Enid, OK, 1990.

8. Kroner-Herwig B, et al: Psychophysiological reactivity of migraine sufferers in conditions of stress and relaxation. Journal of Psychosomatic Research 32(4-5):483-492, 1988.

9. Lapp JE: Music can abort migraines: A one-year follow up. Unpublished manuscript. Muzak.

10. Linoff MG, West CM: Relaxation training systematically combined with music: treatment of tension headaches in a geriatric patient. International Journal of Behavioral Geriatrics 1(3):11-16, 1982.

11. Epstein LD, et al: Music feedback in the treatment of tension headache: An experimental case study. Journal of Behavior Therapy & Experimental Psychiatry 5(1):59-63, 1974.

CHAPTER 117

Composing or Choosing Music for Patient Use During Surgery

Kay Gardner

Music as an accompaniment to surgical procedures has been in use for centuries. Physicians in medieval times were required to study music as one of the seven liberal arts essential to medical training and were taught to feel musical rhythm in pulses.[1] After a hiatus of several generations, music is again finding uses in surgical arenas. Experiments to alleviate the tension of patients undergoing surgery were so successful that the University of Chicago medical research center now uses music with anesthesia in its operating rooms and preparation rooms.[2] When music was used as part of a preoperative teaching session for children, the group of patients receiving music therapy just prior to induction of preoperative medication evidenced less anxiety before and during induction.[3]

As a composer who for almost twenty years has written music specifically for relaxation, meditation, and healing, the author was invited to observe outpatient surgery at the Yale School of Medicine. The nurse-anesthetist who initiated the invitation was interested in how music could diminish the need for dangerous anesthetic drugs, it being felt by many in the field that the anesthesia is more dangerous than the surgery because dosages and patients' reactions to them are so variable.[4]

Based on the observations at Yale, the author believes there are three specific elements of music that may be used in composing or choosing music for patient use before, during, and after surgery. Each of the three elements — repetition, rhythm/pulse and melody — has a specific function.

The function of *repetition* is to bring familiarity, and thus comfort, to the listener. When relaxed, the patient is more receptive to whatever procedure is taking place.[4] When a repetitive pattern is presented, the patient is not required to give it any further direct attention.[5] Composing or choosing music with a repetitive pattern, or *ostinato*, can regulate the even balance of respiration.[6] Since an important part of relaxation is breath flow, regular rhythmic inhalation and exhalation helps to secure complete relaxation.[7]

Hypnotically repetitive music serves as an anesthetic, allowing a patient to enter a receptive, semi-hypnotic state, or trance.[8] Randall McClellan, in *The Healing Forces of Music*, writes: "In cultures where trance is a regular part of spiritual practice, ostinatos predominate in the accompanying music."[6] As relaxation continues, sensory thresholds are lowered,[9] anxiety is reduced and the patient needs lower doses of anesthetics.

The function of *rhythm/pulse* is to duplicate the pulses of the human organism (Fig. 1) through entrainment, a phenomenon discovered by Dutch scientist Christian Huyens in 1665. Also called *mutual phase-locking of two oscillators*, entrainment as it relates to the human body has been shown in the film *The Incredible Machine*, when two individual muscle cells from the heart beat each in its own pulse. As they move together, the rhythm shifts and the two cells are synchronized, beating together as one.[10]

The jury is still out on whether the heartbeat will entrain with musical pulse. Most of the experiments finding no tendency for synchrony between musical pulse and heart rate were carried out before 1955 using recorded Western classical music in which pulse does not predominate.[6] Utilizing modern medical and recording technologies, today's experiments would probably produce different conclusions. Meanwhile, the composer might score a 60 beats-per-minute heartbeat, such as a Spanish tango (Fig. 2), on timpani at forte to entrain the heart.[4]

We do know that evidence exists showing music's entrainment effects on respiratory rates[11] and brain-wave activity.[12] Composers may create music duplicating these pulses, but first, it is essential to know that the music composed or chosen should begin

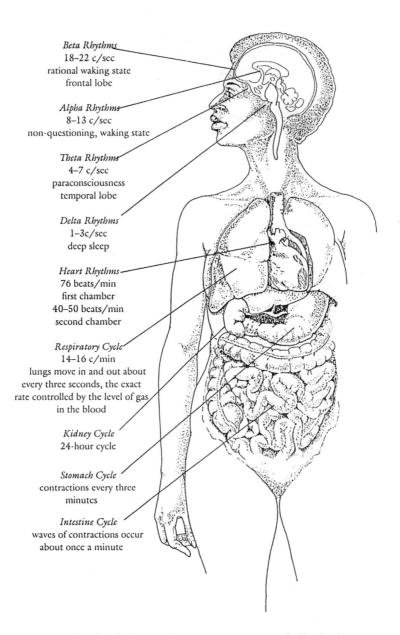

Beta Rhythms
18–22 c/sec
rational waking state
frontal lobe

Alpha Rhythms
8–13 c/sec
non-questioning, waking state

Theta Rhythms
4–7 c/sec
paraconsciousness
temporal lobe

Delta Rhythms
1–3c/sec
deep sleep

Heart Rhythms
76 beats/min
first chamber
40–50 beats/min
second chamber

Respiratory Cycle
14–16 c/min
lungs move in and out about
every three seconds, the exact
rate controlled by the level of gas
in the blood

Kidney Cycle
24-hour cycle

Stomach Cycle
contractions every three
minutes

Intestine Cycle
waves of contractions occur
about once a minute

Sounding the Inner Landscape: Music as Medicine by Kay Gardner
Printed with permission of publisher, Caduceus Publications

Figure 1: *Chart of Body Rhythms*

its pulses according to the *iso* principle,[13] that is, in sync with the patient's pulses, then moving to slower, healthier pulse rates. This maneuver honors the patient's process and serves as a bond between music and patient.

When choosing recordings for patients, slow movements (M.M.=60) from music of the Baroque period are effective for entrainment with respiration.[12] Breathing is a three-part cycle comprised of inhalation, exhalation and still point. During heavy exercise or anxiety, the still point is very short; in deep meditation, sleep, or coma, the still point is long. For the composer who wishes to duplicate the breath cycle, asymmetrical *breathing rhythms*[14] may be most effective (Fig. 3). (Composers: Setting a metronome to M.M.=60, one would take a normal breath cycle of 15 per minute and find that the complete breath cycle occurs in one four-beat measure. A breathing rhythm for this time frame might be 8/8(4/4) with an eighth-note grouping of 3+3+2.[4]

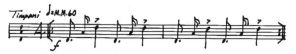

Figure 3: Spanish Tango Heart Pulse

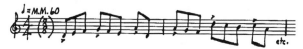

Figure 2: Asymmetrical 'Breathing' Rhythm

One of the principles of biofeedback is that if one is able to slow down one's brain waves, the heart rate and respiration will slow down as well. When the patient is awake and alert, the brain's predominant rhythm is at beta, 14-20 cps (high beta, 23-33 cps occurs with hyperactivity and some types of anxiety). When eyes are closed and awareness moves from external to internal matters, the patient's brain waves move into alpha, 8-13 cps. In deep meditation or sleep, theta waves, 4-7 cps, are most prevalent. Deep sleep and unconsciousness produce delta waves, 0.5-3 cps.[15] There are many New Age recordings claiming to pulse in alpha or theta pulses. For the composer, duplicating the brain waves may be achieved either with vibrato (easily programmed into synthesizers) or by writing long series of repetitive notes[4] (Fig. 4).

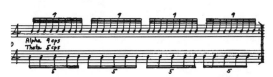

Figure 4: Musical Brain-Wave Rhythms

Pulse duplication as a gradual process starting with the iso principal may be utilized during the pre-surgery period. It then may continue to accompany the actual surgical procedure in order to maintain and regulate patients' pulses.

When the patient moves into the recovery room and begins to regain consciousness, music with melodic content is appropriate. The function of *melody* in medical music is to help relieve pain. In a study by Janet E. Lapp, sufferers of chronic migraine headaches learned to use music not only to enhance their relaxation skills, but to abort their headaches during the prodromal phase.[16] An uplifting, melodious piece of music can sweep a patient so totally into it that, while listening, he/she is unaware of the body. "Anything that moves one away from identification with the body will automatically be calming and reduce awareness of mental attachment to pain."[17]

The post-anesthetic process may be shortened by using music.[18] Music with a high melodic content could minimize postoperative pain.[19] Music of upbeat character in major rather than minor modes would bring the patient back to consciousness in a pleasant frame of mind.

SUMMARY

Slow, repetitive music is best used before surgery to reduce anxiety and to bring patients into relaxation. Music pulsing at alpha and theta brain-wave rates is appropriate during the surgical procedure to help maintain and regulate respiratory and heart rates and to mask extraneous noises and inappropriate surgical staff conversations. Melodious music used after surgery minimizes pain and speeds recovery.

REFERENCES

1. Cosman MP: Machaut's medical musical world. New York Academy of Sciences Journal 23-24, 1978.
2. Assagioli R: Music: Cause of disease and healing agent. *In* Music: Physician for Times to Come, 103. Wheaton, IL: Theosophical Publishing, 1991.
3. Chetta HD: The effect of music and desensitization on preoperative anxiety in children. Journal of Music Therapy 18(2):74-87, 1981.
4. Gardner K: Sounding the Inner Landscape: Music as Medicine, 59,78-96. Stonington, ME: Caduceus Publications, 1990.
5. Clynes M: On music and healing. *In* Music: Physician for Times to Come, 127. Wheaton, IL: Theosophical Publishing, 1991.
6. McClellan R: The Healing Forces of Music, 133-134, 181. New York: Amity House, 1988.
7. Bonny H, Savary L: Music and Your Mind, 94. New York: Harper and Row, 1973.
8. Moreno JJ: The music therapist: Creative arts therapist and contemporary shaman. *In* Music: Physician for Times to Come, 152. Wheaton, IL: Theosophical Publishing, 1991.

9. Guzzetta C: Music therapy: Nursing the music of the soul. *In* Music: Physician for Times to Come, 152. Wheaton, IL: Theosophical Publishing, 1991.

10. Leonard G: The Silent Pulse, 13-15. New York: EP Dutton, 1978.

11. Seashore CE: Psychology of Music, 143. New York: Dover, 1967.

12. Hutchison M; Megabrain, 92-93. New York: Ballantine, 1986.

13. Altshuler IM: Music as a therapeutic agent. *In* Music and Medicine, 269. New York: Henry Schuman, 1948.

14. Sachs C: Rhythm and Tempo. New York: WW Norton, 1953.

15. Goldman J: Sonic entrainment. *In* Music: Physician for Times to Come, 220-221. Wheaton, IL: Theosophical Publishing, 1991.

16. Lapp JE: Music vs biofeedback for migraine headache. Annual Convention of the American Psychological Association, Washington, DC, 1986.

17. Kelly G: *Quoted in* Music facilitates healing: Bodymind coordination. Brain/Mind Bulletin 8 (4), 1982 .

18. McClelland DC: Music in the operating room. AORN Journal 29(2):258, 1979 .

19. Malesky G: Music that strikes a healing chord. Prevention 56-63, 1983.

CHAPTER 118

Use of Music Stimuli in the Neuropsychological Assessment of Head Injury

Bryan C. Hunter

INTRODUCTION

The increase in services to head-trauma patients in the last decade has included music therapy in the interdisciplinary team approach.[1] Standards of practice require that patients be assessed prior to the delivery of music-therapy services.[2] The entry of music therapy into head-injury rehabilitation is recent, and standardized assessments are not yet available. Neuropsychologists, however, have used music stimuli as part of two major test batteries, the *Halstead-Reitan Battery* (HRB)[3] and the *Luria-Nebraska Neuropsychological Battery*,[4] for over 40 years to assess perceptual processing of nonverbal auditory stimuli. In particular, the *Seashore Rhythm Test* (SRT)[5] is included in the HRB as a measure of attention and concentration, and auditory discrimination.[6-10] In addition, some writers credit the SRT with being particularly sensitive to the presence of right-temporal-lobe damage[11,12] Although widely used in neuropsychology, the SRT has a history of problems, including reliability.[13] Music therapy needs accurate assessment tools to document any positive effects it may have in head-injury rehabilitation.

This study sought to determine whether the *Primary Measures of Music Audiation* (PMMA)[14] was a viable addition or alternative to the SRT.[15] The PMMA and the SRT were compared on their ability to discriminate between brain-injured and non-injured persons, and on their ability to predict lateralized brain damage. The relationship between gender, age, education, music training, time since onset of injury, attention/concentration, and auditory-discrimination scores also was examined. Finally, an attempt was made to learn what types of melodic and rhythmic auditory discriminations were most difficult for brain-injured persons.

The study focused on auditory-discrimination skills because they are important for participation in music, an aural art form, and they represent critical adaptive behaviors for everyday living. Music therapy has effected positive change in auditory discrimination in some handicapped populations,[16-18] and may hold similar potential for the head-injured.

Lesions which occur in the temporal lobes can result in deficient auditory-discrimination skills. Consequently, a poor performance on auditory-discrimination tasks such as those on the SRT and PMMA may indicate the presence of brain damage. Neuropsychologists long have been interested in assessing such deficits. Music therapists working with head-injured patients have a vested interest as well.

METHOD

The SRT, PMMA, and the *Digit Span Test* (DST) of the *Wechsler Intelligence Scales*[12] were administered to 80 volunteer Caucasian adults, 40 with traumatic brain injuries and 40 non-injured controls, matched for age and years of education. The injured subjects had suffered traumatic brain injury from blows to the head in motor vehicle accidents or in falls. The brain-injured subjects were functioning at the upper end of the *Rancho Los Amigos Scale*, levels 6-8, and had sought neuropsychological assessment or intervention because of deficits in brain-behavior relationships. All subjects signed approved consent forms before data collection procedures began.

RESULTS AND CONCLUSIONS

1. Discriminant analysis revealed that the brain-injured subjects scored significantly lower than the control group on all auditory-discrimination measures. The analysis further indicated that the SRT and the PMMA both achieved a 72.5% accuracy or "hit" rate in identifying subjects as either brain-injured or control. The binary classification rates, based on cutoff scores, achieved results similar to the discriminant analysis.

2. Discriminant analysis indicated that traumatic-brain-injured subjects classified as having primary right-brain damage, primary left-brain damage, or bilateral damage did not vary significantly in their auditory-discrimination abilities as indicated by scores on the SRT and PMMA. Consequently, neither the SRT nor the PMMA was reliable in classifying injured subjects according to lateralization of brain damage. Thus, the SRT was not sensitive to the presence of right-hemispheric damage in this sample. This result is consistent with other re-search[3,19] which does *not* support the use of the SRT to test for right-hemisphere damage.

3. Multiple regression analysis revealed that gender, age, formal education, music training, and time since onset of injury were not significantly related to auditory discrimination as indicated by scores on the SRT and PMMA. The analysis did show, however, that attention/concentration as measured by DST scores was strongly correlated with the SRT and PMMA, particularly in the brain-injured subjects, and was consistently the strongest predictor of auditory-discrimination scores in both the brain-injured and control groups. Thus, the SRT and the PMMA appear to measure, via nonverbal music stimuli, attention/concentration to some degree.

4. Item analysis of the SRT and the PMMA revealed that the PMMA internal reliability was greater than the SRT in the brain-injured sample (.85 vs. .73). In addition, the brain-injured persons had difficulty discriminating reversals of short rhythmic figures contained in otherwise identical patterns on the SRT. The brain-injured subjects also had trouble discriminating patterns whose first notes differed by a major second on the PMMA tonal subtest. These results may have programming implications for music therapists working with this population.

In conclusion, the PMMA appears to be a viable addition or alternative test to the SRT for assessing auditory discrimination and attention/concentration in traumatic-brain-injured patients. The PMMA matched the accuracy of the SRT (72.5%) in identifying subjects with head injuries, and its internal reliability was higher (.85 vs. .73).

REFERENCES

1. Clayes SM: Personal communication, November 19, 1988.
2. National Association for Music Therapy: Standards of clinical practice. Music Therapy Perspectives 1:13-16, 1983.
3. Reitan RM, Wolfson D: The Halstead-Reitan Neuropsychological Test Battery: Theory and Clinical Interpretation. Tucson, AZ: Neuropsychology Press, 1985.
4. Golden CJ, Hammeke TA, Purisch AD, Berg RA, Moses JA Jr, Newlin DB, Wilkening GN, Puente AE: Item Interpretation of the Luria-Nebraska Neuropsychological Battery. Lincoln, NE: University of Nebraska Press, 1982.
5. Seashore CE, Lewis D, Saetveit JG: Seashore Measures of Musical Talents: Manual. New York: The Psychological Corporation, 1960.
6. Boll TJ: The Halstead-Reitan Neuropsychology Battery. *In* Filskov SB, Boll TJ (eds), Handbook of Clinical Neuropsychology, 577-607. New York: John Wiley and Sons, 1981.
7. Golden CJ, Osmon DC, Moses JA Jr, Berg, RA: Interpretation of the Halstead-Reitan Neuropsychological Test Battery: A Casebook Approach. New York: Grune & Stratton, 1981.
8. Reitan RM: Investigation of the validity of Halstead's measures of biological intelligence. Archives of Neurology and Psychiatry, 73:28-35, 1955.
9. Reitan RM: Theoretical and methodological bases of the Halstead-Reitan Neuropsychological Test Battery. *In* Grant I, Adams KM (eds), Neuropsychological Assessment of Neuropsychiatric Disorders, 3-30. New York: Oxford University Press, 1986.
10. Sheer DE, Schrock B: Attention. *In* Hannay HJ (ed): Experimental Techniques in Human Neuropsychology, 95-137. New York: Oxford University Press, 1986.
11. Kolb B, Whishaw IQ: Fundamentals of Human Neuropsychology (2nd ed). New York: W.H. Freeman and Company, 1985.
12. Lezak MD: Neuropsychological Assessment (2nd ed). New York: Oxford University Press, 1983.
13. George WE: Measurement and evaluation of musical behaviors. *In* Hodges DA (ed), Handbook of Music Psychology, 291-392. Dubuque, IA: Kendall/Hunt Publishing Company, 1980.
14. Gordon EE: Primary Measures of Music Audiation: Manual. Chicago, IL: G.I.A. Publications, 1979.
15. Hunter BC: A comparison of the Seashore Rhythm Test and the Primary Measures of Music Audiation for auditory discrimination assessment in traumatic brain-injured patients. Unpublished doctoral dissertation, University of Kansas, Lawrence, 1989.

16. Grant RE: A developmental music therapy curriculum for the mildly mentally retarded, ages six through twelve. Dissertation Abstracts International, 38, 4009-A (University Microfilms No. 77-29, 760), 1977.

17. Humphrey T: The effect of music ear training upon the auditory discrimination abilities of trainable mentally retarded adolescents. Journal of Music Therapy 17:70-74, 1980.

18. Roskam, K: Music therapy as an aid for increasing auditory awareness and improving reading skill. Journal of Music Therapy 16:31-42, 1979.

19. Steinmeyer CH: Are the rhythm tests of the Halstead-Reitan and Luria-Nebraska batteries differentially sensitive to right temporal lobe lesions? Journal of Clinical Psychology, 40:1464-1466, 1984.

CHAPTER 119

Synchronizing
Music to Heart-Rate

Bradley R. Biedermann

REVIEW of the LITERATURE

Numerous research studies have investigated the effects of music listening on physiological processes. Of these studies, heart-rate has been the most commonly investigated parameter by far (Dainow, 1977). Music research in laboratory settings has attempted to clarify the interactive relationship between bodily and musical rhythms, but has produced variable results (Hodges, 1980).

Within medical settings, the therapeutic effects of music have been noted in several studies (Standley, 1986). Many studies have focused on music's ability to decrease or stabilize heart-rate during medical procedures. These studies have shown that music can have a beneficial effect on heart-rate during various medical treatments, including: intensive coronary care (Bonny, 1983; Guzzetta, 1989); dental procedures (Oyama, et al., 1987); debridement of burn patients (Barker, 1991); bronchoscopy (Metzler & Berman, 1991); childbirth (Brook, 1984); and preoperative conditions (Updike & Charles, 1987). Some other studies in medical settings, however, have failed to demonstrate significant heart-rate differences while listening to music (Davis-Rollans & Cunningham, 1987; Updike, 1990; Zimmerman, Pierson, & Marker, 1988).

The diversity of individual responses while listening to music has led some researchers to attempt to isolate those factors which may influence physiological measures. Researchers have noted the influence of personal factors in the listener which may influence heart-rate responses, including: reactions to variables in the experimental situation itself (Dainow, 1977), and the listener's relationship to the music--e.g., familiarity (Landreth & Landreth, 1974), preference (Davis & Thaut, 1989; DeJong, van Mourik, & Schellekens, 1973), and level of musicianship (DeJong et al., 1973).

Other researchers have isolated specific elements within the music which may influence heart-rate (Edwards, et al., 1991). Although many of the music and physiology studies have compared the relative effects of musical stimuli according to the general classifications of "stimulative" or "sedative," research has shown that these descriptors do not necessarily lead to predictable physiological changes (Taylor, 1973). Several authors have suggested the need for greater definition of musical stimuli during music research, based on individual reactions to specific pieces of music (Hanser, 1985; Hodges, 1980).

Another factor which may influence listener's heart-rate is the principle of entrainment. This principle has been observed during physiological research utilizing music or related elements. Using an audible click over a loudspeaker, Bason & Celler (1972) were able to entrain this auditory stimulus with the listener's heart-rate. By producing this beat at a precise time (within 0.1 second) in the individual's cardiac cycle, it could be used to control heart-rate increases or decreases over a duration of several minutes. In another study, Saperston (in press) achieved significant decreases in listeners' heart-rate using 'physiologically interactive tempo'--music played at a tempo consistently 1-1.9 beats below each subject's ongoing heart-rate.

MATERIALS and METHODS

The present study attempted to isolate the effects of musical tempo on listener heart-rate. The effects of entrainment were also observed. Using a repeated measures design, the heart-rate responses of 19 adult non-musicians were compared under three different 6-minute conditions. Two of these conditions utilized the same music at different tempo settings: a) "entrained"--at a steady tempo equal to the listener's initial heart-rate (for 3 minutes), and then gradually decreased in tempo; and b) "slow"--at a steady tempo of 10 beats per minute below the listener's initial heart-rate. The third was a control condition of silence. Dependent measures included heart-rate (monitored continually at 10-second intervals during the session), and a preference survey for the music (completed after the session).

The three conditions were presented in random order following a 3-minute baseline period, during one 45-minute session. Three-minute periods of silence were also added prior to the baseline period, and following each music condition. These periods were added to allow heart to stabilize between experimental conditions. In addition, the listener's average heart-rate during the final 1 min 40 sec of this time provided the starting tempo for the subsequent music condition.

Each music condition consisted of two baroque pieces--"Largo" from "Winter" of *The Four Seasons* by A. Vivaldi, and "Air" from *Suite No. 3 in D* by J.S. Bach. This particular music was selected for the study for a few reasons. Both pieces contain a continuous and non-syncopated quarter-note bass rhythm, which would provide a steady beat for the synchronization with heart-rate. In addition, both pieces had been utilized in previous physiological studies, and cited for their relaxing qualities.

Digital technology was utilized to allow variations in tempo without altering the other musical elements. The sounds of the musical instruments were reproduced using a digital sampling workstation--Ensoniq EPS-16 Plus. Sampled wind- and string sounds by Ensoniq were utilized to orchestrate the two pieces (English Horn, Flute, Mini-Violin, and Nylon Guitar). The pieces were digitally sequenced using the Performer program for the Macintosh computer. This program was used to generate the pieces during the study and to control the starting tempo and tempo changes.

RESULTS

Figure 1 shows the heart-rate levels for each treatment condition, as averaged across each 1-minute period. Correlated tests were used to analyze the significance of heart-rate changes (averaged across each 1-minute of treatment) from baseline levels. These analyses showed that heart-rate decreased significantly from baseline levels during two 1-minute periods within both music conditions (Table 1). The greatest decreases in heart-rate from baseline levels occurred within the entrained condition during the

third minute (p $\langle$ .01).

Table 1: Mean heart-rate; baseline v. each condition and time period.

Condition	Total	Period: 1	2	3	4	5	6
Baseline	69.2						
Entrained	68.0	68.1	67.7	67.3	68.0	68.6	68.1
Slow	68.1	68.0	68.0	67.7	68.2	67.6	68.5
Silence	68.9	68.8	68.8	68.7	68.7	69.5	69.0

_p< .05_   _p< .01_

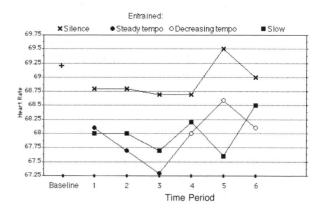

Figure 1: *Mean heart-rate for each time period.*

Comparison of the three conditions using a one-way analysis of variance with repeated measures is given in Table 2. This analysis indicated no significant differences in heart-rate responses between the three overall treatment conditions. Additional analyses using ANOVA for each one-minute period also failed to distinguish the three treatment conditions (p > .1 in all cases).

Regression analysis was used to assess the influence of listener's preference ratings on heart-rate responses during the three treatment conditions (Table 3). For this analysis, individual heart-rate responses were transformed into percentage change scores (from baseline levels) for each 10-second reading. Individual percentage change scores were then grouped according to each musical piece within the two music conditions. A significant interaction was demonstrated between listeners' preference ratings on two scales ("second piece" and "overall sound quality") and degree of heart-rate change during Bach within the slow music condition.

preference ratings on two scales ("second piece" and "overall sound quality") and degree of heart-rate change during Bach within the slow music condition.

A one-factor ANOVA using heart-rate percentage change scores was also used to calculate the variance between subjects across the three conditions. This analysis showed that inter-individual heart-rate responses differed significantly during these conditions ($p < .002$), and indicated diverse individual responses

Source of Variation	SS	df	MS	F	p
Total	6676.26	56			
Subjects	6536.12	18			
Treatments	10.448	2	5.224	1.45	.2479
Residual	129.692	36	3.603		

Table 2: *One-way analysis of variance. Heart-rate by treatment condition*

Table 3: *Regression analysis. Preference x heart-rate change per music.*

Preference Scale	Condition	F	p	r	r-squared
"1st Piece"	No significance during any condition ($p > .3$)				
"2nd Piece"	Entrained (avg.)	.043	.8386		
	Slow-Vivaldi	3.256	.0889		
	Slow-Bach	7.205	.0157	.546	.298
	Silence (1-3 min.)	.83	.3749		
	Silence (4-6 min.)	4.26	.0546		
"Sound Quality"	Entrained (avg.)	.004	.9845		
	Slow-Vivaldi	2.855	.1094		
	Slow-Bach	8.089	.0112	.568	.322
	Silence (1-3 min.)	.294	.5944		
	Silence (4-6 min.)	3.817	.0674		

$p < .05$

to the same stimuli.

DISCUSSION

The results suggested a downward trend in listener heart-rate responses to a steady tempo which had been matched to heart-rate. This occurred during the first 3 minutes of the music--which corresponded with the piece by Vivaldi, and the "A" section of the piece by Bach. Although the greatest decreases in heart-rate occurred during the entrainment condition, these levels were not statistically differentiated from heart-rate levels during the other treatment conditions. Furthermore, when the tempo of the music was gradually decreased (during minutes 4-6 of the entrainment condition) heart-rate levels returned to the initial treatment values or higher. Therefore, this portion of the procedure did not have an apparent effect on heart-rate.

Degree of listener preference did not demonstrate any noticeable impact on heart-rate levels during the entrainment condition. During the piece by Bach within the slow condition, however, degree of preference was significantly correlated with decreases in listener's heart-rate. These findings suggested that the music within the entrainment condition may have influenced heart-rate changes independent of the degree of listener's preference.

In summary, the entrainment procedure using music may offer a mechanism for decreasing listener heart-rate. Additional research is needed to assess the effectiveness of other protocols for entrainment, and the possible usefulness of other musical stimuli with this approach. The investigation of alternative entrainment protocols and music may also help to adapt this procedure to suit the idiosyncratic response tendencies of different listeners.

REFERENCES

1. Barker, L. W. The use of music and relaxation techniques to reduce pain of burn patients during daily debridement. *In* C. D. Maranto (Ed.), Applications of music in medicine (pp. 123-140). Washington, DC: National Association for Music Therapy, 1991.

2. Bason, P. T., & Celler, B. G. Control of the heart-rate by external stimuli. Nature, 238, 279-280, 1972.

3. Bonny, H. L. Music listening for intensive coronary care units: A pilot project. Music Therapy, 3, 4-16, 1983.

4. Brook, E. Soothing music during the active phase of labor: Physiologic effect on mother and infant. Unpublished master's thesis, The University of Florida, Gainesville, 1984.

5. Dainow, E. Physical effects and motor responses to music. Journal of the Acoustical Society of America, 39, 414-416, 1977.

6. Davis, W. B., & Thaut, M. H. The influence of preferred relaxing music on measures of state anxiety, relaxation, and physiological responses. Journal of Music Therapv, 26, 168-187, 1989.

7. Davis-Rollans, C., & Cunningham, S. G. Physiologic responses of coronary care patients to selected music. Heart & Lung, 16, 370-378, 1987.

8. DeJong, M. A., van Mourik, K. R., & Schellekens, H. M. A physiological approach to aesthetic preference-music. Psychotherapy and Psychosomatics, 22, 46-51, 1973.

9. Edwards, M. C., Eagle, C., Pennebaker, J., & Tunks, T. Relationships among elements of music

10. Guzzetta, C. E. Effects of relaxation and music therapy on patients in a coronary care unit with presumptive acute myocardial infarction. Heart & Lung, 18, 609-616, 1989.

11. Hanser, S. P. Music therapy and stress reduction research. J. Music Therapy, 22, 193-206, 1985.

12. Hodges, D. A. Appendix A: Physiological responses to music. *In* D. A. Hodges (Ed.), Handbook of music psychology. (pp. 393-400). Washington, DC: N.A.M.T., 1980.

13. Landreth, J. E., & Landreth, H. F. Effects of music on physiological response. Journal of Research in Music Education, 22, 4-12, 1974.

14. Metzler, R. K., & Berman, T. The effects of sedative music on the anxiety of bronchoscopy patients. *In* C. D. Maranto (Ed.), Applications of music in medicine (pp. 163-178) . Washington, DC: N.A.M.T., 1991.

15. Oyama, T., Hatano, K., Sato, Y., Kudo, M., Spintge, R., & Droh, R. Endocrine effect of anxiolytic music in dental patients. *In* Spintge & Droh (Eds.), Music in medicine (pp. 223-226). New York: Springer-Verlag, 1987.

16. Saperston, B. M. The effects of consistent tempi and physiologically interactive tempi on heart-rate and EMG responses. *In* T. Wigram, B. M. Saperston, & R. West (Eds.), Music and the healing process: A handbook of music therapy. London: Carden Publications Limited, in press.

15. Standley, J. M. Music research in medical/dental treatment: Meta-analysis and clinical applications. Journal of Music Therapy, 22, 56-122, 1986.

16. Taylor, D. B. Subject responses to precategorized stimulative and sedative music. Journal of Music Therapy, 18, 62-73, 1981.

17. Updike, P. A. Music therapy results for ICU patients. Dimensions in Critical Care Nursinq, 9, 39-45, 1990.

18. Updike, P. A., & Charles, D. M. Music Rx: Physiological and emotional responses to taped music programs of preoperative patients awaiting plastic surgery. Annals of Plastic surgery 19, 29-33, 1987.

19. Zimmerman, L. M., Pierson, M. A., & Marker, J. Effects of music on patient anxiety in coronary care units. Heart & Lung, 17, 560-566, 1988.

CHAPTER 120

Schizophrenia and Music:
Research into Nonverbal Communication

Grethe Lund

INTRODUCTION

To be able to communicate, to talk to others, is vital, but since language may be experienced as dangerous by the schizophrenic person, he/she must either deny or transform it — make it less dangerous.[1] This new formation, a so-called formal disturbance of thought or neologism, makes it difficult for relatives and others to communicate with the schizophrenic individual. By using musical sounds as a means of communication, these verbal difficulties can be evaded.[2]

Music as a means of communication has qualities different from those of verbal communication, in that the musical communication takes place through a different set of rules, or absence thereof, and a contact may be established which otherwise had not been possible.[3] The musical communication is not only nonverbal, which is important, but nondiscursive as well, and nonrational in its development of thought, precluding the possibility of metacommunication.[4] While the musical communication is nondiscursive, at the same time, it contains discursive and verbal elements. Verbal communication always contains nonverbal and nondiscursive elements. Music therapy is thus mostly a 'pure' form of interactive psychotherapy.[5]

Inspired by Rosenbaum and Sonne,[6] the author analyzed tapes containing clinical improvisations by schizophrenic patients, recorded during music-therapy sessions at the Viborg Psychiatric Hospital.[7] A clinical improvisation takes place between a patient/subject and the music therapist whereby all the sounds the patient/subject makes by means of percussion instruments are answered by the therapist, who uses the piano as his/her instrument.[8] All improvisations are taped, in order that they may be analyzed later. The patient does not have to study an instrument or have any knowledge of music to be able to participate in music therapy.

MATERIAL

The sample consisted of eight schizophrenic patients and eight normal subjects, age 21-42 years. Each person contributed 10 clinical improvisations (160 total). This does not mean that only these improvisations were taped, but that 10 continuous improvisations from each patient were selected. Selection criteria was that the improvisations gave a picture of the patient's development during the course of therapy. Subjects also participated in 10 sessions corresponding to 10 improvisations. They were told that the author was interested in their musical language and wanted to know if their language was different from that of the schizophrenic patients.[9]

HYPOTHESIS

If a musical language exists, it must manifest itself in the music improvisations in the same way that verbal schizophrenic language manifests itself in writing and speech.[6] Greater knowledge and understanding of a musical schizophrenic language will be important to nonverbal communication unfolding itself in clinical improvisations. This knowledge will pave the way for better interaction, primarily musical. A positive interaction contributes to greater patient confidence with regard to the therapist. This confidence-building may help alleviate schizophrenic symptoms.[10]

METHOD

The basis of the analysis was the use of musical elements[11] and instruments.[12] The elements were chosen only according to the frequency of their occurrence in the improvisations. The analysis partially started with reflections on the occurrence and general use of these elements compared to their occurrence in the improvisations: frequency, duration, loudness of the occurring elements, and use of the instruments. Moreover, it included the attitude of the therapist toward these elements connected with improvisations. The elements were: (1) pulse, (2) repetitions of notes, (3) repetitions of motif, (4) sequences, (5) unstable stepwise movement, (6) glissando, (7) trills, and (8) pauses.

DISCUSSION

There do not seem to be the same differences in nonverbal phrasing between schizophrenics and non-schizophrenics, as in the case of verbal phrasing. Looking at the first element, *pulse*, it is remarkable that not only schizophrenics may lack this element. Lack of pulse in clinical improvisations does not mean lack of a sense of rhythm. It points more towards an existential fear of contact with the therapist. All persons displaying lack of pulse seemed to be more disturbed and frustrated than the others; the interaction was negative in the musical improvisations. The fact that some schizophrenic patients apparently conquer or master this fear, so that it does not express itself in lack of pulse, is striking. It is also noteworthy that three subjects lacked a sense of pulse. This may be due to the fact that subjects were allowed only 10 sessions each. A longer course of therapy sessions may have enabled them to overcome the fear manifesting itself in lack of pulse. Lack of pulse appears to be important to the use of the other elements, and it is not pathognomonic of schizophrenia. Schizophrenia does not always disturb the rhythmical element in a person's musicality or nonverbal manner of expression. The lack of a sense of pulse in the schizophrenic is not directly related to the disease.

Note repetition seems to be the most used form of element development, especially with non-schizophrenics. There appears to be a connection between soft-note repetition and the lack of pulse, which may symbolize a weak self-identity.[13]

Repetitions of motifs and *sequences* are seen more often with schizophrenics than non-schizophrenics. The use of these elements may point towards a tendency to perseveration, but it could also be a way to manifest oneself, to establish oneself as an individual.

Unstable stepwise movements were seen in only one subject. If the element is present, caution is advised. It indicates a lack of security so great it cannot be hidden. It is logical that this element would go together with lack of pulse.

Glissando and *trills*. If we presume that these two elements symbolize happiness and reserve of psychic strength, it is obvious that they hardly ever appear in schizophrenics.

As *pauses* are very short for both schizophrenics and non-schizophrenics, the author does not give them too much importance. Pauses often took place in connection with the change of beaters or instruments.

It cannot be proven that use or non-use of the instruments is of importance in the diagnosis of schizophrenia. The choice and use of instruments in the improvisations indicates something about the patient's *sound-range*. The author became aware that sound range and, in this case, a specific *mutual sound-range* of therapist and patient, was an element of great importance and must be included in the analysis.[14]

MUTUAL SOUND-RANGE

The fact that nonverbal communication seems less dangerous than verbal communication may be one reason that schizophrenic patients initially consider the nonverbal form attractive. Here, they find a possibility of expressing themselves without misunderstandings or paraphrases.

Why, then, do some of these patients want to stop music-therapy sessions after some time? The reason may be that the involvement of primary process material and the flow of associations becomes too overwhelming.[15] Another possibility is that the patient starts to experience contact which is frightening because of the inveterate mistrust and fear of being swallowed up or obliterated as an individual, or because the autism has been broken. A third reason may be that the therapist, unknowingly, frightens the patient because he/she does not respect the patient's sound-range. The therapist does not play, or answer the patient, within his/her sound-range.

SOUND-RANGE, PULSE, AND INTERACTION

The investigation indicates that a mutual sound-range between the patient/subject and therapist may be important to the pulse, which is important to the interaction. The lack of mutual sound-range between patient and therapist affects, presumably, the patient's feelings of security/confidence. The lack of mutual sound-range, therefore, would affect the pulse and, consequently, the interaction. An unstable pulse causes difficulties for the therapist in establishing contact with the patient. Until this contact is established, one is still at the preliminary stage of the therapy course. The therapist's failure to meet the patient in his/her sound-range may be one of the causes of a bad/ negative interaction,[14] which means 'talking past each other.' In musical communication, the patient plays in the treble octave and is answered by the therapist in the great octave; a light sound from the patient is answered by a dark one from the therapist. This chain reaction seems to be important to the result of the therapy course — not only with the schizophrenic patients, but with the subjects as well. The chain-reaction has the following sequence:

Mutual Sound-Range → Pulse → Positive Interaction

CONCLUSION

The use of certain musical elements and not others has not proven that musical improvisations can be used in diagnosing schizophrenia, nor is the use or non-use of the available percussive instruments of diagnostic value. It has not been possible to prove that schizophrenics have a *musical language* different from that of non-schizophrenics. One cannot conclude that there is no difference, but that whatever possible difference exists cannot be proven on the basis of the musical elements and instruments chosen in this study. Moreover, it is possible that the sample size is insufficient.

The final stage of the investigation, analysis of the improvisations in relation to a mutual sound-range, has proven to some degree that a course of music therapy, essentially starting in a mutual sound-range, results in a positive interaction and greater patient confidence in regard to the therapist. A closer examination of a mutual sound-range used by the therapist at the outset may help test the this theory.

REFERENCES

1. Arieti S: Interpretation of Schizophrenia. New York: Basic Books, 1974.
2. Lund G: Music therapy with a schizophrenic patient. British Journal of Music Therapy 15(2):10-12, 1984.
3. Lund G: Music therapy with psychiatric patients. Third International Symposium on Music in Medicine, Education and Therapy for the Handicapped, 139-143. University Press of America, 1985.
4. Watzlawick P: Pragmatics of Human Communication. New York: WW Norton, 1967.
5. Strobel W: Musiktherapie mit schizophrenen patienten. Musiktherapeutische Umschau 6:177-208, 1985.
6. Rosenbaum & Sonne: The Language of Psychosis. New York: University Press, 1986.
7. Lund G: Skizofreni og Musik - en Analyse af Nonverbal Kommunikation. Denmark: Aalborg Universitetsforlag, 1988.
8. Priestley M: Music Therapy in Action. London: Constable, 1975.
9. Cooke D: The Language of Music. Oxford: University Press, 1978.
10. Benedetti G: Skizofreni og Psykoterapi. Denmark: Odense Universitetsforlag, 1983.
11. Seashore CS: Psychology of Music. New York: Dover Publishing, 1967.
12. Sachs C: The History of Musical Instruments. New York: WW Norton, 1968.
13. Hamel MP: Through Music to The Self. Great Britain: Compton Press, 1978.
14. Grinder & Bandler: The Structure of Magic II. Palo Alto, CA: Science and Behavior Books, 1976.
15. Freud S: Metapsykologi 2. København: Hans Reitzel, 1976.

CHAPTER 121

Music Therapy for Hypoacoustic Infants

Isabel Luñansky

The work described herein was begun in Jerusalem in 1973. It is based on affection, and is applied through the sonorous-corporal-musical bond with the patient and his/her family. Treatment is personalized, and the result is the inclusion of the hypoacoustic infant in the social-domestic environment, which often is hostile.

It is generally believed that, since the hypoacoustic individual is unable to hear normally, he is alienated; this alienation increases to the point of *listening autism*. Consequently, the individual loses his connection with the surrounding world.

The author has observed this phenomenon repeatedly. In virtually every case, the alienation resulted from the continuous exclusion from everyday family life. If exclusion of the hypoacoustic is caused by the hearing, it is also the hearing who must initiate the move toward inclusion.

Internal sounds can be felt through sensors throughout the body. If, in this way, one can perceive temperature differences, and can discriminate the agreeable from the disagreeable, the pleasant from the unpleasant, differences of pressure, weight, texture, and shape, one can also distinguish the sound of vibration.

Connection with the external world produces various emotions, which are translated into corporal vibrations. This is common to both the hearing and the hypoacoustic — perhaps aggravated in the latter, whose listening 'alarms' are diminished.

Discussions of these concepts are held with the patient's parents, and are aimed at making this mechanism a conscious one.

METHOD

Starting from a state of relaxation, allowing an enhanced connection with the internal being, the heartbeat is used as the first sound-vibration. The heartbeat is chosen because it provides rhythm and is part of each act of life; it is the source of internal energy and of connection with the exterior. Thus, the basic rhythm for the treatment is the cardiac rhythm.

The following step is designed to establish coordination between respiratory and cardiac rhythms. It corresponds a breathing rhythm to each cardiac one, resulting in a rhythm unique to each individual. This alliance allows the possibility of a language with a distinct rhythm.

This affective-sonorous-corporal bond produces an action, which is to mobilize and musicalize; the result is the discovery of the baby's own potentials. A playful-rhythmic-musical activity is developed, in which body and sonorous-musical objects take part.

Inclusion of the family group is progressive. First, the author works alone with the patient during the activity, although the mother is present. The mother participates in the task when she is able to begin connecting with her own rhythm. The procedure is then followed with the father and any siblings.

Although the cardiac rhythm is the permanent base, recordings are superimposed, according to the rhythm of the language. Sounds of special effects are used — in particular, Stiven Halpern's compositions. To simulate aquatic sounds, the harp is used; in stressful situations, panpipe (siku) works are selected. To enhance the affective mother-child relationship, old Spanish lullabies and songs created by the mother are used.

Finally, the interaction of babies with their mothers is proposed, in a first socializing experience.

RESULTS

The following results have been observed in children who have undergone this therapy during the first months of life:

- improved rhythm;
- less fear of external stimulation;
- greater attentiveness;
- improved equilibrium;

- greater self-confidence and self-esteem;
- language is more melodious and better modulated; and
- stronger connection with the external world.

CHAPTER 122

Melody-Programmed Speech Therapy

Anne-Marie Ferrand-Vidal

DEFINITION

Melody therapy is a part of speech therapy because its purpose is to cure aphasia by way of the melody of the speech delays. Indeed, speech is first a melody — a music of sounds or phonemes to which words are fitted. The meaning of these words is in accordance with the melody.

Oral language can be defined as a combination of two structures (Fig. 1):

■ S1 *melodic* structure (chronologically the first); and

■ S2 *signifying* structure (the word in a spoken sequence).

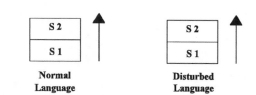

Figure 1: *Language structures.*

When S2 does not exist (e.g. in autism, psychotic states, dysphasia, etc.) or is disturbed (aphasia), it can be reacquired by way of the S1 pre-existing structure.

The method consists of using the prosody of language, i.e. tones, accents, pauses, and intonation, or melodic scheme.

INDICATIONS

Indications for melody therapy include speech- and language disorders (stammering, dyslexia), as well as language delays (dysphasia, absence of language in children aged six years and older, not due to mental retardation or an auditory deficit).

A sample model of corpus must be built by several experts: neurologist, psychologist (or psycho-analyst), phoniatrician, linguist, and musicologist. The

last is absolutely useful to built the "melodies," the "item-sentences," to take into consideration the pauses, the tones, the accents of the melodic schema (Fig. 2).

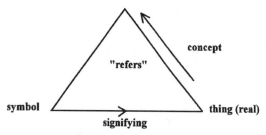

Figure 2: *Model of corpus.*

Melody therapy, by way of rhythm, melody, and a combination of S1 and S2 structures, acts on the symbol and at the same time on the signifying. Thus, it complements traditional speech therapy.

METHOD

Before using melody therapy with children, it is essential to have an active music-therapy session composed of a listening period and an active period, illustrating:

■ rhythm — particularly biological rhythm, since this is experienced before the rhythm of language; and

■ body awareness — especially for autistic children, whose disturbed corporeal diagram disrupts the communication diagram.

Rhythm: The rhythm of the sentence is demonstrated by hand. The therapist takes the patient's hand and strikes the rhythm with him/her. This begins the relationship between the therapist and the patient. The "conveyance" begins here.

Melody: Continuing the rhythm, the therapist introduces the melody by singing softly. The patient accompanies the therapist, who then withdraws his/her input.

Words: The therapist then adds words to the melody, always keeping the rhythm. The patient accompanies him/her, and then sings the *item-sentence* alone.

Communication can be summarized as follows: *what* (afflictions, anguish, joy); *how* (by way of speech, drawing, music, gesture); *to whom* (in this case, the therapist). Thus, the chances of drawing out an autistic or psychotic child are greater when mixing several therapies: relating to music, words, speech, and gesture.

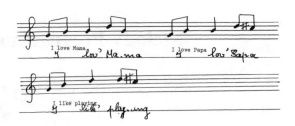

Figure 3: *Example of melody-programmed speech therapy.*

PART IX

NEUROSCIENCES

CHAPTER 123

Listening to Dreams: A Project for
Middle Ear Muscle Activity Audio Level Telemetry

R.I.P. Hayman

Medical sleep research has confirmed what common sense has always known: dreaming is essential to our health and well-being. Without regular dreams our minds know no rest. Numerous studies have indicated the REM (rapid eye movement) stage of sleep as the dream period in which the brain seems to decode information at random and regenerate. To the dreamer it is a period of vivid imagination, yet most often without memory function. Only through effort and training does one gain the ability to have some self-conscious control and remembrance of dream imagery.

People do not usually notice sounds in dreams. Yet voices and background sounds are part of the 'reality' of a dream. Their emotional impact is essential to the power of a dream. Silence is sometimes experienced in an otherwise visually vivid dream and can be more noticeable than the normal hubbub of a scene.

We sleep with our ears open and are quite adept at screening out our usual sounds in order to sleep well. Unusual sounds may alert the listening monitor of the brain and awaken us suddenly. This is a function we share with many animals whose acute hearing is essential to survival. Mothers are particularly attuned to the cry of children in the night, even when others may not notice the sound.

Some sounds enter our dream stage and conjure or transform images. A common experience is the sound of a radio alarm entering morning dreams in distorted images. The intriguing qualities of listening while dreaming have been widely researched and used as suggestive training. The author has developed and performed *Dreamsound,* a night-long event for a sleeping audience based on these phenomena. It is an unusual social context and concert in which the audience provides the imagination. A simple sound may produce a wide variety of dream responses, as related over breakfast.

As a composer who imagines much sound in my dreams, the music I conjure in my sleep is free of the 'real world' constraints encountered while awake. All manners of sound, instruments, and collaborators may appear by chance or by command. The internal high fidelity is unmatched by mere external hearing. But, alas, it is all so fleeting. To roll over in bed can erase the entire experience.

Researchers at Montefiore Medical Center, Bronx, N.Y., performed studies related to a physical phenomenon known as middle-ear muscle activity, or MEMA.[1] This is a function of the brain to the tympanic tensor muscles which control the tension of the eardrums. Usually, these muscles move in response to the level of external sounds, tensing to protect the ears from loud sound and relaxing to allow sensitivity to soft sound. During dream-sleep, phasic discharges pass through the cortex to the sensory area and trigger images. The discharges also trigger simultaneous motor response that produce MEMA and REM. As the eye muscles move in the pattern of the eyes following the imagined vision, so do the middle-ear muscles respond to the imagined sounds. The function is different in that the nerve impulses of REM are a following motion rather than a direct impulse from the dream sound.

The sleep research laboratory at Montefiore was conducting correlation studies of MEMA with the reported sound imagery of volunteer dreamers. The MEMA was recorded by a pressure-strain gauge embedded in a custom plastic ear mold fitted next to the tympanic membrane (eardrum). The movement of the muscles as transmitted through the eardrum was registered on a polygraph alongside simultaneous REM- and brain-wave readings from electrodes. The MEMA was registered at subaudio frequencies, yet clearly showed dynamic variations. The dreamers were awakened at intervals to describe as much as possible the sounds imagined, yielding a close relation to the

MEMA readings. The sounds imagined and correlated were loud - 85 decibels and over, as subjectively estimated by the dreamers.

Based on experience as a volunteer sleeper, the author wondered whether the MEMA could be recorded at audio levels so as to actually hear the sounds imagined in dreams. This would be a remarkable acheivement in a number of ways. There is now no objective record of dream imagery, only the often vague recollections of the awakened dreamer. To actually listen to the 'soundtrack' of dreams could be a valuable tool for the study of the mind. For the musician, such a technique would tap the very fount of imagination.

But is this truly feasible? With the cooperation of the researchers at Montefiore and the support of the ZBS Media Foundation, the author performed a preliminary experiment to make an audio-level recording of MEMA. The ear mold was fitted with a miniature electric condensor microphone. During six hours of sleep in an audio studio, a high-level recording was made of the sounds from the ear mold at my eardrum. A control track was recorded on another channel by an air mike near my head. In subsequent listening and editing, the two channels were compared for sounds emanating from the eardrum. The ear has this ability as a bio-acoustic system. The ringing of tinititus is a common example.

Numerous small murmurs, pops, and brief tones from the ear were compiled. Yet the results were negligible due to the interference of the sounds of respiration, blood circulation, and body movements. The instances of quiet needed to hear the very faint MEMA sounds were very brief between the relatively loud other sounds. A computer analysis of the audio tapes to isolate the signal was discussed, but would be unlikely to succeed. Even if this were possible, the audio dream imagination once transferred via nerve to the tensor muscles to the eardrum would probably be crude dynamics rather than a clear audio 'line out' from the brain.

A signal could be obtained by electrode implantation on the nerve endings to the muscles. This was done on cats, but at their sacrifice. This would be crude intervention for a human, and dangerous to hearing. The nerve would need to be monitored by some telemetric technique. Magnetic resonance imaging provides a possible means, but its most fine focus is of large ganglion, too large for this small nerve. Even this signal, once recorded, may need elaborate decoding to approach a listenable rendition of what is heard by the dreamer.

Perhaps new refinements in medical research technology will provide the way for the realization of MEMA telemetry and listening to dreams. The specifics of what technique may succeed remain to be seen. One might hope that creative scientific minds may someday realize the idea.

Some people have chastised the suggestion as treading on the sacred grounds of the privacy of the mind, as if it were to be a method of control. The idea cannot be so readily realized or abused. It is only the dream-sound imagination which could possibly be accessed. Yet dreams are vital and powerful. A great new frontier could be opened, giving a wondrous wealth of imagination to the waking world.

REFERENCE

1. Roffwarg H, Pessah M: Spontaneous middle ear muscle activity in man: A rapid eye movement sleep phenomenon. Science 178:773-776, Nov 1972.

SUGGESTED READING

1. Hobson JA, McCarley R: The brain as a dream state generator: An activation synthesis hypothesis of the dream process. Amer J Psych 134: 1335-1348, 1977.
2. Dement W, Kleitman N: Cyclic variations in the EEG during sleep and their relation to eye movements, body motility, and dreaming. EEG Clin Neurophysiology 9: 637-690, 1957.
3. Jont A: Cochlear modeling. IEEE ASSP, 3-29, 1985.

CHAPTER 124

Music-Induced Hearing Loss in Norwegian Adolescent Males

H.M. Borchgrevink

INTRODUCTION

Norway has a 15-month compulsory military service for all male citizens over age 18. Since 1981, audiometry of conscripts has been performed at enrollment, at the beginning of military service, during service (according to special criteria) and when ending service.[1,2] First, the recruit is tested for normal hearing, *screening audiometry 20 dB* (whether one hears a tone of 20 dB in each ear for the standard test frequencies 250, 500, 1000, 2000, 3000, 4000, 6000, 8000 Hz). In the event of hearing loss >20 dB for any frequency, pure-tone-threshold audiometry is performed for all the above test fre-quencies. The data are categorized into digit codes to facilitate (computerized) administration procedures. The screening audiometry data recorded at enrollment have been electronically stored since 1981 for each conscript as part of his medical record. The *hearing digit* denotes whether the man has normal hearing, or low-, mid- or high-frequency hearing loss >20 dB >3000 Hz in one or both ears (Table I). Noise exposure leads to selective high-frequency hearing loss. Presbycusis also leads to high-frequency hearing loss, but affects elderly people, and is largely constant for a certain age group. Increasing incidence of high-frequency hearing loss (hearing digits 5 and 4) recorded among Norwegian 18-year-old men at consecutive annual examinations will thus reflect increased incidence of noise-induced hearing loss.

METHOD

Pure-tone *screening audiometry 20 dB* was performed on the entire Norwegian 18-year-old male population (about 35,000 men), each year from 1981 to 1990. Audiometers, method and periodicity of calibration, examination procedure and locations were the same each year. The operators shifted every year, but received exactly the same training and supervision.

Table I: Hearing Digit Code

	Hearing Digit
Normal hearing, threshold <20 dB both ears, or Low-frequency loss >20 dB <500 Hz one ear	9
Low-frequency loss >20 dB <500 Hz both ears	8
Mid-frequency loss >20 dB 1000-2000 Hz one ear	7
Mid-frequency loss >20 dB 1000-2000 Hz both ears	6
High-frequency loss >20 dB >3000 Hz one ear	5
High-frequency loss >20 dB >3000 Hz both ears	4
Mixed hearing loss >20 dB with combined low+mid, low+high, mid+high or low+mid+high	3

Audiometry results were reported for each man in a standard scheme registering whether the person could hear 20 dB on each ear for the standard test frequencies noted above. The *hearing digit* was calculated according to the code in Table I. The audiometry results were stored in an electronic database in terms of hearing digits as part of the medical record for each man. The relative distribution of hearing digits, reflecting the incidence of low-, mid- and high-frequency hearing losses >20 dB, and the incidence of normal hearing were calculated for each enrollment group, 1981-1990.

RESULTS

The results showed that during the period 1981-87 the incidence of pure high-frequency hearing loss (hearing digits 4 and 5) had doubled, increasing from around 15% in 1981-82 to about 35% in 1987 (Table II). Low-frequency hearing loss (digit 8), mid-frequency hearing loss (digits 6, 7) and mixed hearing loss (digit 3) showed no significant increase. Incidence of high-frequency hearing loss stabilized at about 35% in 1988 and 1989, and decreased slightly to 31% in 1990 (Figure and Table II).

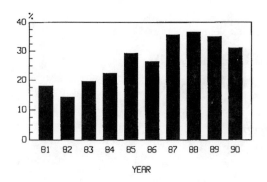

Figure: *Incidence of high-frequency hearing loss.*

DISCUSSION

Selective high-frequency hearing loss is seen in presbycusis, and following noise exposure. Presbycusis produces increasing high-frequency hearing loss with age; thus, it is unlikely to be the major cause of high-frequency hearing loss recorded in 18-year-old-men, and highly unlikely to double its incidence in a young population over a few years' time. Conse-quently, the increased incidence of high-frequency hearing loss recorded above among Norwegian 18-year-old-men at consecutive annual examinations re-flects increased incidence of noise-induced hearing loss.

optimal fitting of headsets may lead to a somewhat higher incidence of high-frequency hearing loss. Both these potential error effects might influence the above data to some extent, but the influence would be expected to be constant each year when examining such large groups of subjects. Accordingly, the incidence *increase* registered for noise-induced hearing loss in 18-year-old males from 1981 to 1987 must be real and valid. The 1987-89 stabilized 35% incidence and slight reduction to 31% recorded in 1990 may be due to information on music-noise hazards, as the 1981-87 incidence increase has been widely published in Norwegian media (television, newspapers, teenagers' programs, and periodicals.

The incidence level might have been somewhat lower if examined under optimal audiometry conditions. Flottorp reported, however, that 50% of a random 1980 selection of normal 15-17-year-old grammar school students exceeded 10 dB high-frequency hearing loss.[3] Many persons with 15 dB loss or more at a university clinic would be expected to show 20 dB loss or more at a military screening, supporting the 15-20% incidence of high-frequency hearing loss found at enrollment around 1980. Buren et al. found no noise-induced hearing loss in a Northern Norway youth sample.[4]

Table II: *Incidence of hearing loss >20 dB in Norwegian 18-year-old males, for years 1981-90*

Hearing Loss	1981	1982	1983	1984	1985	1986	1987	1988	1989	1990
Normal	73.7	77.4	70.6	68.2	61.3	63.9	53.9	51.3	51.3	55.3
Low Hz	1.5	2.7	1.3	1.3	1.5	0.8	0.8	0.8	1.5	1.5
Mid-Hz	1.1	0.9	0.4	0.6	0.5	0.4	0.4	0.4	0.4	0.3
High Hz	18.0	14.3	19.7	22.5	29.3	26.4	35.7	36.6	35.0	31.1
Mixed Hz	5.6	4.0	5.0	4.7	4.8	5.6	5.6	7.1	7.7	6.9
n =	34409	34856	35783	33419	27995	27612	33341	30792	29807	32722

The locations and the procedures for sample selection, audiometry, coding, and storing of data were the same throughout the 1981-90 period. In military audiometric screening, background noise is most likely somewhat higher than in hospital audiometry centers. Background noise characteristically masks the low frequencies, leading to false increase of low-frequency hearing loss. Low-frequency losses did not increase significantly from 1981 to 1990. Non-

The noise-induced hearing losses for many of the subjects are probably small — less than 30 dB; one year later, at the start of military service, threshold audiometry demonstrates that 15% of the conscripts show high-frequency loss of 30 dB or more. Only 5% show substantial losses.[5]

During the period 1981-87, occupational noise exposure was reduced, most likely due to the 1982 regulations on occupational noise exposure under the

1977 Working Environment Act. In Norway, the number of children who continued school/education until age 18 or longer, increased from close to 50% to about 70% during the 1981-87 period. An increasing number of 18-year-old conscripts thus enrolled directly from school without occupational experience. The increased incidence of noise-induced hearing loss in 18-year-old men 1981-87/88/89/90, therefore, is most likely caused by increased *leisure noise*. The only kind of leisure noise that may affect teenagers throughout the country, and influence the hearing of a generation, is *music*. Music-noise from discotheques, rock concerts and increasingly powerful audio/stereophonic devices has obviously increased during this period. Personal audio/stereo equipment shows increased sales/distribution. For example, the "walkman" (headset or insert device listening), introduced around 1979, had sold 600,000 sets by 1987 and is now approaching an estimated one million sets among Norway's four million inhabitants — corresponding to one per person aged 10-30 years.

Music noise in discotheques or rock concerts often fluctuates between 105-115 dBA.[6] *Walkman* headset audio devices can deliver music at 105 dBA level at max. gain 10, and temporary hearing losses 5-25 dB were registered in volunteers after one hour of listening on gain 8 (95 dBA).[3, 7, 8] Susceptibility varies among individuals. A rule of thumb, however, is that noise leading to temporary hearing loss with a feeling of "plugged ears" and tinnitus after exposure tends to produce permanent hearing loss upon repeated exposure.[9] Impulse noise (gunfire, drums) is more hazardous and tends to produce hearing loss after half the noise dose compared with continuous noise.[10] Impulse noises are present in the high intensity *punch* appreciated in rock music. Leisure noise tends to increase the total noise exposure per day, thus reducing noise-free recovery periods and increasing the chance of permanent hearing loss. On the other hand, music noise seems to lead to somewhat less hearing loss than would be expected from corresponding doses of industrial noise.[7, 8] *Walkman* headset devices do not offer any significant hearing protection.[11] Listening levels vary, exceeding 90 dBA in 25%, and 100 dBA in 5% of subjects,[12] and ranging 53-95 dBA among another group of individuals.[13] Some 20% report symptoms of tinnitus.[14] A 1985 review of the literature concluded that non-occupational noise exposure is unlikely to constitute a major source of noise-induced hearing loss in the U.K. population.[15] Symphony orchestra players, however, experience 76-102 dBA (median 90

dBA) levels, and 45% showed noise-induced hearing loss.[16] A military brass band produced a sound level between 80 dBA (pianissimo) and 103 dBA (fortissimo) registered in front of the conductor's ear during outdoor playing.[17]

Noise-induced hearing loss leads to selective death of the particular high-frequency sensory cells in the cochlea needed to discriminate between consonants in speech. The brain gets "blurred" and receives insufficient information. Impaired speech perception is the result, first experienced in background noise, with problems increasing when age-related hearing loss (presbycusis) is added. Hearing aids have limited effect: the sensory cells — the *converter* between mechanical sound waves and nerve impulses — are lost. Restrictions on leisure noise exposure — and music noise exposure — are needed.

NOISE HAZARDS

Below a certain intensity (sound pressure) level, no hearing loss is produced regardless of exposure time. Beyond a certain critical level, hearing loss occurs even after short exposure. In the transition area, the noise hazard roughly follows the *equal energy* rule: equal energy noise doses produce the same hearing loss. Noise may be defined as unwanted sound exposure. The noise hazard is largely the same, however, whether we like the sound or not. As sound appreciation is a brain function, and the brain is situated between the ears, the sound has already passed the ears and caused the potential damage when it reaches the appreciating level. If not, many passionate gunners — and rock musicians — would have preserved their hearing.

Decibel (dB) is a logarithmic sound-intensity measure. Moving away from a noise source, the sound-pressure level decreases by 6 dB for every doubling of the distance to the source. Thus, based on a few registrations, one can estimate sound-pressure levels — and noise hazard or annoyance — at other distances from the source. Hearing a 3 dB increase roughly corresponds to a doubling of the noise hazard. After a 3 dB increase, a given noise dose (intensity level by exposure time) is therefore attained in half the exposure time (the so-called "3 dB rule"). Most people tolerate a daily noise exposure dose of 85 dBA for 8 hours per day without developing hearing loss. A 3 dB increase to 88 dBA is tolerated for only half the exposure time, 4 hours. The tolerated daily noise dose corresponds to 100 dBA for 15 min/day, or 112 dBA for only 1 min/day. Pain is experienced above 120 dB. The "A" in dBA signifies *A-weighting*, a filtering procedure which automatically compensates for man's slight tolerance differences between low frequency (low hazard) and high frequency (high hazard) exposure during the actual sound measurement. Thus, based on dBA and the "3 dB rule," we can estimate the noise hazard without knowing further details of the noise spectrum.

REFERENCES

1. Borchgrevink HM: One-third of 18-year-old male conscripts show noise-induced hearing loss >20 dB before start of military service. Reflecting increased leisure noise? *In* Berglund B, Berglund U, Karlsson J, Lindvall T (eds), Noise as a Public Health Problem, vol 2, 27-32. Stockholm: 1988.

2. Borchgrevink HM: The hearing prophylaxis programme of the Norwegian Armed Forces. *In* Berglund B, Berglund U, Karlsson J, Lindvall T (eds), Noise as a Public Health Problem, vol 2, 33-38. Stockholm: 1988.

3. Turunen-Rise I, Flottorp G, Tvete O: A study of the possibility of acquiring noise induced hearing loss by the use of personal cassette players (walkman). *In* Borchgrevink HM (ed), Effects of noise and blasts. Scand Audiol Suppl 34:133-134, 1991.

4. Buren M, Solem BS, Laukli E: Threshold of hearing in children and youngsters. Brit J Audiol, in press.

5. Borchgrevink, Woxam: In prep.

6. Borchgrevink HM: Unpublished data.

7. Borchgrevink HM: Effects of noise - editor's introduction. *In* Borchgrevink HM (ed), Effects of noise and blasts. Scand Audiol Suppl 34:7-18, 1991.

8. Borchgrevink HM: Effects of noise and blasts - summary and current status. *In* Borchgrevink HM (ed), Effects of noise and blasts. Scand Audiol Suppl 34:173-176, 1991.

9. NATO RSG6 Report. Smoorenburg GF, Borchgrevink HM, Brinkmann H, Dancer A, Forrest MR, Forshaw SE, Papavasiliou A, Patterson JH, Pfander F, Phillips YY, Price GR: Effects of impulse noise. NATO AC/243 (Panel 8/RSG.6) D/9, Bruxelles, 1987.

10. Buck, K: Influence of different presentation patterns of a given noise dose on hearing in guinea pig. *In* Borchgrevink HM (ed), Hearing & hearing prophylaxis. Scand Audiol Suppl 16:83-87, 1982.

11. Skrainar SF, Royster LH, Berger EH, Pearson RG: Do personal radio headsets provide hearing protection? Sound Vibrat, May 1985.

12. Rice CG, Breslin M, Roper RG: Sound levels from personal cassette players. Brit J Audiol 21:273-278, 1987.

13. Bradley R, Fortnum H, Coles R: Research note: patterns of exposure of school children to amplified music. Brit J Audiol 21:119-125, 1987.

14. Rice CG, Rossi G, Olina M: Damage risk from personal cassette players. Brit J Audiol 21: 279-288, 1987.

15. Hughes E, Fortnum HM, Davis AC, Haggard MP, Coles RRA, Lutman ME: Damage to hearing arising from leisure noise. MRCIHR report. Brit J Audiol 20:157-164, 1986.

16. Royster JD: Music and hearing loss: playing deaf? National Hearing Conservation Association annual meeting, Florida, USA, March 2, 1990.

17. Borchgrevink HM (ed): Stoykilder i Forsvaret (Noise Sources in the Norwegian Armed Forces). HQ Defence Command Norway, Oslo, 1991.

PART X

PERFORMANCE STRESS

CHAPTER 125

Psychotherapeutic Use of Metaphor to Release Creative Block

Leslie Weiss • Katherine E.B. Davis • Renée Rocklin

This chapter explores metaphor as the primary representational storage form for human experience. In that role, metaphor allows for profound and efficient mapping of experience both within individuals and between people. Therapeutic techniques which directly capitalize upon metaphor have proven remarkably effective in releasing functional artistic blocks of all kinds, at the conscious, preconscious, and unconscious levels. Our observations of the power of metaphor as a therapeutic tool lead us to speculate on its central role in understanding the powerful reciprocity between art and therapy.

A violinist once said, "I became each note that wafted into the air." Human experience is representational. Knowing begins where physiology leaves off. Events outside our biochemical boundaries, as well as internal biological processes occurring within a perceivable time frame (about 0.1 second), are laid down in experience in a form we call metaphor. The word "metaphor" derives from the Greek *meta*, meaning "over," and *pherein*, "to bear or carry." Metaphors, then, capture information and carry it across a boundary.

Our conceptualization, stimulated by the work of Michael Gazzaniga (1988) and Douglas Hofstadter (1981), is that metaphor serves as the representational locus in human experience where behavior, affect, sensation, and knowing (cognition) converge, the meeting place of body and mind. It is the unit which elegantly and efficiently transfers concepts across the boundaries of experience, both within and between individuals. Art and therapy thus conjoin in metaphorical loci. Metaphor, in our thinking, explains the power of art to function therapeutically, and of therapy to facilitate art.

Metaphors can move like virus particles (David Grove, personal communication) between layers of consciousness and from inside to outside, using any sensory or behavioral medium. They enable us to go from our personal hardware to our own software, from our instrument to our music.

For our own purposes as psychotherapists, treatment capitalizes directly on the key position of metaphor, bypassing conventional language channels to effect directly changes in behavior, affect, sensation, and ways of thinking or knowing. Thus we can often evade conventional lines of psychological defense and other entrenched resistances to change.

We believe that the creative and performance problems posed by artists offer an elegant demonstration of this concept. Most experts on creativity agree that the origin of creativity is in the interface between our genetic endowment and the environment (Mattoon, 1984). The capacity to take control of this process, to generate emotionally involving symbols (metaphors) out of that interaction, is the hallmark of the creative person.

Perhaps artists also have a lower threshold between conscious and unconscious processes and have learned to value contributions of less consciously directed acts, enhancing these impulses with their training and talent. Thus we propose that metaphor is the common denominator of both artistic and psychotherapeutic endeavor.

When the smooth release of energy and information from storage is interrupted, blockage occurs. Interruptions may intrude from outside or from inside, at the conscious or nonconscious levels. Commonly, troublesome events which occur in everyone's lives are buried, often symbolically, meshed into our inner experience world and become new internal sources of interference. Personalized, multi-sensory metaphors, as we understand them, are employed (deployed?) to locate and release blockages.

Keith Johnstone's work (1979), using improvisational theater techniques, emerged out of his own experience with artistic blocks. He identified the key role of the internal critic, analogous to Schiller's "watcher of the gate of the mind," which splits awareness into doer and spectator. The spectator/critic discriminates, evaluates, rewards, and punishes according to learned criteria. This can result in a preoccupation with perfection and fear of failure.

To the extent that an artist starts "spectatoring," performance becomes goal-oriented, tense instead of pleasurable, shadowed by the prospect of failure. Creative impulses are critiqued before they can be fully expressed, if indeed they can be expressed at all. "Instrument" and "music" are disunited.

Cognitive-behavior therapists are quite skillful at intervening in this process and have achieved a high degree of success (Ellis, 1962; Beck, 1976). This treatment is entirely consistent with Johnstone's goals, but is limited to *talking* about change rather than facilitating the *experience* of change, incorporating behavior, affect, and sensation as well as cognition.

Johnstone's acting exercises can be used therapeutically to relieve blocking at the conscious level. These exercises facilitate the creative process by identifying and enhancing personal metaphors (creative impulses) which are offered to others in improvisational skits. Each artist is thus enabled to take risks in a playful, non-critical environment. Creative flow is enhanced in the give and take, decreasing the spectatoring and editing processes which obstruct creative expressing at the conscious level of awareness.

Blockages can also be treated at the preconscious level, using self-directed dream work. Dreaming is a physiological act with psychological content. The functions of dreams are to enlarge our understanding, to yield information that is unavailable from other sources, and possibly to "housekeep" the brain — sweeping it clean of excess or unwanted information (Ullman, 1979). Dreams occur in an environmental context, consistent with life events, thought, and feelings. These elements can trigger unresolved major life themes.

Dreaming also occurs when the need arises to place threatening information in the unconscious. Paradoxically, this may trigger a need to know and grow as a result of such information.

Metaphorical imagery is the language of dreams through which we accomplish both storage and retrieval of information. The visual metaphorical image is the involuntary expression of unknowable feelings and encompasses far more than spoken language can. Yet meanings remain veiled from con-

sciousness, protecting the self-concept, until the manifest meaning can be retrieved safely.

Metaphor is efficient and elegant, a highly distilled form of information. Dream images, whether visual, aural, or kinesthetic, are complex, vibrant, dramatic, and often complete in themselves, like poems. One "symbol" encompasses many words. Because the manifest meaning can remain thus disguised, enfolded in the metaphor, sleep is preserved and the sense of self protected (Ullman, 1990).

Use of metaphor is the common denominator of both artistic endeavor and dream work (Bogzaran, 1990). The capacity to generate emotionally involving symbols (metaphors) out of their interaction with the environment is the hallmark of creative persons. However, artists are subject to the same kinds of conflicts and traumas which afflict other persons and which can result in creative or performance blocks. Changing from their usual "medium" to dream work allows artists to use their talent for retrieving unconscious material through metaphor, while the block remains in the primary artistic "channel." Once the conflict or trauma is resolved metaphorically, the blockage succumbs and a dramatic improvement can occur.

By bypassing linear thought, metaphors can also provide the psychotherapist with a direct route to deeply hidden sources of conflict. Personal metaphors as storage containers for such unconscious material can be manipulated directly using techniques developed by David Grove.

According to Grove, suffering is expressed in language rich in metaphor. Such language provides clues not only to the origin of the problem but to a possible "child within." Early memories, often stored in impressionistic, stylized ways in both body and mind, may present as a wounded "child within" — a fragment of the self frozen in time, which encapsulates toxic experience and also the personal resources necessary to manage it. This results in attenuated adult functioning and blockage.

Psychological access to this phenomenon is achieved through client-controlled spontaneous trance which allows rearrangement of the psychological infrastructure through evolution of highly personalized metaphors (David Grove, 1989a, 1989b, 1990). The goal of treatment is to differentiate and grow the memory out of its original "stuck" form so that it creates another *There*, another *Then*. This allows the client to discover another way to have the memory reformatting his inner, nonconscious world (Grove, 1989a). This quickly frees a reservoir of personal energy.

This approach differs from other therapies using hypnosis, including Erickson's work, in that the therapist's interventions remain entirely content-free. We do not supply symbols, analogies, or "stories" to reframe the client's experience. Rather, we "midwife" the emergence of the person's very own imagery, using special "clean" language techniques. This allows the clinician to move into the matrix of the client's experience without taking control of the process. We work diplomatically within the very personal representations of a client's experience world. David Grove believes that this process adjusts the physiology of memory and experience at the most basic levels.

This reformatting has rapid and profound effects upon bodily sensations, somatic symptoms, affect range, behavioral options, and ways of knowing. It is our belief that these powerful effects result from the key role of metaphor in manifest human experience.

Our clinical experiences with metaphor have taught us that human experience can be profoundly touched at all levels of consciousness, through eyes, ears, and body. This is the task of both therapy and art as we understand them broadly, and account, in our minds, for the powerful reciprocity so often observed.

REFERENCES

Beck, Aaron: Cognitive Therapy and Emotional Disorders. New York: International Universities Press, 1976.

Bogzaran, Fariba: Painting Dream Images. *In* Krippner, Stanley (ed.): Dreamtime and Dreamwork. Los Angeles: Jeremy P. Tarcher Inc., 1990.

Ellis, Albert: Reason and Emotion in Psychotherapy. New York: Lyle Stuart, 1962.

Gazzaniga, M. S.: Mind Matters. Boston: Houghton Mifflin, 1988.

Grove, David; and Panzer, B. I.: Resolving Traumatic Memories: Metaphors and Symbols in Psychotherapy. New York: Irvington Publishers, Inc., 1989a.

Grove, David: Healing the Wounded Child Within. Cassette Training Program, David Grove Seminars: 20 Kettle River Drive, Edwardsville, Illinois 62025, 1989b.

Grove, David: Metaphors to Heal By. Videotape Training Program, David Grove Seminars Edwardsville, Illinois 62025, 1990.

Hofstadter, Douglas; and Dennett, Daniel C.: The Mind's I. New York: Basic Books, 1981.

Johnstone, Keith: Improv. Boston: Faber and Faber, 1979.

Mattoon, Mary Ann: Understanding Dreams. Dallas: Spring Publications, 1984.

Perls, Fritz: Gestalt Therapy Verbatim. New York: Bantam Press, 1969.

Ullman, Montague: Working with Dreams. Los Angeles: Jeremy P. Tarcher, 1979.

Ullman, Montague: Guidelines for Teaching Dreamwork. *In* Krippner, Stenley (ed.) Dreamtime and Dreamwork. Los Angeles: Jeremy P. Tarcher Inc., 1990.

Special acknowledgement is due to Bob Gelbach for editorial support and to David Grove, both for his inspiration and for his personal impact on our creativity.

CHAPTER 126

Stress in the Lives of Musicians —
On Stage and Off

David J. Sternbach

Those who embark on careers as performing musicians expect to live a rich and fulfilling creative life; it comes as a shock for them to realize that the achievement of their career goals may be at the cost of their physical and psychological health. Sadly, this appears to be the case for growing numbers of performers.

It has been reported that the life expectancy of musicians is 20-22% under the national average and that coronary disease accounts for almost five percent more deaths than in the general population.[1] Something is making musicians more ill than they should be; something is killing them too soon. Many observers, the author among them, see the lives of musicians today at a point of crisis with overwhelming concerns generated by their professional lives. Presented herein are some of the author's observations about the sources of these pressures and what can be done about them. In this brief overview of the psychological climate in which performers operate, three main areas of performers' stress — environmental, psychological, and intrinsic — are discussed.

ENVIRONMENTAL STRESSORS

Environmental stressors include the work-place nuisances, abuses, and hazards that players are likely to mention. Many can be alleviated; in this category are working conditions, audition procedures, tenure, salaries, and benefits, which once were universally deplorable in the U.S. and, for many regional orchestras, still are. As musicians have won gains in these areas they have moved on to other issues, addressing tour schedules, adequate rehearsal breaks, chair rotation among the strings, removal of hazards such as asbestos from the work place, and protection from hearing loss, especially for those seated near brass and percussion sections.

Other factors are less amenable to improvement or change but are simply facts of life for musicians which they adapt to if they intend to continue in the profession. There are constant rotating work schedules for orchestras, with rehearsals and concerts mornings, afternoons, and evenings. Add the disruptions caused by tours and the stress increases, particularly for musicians trying to provide constancy in their families' lives. There is physical strain in performance, a constant awareness that even minor injuries can be disabling, and the fact that orchestra players must cede control of their artistic efforts to the conductor. On tours each new hall presents different acoustic problems, a challenge free-lance musicians face two or three times every day.

Players already under the stress of performance pressure may find themselves reacting to uncomfortable chairs, poor ventilation, drafts, poor backstage conditions, halls too hot or too cold, all out of proportion to the causes.

One could mention the extreme competition in an overcrowded profession and the factor most musicians bring up — conflict with conductors. There are many with inappropriate, abrupt, disrespectful temperaments who may also be technically and artistically less capable than the orchestra musicians. There is a legacy of suspiciousness and defensiveness left by such personalities that does little to ease musicians' stress.

While many of these conditions may be shared by non-musicians, it is their total, cumulative effect that contributes to overwhelming stress for performers. Viewed purely from the standpoint of so many stressors in the working environment, it is little wonder that musicians are a population at risk for stress-related physical and emotional problems. And we have as yet made no mention of stage fright.

PSYCHOLOGICAL STRESS

This area of stress has to do with more internal matters, with the maintenance of the ego. Stage fright, a fact of life for nearly all performers, falls in this category — a psychological issue with many contributing factors that exacerbate this syndrome. Musicians work under the constant supervision of the conductor in rehearsals and performances, and this in itself is a factor found in nearly no other calling. Performances take place at a given time and place. There are no second chances. Careers can suffer setbacks or even be destroyed with a single review. Recordings create note-perfect expectancies in the minds of the public, and musicians are well aware that their live performances are measured against these unrealistic standards. There are three aspects to stage fright and while each alone can be stressful, when all three are present the effects can be psychologically crippling.

Pre-performance or anticipatory anxiety is associated with the dread of a future calamity or failure. A musician's life in the hours, days, even weeks or months before an audition or performance can be almost an unremitting purgatory. *On-stage* performance anxiety can range from mild excitement which can serve to enhance performance, to full-blown panic attacks with a host of symptoms including palpitations, dizziness, transient limb paralysis, severe short-term memory loss, blackouts and even cardiac arrest. Finally, there is *post-performance* anxiety, a mental review which can range from an even-tempered appraisal of errors to symptoms resembling post-traumatic stress disorder, especially in the aftermath of auditions or competitions where so much is at stake.

Most musicians develop adaptive coping mechanisms that allow them to contain remarkably high levels of anxiety and still perform consistently at levels sufficient to sustain careers. Many, unfortunately, do so through maladaptive strategies in the defense of the ego. It is these musicians who are at high risk for psychological problems, alcoholism and abuse of both prescription- and street drugs.

Recently, perhaps partly due to the relief beta blockers offer, musicians have begun to speak out more openly about this issue. The traditional concern, however, remains a present-day one: if a player is too frank about this problem, might this not find its way to the ears of management, or worse, the conductor? And then, what consequences for that musician professionally? Musicians used to disguise injuries or illness to avoid summary dismissal. Today an onus still attaches in many players' minds to acknowledging stage fright. This is particularly regrettable since we know that in groups individuals can find consensus and validation of their personal issues that can neutralize the negative charge such emotions carry.[2]

There is increasing evidence that all three aspects of performance anxiety can be treated and to a great extent relieved through a combination of relaxation training,[3, 4] stress reduction training and cognitive restructuring,[5] education about the nature of stress,[6] systematic desensitization and imagery rehearsal.[7] Nevertheless, there persists significant overuse of beta blockers, which have superseded tranquilizers as the drug of choice for thousands of musicians.

Besides performance anxiety, there is the experience of the life cycle itself which poses more complex challenges for musicians than for non-performers, exacting a price that is less well-recognized or understood.

The developmental process which Erikson referred to as the life cycle[8] brings at each level new crises which demand, in turn, more complex reorganization of the psyche. This task is more complicated for performers who possess a second life cycle, that of their artistic growth unfolding throughout a career. This artistic life also possesses stages, and generally these two cycles are in conflict.

Adolescence, for example, is a time when the socialization process has primacy. Dating, consolidation of sexual identity, and the fine-tuning of social skills help individuals develop social confidence. But talented young players have commitments of three, four, even six hours daily in the practice room, leaving them little time to explore and develop social skills and broaden their horizons by developing other interests. Later, in music school, boy pianists date girl pianists, piano being the only thing they can talk about.

The late teens and early twenties see the emergence of the drives for separation and individuation, drives that may collide with the young musician's need for continued financial and emotional support from parents. The process of individuation may also be at odds with the attachment to teachers as both artistic and personal models. Developing young artists seek out the most prominent teachers with whom to study, and it can prove difficult for them to confirm their own identity in close contact with mentors who are more mature artists and who may either inadvertently or intentionally impose their personality styles on their students.

The thirties are a time for the great lunge toward the top. But, especially for women conscious of their biological clock, this time can be experienced as a conflict between the pursuit of career and the urge to begin a family. The costs to women who drop out of business world are well-documented. They are even more severe for performers, who must find the time and mobilize the energy to restore their playing skills to that shining edge before they then struggle to regain their competitive place in the career race.

Perhaps the most affecting crisis comes still later in the course of the normal aging process. In middle age and beyond, performers continue to evolve their personal artist-vision which through the years has developed in richness, clarity, and subtlety. Yet it becomes more evident that one's physical capacities have not remained undiminished through the passage of years. The older artist learns many ways to compensate for those incremental losses, but there is an inescapable realization that the strength and vigor of their twenties is slipping away, even as they judge themselves and are judged by others against just those standards of strength and projection they themselves helped to establish in their youth. More noticeable in wind players than strings, and still more so for brass players, it is an issue every player eventually faces. If their identity has been tied entirely to their career, parting from an active performing career can bring on enormous stress.

Even if the stages of one's life are not at odds with one's artistic development, the simple fact of having to deal psychologically with two life cycles makes for a more complex life. What is self-evident to anyone who is or has been an artist, and especially to the spouses of performers, is that a performing career seems to have a life and a will of its own, and this affects musicians vis-a-vis the social and political concerns of society. How does the ego mediate conflicts between internal drives for success of an artist possessing great talent and society's issues, pressures, and restrictions?

How does a performer deal with civil injustice? What issues to respond to? When? To what degree of commitment? What price to artists in diminished self-respect when they are only spectators of the social issues of the day as they concentrate on their demanding artistic preoccupations? Such conflicts have effects that resonate deeply within the psyche, generating further conflictive processes for the artist.

How can a musician deal with so many complexities? Teachers can play a role here as mentors willing to share their own psychological processes, their experiences of frustration, setbacks and anxieties, and how they cope. This can help students develop a more realistic assessment of the psychological preparation they will need to cultivate to survive and succeed in their difficult profession.

Schools of music can help by establishing required courses on physiology that include exercises for musicians, training in handling stress and performance anxiety and, for that matter, courses in business including marketing, contracts, negotiation skills, time management and promotion, since these are skills most performers will need throughout their professional lives.

INTRINSIC ELEMENTS

This term refers to those psychological factors that are inherent to the life of a performer. How each person lives his or her personal creative vision is an essentially solitary process. This heightened awareness of one's existential loneliness is experienced every hour in the practice room over the years artists take to develop their craft, and never more clear than when they stand alone on a concert stage in a confrontation with the self that requires great resoluteness.

Perfectionism is one of the negative aspects to having creative ideals. Musicians first must find a way to live with their instrument's limitations that can frustrate creativity, but there is a second factor that goes even deeper. This is the adjustment required to tolerate the gap between one's artistic vision and the realization of that vision in actual performance regardless of the limitations of one's instrument.

This tension requires a highly developed capacity to tolerate imperfection. One must find that fine point of balance between a positive obsessive style without which excellence is unlikely to be achieved, and a negative obsessive style. It is this style which leaves an individual vulnerable to excessively self-critical fault-finding that can rob him of any joy in making music, let alone in personal life. The wish to grow artistically and personally has to be constantly balanced with life skills, the capacity to endure limitations with a measure of self-acceptance and contentment with self.

When an individual elects to live the life of a performing artist, there are certain decisions to be weighed in terms of gains and losses. Few, if any, are sufficiently well-informed to make such decisions in advance. It was Freud who said that most of our fundamental life decisions are made from deep within the unconscious, and are only partially subject to mediation by the conscious mind.[9]

Only later, when already deeply committed to their artistic choices, do most individuals discover and begin dealing with the frustrations attached to their decisions. There is a certain psychic price here which must be worked through. Some handle this well, learning to live with limitations as an acceptable price for the opportunity to create. Some handle its price with resentment and remain profoundly ambivalent throughout their lives. Those who remain dedicated to this difficult profession can help themselves by making a lifelong commitment to maintaining and enhancing their physical, emotional, mental, and spiritual well-being. Given the world of today and the steadily increasing number of stressors, it is no longer an option, but a necessity, for musicians to develop psychological awareness and skills equal to their sophistication as performers. This new awareness would be attentive to the progression of the life cycle and its crises, the mechanisms of the psyche, the richness of possibilities in well-developed communication skills, and the ability to control reactivity to stressors.

Western psychology can teach us about stress and neuroses, the life cycle and communication skills. From Eastern meditation teachings we can learn a great deal about controlling the mind's reactions to external events and inner feeling states. The blend of ideas between East and West that we now see occurring promises a new level of integration of the psyche that can provide enormous benefits to performers.

Is there a prescription to offer for the overwhelming stress and isolation of the performer? Address the isolation on all levels, first by reconnecting with resources for renewal and strengthening the vision that originally led the individual to his/her art. Connect with colleagues to develop better conditions as working people and to inspire one another's creativity. Connect with the larger community, not only when on stage, that special area of empowerment for performers, but in other milieus as well. Musicians benefit by giving back something of their art when they perform for those in prisons, hospitals, old-age homes — for any audiences neglected in our society. They are likely to discover that they receive far more than they give; and this is part of the healing process as well.

The musician is a metaphor — we can go a step further by recognizing that we are all, in the complex industrialized societies of today, living under performance pressure. This realization creates a bond between artists and other working people. One of the benefits of arts-medicine conferences is the generation and exchange of information on stress that can be brought back to the general public as they pursue their own 'lives of quiet desperation.' This recognition of the underlying similarities beneath surface differences can stimulate greater support among musicians, their public and larger community.

Finally, what is surprising is not that musicians experience so much physical and emotional damage, but that so many manage to keep their optimism, tenaciously protect their right to exist economically, and find the resources to create — among the distractions, pain, and stress — so much beauty.

REFERENCES

1. Tucker A, et al: Electrocardiography and lung function in brass instrument players. Arch Environ Health 23:327-334, 1971.
2. Yalum I: The Theory and Practice of Group Psychotherapy, 2d ed. New York: Basic Books, 1975.
3. Wolfe M: Coping with musical performance anxiety: problem-focused strategies. Med Probs of Perf Artists 5(1):33-36, 1990.
4. Benson H: The Relaxation Response. New York: William Morrow, 1975.
5. Wolfe M: Correlates of adaptive and maladaptive musical performance anxiety. Med Probs of Perf Artists 4(1):49-56, 1989.
6. Desberg P, March G: Controlling Stage Fright. Oakland: New Harbinger Pubs, 1988.
7. Steptoe A, Fidler H: Stage fright in orchestral musicians. A study of cognitive and behavioral strategies in performance anxiety. Br J Psychol 78:241-249, 1987.
8. Erikson E: The Life Cycle Completed. New York: WW Norton, 1982.
9. Freud S: *In* The Standard Edition of the Complete Psychological Works of Sigmund Freud, vol 21. London: Hogarth Press, 1961.

CHAPTER 127

Mood Enhancement
By Physical Exercise

B.R. Nicholls • *H. Steinberg* • *E.A. Sykes* • *J. Thomas* • *N.N. Ramlakhan*

It is now well established that physical exercise can reduce stress, anxiety and depression, and improve mood. Most studies have assessed the acute effect of one bout of exercise or the cumulative effect of several sessions. Few seem to have monitored mood effects when different kinds of exercise are repeated over several sessions.

SAMPLE

Testing was conducted weekly for 7 weeks in a fitness club with many faithful students (dropout rate only 5%, as compared with up to 70% in the general population) who had often reported that exercise gave them feelings of psychological well-being 'make you feel great!', 'not only does my body feel the benefit of classes but my mind as well' and 'it has given me confidence in every way' - which affected their day-to-day lives.

METHOD

Three types of exercise class ('Aerobic Workout' [introductory and advanced], 'Body Funk', and 'Callanetics') were tested weekly by means of a 48 item adjective check-list,[4] which placed equal emphasis on positive and negative mood. Classes were held in the 'Body Revolution'(BR) fitness club whose methods had been developed by one of the authors (JT). Classes lasted 70 minutes, had 20-25 students, and the adjective lists were presented immediately before and again after the classes. Subjects chose their own class, but were not obliged to attend, and so attendances was apt to fluctuate. According to initial question- naires, subjects' predominant aim was to become or stay physically fit and to loose weight.

About 652 check-lists were collected from 217 subjects. The results were analysed in a preliminary way for 'Improvement', 'Positive difference' and 'Negative difference' in order to obtain measures of overall acute and long-term mood changes:

- 'Improvement' $T = (P2 - N2) - (P1 - N1)$ where $P1$ = positive scores before class, $P2$ = positive scores after class, $N1$ = negative scores before class, and $N2$ = negative scores after class.
- 'Positive difference' $P = P2 - P1$
- 'Negative difference' $N = N2 - N1$

Subjects acted as their own controls over each session's testing.

RESULTS

All mean summary scores changed significantly (two-tailed t-tests, $p < 0.0253$). Thus all groups showed a significant improvement in positive mood and a significant fall in negative mood.

An analysis of variance of the scores from all subjects combined showed a significant effect of the particular week of testing. Both 'improvement' (Fig.l) and 'positive difference' became more positive ($F = 8.19$, $df = 1$-694, $p < 0.004$; and $F = 9.26$, $df = 1$-694, $p < 0.002$ respectively) as testing progressed and the 'negative difference' became more negative ($F = 3.95$, $df = 1$-694, $p < 0.047$). Thus differences in mood before and after class seemed to become larger in successive weeks.

Analysis of variance of results grouped according to the type of class showed effects of both week of testing and type of class. 'Improvement' and 'positive difference' scores were more positive and 'negative difference' scores more negative for the Advanced group than for the Introductory. Similarly, significant differences emerged between the scores of the Introductory and the Callanetics groups ($p < 0.025$), with Callanetics producing more positive 'improvement' and 'positive difference' scores and more negative 'negative difference' scores than the Introductory. The Advanced and the Callanetics

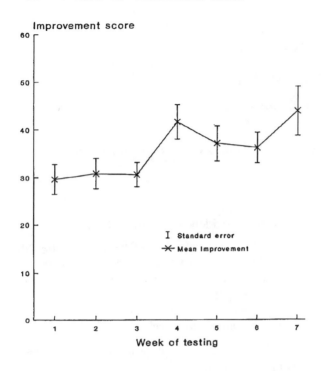

Figure 1: *Mean Improvement score (T) increased significantly after week 4 (p <0.004) and continued up to week 7.*

groups did not differ from each other; the scores of the Body Funk group were more variable.

No correlations were found between the mood scores before and after classes.

DISCUSSION

Exercise produced an immediate overall improvement in mood, resulting from both an increase in positive and a decrease in negative mood. This improvement occurred when classes were repeated weekly for a number of weeks; if anything, the improvements in mood increased with time[5] and after a course of exercise,[2] though it was not long lasting.[3]

When data from classes doing the same sort of exercise but at different levels of competence (Introductory and Advanced) were compared, the summary scores differed significantly. The Advanced group always showed a larger positive improvement in mood and a larger negative decrement. Comparing data from two groups which did different kinds of exercise (Advanced and Callanetics) gave no significant difference. Mood improvement seemed to depend on the cardiovascular content of the exercise, music or fun elements and also on the level of competence reached and the challenge of the exercise

to the student. Body Funk appeared to be more fun but results in this group were very variable and mood improvements were generally smaller than those in the more physically challenging Advanced workout and Callanetics classes.

At least two studies[7,8] found that high intensity exercise generally led to negative moods, while low intensity exercise induced positive moods. This appears to differ from our results, but they used bicycle ergometry as exercise, apparently with one subject at a time; the exercise was relatively brief and uniformly intense. By contrast, the longer workout classes at BR, while incorporating high intensity exercise, fluctuated in their physical requirements and ended with a cool-down period of approximately 4 minutes before the psychological testing. One study[8] compared the effects of music with those of a metronome on perceived exertion and found that subjects with music rated their exertion as less; subjects also found it more pleasant to work to music. All the BR classes involved some music, although this cannot be the sole reason for the difference in results, since the Callanetics classes not only had very little but also different music from that used in the Introductory and Advanced workout classes.

Another study[7] also found some positive mood effects of high intensity exercise, especially in highly fit subjects, who reported more vigour and a small increase in exhilaration after exercise. It seems likely that the students in the Advanced workout and Callanetics at BR were at least 'highly fit' to cope with the demands of those classes and therefore might be more likely to experience mood benefits. Nevertheless, it appears, especially from the Introductory class, that improvement in mood does not depend solely upon high initial physical fitness and may be experienced by the relatively unfit. This is consistent with several reports in the literature.

That no correlations were found between scores before and after classes suggests that beneficial mood effects were not confined only to subjects who began the class with a low mood, as has sometimes been suggested,[6] but our results appear to indicate that exercise can have both acute and cumulative beneficial effects on mood in a 'normal' population.

These preliminary results, and the background literature, together with informal discussions with JT and students of BR, suggest some guidelines for people taking up exercise. It is more beneficial to work in a group with an instructor than alone,[1] and the more congenial the instructor, the lower the dropout rate. A form of exercise should be chosen which presents a realistic challenge and the participant should persevere, since beneficial mood changes will increase with both time and competence.

All the types of exercise tested produced positive moods. However, despite current trends in mainstream exercise teaching, challenging exercises were more beneficial than those which were less demanding.

REFERENCES

1. Dishman RK (ed). Exercise Adherence: its impact on public health. Illinois, Human Kinetics Books, 1988.

2. Dyer JB, & Crouch JG. Effects of running and other activities on moods. Percep. Mot. Skills 67: 43-50, 1988.

3. Frazier SE & Nagy S. Mood state changes of women as a function of regular aerobic exercise. Percep. Mot. Skills 68: 283-287, 1989.

4. Morris M, Salmon P & Steinberg H. The 'runner's high': dimensional structure of mood before and after running. Proc. Sport, Health, Psychology and Exercise Symposium, Bisham Abbey: 147-152, 1988.

5. Roth DL. Emotional and psychological effects of aerobic exercise. Psychophysiol. 26: 593-602, 1989.

6. Simons CW & Birkimer JC. An exploration of factors predicting the effects of aerobic conditioning on mood state. J. Psychosom. Res. 32: 63-75, 1988.

7. Steptoe A & Bolton J. The short-term influence of high and low intensity physical exercise on mood. Psychol. and Health 2: 91-106, 1988.

8. Steptoe A & Cox S. Acute effects of aerobic exercise on mood. Health Psychol. 7: 329-340, 1988.

ACKNOWLEDGEMENTS

This project was supported by a grant from the Wolfson Foundation. We thank Professor Gerta Vrbova and Mr Brian Newman for comments on the manuscript.

CHAPTER 128

Pain and Creation

Marie Sophie Colas

The phrase *Je souffre* (I am suffering) is French — a language which has long since abandoned the old-fashioned use of the verb *douloir* (to pain; be in pain). Nowadays we tend to wrongly use the terms *suffering* and *pain* interchangeably; thus, it is useful to attempt to clarify the difference between the two terms before studying the equally complex relationship between pain and creation and explaining the role of stress mechanisms in the creative process.

We can sense that pain is a much more subtle and infinite feeling than suffering: "It is the unthinkable evil without name or face, nobody's evil."[1]

Suffering also has many connotations, and can be defined as the emotional or personified, moral or psychic experience of pain, itself being more physical or metaphysical. Pain cannot be communicated to others — it takes away any surge of formulation and creation.

Many writers, philosophers, and artists, however, have put forth the idea of creation as a sublime but selective area of pain; this being all the more difficult to bear as the mind as well as the body must suffer the ordeal. In this study, both mind and body are regarded as a whole. Modern medicine finds it difficult to grasp this idea of a whole, be it real or only within the bounds of possibility, and all too often separates illness of the mind from that of the body.

This discrepancy is found in all nineteenth- and twentieth-century literature in which the nominative use of pain carries the idea of suffering. Furthermore, the introduction of the word *stress* in the second half of the twentieth century has not facilitated the description of these "feelings."

Even in the eighteenth century, artistic nostalgia and melancholy were cushioned by the medical term *hypochondria* — illness of the over-sensitive. Goethe, with his hero Werther, began a long list of heroes disappointed by reality, racked with pain, and thwarted due to their own genius. Constant dissatisfaction in addition to a growing obsession with death, a lack of direction, and the search for the absolute, were common among writers of this and the following century.

The biological approach to the role of psychological factors in illness began at the beginning of the twentieth century with the work of American physiologist Walter Cannon and pathologist Hans Selye. By carrying out various experiments not taking into account of the kind of aggression suffered by the subject, these authors noticed the appearance of symptoms such as gastrointestinal ulcers, thymic regression, lymphatic ganglions and hypertrophy of the suprarenal glands. According to Selye, these "symptoms indicate an overloading of the individual's defense capacity."[2] As soon as the internal stability of the system is threatened by psychic or physical aggression, the system itself produces a counterreaction aiming to restore this lost stability.

This is an uncharacteristic reaction, as it is not dependent on the nature of the aggressing agent. The hormones producing this counterreaction are released by the suprarenal cortex and are known as glucocorticoids, due to their effect on sugar metabolism. The mechanism of placing hormones in the nervous system has been explained in the following way: A chain of hormonal agents means that a mental state or an emotion can be expressed as a visceral reaction associated with physical illness.

The term *stress* evolved from these studies. Taken for granted and considered unavoidable today, it does threaten our well-being and can affect us in very serious ways. Many studies have shown the harsh impact of these reaction mechanisms on the system, but they translate using the term *pain*. The pain, sometimes intolerable or invalidating, can make the psychic element unique in human beings with exacerbated emotions. This has often been termed *anxiety* — "this physical anxiety accompanied by painful oppression, this existential malaise."

Did Rimbaud not search for a new language, the words to rid us of the suffering of thought, in the following statement?

"Enough! Punishment is coming. Let's go! Ah! my lungs burn, my temples grind! Night is rolling in my eyes, by this sun! My heart...my limbs! Where are we heading? To battle? I'm weak!"[3]

For those desiring a life different from the routine, the result is that they endure a feeling of emptiness, of desolation and constant confrontation with the anxiety of the human condition. It is important, however, to emphasize the close correlation between the tendency to depression and somatic complaints which often appear in these writings.

"... oh pain! Oh pain! Time eats life away,
And the obscure enemy who devours our heart..."[4]

"Pain like a scissor cut" was the remark from Schiller, while Nietzsche only considers the idea of "great pain, long and slow pain which eats slowly away at us ..." These definitions, in fact, complement each other, and it is appropriate to distinguish between acute and chronic pain in medicine.

It is probable that the pain of artists is either a mixture of acute and chronic suffering or chronic suffering alone. Stoppages, successive deceleration, total silence, over-excitement, blinding acceleration, are shown in the creative path or in the expressive content of the writings themselves. Creative periods go through phases of acute pain followed by melancholic depressions: these are the visceral modifications accompanying stress and which bring with them the production of hormones and the emergence of phases of great pain. Art, the subtle composition of reality and illusion, would serve a cathartic function in transfiguring pain.

The energizing effects of frustration or aggression are recognized, and among the resulting attitudes, two capture our attention:

● *redirected activities*: the appropriate behavior of one of the conflicting tendencies manifests itself, but it reveals itself on an object different from that which initially caused it.

● *substitution activities*: the behavior which manifests itself belongs to a set of behaviors different from that of the tendencies competing with each other.

It took time for stress specialists to understand that it was necessary to distinguish between reaction and action, but to confront the pain caused by this "biological storm," the individual has several options at his disposal; they correspond to adjustment strategies.

As far as the psychologist is concerned, adjustment corresponds to efforts made to solve problems stemming from internal and external demands on the system. The subject may equally regard these as threats to his well-being. The adjustment can be directed either toward the problem itself or toward the emotion it provokes. The variety of adjustment strategies is vast. The hypothesis that creation is a means of releasing pain is probable, however: Artistic composition, in whatever field, is a possible treatment because creativity is never contemplative. Furthermore, knowledge can be acquired about the mechanisms for controlling pain which permit empirical treatment.

"... Be good, oh my pain, and remain quieter ..."[4]

REFERENCES

1. Shneider M: La tombee du jour, Ed. du Seuil, 1989.

2. Danzer R: L'illusion psychosomatique, Ed. Odile Jacob, 1989.

3. Rimbaud A: Une saison en enfer.

4. Baudelaire C: Les fleurs du mal.

CHAPTER 129

Play Attention: The 'How' Experience of Gestalt Psychotherapy — A Clinical Study of Performance Anxiety in Two Guitarists

Michael Kriegsfeld

A Gestalt psychotherapy encounter is viewed by the author as an art form which depends on the joint creative expression of at least two people.[1,2] Communicating is viewed and heard as a musical, dramatic, artistic performance with at least two people acting in concert. This requires on the part of the performers — as well as client and therapist — the readiness and skill to act together, risking open exploration and exchange, making contact through awareness and experimentation. The creative artistic experience of psychotherapy, for which the author uses the musical metaphor of the distinction between the jazz musician and the classical musician, brings into focus the three basic processes: (1) attending, (2) playing, and (3) oscillating.

In the midst of a weekend group psychotherapy retreat, A, a regular group member, leaves the meeting room during the day that D has joined the group. Both are very close in background — music conservatory training, teaching, playing in public (with D limiting himself so that he never plays solo). A has previously suffered with severe performance anxiety. He returns to the group meeting immediately after "undressing" his guitar from its case. As he walks in, he carries his guitar as a performer about to play. He immediately begins sharing his awareness of his professional colleague, his concern about sharp judgment and criticism, and his need to impress the colleague (he fears that he won't), and demonstrates his rising pressure and fumbling. He is unable to tune his guitar to his satisfaction, and comments that he is in trouble already.

Our first process is attending. This is understood as *to care for; to stay with; to be present with; to accompany actions or deeds with the capacity for special consideration, regard, courtesy, and awareness.*[2] A, the old-timer, has brought his problem into the group and begun to work with it, share it, experience it, and express his need for understanding and help. D, first-time member of the group, has been exhibiting a typical role and attitude. He is a watchful, keen observer, passively waiting to see what is going on. He has not made any move to participate, maintaining a receptive "let's wait and see" mode. He withholds, withdraws, and is very cool, giving no outward response.

As therapist, the author plays with both. Both need support and validation — A for his terror and courage, D for his carefulness with the enemy and methodical control.

When A finishes his formal working, he swings into another process of playing. The author had been humming, singing, and whistling a lively tune. A has quickly picked up the tune. Hardly anyone can sit still, as the rhythm and cadence are infectious and captivating, and people tend to hum and tap their feet to the music. The repetitive verse is, "You can't get far without a railroad . . . You gotta have an engine and you've gotta have a track."[3]

Later, D joins in discourse with A and they identify with each other. There is a lull. A retains the guitar; D is more open, but still reserved. The author/therapist asks A, "When will you make the offer?" He is puzzled until reminded that D also plays the guitar. A is affable and hands the guitar to D, who accepts with "Oh shit." A makes excuses for D, sympathizing that D doesn't know the guitar. D excuses himself for not having touched a guitar in two weeks. The author comments that actually, we have been looking for a guitarist to audition who has not practiced. D is anxious, saying he may ruin the strings. He repeatedly tunes the guitar.

Immediacy and improvisation are crucial ingredients for growth as models for self-instruction and self-healing.   In a recent book, Csikszentmihalyi writes, "Even when children are taught music, the crucial problem often arises; too much emphasis is placed on how they perform, and too little on what they experience."[4]

After much explaining about why he cannot perform as expertly as he wishes, *D* plays. He judges his playing as poor. *D* reveals that, as a repressive controller, he forces himself to keep his muscles going in the right places and shares a history of psychosomatic complaints connected with bronchitis and colds. The author/therapist has stimulated this historical review on his part by sharing an observation of the tightness in his body and breathing difficulties. When asked how he feels, he comments, "That was as lousy a performance as I have given and that's not very nice." We immediately try a very old experiment, recently revived and rediscovered. It is *prescribing the symptom*, and asking him to really try for a championship 'lousy' performance. He agrees, but warns that it all will be fake.

Later, when asked to play "the plain old ordinary lousy way," he agrees. Although his body position had been tight and his chest collapsed over the guitar in previous playing, he now opens up his position and frees the guitar. The only talking the author/therapist does is to say "breathe." *A*, who has been very alert and attentive, picks this up and we are softly saying "breathe" in cadence. *D* has performed solo beautifully. His wife, also a musician, is present and comments on how well he played. She informs us that she has never heard him play better — ever! The video tape reveals body movements, facial expressions, gestures, and organismic responsiveness that give vitality to the interactions among *A*, *D*, the group, and the leader.

The leader leads the follower by following the follower's lead. The follower follows the leader by leading the leader in the way he will follow. They attend to each other and to themselves simultaneously without thought, without judgmental injunctions, without obligations, without stops, and without plans.

In the exchange, we both grow and become more in tune with ourselves, and with each other. I am attending and playing with all my skill, awareness, and interest in myself as well as in the other person. The patient in turn is attending, playing with his/her skill, awareness, and interest in himself/herself as well as in me. What we interrupt, how we interrupt, how we create dissonance, how we create harmony, what we leave over for another session, bubble up in ever-changing flow from our individual figures and grounds as we discover infinite gestalts in ourselves and in the other.[2]

REFERENCES

1. Kriegsfeld M: Play Attention: The How Experience of Gestalt Psychotherapy. First International Symposium on Nonverbal Aspects and Techniques of Psychotherapy. World Psychiatric Association, Canadian Psychiatric Association, University of British Columbia, 1974.
2. Kriegsfeld M: Play Attention: The How Experience of Gestalt Psychotherapy. *In* Grayson H, Loew C (eds), Changing Approaches to the Psychotherapies. New York: Spectrum Publications, 1978.
3. Washington N, Tiomkin D: You Can't Get Far Without a Railroad. New York: Northern Music Corporation, 1957.
4. Csikszentmihalyi M: Flow, The Psychology of Optimal Experience, 112. New York: Harper & Row, 1990.

CHAPTER 130

Musical Performance Anxiety and Depression, Performing Experience and Personality Traits: A Correlational Study

Karin S. Naimark • *Paul M. Lehrer*

The purpose of this study was to attempt to determine whether depression is a dimension of musical performance anxiety (MPA), explore anxiety and depression patterns before a major performance, and assess possible relationships of MPA and depression with personality traits.

Approximately 125 questionnaires were mailed or distributed to musicians, students, teachers, schools, and conferences throughout New York, New Jersey, and Pennsylvania. Participants were either music students, music teachers, or professional musicians, and were preparing for a major performance that was primarily solo in nature.

Questionnaires included Speilberger's State-Trait Anxiety Inventory (STAI), Beck's Depression Inventory (BDI), Cattell's 16 Personality Factor Inventory (16PF), and a music questionnaire developed by the researchers assessing performance experience and asking for a 1-100 rating of anxiety at the concert.

Participants completed the STAI and BDI one month prior to the concert. The state portion of the STAI and the BDI were completed weekly through the week prior and again on the day following the performance. The 16PF and the music questionnaire were completed shortly after the concert.

Twenty-one musicians responded (11 female and 10 male). The mean age was 25.8 ± 5.64. There were six vocalists, four pianists, four organists, two tubists, and one each of the following: bassoonist, double bassist, flutist, guitarist, and conductor. The mean number of years of study was $10.9 \pm SD = 5.2$. Primary status included 16 full-time music students, one part-time music student, one college faculty member, one music teacher, two private music teachers, two soloists, and one music director (several participants listed more than one status).

RESULTS

Pearson correlation analysis revealed significant positive correlations for three of the four weekly pre-concert STAI and BDI scores ($r = .66^{**}$, $n = 19$ to $.79^{***}$, $n = 19$).

STAI and BDI mean scores showed a significant drop from pre- to post-concert times as determined through a repeated-measures analysis (STAI: $F(4,19) = 5.75$, $p < .0005$, BDI: $F(4,19) = 3.85$, $p < .007$).

Of the 20 subjects who completed the BDI at least three times, nine registered at least one score within the clinical depression range during the pre-concert month.

Pre-concert STAI measures correlated positively with 16 PF scales of Insecurity, Tension, Anxiety, and Neuroticism, and negatively with Intelligence and Leadership.

Experience (number of performances) correlated negatively with STAI measures of anxiety before the concert ($r = -.78^{**}$, $n = 12$), and with MPA 1-100 ratings for anxiety immediately preceding the concert ($r = .62^{*}$, $n = 12$).

Experience (number of performances) and 16 PF t-tests revealed that musicians with greater experience tended to score higher on scales of Intelligence, Dominance, Boldness, Independence, and Leadership, and lower on Insecurity and Neuroticism.

Age at first performance showed significant positive relationships with depression measures ($r = .69^{***}$, $n = 20$ with BDI scores one week before concert; and $r = .65^{**}$, $n = 21$ with highest pre-concert BDI scores) and, to a lesser extent, with anxiety measures ($r = .63^{**}$, $n = 20$ with state STAI scores one week before the concert).

CONCLUSIONS

1)   Depression is a common manifestation of musical performance anxiety, and may reach clinically significant levels.

2)   Performing experience is negatively related to stage fright, and positively related to "healthy" and assertive traits. This contradicts the popular notion that successful artists are retiring and neurotic.

3)   People who begin their performing careers earlier in life experience less stage fright than others. Early experience may produce greater performing security later in life.

CHAPTER 131

Music Performance and Cognitive Modulation

Andre Picard

INTRODUCTION

Many studies suggest that psychological factors such as apprehension[1,2] might be implicated to some extent in the attenuation of artistic quality in musical performance.[3-5] However, the role of cognitive factors such as the performer's evaluation of the importance of the event and his/her evaluation of his/her own coping capabilities have not yet been investigated in real performance situations.

The aim of this research was to explore the concepts that could be related to the emergence of performance anxiety among undergraduate music students in real performance situations.

MATERIALS and METHODS

The pretest and posttest of this naturalistic multiple-case study consisted of two successive semestrial music instrument examinations held five months apart. Eight undergraduate music students (5 females, 3 males; age 20-24, mean 21.6 years) at the Laval University School of Music (Quebec, Canada) volunteered to participate in the experiment. In the beginning of the study the subjects were given:

1) the Spielberger et al's STAI, Trait Scale[6];
2) the Sweeney's Maladaptive Anxiety Screening Questionnaire[7]; and
3) Picard's *Questionnaire Relatif l' Elaboration de Concepts*.[8]

The psychological tests used one hour prior to the subjects' musical performance were:

1) Spielberger et al's STAI, State Scale[6];
2) Horowitz et al's Positive States of Mind Scale[9];
3) Lemyre et al's[10] *Mesure du Stress Psychologique*, Short version A at the pretest, and Short version B at the posttest; and
4) Riffe's Stage Fright Index.[11]

Immediately after their performance the subjects were asked:

1) to rate their satisfaction about themselves,
2) to rate their satisfaction about their performance;
3) to rate in percentage their musical performance;
4) to answer the Lehrer et al's Musical Performance Anxiety Questionnaire;[4] and
5) to answer a questionnaire about the absorption of alcohol, medicine, drugs, caffeine, and tobacco.[12]

The physiological parameters measured at the pretest and at the posttest were:

1) heart rate, measured for a whole minute;
2) blood pressure; and
3) middle finger temperature, measured over a three-minute period.

These three measures were taken by a registered nurse 15 and 5 minutes before the performance, and 5 and 15 minutes after the performance.

The behavioral measures consisted of the official marks given by each member of the subjects' self-evaluation and with the scores of four professional musicians who rated each performance independently.

Five weeks after the pretest the subjects were given:

1) Spielberger et al's STAI, Trait Scale[6]; and
2) Lemyre et al's[10] *Mesure du stress psychologique*, Short version A as a control measure.

Between the pretest and the posttest the researcher conducted a series of seven individual semi-structured interviews with each subject. Blood pressure and finger temperature were taken by the researcher at the beginning of six successive weekly sessions. At the first meeting the researcher and the subjects reviewed the results of the pretest, including the final mark of the musical performance itself. The remaining weekly meetings were initiated with discussions upon short texts in the fields of music history, sociology, music education, psychology, as well as biographies of musicians. The subjects had to spend 10 to 15 minutes reading these excerpts prior to the meeting.

These readings were grouped under six themes as follows: 1) the social role of the musician; 2) the social role of the musical formation; 3) the role of the musical instrument examination; 4) the social role of the subject as a musician; 5) the role of his/her own musical formation; and 6) the role of his/her impending semestrial musical instrument examination. The goal of these interviews was to explore the personal concepts of each subject concerning his/her evaluation of the importance of the musical instrument examination and each subject's evaluation of his/her coping strategy/ies. Throughout these 56 individual interviews the researcher based his approach on the hypothesis that the psychological appropriation of the event and of the performer's coping capabilities might counterbalance his/her psychological apprehension when placed in a real performance situation. However, every interview was conducted with a view to respect each subject's own coping strategy/ies, the researcher suggesting psychological appropriation rather than imposing it. Each interview was audio taped, transcribed, and analysed.[13-18]

RESULTS AND DISCUSSION

Many statistical tests were performed (Statview 512+, 1986). Product moment correlations were obtained from each pair of psychological tests and behavioral measures ($n = 8$; $r_{.01} \geq .707$; $r_{.01} \geq .834$).[19,20] Over a 40-day period the retests of Spielberger et al's STAI, Trait Scale[6] and of Lemyre et al's[10] *Mesure du stress psychologique*, Short versionA gave a highly significant correlation respectively of .969 and .835. The test-retest correlation over a five month period yielded a statistically significant correlation of .822 for the Lehrer et al's Musical Performance Anxiety Questionnaire,[4] and of .831 for the Horowitz et al's Positive States Of Mind Scale.[9] The correlation between the official juries' evaluations of the musical performance at the pretest with those at the posttest (where the raters were not the same as at the pretest) reached .846. No significant correlation was obtained between any of the scores of the psychological measures and the performance ratings, neither at the pretest nor at the posttest.

According to a series of t tests for repeated measures applied to the psychological tests,[21-24] a significant statistical difference between the pretest and the posttest appeared only in the case of Horowitz et al's Positive States Of Mind Scale[9] and Lemyre et al's[10] *Mesure du stress psychologique*, Short version A at the pretest and Short version B at the posttest.

Among all the measures of the three physiological parameters only the measures of heart rate taken five minutes after the musical performance at the pretest yielded a significant correlation of .777 with the scores of the musical performances (i.e., 1 significant correlation out of a total of 32). ANOVAs showed significant differences of mean scores during the measurement procedures of each physiological parameters at the pretest and at the posttest while t tests for repeated measures yielded statistically significant differences only in the case of the systolic blood pressure.

The correlations between the marks of the official jury and those of the blind jury were highly significant both at the pretest (.890) and at the posttest (.868) but no significant t value (repeated measures) were obtained for these scores.

The preliminary qualitative data yielded by the responses of the subjects to open-ended questions of different tests and the recorded conversations between the subjects and the researcher suggests that most of the subjects never thought of planning their musical examinations on a cognitive basis, nor were they taught to do so. These data also suggest that a possible psychological appropriation aimed at counterbalancing psychological apprehension might be positioned in a theoretical model with respect to acceptation 1) of the event, and 2) of the personal coping capabilities, with 3) motivational implications. Throughout this real musical performance quasi-experimental context conviction (or lack of it), the affective ground of psychological modulation, seemed to produce a greater impact on the artistic quality of musical performance than did conception, the intellectual ground of psychological modulation, yet this impression came after an exploration of the subjects' cognitive field.

CONCLUSIONS

It would certainly be hazardous to offer here conclusions on significant issues since data are presently in the process of analysis. It is possible that external factors (to be investigated) had some effect on the variables of the study. The length of the meeting period might also be questioned. The results of the t tests for repeated measures should be interpreted cautiously, for there might be a significant difference between the means of the same repeated tests, even if the statistical figures lead us to maintain the null hypothesis. The opposite is also true.[25-27] The fact that little information came out of the physiological measures should be more fully investigated. If this phenomenon is replicated in other naturalistic settings, it would emphasize factors involved in musical performance anxiety.

Since this research was exploratory in nature, generalization of the findings should be still investigated on more practical grounds. The knowledge gained from a better understanding of the psychological components of music performance anxiety may very well lead to pedagogical implications such as the emergence of the need to prepare the students on cognitive, affective, and psychomotoric basis.

REFERENCES

1. Lemyre, l. (1986). Stress pschologique et apprehension cognitive. Thèse de doctorat. Université Laval.
2. Litt, M. D. (1989). Cognitive mediators of stressful experience: self-efficacy and perceived control. Cognitive therapy and research, 12, 3: 241-260.
3. Salmon, P.G. (1990). A psychological perspective on musical performance anxiety: a review of the literature. Medical Problems of performing artists, 5, 1: 2-11.
4. Clark, D.B. (1989). Performance-related medical and psychological disorders in instrumental musicians. Annals of behavioral medicine, 11, 1: 28-34.
5. Lehrer, P. M.; Goldman, N.S.; Strommen, E.F. (1990). A principal components assessment of performance anxiety among musicians. Medical problems of performing artists, 5, 1: 12-18.
6. Spielberger, C.D., Gorsuch, R.L., Lushene, R.E. (1970). STAI manual for the state-trait anxiety inventory. Palo Alto, CA.: Consulting Psychologists Press. Form Y-1 translated (in French) and adapted by Dr. J. Gauthier.
7. Sweeney, G.M. (1981). The separate and combined effects of cue controlled relaxation and cognitive restructuring in the treatment of musical performance anxiety. Doc. Thesis, Penn. State U.
8. Picard, A. (in press) Utilization de l' analyse de contenu dans une recherche en education musicale.
9. Horowitz, M., Adler, N., Kegeles, S. (1988). A scale for measuring the occurence of positive states of mind: a preliminary report. Psychosomatic medicine, 50: 477-483.
10. Lemyre, l., Tessier, r., Fillion, l. (1990). Mesure du stress psychologique. Brossard, Quebec: Behaviora.
11. Riffe, J.B. (1987). The effects of diaphragmatic breathing on stage fright and musical performance in college music students. Doctoral disseration. West Virginia University.
12. Picard, A. Execution musicale et modulation cognitive: une approche pedagogique. Laval University, Doctoral dissertation, in preparation.
13. Krippendorff, K. (1980). Content analysis: an introduction to its methodology. Beverly Hills, CA.: Sage publications.
14. Ghiglione, R., Beauvois, J.L., Chabrol, C., Trognon, A. (1980). Manuel d' analyse de contenu. Paris: Librairie Armand Colin.
15. Merriam, S.B. (1988). Case study research in education, a qualitative approach. San Francisco: Jossey Bass Publishers.
16. Bardin, L. (1989). L' analyse de contenu (5e ed.). Paris: Presses Universitaires de France.
17. Weber, R.P. (1990). Basic content analysis (2nd. ed.). Newbury park, california: Sage publications.
18. Grange, A. (1990). Reussir l' analyse d' un texte. Lyon: Chronique social.
19. Pfeiffer, K., Olson, J.N. (1981). Basic statistics for the behavioral sciences. New York: Hoit, Rinehart and Winston.
20. Triola, M.F. (1989). Elementary Statistics (4th ed.). Redwood city, CA.: Benjamin/Cummings.
21. Kiess, H.O., Bloomquist, D.W. (1985). Psychological Research methods. Boston: Allyn and Bacon.
22. Heyes, S., Hardy, M., Humphreys, P., Rookes, P. (1986). Starting statistics in psychology and education. London: Weidenfeld and Nicolson.
23. Shontz, F.C. (1986). Fundamentals of research in the behavioral sciences: principles and practice. Washington, D.C.: American Psychiatric Press.
24. Mason, R.D., Lind, D.A., Marchal, W.G. (1988). Statistics, an introduction (2nd ed.). San Diego: Harcourt, Brace, Jovanovich.
25. Cohen, J. (1977). Statistical power analysis for the behavioral sciences (rev. ed.). New York: Academic Press.
26. Agras, W. S. (1989). Treatment outcome

evaluation methodology: an overview. Advances in behavioral research and therapy, 11, 3: 215-220.

27. Rossi, J.S. (1990). Statistical power of psychological research: what have we gained in 20 years? Journal of consulting and clinical psychology, 58, 5: 646-656.

ACKNOWLEDGEMENTS

The researcher wishes to thank Professors David Bircher, D.M.A., and Jean-Paul Des Pins, Ph.D., respectively Chairperson and Co-Chairperson of his Dissertation Committee at Laval University for their invaluable help.

CHAPTER 132

Synchronizing Body and Mind:
The Key to Creative Process

Joan Whitacre

Abstract

For a person to give herself completely to creative activity, her whole body and mind must be saturated with the process. She feels the action, e.g. the music-making or movement, throughout her whole being, opens to this felt experience, and attunes her action, allowing herself to be guided by the intelligence of this felt experience to the intelligent guidance of this felt experience. The manner of creative work emerges from and expresses the synchronizing of body and mind.

How can the intentions and demand of creative work be embodied in a manner that enhances the artist's potential for inspiration, excellence, and fulfillment? Intentions arise in the artist's mind, in response to her experience of herself and the world. Specific demands arise out of the constraints of the creative task, e.g. the texture and density of the materials being used, the shape and size of the instrument being played, the rhythmic dynamics of the piece being played or danced to. These "real" demands, however, are often exaggerated by other qualifying conditions such as the techniques being utilized, the ambitions of the artist or her teachers, or a fear of criticism. it would be well to ask whether the body must be forced into the mold of a particular school of dance or aggressively patterned according to a specific technique for a particular instrument. Must the artist stoically endure the anxiety of performing or the loneliness of painting? Finally, is arts medicine limited to aggressive interventions, which tend to treat the problem as belonging to a disembodied object, and coping strategies which help artists to merely manage stress?

The author presents the predicament of creative artists as a creative challenge to the artists themselves, their educators, and therapists. We are challenged to support the process and transmit the means by which creative-arts students and professionals recognize their unique creative vision and capabilities, and cultivate all of their inner resources. The creative process will first be addressed from a philosophical perspective built on clinical experience and supported by theoretical study in Buddhist psychology and philosophy, phenomenological psychology, somatics, and motor learning. Practical ramifications for re-education are discussed.

Despite a recent loosening of dogma, the current, predominant medical model still regards the body as the only viable domain for physical intervention and the mind as the sole purview for psychological investigation.[1] However, the clinical experience of somatic educators and movement therapists, among others, has given rise to the observation that the more fully a person is engaged in a creative process, the more fully that person embodies the creative process. All faculties and activities, be they considered 'physical' or 'mental' from a conventional dualistic point of view, contribute appropriately to the process. Creative action is regarded as *an activity of the whole body-mind organism, requiring the alert, attuned presence of perception, cognition, emotion, and movement ... of the whole interconnected structure of skeletal, muscular, neurological, glandular, and organic units, requiring harmonious coordination of support and movement processes.*[2] It is not just a dancer's form that is involved in a pas de deux; it is not just a writer's hands and linguistic ability that are engaged in writing. The whole person is, and desires to be, present for the task.

According to Buddhist philosophy, our conception of body and mind as two separate entities is an artificial construct, as is a conception of body and mind as one simplistic. Body and mind, in fact, are not entities. They are the common reference points used to delineate, and inaccurately to divide, an individual's embodied being. *Body* describes the whole field of our experience, and *mind* refers to that which experiences this field and reflects upon it. Body is not a solid, fixed thing, but rather a continually changing aggregate of phenomena, a field of attention. Mind is not an entity that 'decodes' messages received through the bodily organs, but rather an "originative form of activity."

During the creative process, when the *mental* activity of experiencing and reflecting upon the experience is *in sync* with, or synchronizes with, the *bodily* activity of creating, the distinction between mind and body dissolves. Mind does not hold the field of attention, nor does body get *in the way*. Expressive action results from this synchronization; creative work can emerge wholesomely, without self-castigation or struggle. When reflection becomes judgmental, however, it dominates the field of attention and sees the field as a disembodied object, a *body*. The artist feels that she is in her own way or that she is, disconnectedly, watching he body or activity. She judges physical disharmony, evidenced in pain, fatigue, or strain, as an obstacle to be conquered, rather than an intelligent voice to be heard.

Phenomenological psychology espouses the therapeutic necessity of focusing on the phenomenon of one's own life, as the living of it is experienced by the person.[1] Analysis of its meaning proceeds from this inner focus, rather than from interpretation imposed by an external system. This focusing engages all of the senses, enhancing a person's awareness and physical experience of being in the world.[1] This awareness has been identified as a *bodily felt sense*.[4]

David Levin states that this awareness allows one to "retrieve . . . an experience of Being in its more hospitable, more wholesome dimensionality." He calls this therapeutic process a recollection, whereby one regains a sense of body-mind integrity.[5]

Recollection is actually a term used to describe basic Buddhist meditation practice. It refers to a recollection of the present, i.e. a recollecting of one's mind into the present, accomplished by letting go of regret and clinging to the past and hope and fear for the future. The artist comes face to face with her disharmonious behavior towards herself and her creative endeavor — her patterns of being out of sync. Recollection also opens her to recreating her behavior, as a manifestation of synchronizing. Thomas Hanna, a spokesperson for the field of somatics, states that somatics studies the body as perceived from within. Thus, it takes a first-person viewpoint, seeing the body from the outside, as an objective, analyzable, and measurable entity. Rather than rejecting the third-person viewpoint, he regards each view as co-equal.[6]

Simultaneously, each potential artist is endowed with a unique intelligence and passion, and possesses a singular vision. While somatics recognizes the objective generalities of structure and function which apply to all human beings, and the general processes and issues which apply to all artists, its distinct modus operandi is to investigate and support the artist's unique experience and expression of her sensed life.

Somatics provides a definitive vision and practical methodology for the process of recollection. It recognizes that human beings are able to modify their functioning by giving attention to the sensory qualities of their bodies' structures and functions.[7] This attending activates an ever-increasing responsiveness to internal needs, desires and interests, and an ever-developing ability to move towards those needs, etc.

This process of attending and responding cultivates inner resources in certain vital areas of functioning. It attunes those resources to the varying demands of the creative work. These resources manifest in the release of unnecessary tension, the restoration of well-being, the establishment of a dynamic base of support, the focusing of attention, and expressive communication. According to Hanna, the goal of somatic process is an ever-enhanced understanding of the somatic process and an ever-revised set of guidelines for its enhancement.[8]

How can creative artists, their educators, and therapists utilize this approach? The artist or arts student undertakes and makes a commitment to the process or recollection as a discipline. This process learns to focus attention on the sensory-motor details of required skills and tasks. In the course of this process, she becomes aware of her use of unnecessary tension in performing various tasks, and is enabled to release those tensions. As her ability to focus stabilizes, she becomes aware of relationships across various levels of her functioning. She gradually becomes skilled in understanding the meaning of the various sensations which she has learned to discriminate, such as pressure, stretching, or pain. Finally, she develops sensitive responsiveness to this ongoing feedback of her sensory-motor functioning. She is thereby continually able to adapt her movement to changing task requirements and changing internal states. Such an artist acquires a repertoire of corrective responses which she is able to apply appropriately and confidently. She also is able to discern and willing to acknowledge when she requires professional assistance.

This process can be elucidated in the language of motor-learning. Acquiring skill necessitates a structural compatibility between the student of a particular art and the required tools or given instrument. It also requires the student's commitment of attention and awareness. In the beginning stages of learning to play the violin, for example, attention must be given to various basic factors such as the way in which the violin and one's arm are supported, and standing with ease while holding the violin. The musician gradually develops a thorough kinesthetic awareness, a bodily felt sense, of her own bodily instrument in its relationship to the violin, its structure, range of action, ability to support, express, and resonate forces. The violin then becomes a flowing extension of the body rather than the source of stressful demands *on* the body. As the violin student matures in this regard, control of these fundamental aspects of he violin playing shifts to more automatically functioning levels. Her focal attention and awareness concomitantly shift to other fields of attention, becoming more fully occupied with the felt bodily sense of the music in its dynamics, rhythms, and colors — the emotional content of the music.

What results occur in response to this approach? Artists and arts students report relief from discomfort and pain, greater mobility, increased confidence, enhanced capacity to deal creatively with problems, and attendant emotional satisfaction. Indeed, the body-mind explorations that constitute the recollective process can become a source of inspiration and creative expression.[7]

REFERENCES

1. Seem M, Kaplan J: Bodymind Energetics. Vermont: Healing Arts Press, 1989.
2. Whitacre J: Synchronizing body and mind: The key to creative process. New York University Conference Proceedings: Mind, Body, and the Performing Arts, 1985.
3. Guenther HV: Buddhist Philosophy in Theory and Practice. Baltimore: Penguin Books, 1972.
4. Gendlin ET: Focusing. New York: Bantam Books, 1981.
5. Levin DM: The Body's Recollection of Being: Phenomenological Psychology and the Deconstruction of Nihilism, 53. London: Routledge & Kegan Paul, 1985.
6. Hanna T: The field of somatics. Somatics 1(1): 30-34, 1976. As quoted in Gomez N: Movement, Body and Awareness, 1988.
7. Gomez N, Bolster G: Movement, Body and Awareness. Montreal: On deposit at National Library of Quebec, 1988.
8. Hanna T: What is Somatics. Somatics 5(4):4-8, 1988. As quoted in Gomez N: Movement, Body and Awareness, 1988.

SUGGESTED READING

1. Arend S: Developing the substrates of skillful movement. Motor Skills: Theory into Practice 4(1):3-10, 1980.
2. Bartenieff I, Lewis D: Coping with the Environment. New York: Gordon & Breach Science Publishers, 1980.
3. Brooks CB: Sensory Awareness: The Rediscovery of Experiencing. Santa Barbara, CA: Ross Erickson Publishers, 1982.
4. Brooks VB: The Neural Base of Motor Control. London: Oxford University Press, 1984.
5. Cohen BB: The training problems of the dancer. Contact Quarterly 7(3/4):9-15, 1982.
6. Cohen BB: Perceiving in action. Contact Quarterly 9(2):24-39, 1984.
7. Cohen BB: The Mechanics of Vocal Expression. Unpublished manual, 1985.
8. Davis M: Movement as patterns of process. Main Currents in Modern Thought, Vol 31, 1974.
9. Dell C: A primer for movement description. New York: Dance Notation Bureau, 1970.
10. Evarts EV: Brain mechanisms in movement. Scientific American 229(1):96-103, 1973.
11. Gallistel CR: The Organization of Action. Hillsdale, NJ: Lawrence Erlbaum Assoc, 1980.
12. Gendlin ET: Experiencing and the Creation of Meaning. Glencoe, NY: Free Press, 1962.
13. Gentile AM: A working model of skill acquisition with appreciation to teaching. Quest 17:3-23, 1972.
14. Hanna T, Higgins JR: Human Movement: An Integrated Approach. St. Louis: CV Mosby Co, 1977.
15. Higgins SA: Movement as an Emergent Form. Pre-publication manuscript, 1982.
16. Laban R: The Mastery of Movement. Boston: Plays Inc, 1950.
17. Masao I: The Cerebellum and Neural Control. New York: Raven Press, 1984.
18. Merton PA: How we control the contraction of our muscles. Scientific American 226(5)-30-37, 1972.
19. Smith NS, Nelson L: Interview with Bonnie Bainbridge Cohen. Contact Quarterly 5(2):20-28, 1980.
20. Sweigard L: Human Movement Potential. New York: Harper & Row, 1974.

PART XI

VISUAL ARTS
MEDICINE

CHAPTER 133

Children's Art Safety: A Survey of Canadian Elementary-School Art Programs

Shalini Gupta • *John R. Harrison*

INTRODUCTION

In 1982, Canada's Department of National Health and Welfare initiated a Safer Arts Program directed at promoting awareness of health hazards in arts-and-crafts materials and the adoption of good work practices.[1] The goal was to inform and educate professionals, artists, or hobbyists through published materials, lectures, and advice.

The first project was a series of posters and a booklet, *The Safer Arts* (published in English and French), on a variety of arts-and-crafts media such as painting and printmaking, dyes and fibers, pottery and ceramics, stained glass and glass blowing, sculpture, wood, photography, metal working and jewelry, and enamelling.[2] The response to these items was so large that a second printing was necessary.

ELEMENTARY-SCHOOL SURVEY

The current focus of the Canadian Safer Arts Program includes emphasis on health and safety awareness in children, parents, and teachers regarding art programs. A booklet on children's art safety is in preparation. The first phase of this project, a survey of school art programs from grades one to eight, was initiated in January 1991. A questionnaire was mailed to the principals of 3,970 randomly selected schools in Canada. It was designed to study the use of art materials and processes in art programs and was completed by art teachers.

Art was defined for this survey as any program or class exercise that works with paints, dyes, fibers, stained or blown glass, metal, wood, or enamel, or makes prints, photographs, sculptures, jewelry, pottery, or ceramics.

The main objective of this national survey, and the children's art-safety booklet to be produced as a result of it, is to provide information about the safe use of arts-and-crafts materials by children and teachers in schools. The booklet will also include information about the hazards of excessive exposure to toxic products.

SURVEY METHODOLOGY

Questionnaire Categories

The categories used in the questionnaire were: students, art activities, purchasing procedures, art products, clean-up, disposal, inventory, storage, student awareness, general safety and personal protective equipment, health and safety emergency procedures, teacher and student health, teachers, legal matters and regulations, and health and safety programs. Under each of these categories, a series of questions were posed. For instance, under art activities, fifteen different art processes were listed to determine whether (a) a specific process was used, (b) the work occurred in a regular or separate art room, and (c) determine the grade level in which the process was used.

Sample Design

The sample design consisted of stratifying the sample by five regions (Atlantic, Quebec, Ontario, Prairies, and British Columbia), two grade levels (1-6, 7-8), and school types (private, public, special needs, and native).

The first stratification, the provinces and territories, follows from the fact that education is a provincial responsibility in Canada and the provincial governments control budget, curriculum design, and teacher-training requirements, as well as health and safety regulations. The second stratification, grade level, was chosen because of the different types of materials used in these grades and the physiological sensitivity of children of various ages. The third stratification was school type. While public and private school are the most common types of schools, special-needs schools were incorporated because of their traditional heavy emphasis on art materials for these children. Native schools were also chosen because of their distinct situation in Canada.

Sample Requirements

The sample size requirement for the study stratification was calculated and the sample sizes were based on the following criteria:

■ *Desired Precision of Results*: The sample sizes are sufficiently large so that if p is a proportion estimated from the sample results, then the true population percentage will lie in the interval p + 10%, except for a 1-in-20 chance. The interval p + 10%, except for a 1-in-20 chance, is referred to as a 95% confidence interval.

■ *Expected Response Rate*: The sample sizes included an adjustment for an expected response rate of 50%. With a final response rate higher than 50%, the results would be more precise than required; with a response rate lower than 50%, the results would be less precise than required.

Response rates in mail surveys often are very low, and it is not uncommon to see rates much lower than 50%. It was felt, however, that teachers who are involved in art programs are very concerned about health and safety practices, and would therefore be motivated to respond. In addition, to increase the response rate, a second set of questionnaires was mailed to those who had not responded to the first.

■ *Variability of Characteristics in the Population*: It was assumed for this survey that most of the estimates would be proportions or percentages. The sample size required depends on the variability of characteristics in the population being surveyed. Essentially, the smaller the variability in the population, the smaller the sample size required to have good estimates of the characteristics of interest. For example, for a proportion p being estimated, the closer p is to 1 or to zero, the smaller the sample size required to provide good estimates. The point of maximum variability is when the proportion p in the population is 0.5. In order to estimate p from a sample when this is the case, the sample size required is greatest — i.e. this is considered a worst-case scenario.

As little is known about the distribution of characteristics relevant to health and safety practices in Canadian school art programs, sample sizes have been calculated for a p = 0.5, i.e. these sample sizes are the maximum required.

Sample Distribution

The table below shows the distribution of the samples within Canada. The sample sizes have been distributed proportionally based on the number of schools in each province I territory.

Survey Collection

The collection and capture of the questionnaires were completed on June 11, 1991, with a 62.8 % recovery. These results produce a higher statistical precision than was initially expected. The table below summarizes the total mailout and response rates by grade level and province, respectively.

Few national surveys produce a response rate as high as in this study. Questionnaire results are being analyzed and will be published separately.

Children's Art Safety Questionnaires — Total Mailout and (Total Response as of June 11, 1991)

SCHOOLS	ATLANTIC	QUEBEC	ONTARIO	PRAIRIES	BRITISH COLUMBIA	TERRITORIES	TOTAL MAILOUT	PERCENTAGE OF TOTAL MAILOUT
Public								
1 - 6	247 (170)	232 (145)	192 (148)	176 (125)	198 (139)	83 (51)	1,128 (778)	69.0
7 - 8	239 (161)	182 (113)	151 (128)	190 (143)	158 (116)	76 (36)	996 (697)	70.0
Private								
1 - 6	47 (18)	74 (39)	177 (102)	189 (101)	118 (63)	- (-)	605 (323)	53.4
7 - 8	53 (20)	198 (137)	198 (100)	108 (53)	134 (88)	- (-)	691 (398)	57.6
Special Needs	20 (10)	164 (72)	135 (92)	90 (56)	85 (46)	- (-)	494 (276)	55.9
Native	- (-)	1 (1)	3 (1)	50 (19)	2 (-)	- (-)	56 (21)	37.5
Total	606 (379)	851 (507)	856 (571)	803 (497)	695 (452)	159 (87)	3,970 (2,493)	62.8

REFERENCES

1. Harrison J: Art-related health hazards: Artists should be put in picture. CMAJ (140):702-703, 1989.

2. Department of National Health and Welfare, Canada. The Safer Arts: The Health Hazards of Arts and Crafts Materials, 1990.

CHAPTER 134

Safety in the Theater Working Environment:
A Study on Incidence and Causes of Reported Injuries and Accidents Among Workers in Swedish Public Theaters

Walter Ruth • *Lars I. Persson*

Abstract

The causes of accidents have been studied using a systems approach to theater work. An early finding of this research was that holistic descriptions of the theater as a production system, including all kinds of activity, hardly existed. Such a model, as a basic concept for studying the interaction between artistic and technical production work in theaters, was developed. It is concluded that the production system of a theater is characterized by the conflict between two parts of the production process which have the same goals but with different needs. On one hand, the artistic process developing the scenic interpretation of the text; on the other, the physical, technical processes of manufacturing the set decorations, props, costumes, lighting, and sound that are needed to perform the scenic interpretation. On one hand, the need for a certain amount of *chaos* and late decisions, as fuel for creativity; on the other, the need for *order* and a time schedule that allows the planning of rational production, and the craftsmen to use their skill. Since the artistic result is the product of the theater, the technical part of the production often has a considerably lower status, which is an important cause of accidents, not only among technical staff.

A pilot study begun in 1985, entitled *The Theatre's Working Environment and its Future Development*,[1] has developed into an ongoing research project at Luleå University on working conditions, accidents, and organizational and technological development in all Swedish municipal-, county- and state supported theaters.[2] Its major aim is to study the total production process of the theater, especially the influence of artistic production on the working conditions of the technical production, and vice versa.

In a parallel project at Lund University, the reactions of artists to physical and psychological strain are studied. In an investigation by the present authors, overlapping both projects, reported injuries and accidents among different professions working in Swedish public theaters have been studied over the period 1980-88, and the study is ongoing.

ACCIDENTS AND INJURIES

The risk of work injury as a result of an accident or physical strain is high within the theater (Fig. 1). One-third of the employees have had some type of reported injury within a five-year period. Dancers are most at risk, with an incidence of reported injuries as high as 1.1, followed by carpenters, blacksmiths, and stage hands, with incidences around 0.5-0.7, and actors 0.25. The few low-risk professions in the theater include tailors, wig-makers, and administrators.

In Sweden, many traditional risks, such as the use of hazardous agents, are restricted by law. All work injuries must be reported. Yet, injuries are still neglected (particularly among artists), especially if they do not directly hinder performance. It is suspected that this occurs more often in the theater than in industry, which often has routine procedures for reporting of injuries. In general, preventive measures and the planning for better environmental conditions are much more developed in industry.

A detailed study of injury- and accident reports reveals that, especially among artists, there often is a delay of several months before the accidents report is filled out. Actors and dancers tend to delay reporting until they feel chronic pain or can no longer perform. A considerable number of reports also mention several separate incidents where the previous accident might have caused some injury which enhances vulnerability and risk of further damage. In industry, such incidents would have resulted in a number of separate reports. There also was a tendency in several theaters for actors to delay taking sick leave until the play is in a break period.

In a survey of 146 Swedish ballet dancers, it was revealed that only seven (out of 128 responding) did

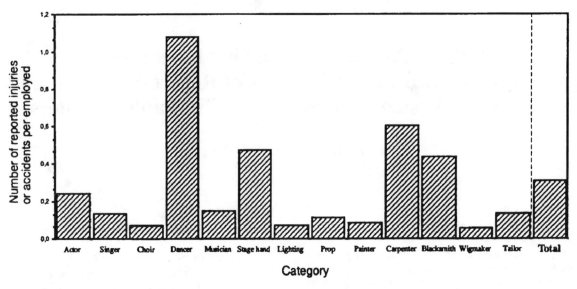

Figure 1: *Incidence of reported in juries and accidents over five years (1984-88) for 1363 employees of different categories in a representative sample of Swedish public theaters.*

not suffer from any kind of injury during the latest 12-month period.[3] A large number of dancers' injuries are never reported, since there is an emphasis on not giving up too easily and not complaining. If they do, their careers might be terminated. Some choreographers reject complaining dancers. The result is that a number of very talented dancers have had to quit because of chronic injuries resulting from continuous dancing under pain.

CAUSES OF ACCIDENTS AND INJURIES

Between 50% and 80% of the injuries among actors, dancers and musicians involve heavy physical load (Fig. 2). In musicians, this is a major cause of tendinitis and other musculoskeletal disorders. Long periods of monotonous, repetitive arm movements while the body is rigidly seated is the predominating situation described in these reports. In the case of

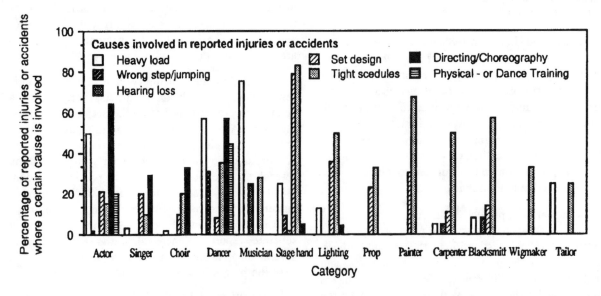

Figure 2: *Causes of reported injuries and accidents during a five-year period among various personnel categories in Swedish public theaters. The accident- and injury reports were examined with regard to the extent to which different properties of the theater as a production system were involved in the chain of events leading to hazard formation.*

actors, the total injury rate has increased to 0.24 during the five-year period 1984-88, as compared to 0.17 in the previous 1980-84 period.[4] Comparing the descriptions of *what happened* in the reports from the earlier and later periods, it is possible to form a hypothesis that the artistic trend towards a more *physical* theater might be a major cause of the increased accident rate. In more than 50% of the *heavy load* cases among actors, they have been involved in some violent physical activity, either during performance on stage or during training for such activities. Catch-as-catch-can wrestling or other types of simulated fights and acrobatic hazardous movements are typical examples of what was going on. Many of these cases belong to the above-mentioned group who tend to report several repeated injuries in one report.

Training was responsible in 20% of the artists' injuries and in 50% of the dancers'. One reason, as noted by Ramel,[3] is inadequate warming up at the beginning of the compulsory *morning school*. Our study of the injury reports revealed that the morning school certainly is a dangerous activity. Many of these cases also show injury patterns where the lack of warming up could be a major cause. The authors can also confirm the findings of Ramal that dancers who respond inadequately to their body signals tend to have injuries. Dancers report that they tend to suffer pain for a long time before reporting injury or taking sick leave. Bad landings after high or difficult jumps also is a significant cause of dancers' injury (25%).

In both actors' accidents with *physical theater* and dancers' jumps and heavy loads, the artistic concept of the director or choreographer has a strong influence (65% in actors' injuries and nearly 60% in dancers'. This is also an important factor among other groups, such as opera- and choir singers (30-40%), or even stage hands and lighting technicians.

Cuts, broken bones, and crushing are relatively common among stage hands; cuts of varying severity also dominate injuries reported by carpenters. The latter also suffer sprains, dislocations, and pulled muscles. Many of their injuries are related to the construction and design of set decorations (10-80%). Often, little consideration is given to the way it should be handled, carried, or manufactured when the set designer conceptualizes his work. Actors also have accidents related to set design. One important factor might be the lack of communication in most theaters between artists and technical staff manufacturing the decorations (Fig. 3). Preliminary results show a lower incidence of accidents related to set design in theaters with better communication between different personnel categories.

The predominant cause of accidents for technical staff is tight time schedules. They must hurriedly adapt to the terms of the artistic production. This brings us back to the status of technical staff and the concept of balance between order and chaos.[5]

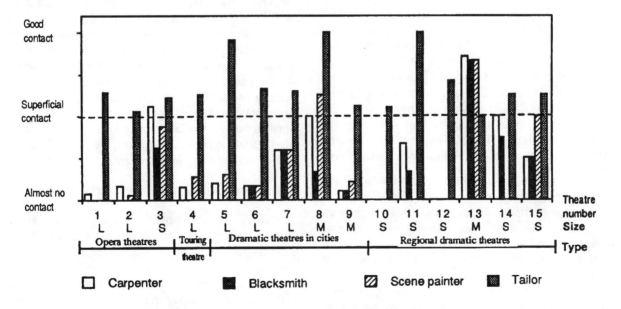

Figure 3: *How much contact (during work) do artists have with technical staff in the theater? Communication is poor in most theaters. Data from a large-scale (unreported to date) survey of Swedish artists.*

THREE PARALLEL PRODUCTION PROCESSES IN ONE HOLISTIC SYSTEM

Theater production can be looked upon as three parallel production processes: artistic, technical, and administrative. They all use different production methods, different technology, different management, different staff with different education and backgrounds, and different premises. Due to the shortage of space in most theater houses, there is often a considerable geographic distance between locations of the three processes. Often, they also have different economic budgets. It is important to remember, however, that the three different production processes shall produce one, and only one, product: the *performance* — or, rather, a series of performances: the *repertoire*. It is no easy task, therefore, to be managing director of a theater — or, as the Swedish playwright August Blanche puts it in his comedy *A Travelling Theatre Company*: "The devil should be theater director!"

To safeguard all three processes, interaction is key. Theater production must occur within a holistic system. But it is a difficult balancing act between independence sufficient to maintain a rational production in each of the three processes, and integration necessary to avoid sub-optimizing and conflicting objectives. Again, it is a matter of balance between *order* and *chaos*. The key roles in solving these problems must be played by people taking part in decision-making and production in each of the three processes. Effective interaction requires a high level of awareness of the consequences that actions taken in one part of the system will cause in other parts of the system.[6] This requires that all participants in the system have adequate knowledge of what is important matters for the others. To understand this, they must know fairly well how the work of others is done. The theater director is responsible for fostering this enhanced awareness. This also happens to be the most effective way to promote the basic objectives of art.

The famous Russian theater theorist and director Stanislawskij wrote, in his essay *Etika*: *All those of different professions working in the theatre — from the receptionist, the cloak room attendant, the auditorium attendant, and the box office personnel, who are those which our spectators first meet when they come to us, to the administrative staff, the accountants, the director, and ourselves the actors, who perform the creative work together with the play writer and the composer, and for whose sake people fill the auditorium — all are servants to Art and have to be subjects to the basic objectives of*

Art. Without exceptions, all of them participate creating the performance ... The theater worker's cooperative slavish dependence upon the objectives of Art does not only concern the performance but all the day's work ... If a rehearsal by some reason becomes nonproductive, it means that those who disturbed the work harm the objectives of Art.[7]

Stanislawskij's perspectives are of great interest. He has had a major influence on the view of theater as art in the western hemisphere. Although several of his theories, e.g. the *fourth wall*, were strongly rejected by later theater theorists, his ideals regarding the relationship between the *actor and his art*, like those cited above, still live in modern theater, as studies have confirmed.[2, 8]

Stanislawskij's field of vision is narrow, focusing primarily on the actors and seemingly ignoring the technical staff. Translated to the work organization of larger modern theaters, his ideals lead to status differences between various categories of personnel. Stage hands of large theaters have described themselves as "the coolies." This can pose a threat to effective interaction. The situation is better in smaller, regional theaters.

Outside the theater, there is a tendency to focus on performance and forget that 90% of theater work is not performance! The fact that theater production involves a massive contribution of work by professions normally found in industry, like blacksmiths, carpenters, welders, electricians, upholsterers, painters, tailors, and dressmakers, to mention just a few, is little known. Since decisions about theater building plans are primarily the products of these ill-informed outsiders, a typical result is a luxurious lobby area for the audience, reasonably good stage facilities for performances, and disastrous lack of space for rehearsals, workshops, storage, and transports. This outsider view of what theater is, combined with a quasi-exclusive focus on the actor, are the basic causes behind bad working environment.

ORGANIZATION AND NEW TECHNOLOGY

There are also organizational problems in the theater, comparable to those in industry. As in industry, there is an ongoing high-tech development in the theater. The transfer of know-how from industry, however, is lacking. Theaters now tend to make the same mistakes industry did some ten years ago, e.g. taking too much of the system's control away from man and giving it to machines. A typical result is computerized handling of decorations, without utilizing the knowledge of skilled stage workers, causing accidents, monotonous work, and artistically poor visual effects. An approach to solving these problems has been developed for the new fly machinery system of the old opera house in Gothenburg. Knowledge from industrial hydraulic transport technology has been combined with sophisticated theater technology and ergonomics, to form a computerized system where all advantageous properties of the old manual system, such as manual controllability, remain.[9] By involving the stage workers in the planning, and by forbidding the system engineers to deliver a completed version of the software, the new way of running the system closely resembled the old way, except that the heavy manual handling of counterbalances and pulling of ropes was substituted by the use of a joystick. But the same *feeling* and direct contact was there. Gradually, during a period of more than a year, more sophisticated software properties were developed, involving the workers. They have also been trained to understand the entire system and to perform maintenance and service work. As a result, the status of these "coolies" has risen considerably.

REFERENCES

1. Lindström KG, Persson LI, Ruth W, Svenstam Å: A study of the theater working environment and its future development. Lund University, Research Report PU 87:159 (in Swedish), PU 89:172 (in English, abbreviated), 1987, 1989.

2. Ruth W: The theater working environment. Project Plan, Swedish Work Environment Fund, Project #87-0109 (Stockholm), 1987.

3. Ramel E: Working conditions and troubles in the locomotive organs in ballet dancers at three Swedish theaters. Project Report (in Swedish), University of Lund, 1991.

4. Ruth W, Persson L: Arbetsskador och olycksfallsanalys inom teaterverksamhet. Luleå University of Technology, Research Report, TULEA 1987:25, 1987.

5. Ruth W: The balance between order and chaos. On the working environment and organisation of work in theaters. *In* Quinnec Y, Daniellou F (eds): Designing for Everyone: Proceedings from the 11th IEA Congress, Paris, July 1991, 1196-1198. London: Taylor & Francis, 1991.

6. Ruth W: New technology in old culture. An action theory for working environment planning in the introduction of new technology in production systems of tomorrow. *In* Karnowski W, Yates SR (eds), Advances in Industrial Ergonomics and Safety, Volume 3. Proceedings of the Annual International Industrial Ergonomics and Safety Conference, Lake Tahoe, June 1991, 753-760. London: Taylor & Francis, 1991.

7. Ludawska J (ed): Att vara äkta på scén — Selections from Stanislawskij. Stockholm: Gidlunds-Theatron, 1986.

8. Lindén J, Torkelson E: 1990, Yrke skådespelare. Kritiska moment i arbetslivet. Lund University, Research Report, preliminary version, 1990.

9. Ruth W, Nyström M: The human work as basis for the development of high-tech systems for materials handling and transports in theater production and in the planning of theater buildings. Invited lecture at NOTT-89, Third Nordic Conference of Theater Technology, Copenhagen, June 1989.

SUGGESTED READING

1. Ritter S: Die Bühnentechnik und die Bühnensysteme als Bestandteile des Transport-Umschlag- und Lagersystems Theaterbühne/ Technische Universität Dresden, Dissertation Doktor-Ingenieur 02.02.1988, (Dresden).

2. Ruth W, Kull G, Nyström M, Olsson G, Thorell B, Westerlund E: Materialhantering och transporter inom teaterverksamhet, Luleå University of Technology, Research Report TULEA 1986:24, 1986.

3. Ruth W: We are prosperous: On the socio-economic effects of culture production. Invited lecture at Development Seminar 28-29.5, Östergötlands Regionteater (Norrköping), 1990.

CHAPTER 135

Visual Artists with Physical Disabilities

Lois Kaggen

Professional visual artists with physical disabilities face many career obstacles that severely limit their access to exhibition opportunities. Artists with impaired hearing, speech, vision or mobility are unable to compete equally with able-bodied artists because of the physical inaccessibility of numerous galleries and negative attitudes towards persons with disabilities. Wheelchairs or prostheses, along with communicative impairments of disabled artists, contribute to museum- and gallery directors' prejudiced and biased judgments about art created by the physically disabled.

Resources for Artists with Disabilities, a not-for-profit, tax-exempt corporation, promotes public awareness of and organizes exhibition opportunities for professional visual artists with physical disabilities. Such exhibits, juried by art professionals, offer the public and the arts community direct access to the visual statements of this disenfranchised minority of visual artists who are physically impaired.

Disabled artists throughout the United States have submitted slides of their art work for inclusion in Resources for Artists with Disabilities' slide-library, which is available for viewing by exhibition curators and directors.

The physical disabilities of these artists include multiple sclerosis, cerebral palsy, polio, retinitis pigmentosa, severe traumatic brain injury, and peripheral neuropathy. Their visual, auditory, and motor dysfunctions, such as deafness and quadraplegia, necessitate specific services that help to mainstream these artists into the very competitive New York art world.

To enable them to be able to compete more equaly for art-world recognition, Resources for Artists with Disabilities offers disabled artists barrier-free exhibition sites, transportation and hanging of their art work, interpreters for the deaf at symposia and receptions, transportation for disabled artists to these events, and attendant care at receptions when needed. These services enable the disabled artists to gain exhibition experience and publicity for their art work, to attend and participate in art events and receptions sponsored by the organization, and to gain public exposure and competitive recognition, thus enhancing their ability to function independently in the art world.

Since its founding in 1987, Resources for Artists with Disabilities has organized and coordinated twelve art exhibits in public exhibition spaces in New York City, a world-renowned art center. In addition, at the request of the United States Information Agency, Resources for Artists with Disabilities has organized meetings with, and the demonstration of painting techniques by, a delegation of physically disabled artists from Jilin Province in the People's Republic of China. The organization has also coordinated and participated in five panel discussions and symposia concerning disabled artists, including a 1990 symposium at the Edward John Noble Education Center at the Museum of Modern Art in New York City. A 32- minute video documentary of this symposium has been professionally produced.

For further information, contact: Resources for Artists with Disabilities, Inc., 77 Seventh Avenue, Suite PH-G, New York, NY 10011-6645

CHAPTER 136

Van Gogh as Replacement Child

J. G. M. van Rossum

In the 862 letters which have been preserved and which Vincent van Gogh sent to his brother, Theo, no mention is made by the painter of his namesake/ brother, born exactly a year earlier. On March 30, 1852, the first Vincent Willem, the eldest child, was (still)born. On March 30, 1853, the second Vincent Willem was born. Both Vincents were recorded under the same number (No. 29) in the parish birth register of Zundert. It is obvious, therefore, that there are a number of similarities between the two brothers: the same day of birth (March 30, whereby the day of birth is also the day of death), the same name, the same registration number in the parish birth register. Until 1871, Vincent's parents lived in Zundert (he was then 18 years old), and the elder Vincent Willem lay buried in the graveyard of the Reformed Church, where his father was a minister. Frequently, Vincent passed his dead brother's grave.

Although nowhere does Vincent mention his predecessor consciously or directly, it appears from his letters that he was frequently preoccupied with his brother, both associatively and subconsciously, as seen in the following examples:

Letter No. 79: About his first sermon in England he writes, "When I was in the pulpit, I felt like someone who emerges from a dark cavern under the ground into the friendly light of day." Another excerpt, from No. 116: "... because it makes someone feel good to know that another brother of his is alive and walking around on this earth ... that as it were one can feel solid ground under one's feet." In Letter No. 132, the last letter before his nine-month period of silence from the Borinage: "Yet it is better that men can mean something to one another, than that men should stand opposite each other as corpses, more so because as long as one does not have the right to the title of the corpse by legal death ... that both are still in the land of the living ..." and, further, "that one feels incomplete and unworthy and superfluous ..." and "I am considered an intruder and

superfluous, so that it would be better if I were not here." Lastly, from Letter No. 564: "... in the portrait by Delacroix there is a gentleman with reddish hair and beard who resembles both you and me very much, and who reminded me of this poem by De Musset: 'Everywhere I have been on earth, there was an unhappy one, dressed in black, who came and joined us and looked at us like a brother.'"[1]

In *Broers en Zussen*[2] ("Brothers and Sisters"), Gerritsma mentions the indirect influence of the death of a sibling. Parents frequently try to rediscover the dead child in one of the remaining children. When the child's death has occurred before his or her birth, that child will have to learn to live with two identities: his or her own and that of the dead brother or sister. The parents unwittingly identify the two (the dead child and the replacement child). They are compared continually. Negative feelings toward the dead child are repressed and an image of the dead child is created which is over-idealized and, therefore, unrealistic, even if the child was stillborn. The replacement child is burdened with the impossible task of having to compete with his dead rival and, in the fantasy created by the parents, becomes responsible for the death of the other child. He has taken his place but will never be able to live up to the expectations of his role: there is little space for the development of his personal identity. A great discrepancy exists between a high ideal which cannot be reached and reality. This can lead to depression.

Depressions which occur during the Christmas season are primarily the result of awakened conflicts related to unresolved sibling rivalries ... partly because the holiday celebrates the birth of a Child so favored that competition with Him is futile, earlier memories, especially of oral frustrations, are rekindled.[3]

Replacement children are strongly attracted to and are sometimes preoccupied with death, graveyards and houses of mourning, and they often feel they will die young.

These themes can be found in van Gogh's letters and visual art, e.g. in Letter No. 91, in which he describes his visit to Zundert. Consider his stay in the Borinage, where he went down into the coal mines, nicknamed "the mass grave" or "Coffin." Call to mind paintings and drawings with the sower and reaper, with the sunrise and sunset, or with heaven and earth; the earth dug as he had seen grave-diggers doing countless times in the graveyard next to his parental home; the earth in which people are buried and which contains rotting tree trunks, but which also nourishes and brings forth the *potato*. The significance of this word can be found in the translation of the Dutch word, which means *earthapple*. The potato, with its association with earth, is found in his still-life paintings of the potato and in his masterpiece *The Potato-eaters*, painted in May 1885.

REFERENCES

1. DeMusset: Verzamelde Brieven van Vincent van Gogh. Amsterdam: BV 't Lanthuys, 1974.
2. Mettrop-Wurster I, et al: Broers en Zussen, 30-43. Meppel/Amsterdam: Boom, 1989.
3. Boyer BL: Christmas neurosis. J Amer Psy Assn 3:467-488, 1956.
4. Lubin AJ: Stranger on the Earth. New York: Holt, Rinehart and Winston, 1972.
5. Van Rossum JGM: Van Gogh's Kerstmis, 2-6. Venlo/Riagg: Bij de Tijd, 1990.

PART XII

VOCAL ARTS
MEDICINE

CHAPTER 137

The Professional Voice:
The Science and Art of Clinical Care
An Outline

Robert Thayer Sataloff

The author combines his experience as a professional singer, university choral conductor, and laryngologist in a didactic presentation of clinically relevant vocal pedagogy and laryngology. The objective of this outline is to provide comprehensive understanding of voice and a systemic approach to the problems of professional voice users. Although centering primarily on singers, the principles presented are relevant to professional speakers, as well. Special emphasis is placed on unique aspects of the history, on environmental and physical factors that have a direct effect on vocal function, and on medical conditions outside the head and neck that may be responsible for voice dysfunction. Specific guidelines for the management of acute and chronic vocal dysfunction are presented.

I. ANATOMY OF THE SINGING VOICE

   A. Larynx
      1. Mucosa
      2. Intrinsic muscles
      3. Extrinsic muscles

   B. Supraglottic vocal tract

   C. Tracheobronchial tree, lungs and thorax

   D. Abdomen

   E. Musculoskeletal system

   F. Psychoneurological System

II. HISTORY

   A. Age

   B. Complaint(s)
      1. Duration
      2. Associated illness
      3. Nature
         a. Hoarseness
         b. Fatigue
         c. Volume disturbance
         d. Prolonged warm-up time
         e. Breathiness
         f. Loss of range
         g. Tickling or choking
         h. Pain

   C. Date of next important performance

   D. Professional singing status and goals

   E. Amount and nature of voice training
      1. How many years singing?
      2. How many years of training?
         a. Continuous
         b. Interrupted
      3. How many teachers?
      4. How long with current teacher?
      5. Any training of the speaking voice?

   F. Type of singing and environment
   (*Lombard effect*)
      1. Classical
      2. Pop
      3. Amateur
      4. Choral

   G. Rehearsal
      1. Vocal practice: When, how, how long?
      2. Performance rehearsal

   H. Voice abuse
      1. Singing
         a. Technique
         b. Preparation
         c. Environment
         d. Health
         e. Other

2. Speaking
    a. Dissociation of speaking and singing voice
    b. Cars
    c. Backstage greetings
    d. Post performance parties
    e. Cheerleading
    f. Conducting

I. General health
    1. Physical condition
    2. Amount of sleep
    3. Weight changes

J. Medical condition
    1. Upper respiratory infection
    2. Allergy
    3. Post nasal drip
    4. Sinus disease
    5. Dental
    6. Reflux
    7. Endocrine including menstruation
    8. Constipation of diarrhea
    9. Hearing loss
    10. Anxiety
        a. Performance anxiety
        b. Outside stress (agents, etc.)
    11. Hypochondriasis

K. Exposure to irritants
    1. Allergy
    2. Dust
    3. Cold
    4. Dry heat
    5. Recent travel
    6. Other

L. Smoke
    1. Tobacco
    2. Marijuana
    3. Other

M. Drugs
    1. Alcohol
    2. Antihistamines
    3. Antibiotics
    4. Diuretics
    5. Hormones (especially birth control pills)
    6. Cocaine
    7. Vitamin C

N. Foods
    1. Milk
    2. Ice cream
    3. Alcohol
    4. Nuts
    5. Chocolate
    6. Fad diets
    7. Spices
    8. Herbal teas
    9. Lemon

O. Surgery
    1. Laryngeal
    2. Tonsillectomy
    3. Neck
    4. Abdominal or thoracic
    5. Other
        a. Intubation
        b. Musculoskeletal

III. PHYSICAL EXAMINATION

A. Complete ear, nose and throat examination
    1. Ears and hearing
    2. Conjunctiva
    3. Nose
    4. Oral cavity
    5. Nasopharynx
    6. Neck

B. Special laryngeal examination
    1. Speaking voice
    2. Laryngoscopy
        a. Indirect
        b. Stroboscopic
        c. Fiber optic
        d. Rigid direct
    3. Singing voice
        a. Stance
        b. Support
        c. Muscles of neck and face
        d. Position of larynx
        e. Tongue
        f. Voice quality
        g. Range
    4. Special tests
        a. tape recording
        b. spectrography

C. Other appropriate examinations
    1. General physical examination
    2. Abdominal
    3. Musculoskeletal
    4. Neurologic

IV. COMMON DIAGNOSES AND TREATMENTS

A. Reflux laryngitis

B. Anxiety

C. Muscle problems
   1. Minor technical errors
   2. Major technical errors
   3. Distant source
   4. Dental

D. Voice abuse

E. Upper respiratory infection without laryngitis

F. Laryngitis
   1. Visible serious damage
   2. Mild to moderate edema and erythema
      a. Inflammation vs. infection
      b. Glottic or supraglottic vs. subglottic
   3. Voice rest
      a. Larynx
      b. Economic effect
      c. Reputation
      d. Stress factors
   4. Voice lessons
   5. Steam

6. (Nasal irrigations)
7. Treatments
   a. Ultrasonic
   b. Local massage
   c. Psychotherapy
   d. Biofeedback
8. Drugs
   a. Steroids
   b. Antibiotics
   c. Antihistamines
   d. Diuretics
   e. Entac
   f. Organidin
   g. Adrenocorticotropic hormone
   h. Proteolytic enzymes
      1. Papase
      2. Thymorel
   i. Aspirin
   j. Analgesics
   k. Anti-anxiety

V. PREVENTION THROUGH VOICE MAINTENANCE

CHAPTER 138

Preventing Vocal Abuse in Non-Classical Singers

Jeannette L. Lovetri

The single most significant difference between classical and non-classical vocal technique, and the one which causes the most difficulty, is tonal texture or quality, referred to herein as *register*. Tonal texture largely determines what the average listener *hears* as the difference between classical and non-classical singing.

A register is a group of sounds which are homogeneous and distinct from other groups of sounds.[1] The voice may be divided into two registers: *head*, for soft, clear sounds which resonate primarily in the mouth and face, and *chest*, for loud, steady sounds which resonate primarily in the lower throat and chest. In beginners, head register is associated with high notes, and chest register with low notes of any given singer's range. In skilled singers this distinction dissipates.[2] While other factors are certainly involved in the production of tone, a singer's ability to control register makes or breaks the ability to control style. Misunderstanding what the word *register* means is a common, but not serious, problem. *Misusing* a register — that is, misunderstanding how it functions — is another matter, as this can cause anything from small musical distortions to severe vocal fold pathology.

The chest register comes into action at medium-to-loud volume levels. In chest register, the vocal folds meet with greater speed and force. Because the folds are shorter and denser, there is greater surface area making contact with each vibratory wave. It could be stated, therefore, that using the chest register incurs greater vocal fold activity. The higher in pitch this register is sung, the more activity takes place in the folds.[3] These factors taken together increase the probability that vocal-fold pathology will occur. Singers quickly discover that chest register can cause problems, because all non-classical singing is done predominantly in the chest register. Non-classical singers want to know how to stay healthy while sounding *commercial*. Most often it is female

singers who are asked to sing higher in the chest register than is safe for the vocal folds. Non-classical male singers also suffer from overuse of the chest register, but are at less risk than females because it is a more natural function in males, given that their range is usually about one octave lower than women's, and the transition between chest and head registers occurs near the top of their range.

The basic principles of classical vocal training, when applied to beginning singers in any style of music, will be helpful. Development of breath control, evenness of tone quality throughout the range, strengthening of the intrinsic vocal muscles and relaxation of extrinsic ones, are useful to *all* singers. It is important to note, however, that the primary textural component in classical singing is *head* register, and head register can be developed *only through training*.[4] Classical singers, therefore, *must* study technique *in order to become classical singers*. Non-classical singers are under no such constraint. If they choose to study voice at all, they do so primarily to maintain vocal health and to develop greater expressive capability, extending whatever technical tendencies they come by naturally.

Non-classical music includes rock and roll, gospel, country, Broadway, rhythm and blues, jazz, ethnic, and experimental theatre pieces. Each of these styles demands a different vocal technique. Some employ more physical movement than others, some are more musically complex, some require greater vocal range, others are quite contained. It is unwise to generalize about non-classical styles. Rather, when training a non-classical singer, the teacher must ascertain the needs of the individual performer and know the professional demands of the style of music he or she chooses to sing, and adapt the process accordingly.

Because they incur problems more often, each of the following examples is of a female singer. The singers were already performing when vocal abuses began and were unable to correct the problems on their own. In each case, basic principles of classical vocal technique were either given for the first time, or re-established if they had been present previously. Then, each singer was guided to solve the problems occurring in her own voice, and apply the solutions to specific songs and/or performances.

Student A, a true contralto in her early thirties, was singing with a rock-and-roll band. Her range was limited to just over one octave and her problems were consistent flatting and inability to sustain singing over a whole evening's performance. Her voice would tire easily and she would occasionally lose it entirely after a singing engagement. The vocal folds were diagnosed by her physician as being normal, i.e. without pathology.

Ms. A had not had any prior vocal or musical training. She nevertheless composed her own songs. Her musical ear was good, since she was aware of the flatting. Ms. A was on her way to severe problems and had already experienced career disruption due to her lack of vocal reliability. The corrective exercises were focused on promoting greater activity in the head register. This was done by using exercises which worked on the face, soft palate, tongue and jaw, to help indirectly stretch (lengthen and thin) the vocal folds. In head register the vocal folds meet more rapidly but with less speed and force. Because the vocal folds are stretched at their edges, there is less surface area making contact with each vibratory wave. These are two factors which decrease the probability that there will be vocal-fold pathology in head register. Also, by changing position and behavior of these body parts (alternately stretching then moving them), it became possible to gradually relax and then reposition the inner or pharyngeal space in Ms. A's throat.[5] The space increased, which changed the vocal acoustics and allowed higher resonant frequencies to be amplified, which, over time, corrected the flatting, even in her highest notes. That was the first improvement.

The second improvement was in vocal stamina. Ms. A stopped getting tired and hoarse after performances within two months of beginning training. The third improvement was a lengthening upward of her range by a minor third. The fourth improvement was increased clarity, resonance, and flexibility of the voice in general, including her speaking voice. At no time did she change the material she was singing. Ms. A did not sound different, just "better." From a psychological standpoint, she had not lost that part of herself which she identified as "the rock singer."

Rather, she had gained awareness of other possibilities available to her voice and body which enhanced what she had been striving to achieve. After two-and-one-half years, she stopped studying, satisfied that her goals had been reached. She maintains her vocal technique through regular practice and has had no further difficulty in the ensuing three years since study ceased.

Ms. B, a dancer in her late twenties, was understudying the star in a Broadway show. Ms. B had never sung solo, and was a light soprano with a weak chest register. The star was an older women with a low range. The producer would not put the understudy's music in a higher key, so Ms. B was forced to sing in keys which were too low, a very dangerous situation. Ms. B knew the star was to take vacation for four days. The knowledge that she would be making her singing debut, as the lead of a show, on Broadway, in front of critics, made her very nervous.

Ms. B's chest register was slowly and carefully strengthened through gentle, repetitive exercises on low pitches, which allowed the thyroarytenoid or vocalis muscle (the body of the vocal fold)[6] to develop resilience and muscle tone. Attention was paid to maintaining relaxation of external neck and throat muscles and to maintaining strong breathing at all times. Over a period of four weeks, Ms. B prepared diligently, and all her solo performances were a personal and critical success.

Ms. C is an international performance artist with a three-octave range. She has been singing her own compositions for 25 years. Her music often uses sounds and noises rather than words. She had been experiencing uncharacteristic pitch problems, particularly in her much-used middle range. She had studied singing with several teachers. At the time difficulties occurred she was in her early forties, and was experiencing flatting and vocal fatigue. Three throat specialists had diagnosed her vocal folds as being healthy. She was in a state of anxiety about her voice, her abilities as a composer, her musical expression, and her career commitments, which extended several years into the future.

Ms. C's lower- and middle-range notes had been pushed by training until the chest register was very loud. The tongue, jaw and neck muscles had been allowed to stiffen. She had gradually lost the ability to make the small adjustments necessary to maintain vocal balance. In working to re-balance the middle range, exercises which stimulated head register were chosen.

Within three sessions, dysfunction decreased. Ms. C returned from a two-week tour reporting that she had experienced no flatting, and no fatigue. Continued work released tongue-, jaw- and neck tension, and improved breath management. Ms. C was pleased that she did not have to edit or change her material, and felt she could continue composing in her well-known style without further risk. She has maintained her technique through regular practice with taped exercises and is now able to go for extended periods of time without lessons while touring, and has had to perform several times while under stress or while ill, with no negative results.

CONCLUSION

It is necessary to cultivate the head register in all non-classical singers in order to avoid vocal abuse. Doing so produces a third register,[3] which is a mix-

ture of the two, having the best of both qualities. The sounds are vigorous and energetic, yet more relaxed and free, which allows the non-classical singer to be commercially successful without sacrificing health, either physical or psychological.

REFERENCES

1. Reid CL: The Free Voice, 58. New York: Patelson Music House, 1965.
2. Bunch M: Dynamics of the Singing Voice, 69. Vienna New York: Springer-Verlag, 1982.
3. Vennard W: Singing, the Mechanism and the Technic, 66, 69. New York: Carl Fischer, 1967.
4. Reid CL: Voice: Psyche and Soma, 48. New York: Patelson Music House, 1975.
5. Sundberg J: The Science of the Singing Voice, 22. Dekalb, IL: Northern Illinois University Press, 1987.
6. Sataloff RT: Professional Voice: The Science and Art of Clinical Care, chapter 3, 29. New York: Ronald J. Baken, Columbia University/ Raven Press, 1991.

CHAPTER 139

Treating Voice Disorders with Acupuncture of Acupoint 'Li'

Youxia Li

Extensive study of the literature, research, and clinical experience led to the discovery of *acupoint Li*, which has remarkable therapeutic implications in phonetic ailments. Moreover, the author went beyond the restrictions of ancient physicians, and systematically studied needling technique, needle specification, and intensity of stimulation; and summarized the theory of laryngeal acupuncture.

SELECTION OF ACUPOINT AND METHOD OF NEEDLING

Locating acupoint Li is based on the theory of channels and collaterals, clinical practice, and extensive knowledge of the anatomy of muscles, bones, and joints around the point. The author first punctured acupoint Li on a cadaver, took anatomical films of the different layers of local tissues, observed the needle trajectory through the subcutaneous tissue, platysma, musculus omohyoideus, and musculus constrictoris pharyngis inferioris, and reached the border of the superior angle of the thyroid cartilage.

METHOD

For locating the point, patients were seated with the head slightly tilted up, or supine with the neck exposed. The point is located at the junction between the anterior border of the sternocleidomastoideus muscle and the border of the superior and inferior angle of the thyroid cartilage. The needle should avoid the carotid artery, identified by its pulse. A 1.5-cun needle (40 mm), gauge 32 (0.26 mm), was used.

During insertion, the needle should form an angle of 45°-60° with the sagittal plane. Before insertion, the point is palpated and pressed with the tip of the left index finger to ascertain the location and assess the condition of the channel (excess or deficiency) and the thickness of the muscle, so as to determine the depth and method of insertion as well as push away the sternocleidomastoideus and carotid artery. The local muscle is vibrated with the left index finger at a frequency of 4-5 Hz while the needle is inserted into it evenly with the right thumb, index and middle fingers. After insertion, the left index finger is kept on the point to help induce and stimulate the *qi* of the chan-nel. The needle then reaches the depth required and *qi* arrives, causing the patient to feel a fishbone-sticking sensation, a positive sign. The point is either reduced or reinforced with rotation. Mild stimulation is advisable, usually about 1/6-1/2 that of the traditional body points.

During treatment of phonetic diseases by needling point Li, arrival of *qi*, *qi* activating, and *qi* radiating towards the affected area are the three keys to obtaining therapeutic results. Circulation of *qi* relies on the function of the channels in transmission. Under normal physiological conditions, the transmission is normal. Under pathological conditions, transmission is low or blocked. As long as the transmission function of the diseased channel is normalized, pathological changes are regulated and normal physiological function recovered. The transmission of *qi* during needling relies on the arrival of *qi*. Once the *qi* is obtained after insertion, the tip of the needle cannot be moved back and forth, or the *qi* will be lost. When the *qi* arrives, therefore, it should be maintained by rotating the needle clockwise or counter-clockwise 3-5 times until stuck and a sensation of heaviness is felt by the practitioner and the needling sensation (*qi*) radiates into the throat and reaches the focus. This is known as *qi* radiating towards the affected area. The *qi* should be maintained not only during retention of the needle, but also after the needle is removed, with the fishbone-sticking sensation possibly lasting for 10 hours or more, due to differences in manipulation.

MATERIALS

A total of 1,438 (721 males, 717 females) patients received simple acupuncture treatment of point Li from 1983 to 1990. Age range was 9-74 (Table I).

Table I: Age Distribution

Age	9-20	21-30	31-40	41-50	51-74
# of Cases	124	379	478	289	168

The shortest duration of symptoms was 1-2 days; the longest was 17 years (Table II). Acute cases numbered 671, while 767 were chronic (Table III).

Table II: Duration of Symptoms

Duration	> 1 Month	> 1 Year	1-3 Years	3-17 Years
# of Cases	671	426	213	128

Of the total number of patients, 612 were professional singers (406 females, 206 males). The remaining 826 patients (311 females, 515 males) had different occupations (Table IV).

Phonetic problems often result from the simultaneous existence of several pathological changes in the vocal cords. Patients suffered primarily from acute and chronic congestion, vocal-cord edema, vocal nodules, local prominence caused by vocal hypertrophy, vocal-cord polyps, submucous bleeding of the cords, various types of poor vocal occlusion, and tumor.

RESULTS

Table III: Therapeutic Effect by Chronicity of Symptoms

	# of Cases	Cured #	Cured %	Improved #	Improved %	Ineffective #	Ineffective %	Effective #	Effective %
Acute	671	654	97.5%	17	2.3%	0	0.0%	671	100.0%
Chronic	767	179	23.3%	438	57.0%	150	19.6%	617	80.4%
Total	1438	833	58.0%	455	32.0%	150	10.0%	1288	90.0%

Table IV: Therapeutic Effect by Professional Group

Occupation	# of Cases	Cure	Improved	Ineffective	Effective Rate	Ineffective Rate
Professional Singer	612	421	168	23	96.24%	3.76%
Other	826	412	287	127	84.63%	15.37%

Criteria were defined as follows:

□ *Cure*:   After 1-30 treatments with acupuncture only, all subjective symptoms disappear, voice recovers completely, and the patient can perform normally. Laryngoscopic examination shows that pathological changes of the vocal cords disappear.

□ *Improved*: After 1-30 acupuncture treatments, the subjective symptoms are obviously improved, with normal or improved phonation, and the patient can keep up with performance. Laryngoscopic examination shows that vocal pathological changes are almost back to normal.

□ *Ineffective*: After 1-30 acupuncture treatments, subjective symptoms are not changed to any significant degree, phonation is not improved, and pathological changes are not alleviated.

CASE STUDY

Jiang, a 28-year-old actress in the Ji Ning Bang Zi Opera Troupe of Shandong Province, suffered from hoarseness and weak phonation for several months and could not sing opera. Diagnosis of a right vocal polyp was made at a phonetics clinic, and various treatments were administered for more than two months, with no improvement. The patient was afraid of surgery and came to the author's clinic for help. Laryngoscopy revealed that the vocal cord was pale with local light red color, and there was a granular polyp prominence at the posterior border of the anterior third of the vocal cord with a larger base, semi transparent edema, and exposure of few vessels around it. The occlusion was poor. Adduction and abduction were normal. The right vocal cord functioned slowly in subsultory phonation. After 24 treatments with acupuncture of point Li, the patient recovered her ability to sing opera. Laryngoscopic examination confirmed that local pathological change completely disappeared.

DISCUSSION

Point Li is located at the throat where many channels meet, including the eight channels which have the coordinative function vis-à-vis the regular channels, playing the guiding role and regulating the volume of *qi* and blood in the channels. Point Li, therefore, located at this pivot, plays a governing role with regard to the other local points selected for treating phonetic diseases. In comparison to the points mentioned in ancient classics for treatment of phonetic diseases, puncturing point Li may present more advantages — dredging the channels, and invigorating the *qi* activity so as to activate blood circulation, promoting subsidence of local edema and congestion, and restoring the normal functions of the laryngeal muscle and vocal cord.

Intensity of stimulation is closely related to the reduction or reinforcement method, and can be taken as a parameter for the entire course of manipulation in either. Any kind of needling must have its intensity of stimulation. When needling point Li, clockwise and counterclockwise rotations of the needle cause different intensities of stimulation. Generally, clockwise rotation of the needle produces stronger stimulation. The reduction and reinforcement methods produce different intensities of stimulation. Selection of either depends upon the condition of the body. It must be adapted to the patient's physiological and pathological condition.

Point Li is the nearest sensitive point to the vocal cords. Selection of this point is in keeping with the theory, 'the nearer, the better.' Puncturing this point may give rise to a bone-sticking sensation, increase the secretion of saliva, and relax the throat, leading to favorable results. In a case of acute congestion and edema, for example, obvious improvement may be observed after needling, and the patient may be cured with 2-5 treatments. In the case of a polyp at the early stage, about 10 treatments may cure or improve the condition. It would be difficult, however, for acupuncture to eliminate a large polyp. Still, it can assist in eliminating local congestion and edema before and after surgery, and promote postoperative recovery.

Clinical application of point Li forced the re-evaluation of the rule that depth of insertion for neck points cannot go beyond 4 fen, or it will cause an accident. Having inserted the needle at a depth of 1.2-1.5 cun, the author believes that if the practitioner is familiar with the anatomy, and strictly controls the selection of needles and method of insertion, the greater depth will remain safe and help obtain relief.

Point Li is the closest point to the vocal cords, located symmetrically on both sides of the neck. The point on either side has the function of exciting or inhibiting the vocal cord on that same side. Puncturing this point may simultaneously treat different pathological changes on both sides. In the case of a hypertrophic vocal cord on one side, the point can be punctured bilaterally with different manipulations to eliminate pathological changes from the diseased side while protecting the healthy side. The therapeutic adaptability of this method is much more extensive than any other. During treatment, needling this point may make throat secretions more fluid, relax the neck, and improve the tension of laryngeal muscles. This method, therefore, can be used routinely to keep an actor in top form before performance, so as to enhance the potential of the laryngeal muscle. It is a simple, safe, and effective method for care of the artist's phonation.

SUGGESTED READING

1. Shanghai College of Traditional Chinese Medicine: Acupuncture and Moxibustion. People's Health Publishing.
2. Lu Shoukang, Hu Bohu, et al: 100 Acupuncture Techniques. China Medical Science and Technology Publishing.
3. Hebei Medical College: Anatomy of the Human Body. People's Health Publishing.
4. Li Baoshi, et al: Laryngology. Shanghai Science and Technology Publishing.
5. China Medical University: Local Anatomy. People's Health Publishing.
6. Zhejiang Medical University, Zhejiang College of Traditional Chinese Medicine: Anatomical Illustration for Acupuncture. Zhejiang People's Publishing.
7. He Zongde, Yu Yangju, et al: Modern Otorhino-laryngologic and Stomatologic Science in Chinese Medicine. Anhui Science and Technology Publishing,.
8. Huang Fumi: A-B Classic of Acupuncture and Moxibustion. Jin Dynasty Commercial Publishing.
9. Gao Wu: A Collection of Germs in Acupuncture and Moxibustion. Ming Dynasty Shanghai Science and Technology Publishing.
10. Zhou Jifu: A Practical Complete Book of Treatment of Phonetic Diseases. Academic Publishing.

CHAPTER 140

Acupuncture Treatment
of Vocal Fold Hypertrophy

Jian Pi • Yonjun Zhang

The authors treated and observed 50 singers suffering from hypertrophy, for one month, by puncturing the Renyin (St. 9) and Shuitu (St. 10) acupoints. The cure rate was 90%, with fully recovery in 20%. In the control group, the same kind of patients were treated with comprehensive methods, yielding a cure rate of 86% with full recovery in 14%. Statistical analysis showed the difference to be non-significant, thus proving that the sole use of acupuncture treatment can achieve satisfactory results.

INTRODUCTION

Vocal folds hypertrophy is a common disease of the throat. It is often considered as one of the types of chronic laryngitis. It includes swelling, hypertrophy and nodular formation of the whole vocal fold, as well as dissociated edges. The above pathological symptoms lead to an increase in the size of the vocal fold and a decrease in the frequency of vibration, so the voice becomes low and deep. The accumulation of fluid within the fold results in the loosening and softening of tissue structure. This is characterized by a stuffy and dark tone color. If the hypertrophy is confined to only one side of the fold, the tone quality will become unharmonized, because of size difference of the two vibrators and closure hinderance. The stable and regular airflow, which is needed to produce normal sound, turns into turbulent airflow, forming some random and irregular vibration noise. As a result, the voice becomes hoarse. The above mentioned are generalized as 'mute of the throat' (*Nei Jing*) by traditional Chinese medicine. This disorder is a great threat to professional voice. So a controlled clinical study was performed by puncturing the acupoints Renyin and Shuitu.

MATERIALS and METHODS

Two groups of patients with vocal folds hypertrophy of vocal folds were selected. Their ages ranged between 20 and 40 years. Most of the them were 30 years of age (Table 1).

The patients under treatment were randomly

Table 1: Acupuncture (A) and Control (C) male (m) and female (f) distribution of vocal fold pathological categories.

	A-m	A-f	C-m	C-f
Bilateral Diffuse Vocal Fold Hypertrophy	6	3	3	3
Whole-length Hypertrophy of Edges	9	19	18	15
Local Nodular Hypertrophy of Edges	5	8	6	5
TOTAL	20	30	27	23

divided into two groups, according to their order of arrival. There were 50 cases in the acupuncture group. Patients of this group were treated by puncturing the acupoints of Renyin and Shuitu once daily in six-day courses with a one-day interval between courses. During treatment, the patients sat straight. The practitioner inserting the needle used an extremely tiny needle called 'filliform needle' and was careful to avoid the pulsating area of the carotid artery. The needle is inserted step by step, at a pace just like the pecking of a sparrow. After insertion, the range of nonification or purgation according to the strength of twirling the needle should be gentle and small. This process should continue until the patient has a sensation of 'fishbone' or feels slightly bloated at the throat. The needle is then retained for 15-30 minutes. This group was observed for four weeks. As for the 50 cases of the control group, patients were treated with usual comprehensive methods (antibiotics, prednisone, and physical therapy).

CRITERIA OF CURE

1. *Full recovery:* symptoms of hoarseness of the singer's voice have disappeared as noted by the singer him/herself and by others. Under laryngoscopy, the pathological changes of vocal cord hypertrophy have vanished. Through follow-up visits, the singer was able

to give ten consecutive performances without suffering any relapse.

2. *Significant improvement*: symptoms of hoarseness are greatly mitigated as noted by the singer him/herself and by others. Under laryngoscopy, there was an obvious subsidence of the pathological changes of hypertrophy. The singer was able to give daily performances.

3. *Improvement:* The voice has become moist as noted by the singer him/herself and by others. The symptoms of hoarseness have been mitigated. the singer was able to give performance on stage. Under laryngoscopy, the pathological changes of hypertrophy are unaltered.

4. *Ineffectiveness*: symptoms of hoarseness were unaltered as noted by the singer him/herself and by others. under laryngoscopy, the pathological changes were either unaltered or worsened.

RESULTS

1.   In the acupuncture treatment group, the cure rate was 90%; with full recovery and significant improvement in 54%. In the control group, the cure rate was 86%; with full recovery and significant improvement in 44%.

2. Through contrast, the difference between the ratio of internal formation was not significant (x^2 = 1.176, p)0.1) (Table 2).

Table 2: Results Distribution Between Acupuncture and Control Groups by Vocal Fold Pathological Categories.

	Dif. Bil. Hyper.	Whole Edges	Local Nodular	T
ACUPUNCT				
Full Recov.	1	6	3	10
Sig. Improv.	2	13	2	17
Improv.	4	9	5	18
Ineffect.	2	0	3	5
Total	9	28	13	50
CONTROL				
Full Recov.	2	3	2	7
Sig. Improv.	2	8	5	15
Improv.	2	17	2	21
Ineffect.	0	5	2	7
Total	6	33	11	50

3. After statistical processing of the cure rates of the two groups, the difference was not significant. This demonstrates that the curative effect of both treatments are similar.

4. Acupuncture treatment is rather easy to adapt, so it has a great significance in application, but acupuncture techniques need to be very light and gentle, and it is rather difficult to master the proper touch. Accuracy in handling the needle directly affects the curative effect.

DISCUSSION

According to the traditional Chinese medical theory of channels and collaterals, all the channels are stretched all over a person's body, through which Qi (vital energy), blood and body fluids travel. Unobstructed channels result in unimpeded mechanism of Qi and moist voice. However, the chronic disease of vocal fold hypertrophy and swelling are closely related to the blockade of channels, which is caused by blood stasis and sludge due to the stagnation of Qi and turbid dampness and sputum condensation. To explain this in modern medical theory, the blockade of the throat microcirculation results in the hypertrophy and swelling of the vocal fold. The blockade of the lymphatic microcirculation may easily result in the swelling or local cysts of the vocal fold. The obstruction of blood capillary can easily cause blood stasis of the vocal fold and the expansion of blood vessels. At this stage, if there is an inflammatory trauma, such as a bacteriogenic infection following a cold; or a non-inflammatory trauma, such as overuse and inproper use of the throat, a person is more likely to suffer from this disorder. As for the singers, the degree of intensity in their use of the throat is several times higher than that of ordinary people. As a result, the blood capillary within the vocal fold and the microlymphatics of the vocal fold are temporarily blocked due to high pressure. Any person who has an harmonized relationship between Qi and blood and an abundant visceral Qi generally has a self-adjusting ability. But if a person's relationship between Qi and blood is disturbed, s/he may worsen the degree or prolong the time of the blockade. Finally, some parts of the vocal fold will suffer from chronic physical damage due to to lack of blood, decay, necrosis, hyperplasia, and bacterial invasion.

The acupoints of Renyin and Shuitu adapted in this paper belong to the stomach channel of foot Yangming which are the 'sea of grain and water' (Figure 1, Table 3). The viscera receive Qi from

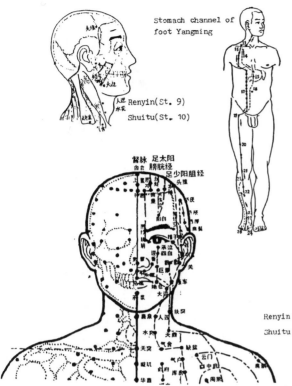

Figure 1: Stomach Channel of Foot Yangming, the 'sea of grain and water'.

Table 3: Stomach Channel of Foot Yangming.

中 文	英 文	中 文	英 文
承 泣	(St. 1) Lacrimation Receiver	滑肉门	(St. 24) Slippery Flesh Gate
四 白	(St. 2) Four Whites	天 枢	(St. 25) Upper Pivot
巨 髎	(St. 3) Huge Crevice	外 陵	(St. 26) Outer Mound
地 仓	(St. 4) Terrestrial Granary	大 巨	(St. 27) Super Great
大 迎	(St. 5) Great Welcome	水 道	(St. 28) Water Channel
颊 车	(St. 6) Mandibular Joint	归 来	(St. 29) Return
下 关	(St. 7) Lower Pass	气 冲	(St. 30) Rushing Energy
头 维	(St. 8) Head Corner	髀 关	(St. 31) Femoral Pass
人 迎	(St. 9) Man's Pulsation	伏 兔	(St. 32) Prostrate Rabbit
水 突	(St. 10) Water Projecting	阴 市	(St. 33) Yin Market
气 舍	(St. 11) Energy Room	梁 丘	(St. 34) Hill Ridge
缺 盆	(St. 12) Supraclavicular Fossa	犊 鼻	(St. 35) Nose of Calf
气 户	(St. 13) Energy Gate	足 三里	(St. 36) Foot Three Li
库 房	(St. 14) Storage House	上巨墟	(St. 37) Upper Huge Passage
屋 翳	(St. 15) Chamber Roof	条 口	(St. 38) Narrow Mouth
膺 窗	(St. 16) Chest Window	下巨虚	(St. 39) Lower Huge Passage
乳 中	(St. 17) Breast Centre	丰 隆	(St. 40) Rich and Prosperous
乳 根	(St. 18) Breast Base	解 溪	(St. 41) Opened Hollow
不 容	(St. 19) No Containment	冲 阳	(St. 42) Rushing Yang
承 满	(St. 20) Full Receiving	陷 谷	(St. 43) Sinking Valley
梁 门	(St. 21) Beam Gate	内 庭	(St. 44) Inner Court
关 门	(St. 22) Closed Gate	厉 兑	(St. 45) Sick Mouth
太 乙	(St. 23) Grand Yi		

Yangming via their own individual channel. Since the throat is the point where channels are circulated through and meet, acupuncture treatment by way of selecting the acupuncture points of the corresponding channel can unblock the mechanism of *Qi*, promote the absorption of the accumulated fluid within the vocal fold, thus eliminating swelling, resolving nodes and restoring the singer's voice. However, if the patient has a relatively longer case history and severe hypertrophy and swelling, hyperplasia of the epithelium on the surface of the vocal fold is obvious and the mucous membrane has also overgrown due to swelling. In this case, even if the accumulated fluid has been absorbed, the stretched tissue still remains. Under laryngoscopy, it can be seen that the hypertrophy has not been completely mitigated. The lower layer of the mucous membrane, expanded by fluid tends to accumulate it again. So, it is necessary to have frequent follow-up visits and close medical monitoring.

With regard to the course of treatment, generally it is possible to estimate the curative effect after four consecutive courses. The curative effect is most obvious in those patients whose hypertrophia and swelling have affected the complete brim area of the vocal fold. Nevertheless, those patients who suffer from diffuse or nodular hypertrophy need more courses.

Because it was impossible to apply double-blind method in the process of comparing the two groups, psychological factors could not be excluded. Quantification of targets could not be realized due to the limitations of this setting. As for those cases with irregular follow-up, the last observation was selected as the criteria. Despite all these, acupuncture treatment has great potentials in application, because it is convinient to adapt, has no side effects and can easily be accepted by the patients.

CHAPTER 141

Vocal Abuse in University Cheerleaders

Florence B. Blager • *Ronald C. Scherer* • *Jon N. Lemke*

INTRODUCTION

Cheerleading — the "all-American" sport image — has been described as extremely damaging to the voice.[1-5] Even among those who have described this voice use as damaging, however, attempts to establish the factors in cheerleading that have a destructive impact on the vocal mechanism have been inconclusive. Factors that have been discussed which differentiate cheerleaders with and without laryngeal pathology or dysphonia include marked pitch elevation,[3] hard vocal attack,[1] depressed pitch range,[6] and constitutional vulnerability.[7] Methods of evaluation of voice change have included voice intensity measures,[7, 10] respiratory volumes,[9] and questionnaires.[2, 4] Training in appropriate breath support and voice production techniques has been suggested to prevent damage to the voice and larynx.[1, 5, 8, 10]

This study was an attempt to measure the acoustic characteristics of cheerleaders' voices throughout the cheerleading season, give training in appropriate voice techniques and vocal hygiene, and evaluate the impact of the training on voice quality.

MATERIALS AND METHODS

Sixteen cheerleaders, eight male and eight female, comprised the cheerleading squad at the University of Colorado at Boulder during the 1990-1991 sports season. They cheered from September 1990 through April 1991.

History questionnaires were completed at the beginning of the study and follow-up questionnaires at the end. Voices were recorded at four different times: (1) before cheerleading season started; (2) after cheerleading camp and first game; (3) after voice training and cheering; and (4) after the last game. Voice training between Times 2 and 3 was held in two sessions: Session 1 covered techniques to warm up the voice and to relieve vocal tension; Session 2 covered structure and function of the voice, prevention of abusive vocal habits, use of breath support, developing vocal resonance, and medical care of voice problems.

Laryngoscopic examination was performed between Times 2 and 3, using recorded stroboscopy.

Acoustic recordings at Times 1, 2, and 3 were made at the Recording and Research Center, Denver Center for the Performing Arts. Subjects stood within an IAC booth. Their voices were recorded using an AKG microphone, Digital Sound Corporation amplification, and a Sony PCM-plus videotape recorder. Time 4 was recorded at the University of Colorado in Boulder in an IAC booth. Voices were recorded on a TEAC MDX-3R reel-to-reel tape recorder using a Sennheiser MD-44IU microphone. The subjects stood two feet from the microphone.

Each person was instructed to produce 15 sustained /a/ tokens in a normal, steady voice. They also performed the cheer "Go Buffs, Go!" at least four times in a loud voice, and then in a loud voice using cheering gestures.

Acoustic analyses of the sustained /a/ vowels included the "short-term" (cycle-to-cycle perturbation) measures jitter and shimmer, and the "long-term" perturbation measures called the coefficient of variation for frequency (CVF) and for amplitude (CVA). The harmonics-to-noise ratio,[12] the harmonic spectral slope (HSS, the slope in dB per octave of the average calculated microphone cycle), and the average fundamental frequency (Fo) were also calculated.

A repeated measures analysis of variance was performed on the group of five males having recordings at Times 2, 3, and 4. Only two females returned for the final recording, which gave insufficient data to control for gender differences.

To evaluate the impact of training, comparison was made with the results of a follow-up study the senior author conducted with high-risk voice users in a health-care setting.[13]

RESULTS

Only two measures showed significant change over time: a decrease in slope of the HSS and a drop in the fundamental frequency for the five males (Fig. 1). There were no significant changes in voice perturbation measures. Although the power may have been inadequate to find significant changes in voice perturbations, there were no consistent trends across subjects.

HSS

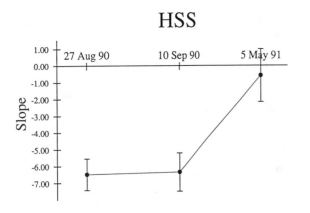

MEAN Fo

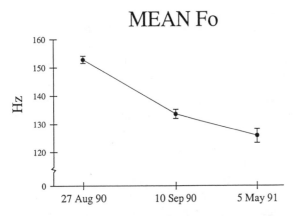

Figure 1: *Harmonic spectral slope (HSS) and fundamental frequency (Fo) across three recording dates for 5 male cheerleaders, significant at p<.05.*

Information from the history and follow-up questionnaires is shown in Charts 1, 2 and 3. No statistical treatment was used with this information.

DISCUSSION

Cheerleaders are at great risk for voice damage because of the required use of a loud voice during sports games and squad practices. It could be expected that the voice quality may deteriorate during the sports season. The acoustic voice analyses of the group did not support general voice quality deterioration, and laryngoscopic examination did not reveal laryngeal damage.

The perturbation analyses were not statistically significantly different over time. The significant findings of the fundamental frequency decrease (by about 3 semitones) between August 27, 1990 and May 5, 1991 may reflect greater comfort with the cheerleading task, and the decrease in spectral slope may reflect use of slightly louder voices, neither finding suggestive of a significant change in the cheerleaders' voices. The voice sessions and attention to the voices of the cheerleaders may have contributed to the prevention of voice deterioration. It may be an exaggeration to ask to assume that a few sessions during which the cheerleaders strongly attended to voice would have the effect of improving the voice over the duration of their sports season. Thus, the finding of no significant change in voice perturbations may be thought of as a positive finding.

Those cheerleaders who had had previous voice training appeared to have clearer voices than those without training with respect to the "long-term" perturbation measures HNR, CVA, and CVF (Fig. 2). The perturbation separation for the two groups suggests that future designs may wish to control for prior singing and speaking voice training.

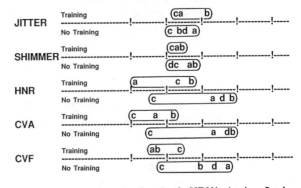

Figure 2: *Cheerleaders' voice profiles, with and without voice training. Perturbation measures are for the last recording time.*

```
┌─────────────────────────────────────────────────────────────────────────────┐
│ CHART 1                                                                       │
│                        FROM HISTORY QUESTIONNAIRE                             │
│                        (Before Cheerleading Season)                           │
│                                                                               │
│ Number                              16 (8 male, 8 female)                     │
│                                                                               │
│ Mean Age                            20                                        │
│                                                                               │
│ Mean Number Residences before college  4.56                                  │
│                                                                               │
│ Training in Body Work               12-yes, 4-no                              │
│                                                                               │
│ Types of Training                   Males-Athletes (3)     Females-Dance (5)  │
│                                           Martial Arts (2)      Gymnastics (6)│
│                                                                               │
│ Most Significant Training for Cheerleading  Males-Athletes (4)  Females-Gymnastics (5) │
│                                                                               │
│ Currently Weightlifting             yes-15                                    │
│                                                                               │
│ Learned Voice Warm-Ups in the Past  yes-5                                     │
│                                                                               │
│ Present Health                      Excellent-10                              │
│   (August 15, 1990)                 Good-5                                    │
│                                     No answer-1                               │
│                                                                               │
│ Alcohol Use                         yes-13                                    │
│   Mean Age Started                  Males-17.76            Females-16.5       │
│   Amount/week                       Males-10.5             Females-3.77       │
│                                                                               │
│ Cheered with Laryngeal              yes-11                                    │
│   Problems in the past                                                        │
│   Afflicted Voice Quality           yes-9                                     │
└─────────────────────────────────────────────────────────────────────────────┘
```

```
┌─────────────────────────────────────────────────────────────────────────────┐
│ CHART 2                                                                       │
│                      FROM FOLLOW-UP QUESTIONNAIRE                             │
│                      (After Cheerleading Season)                              │
│                                                                               │
│ Number                           9 (6 male, 3 female)                         │
│ Mean Cheering/week               6 hours                                      │
│ What do you remember from        Vocal Hygiene:        Voice Quality:         │
│   the voice workshop             Drink Water-6         Warm up voice-7        │
│   presentations?*                Use water for phlegm-6  Other voice exercises-4 │
│                                  Don't clear throat-4                         │
│                                  Other hygiene points-2                       │
│ What information have you used?* Drink water-4          Various Voice exercises-8 │
│ How much water do you drink?     Average of 6.27                              │
│                                    glasses/day                               │
│ Has voice changed since cheerleading  Males             Females              │
│   season began?                    no-2                  no-3                 │
│                                    yes-4                                      │
│ If so, how would you describe the change?*  Improved-3   Use stretches-1      │
│                                                                               │
│ What changes have you made?      Male                  Female                 │
│     Don't scream; yell loud enough  1                                         │
│     Direct voice                 1                                            │
│     Deeper, more forceful sound                        1                      │
│     Lower, more constant tone    1                                            │
│     Tone vibrates in nose and face  1                                         │
│     Use diaphragm                2                                            │
│     Sound with breath support                          1                      │
│                                                                               │
│ What has been the effect on your voice?*                                      │
│     Voice not as gone after game  2                                           │
│     Voice fatigued, but still have it  1                                      │
│     Stronger, louder                                   1                      │
│     Sounds better                                      1                      │
│     Lasts longer                                       1                      │
│     Don't get hoarse as much     1                                            │
│     Much improvement             1                                            │
│     Feels better                                       1                      │
│     Voice rarely feels tired or strained               1                      │
│     Don't get sore throats like before  1                                     │
│                                                                               │
│ *Open-ended question                                                          │
└─────────────────────────────────────────────────────────────────────────────┘
```

CHART 3

FROM FOLLOW-UP QUESTIONNAIRE

Sensations in Throat and Voice Quality.
Which of the following do you experience?

(1= Never, 2= Sometimes, 3= Frequently, 4= Always)

	Males (6)		Females (3)	
	End of Practice Day	End of Cheerleading Day	End of Practice Day	End of Cheerleading Day
a. Throat feels tired	1.16	1.66	1.33	1.66
b. Throat is painful	1.16	1.42	1.33	1.66
c. Phlegm in throat	1.33	1.83	2.33*	2.66*
d. Feel "something" in throat	1.2	1.2	2.0*	2.0*
e. Clear throat a lot	1.5	1.66	2.0*	2.0*
f. Voice is hoarse	1.5	2.42*	1.33	1.33
g. Can't speak loudly	1.0	1.50	1.33	1.33
h. Lose voice	1.0	1.33	1.0	1.0
	* Represents an average score of 2 or more.			
	1.22	1.73	1.58	1.71

Information from the follow-up questionnaires suggests that the subjects recalled and used information on voice techniques as well as vocal hygiene. This is in contrast to a follow-up study the senior author conducted with high-risk voice users in a health-care setting whose recall and use of information was focused on vocal hygiene, not voice techniques.[13]

In future designs, use of a simultaneously studied, instead of a historical, control group that does not receive voice training would strengthen the results. Using identical questionnaires for pre- and post-tests would define the parameters of voice change more specifically.

It was difficult to get consistent attendance at the recording sessions, resulting in limited data. The related factors for this — distance, scheduling, more encouragement, etc. — need to be controlled more rigorously in future studies.

It has been suggested that knowledge of voice care and vocal training would help prevent vocal abuse in cheerleaders. The findings of the present study appear to support this. Such intervention may help prevent what at present can be a source of serious and, at times, long-term damage to young voices.

REFERENCES

1. Case JL: Clinical Management of Voice Disorders. Rockville, MD: Aspen Systems Corp, 1984.

2. Gillespie S, Cooper B.: Prevalence of speech problems in junior and senior high schools. Journal of Speech and Hearing Research 16:739-743, 1973.

3. Wilson KD: Voice Problems of Children. Third Edition. Baltimore: Williams & Wilkins, 1987.

4. Campbell S, Reich A, Klockars A, et al: Factors associated with dysphonia in high school cheerleaders. Journal of Speech and Hearing Disorders 53:175-185, 1988.

5. Andrews M, Shank KH: Some observations concerning the cheering behavior of school-girl cheerleaders: Language, Speech and Hearing Services in Schools 14:150-156, 1983.

6. Sander E, Ripich D: Vocal fatigue. Annals of Otology, Rhinology and Laryngology 92:141-145, 1983.

7. McHenry MA, Reich AR: Effective airway resistance and vocal sound pressure level in cheerleaders with a history of dysphonic episodes. Folia Phoniatrica 37:223-231, 1985.

8. Aaron VL, Madison CL: A vocal hygiene program for high school cheerleaders. Language, Speech, and Hearing Services in Schools 22: 287-290, 1991.

9. Reich AR, McHenry MA: Respiratory volumes in cheerleaders with a history of dysphonic episodes. Folia Phoniatrica 39:71-77, 1987.

10. McHenry MA: Vocal SPL control in cheerleaders with a history of frequent acute dysphonic episodes. Doctoral dissertation, University of Washington, 1983.

11. Scherer R, Gould WJ, Titze I, et al: Preliminary evaluation of selected acoustic and glottographic measures for clinical phonatory function analysis. Journal of Voice 2:230-244, 1988.
12. Yumoto E, Gould WJ, Baer T: Harmonics-to-noise ratio as an index of the degree of hoarseness. Journal of the Acoustics Society of America 71:1544-1550, 1982.
13. Blager FB: Follow-up study of high-risk voice users. ASLHA Natl Conv, Seattle, WA, 1991.

ACKNOWLEDGEMENTS

The authors would like to thank Marilyn A. Hetzel, Ph.D., and Raymond P. Wood II, M.D., for their work in the Voice Workshops; Larry Brown, D.M.A., for his work on the voice analysis; and Yoshiyuki Horii, Ph.D., for his help in recording the subjects during Time 4.

Support from NIDCD Grant 1 PG0 DC00976-01 is gratefully acknowledged.

CHAPTER 142

Singing Exercises and Their Effect on Pathological Voice Conditions

Barbara Mathis

INTRODUCTION

Good vocal health is a vital concern for those who use the voice in a professional capacity, e.g. teachers, singers, actors, clergymen, and lawyers. Research in the area of vocal health reveals the need to determine whether specific exercises are beneficial to the voice[1] and whether exercises used to train the singing voice might be beneficial in alleviating pathological and/or dysfunctional voice disorders. Exercise as training or treatment for the voice has been around since ancient times,[2] and extensive training for the singing voice through exercise may be traced from the seventeenth and eighteenth centuries to the present.[3]

The benefits of therapeutic and conditioning exercise have been well established in fields such as medicine[4] and sports,[5] and, to a certain extent, in the voice professions. Sources in vocal fields disagree, however, about the benefits of various techniques and the extent to which exercise is beneficial to the voice.[6]

The purpose of this study, therefore, was to describe the response of a variety of pathological voices to a selected set of singing exercises. Specific problems were to describe (before, during, and after exercise) the laryngeal conditions of patients diagnosed with muscle-tension dysphonia (laryngeal hyperfunction), nodules, recurrent laryngeal nerve paralysis, or iatrogenic dysphonia.

METHODS

Subjects were selected from the private practice of cooperating physicians who felt that the vocal instruction and exercise program might be helpful. Among the patients selected were two males and five females whose ages ranged from 24 years to 67 years. Occupations of those involved included teachers, students, housewife-singers, and professional pop singers.

This study used an individual subject research design (case studies) to report the effects of specific vocal exercises on pathological voice conditions. Instrumentation for assessing conditions before, during (where applicable), and after exercise included a brief case history, subject interviews, attending physicians' medical charts, flexible fiberoptic video naso-laryngoscopy, video cassette recorder and video tape segments, three physician/observers, and a specific diagnostic procedure, which provided a method of assessing organic, functional, and perceptual variables. Three physician/observers rated the general condition of the laryngeal area and the condition of the right and left vocal folds; seven functional variables[7] (Table I); and pitch range, intensity range, breath volume, and flexibility. Estimates of inter-observer reliability were calculated by using a Generalizability Coefficient[8] for the physicians' initial and final ratings for each variable for all subjects (Table II).

For the exercise program, the researcher chose seven vocalises from the routine designed by Allan R. Lindquest, whose techniques combined those of the Italian school with those of Swedish studios which produced such singers as Flagstad and Bjoerling.[9] The seven vocalises included a warm-up *massage* and exercises for separation and blending of the registers, vowel clarity and modification, tone focus, vocal attack, and flexibility. In addition to the exercise routine, subjects received basic instruction in breathing techniques, proper body- and facial posture,[10, 11] and relaxation. No attempt was made to alter subjects' normal life patterns or amount of voice usage, except in the following manner: Subjects were asked to perform the exercise routine at least once each day; to use the instruction received from the exercise routine as much as possible in daily voice use; and to recall and use the physical sensations and habits established by the exercises in other voice usage.

Table I: Functional Variables

---

1. Cord closure   (visual and perceptual)

Rating scale   0   normal
                     hypertension: +1 +2 +3
                     hypotension: -1 -2 -3

2. Arytenoid cartilage closure angle

Rating scale   0   normal
                     hypertension: +1   +2   +3

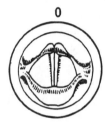 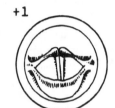 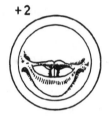 

3. Length of vocal folds visible during phonation

Rating scale   0   normal
                     hyperfunction:
             +1   (2/3)   +2 (1/2)   +3 (1/3 or less)

4. Width of vocal folds visible during phonation:
    directly related to action of the ventricular folds

Rating scale   0   normal (full width of folds in view;
                         little or no action of v. folds)
                +1   anterior 1/3 covered by v. folds
                +2   anterior 2/3 covered
                +3   nearly or completely covered

5. Position of epiglottis

Rating scale   0   normal (against tongue base)
                     hyperfunction (overhang indicating
                     tension):   +1   +2   +3

6. Laryngeal introitus

Rating scale   0   normal space
                     hyperfunction (constriction indicating
                     tension):   +1   +2   +3

7. Pharyngeal circumference diameters
    Use same rating scale as for laryngeal introitus.

Table II: Estimates of Interobserver Reliability

Variable	First Video Segment	Final Video Segment
Organic Variable 1 (general laryngeal condition)	.9915	.9999
Organic Variable 2 (right vocal fold)	.9936	.9818
Organic Variable 3 (left vocal fold)	.9779	.9635
Functional Variable 4 (cord closure)	.8746	.9082
Functional Variable 5 (arytenoid cartilage closure angle)	.9712	.9460
Functional Variable 6 (length vocal folds visible)	.9547	.9544
Functional Variable 7 (width vocal folds visible)	.9588	.8150
Functional Variable 8 (position of epiglottis)	.9709	.9999
Functional Variable 9 (laryngeal introitus)	.9267	.9417
Functional Variable 10 (pharyngeal circumference diameter)	.8977	.8920
Perceptual Variable 11 (pitch range)	.9425	.9020
Perceptual Variable 12 (intensity range)	.9821	.9811
Perceptual Variable 13 (breath volume)	.9602	.9999
Perceptual Variable 14 (flexibility)	.9852	.9812

RESULTS

The subjects in this study showed improvement in the variables selected for assessment during and after the time period when they allegedly were using the exercise program and techniques. Two case studies of teachers diagnosed as having muscle-tension dysphonia revealed positive change after exercise in organic, functional, and perceptual conditions. A case study diagnosed with nodules revealed positive change after three months on the exercise program while continuing extensive voice usage as a professional rock singer. Two case studies of singers with paralytic vocal fold showed dramatic improvement in all areas of assessment after exercise, thus enabling them to return to solo singing, although one retained the paralytic fold (paramedian position). This study also reported two cases of singers diagnosed as having iatrogenic dysphonia after vocal-fold surgery and their attempts to rehabilitate the speaking and singing voice

through speech therapy and exercise. Positive change occurred in all areas of assessment, but some conditions remained below normal.

DISCUSSION

Therapeutic results are often difficult to assess accurately due to the nature of the healing process, differences among individuals and their specific pathologies, and the presence of uncontrollable outside factors; therefore, it is with caution that these conclusions are presented. Descriptions of the vocal conditions, based on subject interviews (Table III), reading the attending physicians' medical charts (Table IV), and obtaining diagnostic results from three physician/observers supplied objective and subjective assessments of changes which occurred during the time subjects claimed to be using the exercise routine. In all case studies, the patient, attending physician, and the three physician/observers noted change in laryngeal conditions and/or behavior after using the exercise routine designed by Lindquest.

Table III: Examples from Patient Interviews

Case Study No. 2:   Muscle-Tension Dysphonia

"The results of using the vocalises and medical analysis by use of laryngoscope and video tape have been extremely beneficial. Within a period of four or five months, the health of the vocal cords, and the ease of tonal production, improved dramatically. The ulcers have not recurred, and a freedom from tension in both the singing and speaking voice is now evident to me."

Case Study No. 5   Paralyzed Vocal Fold

Before beginning the exercise routine, the patient complained of having no endurance in her speaking voice. Although she had been a soprano soloist before the paralysis, she had recently begun to sing in her church choir as an alto with limited range, breathiness, and uncontrollable vibrato. After 8½ months, the patient reports from her diary: "Sang *Pie Jesu* from Faure's *Requiem*. Went well. Have been so pleased at the stamina through the long, extra rehearsals. The next goal is to sing in July for a national convention in front of 20,000 people. All this, in just one year. Another plus is the speaking voice is much stronger. At the beginning, I could not speak to my husband in another room."

Case Study No. 6   Iatrogenic Complications

When examined before beginning the exercise program, the patient was singing five nights a week for five hours with about four solid hours of singing. Even though she complained of severe problems with hoarseness, she was unable or unwilling to stop her job temporarily for vocal rest. After five months of exercise, she comments: "I can now do songs I was never able to sing before. I have a wider range and clearer tone. I can hold notes longer."

Table IV: *Examples from Medical Charts*

Before Exercise	After Exercise
	5 Months
Vibratory margins of vocal folds irregular in outline	60% better; swelling less on left fold
Laryngeal posture squeezed	Laryngeal posture good while doing exercises
False cords meeting	
Some hyperkeratosis on both folds	Less hyperkeratosis
	3 Months
Nodular swelling, larger on right vocal fold	Left vocal fold clear
Incomplete glottal closure with air gaps anterior	Nodule on right fold ⅛ smaller
and posterior to nodular swellings	Air gap and breathiness 50% better
Producing breathy singing tone and raspy speech	Clearly on the right track
Inefficient phonation	
	10 months
Paralysis of left vocal fold	Paralysis remains unchanged
Breathy vocal quality	Singing voice excellent, even without considering patient's age
Uneven vibrato	and unilateral cord paralysis
	2 Months
Paralysis of right vocal cord	Normal condition: two functioning folds
Weak, breathy quality	Clear quality
Hypertension	Normal laryngeal posture when singing
	6 Months
History of vocal polypectomy and resulting	Dramatic improvement!
hoarser voice due to scar tissue	Gold laryngeal posture in singing
Vocal fold edema	Would like to see further improvement in speaking voice

Although the positive changes could have been due to unknown factors, it is the opinion of the researcher that the exercise routine was beneficial in alleviating pathological and dysfunctional conditions found in the subjects. Just as gentle stretching exercises benefit muscles in other parts of the body, as demonstrated in sports, medicine, and other fields, vocalises may have the same effect on laryngeal health. Designed to train the healthy singing voice, Lindquest's routine employed vocalises to warm up and gently stretch the muscles of the larynx, to separate and practice vowel clarity and modification, to encourage tone focus and a good vocal attack, and to develop flexibility and strength. The routine seemed effective in alleviating subjects' pathological conditions and/or dysfunctional behavior; however, since this research used a single case study design, more research is needed to determine the effects of the exercise program on additional subjects. The voice profession should further investigate the efficiency of this and other techniques, exercises and musical vocalises which might bring about positive changes in vocal conditions and behavior.

REFERENCES

1. Sundberg J: The Science of the Singing Voice, 193. Dekalb, IL: Northern Illinois University Press, 1987.
2. Finney G: Medical theories of vocal exercise and health, Bulletin of the History of Medicine 40(5):395-406, 1986.
3. Thomas BA: A History of Instruction in 'Bel Canto' Singing. Research study for MUED 5500, North Texas State University, Denton, TX, 1984.
4. Colson JHC, Collison FW: Progressive Exercise Therapy, 3-4. Boston: Wright Publishing, 1983.
5. Allman FL: Exercise in sports medicine. *In* Basmajian JW (ed), Therapeutic Exercises, 456. Baltimore: Williams & Wilkins, 1978.
6. Mathis BA: Selected Vocal Exercises and Their Relationship to Specific Laryngeal Conditions: A Description of Seven Case Studies, 111-135. Ann Arbor, UMI, U. North Texas, 1990.
7. Lawrence VL: Suggested Criteria for Fiberoptic Diagnosis of Laryngeal Hyperfunction (video tape). Houston, TX, 1985.

8. Crocker L, Algina J: Introduction to Classical and Modern Test Theory, 167.   New York: Holt, Rinehart and Winston, 1986.

9. Lindquest AR: Taped lessons and interviews (1971, 1972, 1977, 1983).

10. Bunch M: Dynamics of the Singing Voice, 103-109. New York: Springer-Verlag Wien, 1982.

11. Sataloff RT: The professional voice: Part II. Physical examination. Journal of Voice 1(2):198, 1987.

ACKNOWLEDGEMENTS

This study was made possible through the cooperation, expertise, and generosity of the late Van L. Lawrence, M.D., past editor of The Voice Foundation publications and physician for the Houston Grand Opera. The author also extends personal gratitude and appreciation to the late Allan R. Lindquest for his knowledge of the singing voice and his techniques and exercise design.

CHAPTER 143

Effect of the Menstrual Cycle on the Singer's Voice

Peifang Chen

The author has studied 80 female singers. Careful observation was made of their voices and vocal cords during their menstrual cycles. Observations and comparisons were made over a period of more than three cycles. The results are as follows:

Table I: *Age Range of Singers*

Age	17-20	21-25	26-30	31-40	41-48
Number of Cases	17	39	12	10	2

Many female singers complained that their voices changed before menstruation — 69 cases, or 86.3%. The main symptom was husky voice (55 cases), including change of quality of tone color (38 cases) and hoarseness (17 cases). Other symptoms were change of tone, difficulty in top voice, decreased volume, difficulty in changing tone, and lack of control during singing (Table II). Many symptoms were often present simultaneously.

In 14 cases (17.5%), the singers' voices began to change about one week prior to menstruation. At the earliest, their voices began to change 9 days before menstruation. Change of voice occurred primarily 1-4 days before menstruation. Duration of voice changes are indicated in Table III.

The main symptom *during* menstruation is a husky voice. Among 41 cases, 31 changed in tone color and 10 presented hoarseness, primarily in speaking and in mid-range. In addition, several symptoms might appear simultaneously, such as lowering of tone and difficulty in producing sound at high pitch, or sound bursting. In one case, the voice was becoming dull, which occurred most often during ovulation, and then became remarkably hoarse 10-15 days after menstruation (Table IV).

Table II: *Symptoms of Voice Change Prior to Menstruation*

Total	No. of Cases	Symptoms
55		*Change in Quality of Tone Color and Harshness*
	19	Dull
	4	Dry
	8	Not clean
	7	Bright
	17	Husky
13		*Change of Tone*
	10	Reduced by 1-2 pitches
	2	Reduced by 3-4 pitches
	1	Increased by 1 pitch
8	8	Reduced volume
10	0	Difficulty in high-pitch tones; tightness
6	6	Lack of control and difficulty adjusting voice
9	9	Sing with great effort; voice cannot last long
11	11	No symptoms

Table III: *Duration of Voice Change Before Menstruation*

%	No. of Cases	Duration
22.5%	18	1-2 days
21.2%	17	2-3 days
12.5%	10	3-4 days
8.75%	7	4-5 days
3.8%	3	5-6 days
17.5%	14	Over 7 days
13.8%	11	No change

The vocal cords vary in different ways during the menstrual cycle: mainly hyperemia, edema, and vigorous expansion of blood vessels (Table V). At times, several symptoms might occur simultaneously.

Table IV: *Symptoms of Voice Changes During Menstruation*

Total	No. of Cases	Symptoms
41		*Change in Quality of Tone Color and Husky Voice*
	20	Dull
	2	Dry
	6	Not clean
	3	Bright
	10	Hoarse
13		*Lowering of Tone*
	2	½ pitch
	9	1-2 pitches
	2	3-4 pitches
14		*Difficulty in Top Pitch*
	1	Bursting
	12	Tightness
	1	No falsetto tone
7	7	Reduced volume
11	11	Difficulty controlling voice
7	7	Greater effort needed to sing; difficulty breathing
1	1	Easy to produce a sound
21	21	No change

Table V: *Examination of Vocal Cords During Menstruation*

Total	# of Cases	Local Examination
58		*Vocal Cord Hyperemia*
	7	Slight hyperemia and pinkish white
	51	Pronounced hyperemia
28		*Varying Degree of Edema*
	8	Greater surface reflection
	20	Pronounced edema
9		*Inadequate Vocal Cord Closure*
	6	Long seam
	3	Triangle seam
20		*Pathological Blood Vessel Change*
	10	Strip shape
	8	Small red spots;
	2	with hemorrhage
5	5	Pronounced hypertrophy
12	12	Vocal cords without luster; dull
27	27	Increased secretion
2	2	No changes

Based on observation of 80 singers over several menstrual cycles, it was found that their voices changed in varying degrees both before and during menstruation. Most changes occurred 1-2 days before menstruation. The change of voice was remarkable. Changes in tone color before menstruation were even greater than during menstruation. Although the voice changed during menstruation, hyperemia and edema of the vocal cords sometimes made singing easier. After 3-5 days, hyperemia and edema abated, and the voice could recover gradually. Change was mainly in the quality of tone, such as heavy and dull voice, dry and unclean voice, bright voice or hoarseness in speaking and singing, especially in mid-range. In addition, the tone also changed. In general, the tone was reduced by 1 to 2 pitches, sometimes by half a pitch or up to 4 pitches. Singers experienced difficulty in high pitch, and volume was low. They had to exert great effort to sing, and the voice was not easy to control.

Symptoms throughout the body during menstruation — breast pain, lower abdominal pain, lumbago, aching in lower limbs, insufficient or excessive bleeding, insomnia, emotional fluctuation — local change of vocal cords and voice change are closely related. Local changes of voice and vocal cords in each cycle varied among subjects. This was closely related to their general health and external factors. Some performers never experienced voice change. However, vocal cords and voice may also change with local hyperemia and edema, and inadequate closure may occur during menstruation due to factors such as a recent busy schedule, excessive performance, performance anxiety, poor health conditions, fatigue, etc.

During menses, the performing schedule should be adequately reduced or even stopped for some performers. Excessive exercise will change the voice. Care should be taken to limit daily singing.

CHAPTER 144

Relationship Between 'Sound Brilliance' and Sensomotoric Phenomena in Singing and Instrument Playing

Gisela Rohmert

Singing and instrument-playing are based on sensomotoric activity, the pursuit of which requires a high level of sensomotoric coordination.[1, 2] The author's research demonstrates a clear connection between the appearance of *sound brilliance* and sensomotoric phenomena.[3, 4]

In this connection, it is necessary to define more precisely the term *brilliance*. A sound that the human ear perceives as *brilliant* is characterized by a profiling of certain frequency areas in the sound spectrum. The term *singer formant* is used in the literature to describe a highly capable and brilliant voice.[5, 6]

The word *formant*, in regard to the sound spectrum, describes an area of greater amplitude in the frequency range. This singer formant, however, this sign of a highly qualified voice, is seen in general discussion only as a positive byproduct, not a specific theme of traditional voice training.

There are still questions regarding the tolerance of the shifting of the frequency areas and the amplitude and number of overtones enveloped in the area of the singer formants. Also, the idea that for females' voices the singer formant lies at 4000 Hz must, as a result of recent discoveries, be seen as questionable.[4]

With functionally advanced voices, the appearance of two additional singer formants around 5000 and 8000 Hz has also been documented, but these two formants have not, until now, appeared as a topic of scientific discussion. The reason for this may be that these formants can be found and measured only in unusually well-balanced voices.

With this information, we can establish four definite parameters for the human voice: the basic or fundamental pitch, the vowel, the vibrato, and the singer-formant group. The last has a direct connection to specific areas of sensitivity in the human ear.[7, 8] Tomatis discovered the importance of high frequencies for brain and muscle tone, and emphasizes the role of the ear in supplying energy to the brain through the reception of high frequencies.[9]

Because the singer formants bring structure to these generally diffuse high frequencies, their effect on the energy-charging of the cortex is likely to be greatly increased. The affinity of the ear for the singer formants indicates the readiness of the organism, the preference to make use of these frequency areas.

Research shows that the singer formants can take on the role of teacher for the voice and bring about astonishing phenomena in physiological coordination. In a *synergetic* sense,[10] the singer formants act as an *organizer* for the vocal function. In their position as a developed guide for the voice, they give the sound the character of a comprehensive sensory stimulus.

This sound also has a positive effect on muscle tone through its influence on the gamma-nervous system. With sensomotoric work, the muscle spindles innervated by the gamma-nervous system have central importance to coordination of movements.[11, 12]

Muscle tone as an indicator of the entire neuromuscular apparatus determines the quality of the coordination of movement, which is a requirement for the effective realization of music. An optimal body tone in this respect is referred to by Glaser as *Eutonus*.[13]

The stimulation of the gamma-nervous system originates from the higher systems, principally from the *reticular formation* and the *vestibular apparatus*. The importance of the vestibular apparatus for the processing of frequencies has been emphasized.[9]

Connected with the body tone-regulating function of the reticular formation is the reflex arch of the *tensor tympani* muscle which, according to current opinion, is directly controlled by the reticular formation.[14] This is of particular interest in regard to the influence of the singer formants on sensomotoric systems. Also controlled by the third branch of the trigeminus nerve is the *tensor veli palatini* muscle, which enables the eustachian tubes to open laterally. This connection provides for a very fine differentiated opening of the eustachian tubes. The equipping of the tensor tympani with muscle spindles, in contrast to the *stapedius* muscle, substantiates this theory.[14]

Since the sensoric stimulus of the second and third singer formants coincides with impedance minimums in the middle ear,[7] it can be presumed that the human voice on a higher artistic level complies with a biological code. This *sound code* has a greater influence on the economy and efficiency of vocal function than the attempt at voluntary muscle differentiation. This is demonstrated by the effect of sound with singer formants on the suspension apparatus of the larynx. Beyond that, there are other observed effects of the singer formants on the body. The first singer formant (ca. 3000 Hz), for example, has a direct structural influence on the laryngeal musculature. It helps to differentiate the medial compression of the vocal bands and to economize the effort. Without the second singer formant (ca. 5000 Hz), however, its influence is restricted. In many cases, it forces the laryngeal musculature and thereby indirectly increases the subglottal air pressure.

The second singer formant stimulates a fine controlling of the vowel tract, thereby relieving the workload of the larynx. The author's initial tests and observations lead to the belief that this second formant (ca. 5000 Hz) also has a direct influence on the freedom of movement in body joints. It does not automatically appear as a satellite of the first singer formant, but instead develops itself freely and spontaneously.

The third singer formant (ca. 8000 Hz) may appear earlier, later, or at the same time. Its influence has far-reaching effect at all levels of the body, particularly in the higher systems — brain hemisphere coordination, rhythm of the brain and spinal fluid, glandular system function, coordination of the over- and under-pressure systems in the larynx and the ears, gamma-nervous system, and the diaphragm chain. Above all, the third singer formant refines the *brilliance* characteristic of the voice.

Despite the specific individual effects of the three singer formants, they form a unity and begin to unfold their effectiveness when they work in coordinated harmony.

The author's research has demonstrated the impressive capability to influence the brain liquid rhythm with the singer formants, especially the third at 8000 Hz. The regulation of this fluid rhythm is the focus of cranio-sacral therapy, a branch of osteopathic medicine that, through this movement of the spinal and brain fluid, can influence the whole body.

A singer who produces a well-developed 8000 Hz formant demonstrates an especially strong and well-balanced cranio-sacral rhythm. Conversely, through the use of this technique, it is easier to attain the conditions necessary for producing these formants.

Based on work with tinnitus patients[15] and tests on the reaction of the ear to high decibel sounds,[16] it is obvious that, in a voice with this brilliance developed to a high artistic level, there is a potential for medically verifiable healing power. Ancient stories telling of the healing power of the human voice can possibly be explained here in the secret of the singer formants.[17]

The prerequisite for the previously described phenomena is an exceptionally high-quality sound. It must have enough high-quality energy to stimulate the reticular formation into bringing about a change in the tone of the whole neuromuscular apparatus. This effects an extraordinary economy and efficiency of the sensomotoric processes. The author's research supports the theory that the reticular formation reacts preferentially to the higher frequencies of the singer formants.

Based on these experiences, we see important consequences for vocal training. It is interesting, for example, to observe the interdependence of the singer-formant group with the operation of the diaphragm chain.[4] These principles would seem equally important and applicable for instrument-playing. Initial results show that the instrumentalist can and should develop at least one of these singer-formant areas on his/her instrument. This can be accomplished only by working on vocal training, whereby the changes in the voice with regard to effortlessness, efficiency, and *sound brilliance* can be directly carried over to the instrument.

In summary, the importance of the singer formants for singing and instrument-playing and the high frequency needs of the human ear have not yet been sufficiently recognized in the scientific and music communities. At the Lichtenberger Institute for

Functional Voice Training, we are dedicated, in cooperation with the Institute for Work Science and Ergonomics at the Technical College Darmstadt, to daily research, development, practice, and teaching of these principles. Through these activities, we hope to prove and demonstrate the actual potential of the human voice, which lies far beyond what has been, until now, thought unattainable.

REFERENCES

1. Rohmert W (Hrsg): Grundzü des funktionalen Stimmtrainings. Köln: Schmidt, 5 Aufl, 1989.
2. Balser D: Untersuchung funktionaler Ablaufbedingungen komplexer sensumotorischer Fertigkeiten am Beispiel des Streichinstrumentenspiels. Frankfurt: Lang, 1990.
3. Rohmert G: Sängerformanten. *In* Rohmert W (Hrsg), Beiträge zum 1. Kolloquium Praktische Musikphysiologie, 77-80. Köln: Schmidt, 1990.
4. Rohmert G: Der Sänger auf dem Weg zujk Klang: Lichtenberger Musikpädagogische Vorlesungen. Köln: Schmidt, 1991.
5. Sundberg J: Articulatory interpretation of the "singing formant." Journal of the Acoustical Society of America 55:838-844, 1974.
6. Winckel F: Physikalische Kriterien für objektive Stimmbeurteilung. Fol Phoniat 5:232-250, 1953.
7. Lenhardt E: Physiologie der Schalleitung einschließlich Ohrtrompete. *In* Berenden J, Link R, Zöllner F (Hrsg), Hals-Nasan-Ohrenheilkunde in Praxis und Klinik, Band 5: Ohr I. Stuttgart: Thieme, 1979.
8. Borchard JM, Irrgang E, Abdresen B: Die Funktion der menschlichen Ohrmuschel. *In* Spektrum der Wissenschaft, 66-74, 1987.
9. Tomatis AA: Der Klang des Lebens; vorgeburtliche Kommunikation — die Anfänge der seelischen Entwicklung. Hamburg: Rowohlt, 1987.
10. Haken H: Erfolgsgeheimnisse der Natur; Synergetik: Die Lehre vom Zusammenwirken. Stuttgart: Deutsche Verlagsanstalt, 1981.
11. Haase J: Haltung und Bewegung und ihre spinale Koordination. *In* Haase J, Henatsch HD, Jung R, Strata P, Thoden U (Hrsg), Sensomotorik: Physiologie des Menschen, Band 14, 99-192. München: Urban & Schwarzenberg, 1976.
12. Henatsch HD: Zerebrale Regulation der Sensomotorik. *In* Haase J, Henatsch HD, Jung R, Strata P, Thoden U (Hrsg): Sensomotorik: Physiologie des Menschen, Band 14, 265-420. München: Urban & Schwarzenberg, 1976.
13. Glaser V: Eutonie. Das Verhaltensmuster menschlichen Wohlbefindens. Heidelberg: Haug, 1990.
14 Rauchfuss A, Hiller E, Leitner H, Wöllmer W: Reaktion des M. tensor tympani — ausgelöst durch nasal applizierte Trigeminus-reizstoffe. Laryng Rhinol Otol 66:131-132, 1987.
15. Heimers S: Die Wirkung des Sängerformanten bei Tinnitusleiden. *In* Rohmert W (Hrsg), Beiträge zum 2. Kolloquium Praktische Musikphysiologie, 250-255. Köln: Schmidt, 1991.
16. Fischer J: Kurzmitteilungen. *In* Rohmert W (Hrsg), Beiträge zum 2. Kolloquium Praktische Musikphysiologie, 256-259. Köln: Schmidt, 1991.
17. Rohmert G: Der Fall Orpheus. *In* Rohmert W (Hrsg), Beiträge zum 2. Kolloquium Praktische Musikphysiologie, 267-281. Köln: Schmidt, 1991.